Cardiovascular Plaque Rupture

FUNDAMENTAL AND CLINICAL CARDIOLOGY

Editor-in-Chief

Samuel Z. Goldhaber, M.D.

*Harvard Medical School
and Brigham and Women's Hospital
Boston, Massachusetts*

Associate Editor, Europe

Henri Bounameaux, M.D.

*University Hospital of Geneva
Geneva, Switzerland*

ADDITIONAL VOLUMES IN PREPARATION

Cardiovascular Plaque Rupture

edited by

David L. Brown

Albert Einstein College of Medicine
and Montefiore Medical Center
Bronx, New York

MARCEL DEKKER, INC.   NEW YORK · BASEL

ISBN: 0-8247-0276-X

This book is printed on acid-free paper.

Headquarters
Marcel Dekker, Inc.
270 Madison Avenue, New York, NY 10016
tel: 212-696-9000; fax: 212-685-4540

Eastern Hemisphere Distribution
Marcel Dekker AG
Hutgasse 4, Postfach 812, CH-4001 Basel, Switzerland
tel: 41-61-261-8482; fax: 41-61-261-8896

World Wide Web
http://www.dekker.com

The publisher offers discounts on this book when ordered in bulk quantities. For more information, write to Special Sales/Professional Marketing at the headquarters address above.

Current printing (last digit):
10 9 8 7 6 5 4 3 2 1

PRINTED IN THE UNITED STATES OF AMERICA

To my wife, Nancy

My children, Noah and Erin

And the memory of my father

Series Introduction

Marcel Dekker, Inc., has focused on the development of various series of beautifully produced books in different branches of medicine. These series have facilitated the integration of rapidly advancing information for both the clinical specialist and the researcher.

My goal as editor-in-chief of the Fundamental and Clinical Cardiology series is to assemble the talents of world-renowned authorities to discuss virtually every area of cardiovascular medicine. In *Cardiovascular Plaque Rupture*, David L. Brown has edited a much-needed and timely book. Future contributions to this series will include books on molecular biology, interventional cardiology, and clinical management of such problems as coronary artery disease.

Samuel Z. Goldhaber

Foreword

Cardiovascular Plaque Rupture provides a thorough discussion of the background and pathophysiology for the development of atherosclerotic plaques, mechanisms responsible for their progression, and those critical events that lead to the development of unstable or vulnerable atherosclerotic plaques, i.e., ones prone to ulceration/fissuring, thrombosis, and the sudden developments of the acute coronary syndromes.

Molecular mechanisms and epidemiological evidence for inflammation playing a causal role: the role of mechanical stress; and the potential triggers responsible for coronary plaque rupture and determinants of thrombosis after plaque rupture are discussed in detail. The clinical manifestations and arteriographic appearances of plaque rupture are identified.

Techniques to assess plaque vulnerability are also discussed in detail, including intravascular ultrasonograpy, intravascular palpography, optical coherence tomography, magnetic resonance imaging, and in vivo thermography. Finally, experimental animal models and clinical studies directed at preventing atherosclerosis progression and plaque rupture are reviewed, including animal models of coronary heart disease, clinical trials using potential inhibitors of cardiovascular plaque rupture, the results of cholesterol-lowering, antibiotic therapy, plaque sealing techniques, serine protease inhibition, and gene therapy.

The unstable atherosclerotic plaque is a major problem in contemporary cardiology. It causes the abrupt development of unstable angina, acute myocardial infarction, and probably acute cerebrovascular accidents in many patients without prior warning of its presence. It is very important that we develop the insights related to mechanisms of development, the methods to detect, and protective therapies that prevent ulceration and fissuring of unstable plaques and their contribution to the progression of atherosclerosis.

Cardiovascular Plaque Rupture provides a timely review of a clinical problem of immense importance. It provides up-to-date information concerning the development and risks of, and potential treatment for, this problem. The insights provided in this book are important to everyone involved in the care of patients with cardiovascular diseases. I recommend it with enthusiasm to all who are engaged in the war against cardiovascular disease.

James T. Willerson, M.D.
President, The University of Texas Health Science Center at Houston
Houston, Texas

Preface

Plaque rupture is the common pathophysiology of the acute ischemic syndromes of sudden cardiac death, acute myocardial infarction, and unstable angina. As such it is responsible for 700,000 deaths per year and approximately $50 billion in costs in the United States alone. Although the mortality from these diseases is decreasing in the United States, in many parts of the world it is rapidly increasing. Thus, plaque rupture represents one of the major public health hazards of the new millennium.

Until recently very little was known about plaque rupture. In the past decade its relationship to the acute ischemic coronary syndromes has been established by careful pathological studies by many investigators. In addition, through study of human tissue and cultured cells much has been learned about the mechanisms of plaque rupture. The distribution and effect of physical stresses on plaque have been elucidated, as have a number of proteolytic processes that cause degradation of the collagenous and non-collagenous components of plaque. Inflammation has been identified as playing an important role in the pathogenesis of plaque rupture. However, the triggers of the inflammatory response are not well understood. Infectious agents have been identified in atherosclerotic plaque and are proposed as one possible initiator of the inflammatory response.

In addition, relatively little is known regarding the ability to detect and treat plaque at risk of rupture. Intensive efforts are underway to characterize and identify vulnerable plaque using invasive and noninvasive approaches. Methods being investigated include both new imaging modalities and modifications of existing technology for use in the coronary arteries.

Treatment to prevent plaque rupture by stabilizing the vulnerable plaque is in its infancy. Dramatic success has been achieved with the use of HMG-CoA reductase inhibitors to lower cholesterol. However, these powerful agents reduce the risk of plaque rupture by only about 30%. Additional therapeutic strategies are therefore urgently needed. Because of the possible link to infection, antibiotics for prevention of plaque rupture are under intense investigation. Other drugs are being developed that may prevent plaque rupture by inhibition of the inflammatory reaction or the enzymes responsible for plaque degradation.

It is the goal of *Cardiovascular Plaque Rupture* to present a timely review of these findings and to stimulate further research into this important topic. Many of the leading investigators in this emerging new field of investigation have contributed to this project. I am deeply grateful to them for their time and expertise. I would also like to acknowledge the critical contribution of the professionals at Marcel Dekker, Inc., in particular Sandra Beberman and Barbara Mathieu. They have kept this project moving despite the untimely death of their colleague Graham Garratt (who immediately grasped the importance of a book on this subject when I presented it to him) and the birth of my twins and the resultant inertia caused by a year of sleep deprivation. It is my hope that this text will serve to stimulate interest in this field, present the fundamentals, and lay the groundwork for understanding and contributing to the many important advances that are yet to come.

David L. Brown

Contents

Techniques to Assess Plaque Vulnerability

Prevention of Plaque Rupture

Contributors

Robert J. Applegate, M.D.   Cardiology Section, Department of Internal Medicine, Wake Forest University School of Medicine, Winston-Salem, North Carolina

Ergin Atalar, Ph.D.   Associate Professor of Radiology and Biomedical Engineering, Johns Hopkins University, Baltimore, Maryland

Juan Jose Badimon, Ph.D., F.A.C.C.   Associate Professor, Department of Cardiology, Zena and Michael A. Wiener Cardiovascular Institute, Mount Sinai School of Medicine, New York, New York

Lina Badimon, M.D.   Cardiovascular Research Center, CSIC–Hospital Santa Cruz y San Pablo, Universidad Autònoma de Barcelona, Barcelona, Spain

Anton E. Becker, M.D., Ph.D.   Professor, Department of Cardiovascular Pathology, Academic Medical Center, University of Amsterdam, Amsterdam, The Netherlands

Michael Berlowitz, M.D.   Senior Fellow, Division of Cardiovascular Medicine, Department of Medicine, Albert Einstein College of Medicine and Montefiore Medical Center, Bronx, New York

Joan W. Berman, Ph.D.   Professor, Department of Pathology, Albert Einstein College of Medicine, Bronx, New York

Mark E. Brezinski, M.D., Ph.D.   Brigham and Women's Hospital, Boston, Massachusetts

David L. Brown, M.D.   Associate Professor of Medicine, Epidemiology, and Social Medicine, and Associate Director, Division of Cardiovascular Medicine, Department of Medicine, Albert Einstein College of Medicine and Montefiore Medical Center, Bronx, New York

Allen P. Burke, M.D.   Department of Cardiovascular Pathology, Armed Forces Institute of Pathology, Washington, D.C.

E. Ignacio Céspedes, Ph.D.   Jomed Inc., Rancho Cordova, California

James H. Chesebro, M.D.   Zena and Michael A. Wiener Cardiovascular Institute, Mount Sinai School of Medicine, New York, New York

Aram V. Chobanian, M.D.   Professor of Medicine, Whitaker Cardiovascular Institute, and Dean, Boston University School of Medicine, Boston, Massachusetts

Erbin Dai, M.D.   Research Assistant, Vascular Biology Research Group, Robarts Research Institute, University of Western Ontario, London, Ontario, Canada

Chris L. de Korte, Ph.D.   Experimental Echocardiography, Thoraxcentre, Rotterdam, The Netherlands

Leonidas Diamantopoulos, M.D.   Department of Cardiology, Athens University, Athens, Greece

Andrew Farb, M.D.   Staff Cardiovascular Pathologist, Department of Cardiovascular Pathology, Armed Forces Institute of Pathology, Washington, D.C.

Michael S. Feld, Ph.D.   Professor, George R. Harrison Spectroscopy Laboratory, Massachusetts Institute of Technology, Cambridge, Massachusetts

Carl M. Fier, M.D.   Department of Cardiology, Mount Sinai School of Medicine, New York, New York

Peter J. Fitzgerald, M.D., Ph.D.   Center for Research in Cardiovascular Interventions, Stanford University School of Medicine, Stanford, California

James G. Fujimoto, Ph.D.   Department of Electrical Engineering and Computer Science and the Research Laboratory of Electronics, Massachusetts Institute of Technology, Cambridge, Massachusetts

Valentin Fuster, M.D.   Zena and Michael A. Wiener Cardiovascular Institute, Mount Sinai School of Medicine, New York, New York

Zorina S. Galis, Ph.D.   Assistant Professor, Division of Cardiology, Departments of Medicine and Biomedical Engineering, Emory University School of Medicine, Atlanta, Georgia

Enrique P. Gurfinkel, M.D., Ph.D.   Director, Coronary Care Unit, Favaloro Foundation, Buenos Aires, Argentina

Victoria L. M. Herrera, M.D.   Associate Professor of Medicine, Whitaker Cardiovascular Institute, Boston University School of Medicine, Boston, Massachusetts

Allen Jeremias, M.D.   Center for Research in Cardiovascular Interventions, Stanford University School of Medicine, Stanford, California

Marwan Kazimi, B.S.   Department of Pathology, Albert Einstein College of Medicine, Bronx, New York

Frank D. Kolodgie, Ph.D.   Department of Cardiovascular Pathology, Armed Forces Institute of Pathology, Washington, D.C.

John R. Kramer, Jr., M.D.   Staff, Department of Cardiology, Cleveland Clinic Foundation, Cleveland, Ohio

Richard T. Lee, M.D.   Cardiovascular Division, Department of Medicine, Brigham and Women's Hospital, and Associate Professor, Department of Medicine, Harvard Medical School, Boston, Massachusetts

William C. Little, M.D.   Chief of Cardiology and Professor of Medicine, Cardiology Section, Department of Internal Medicine, Wake Forest University School of Medicine, Winston-Salem, North Carolina

Li Ying Liu, M.D.   Research Assistant, Vascular Biology Research Group, Robarts Research Institute, University of Western Ontario, London, Ontario, Canada

Alexandra Lucas, M.D., F.R.C.P.(C.)   Associate Professor and Scientist, Departments of Cardiology and Medicine and Vascular Biology Research Group, Robarts Research Institute, University of Western Ontario, London, Ontario, Canada

Harry Ma, M.S.   Department of Pathology, Albert Einstein College of Medicine, Bronx, New York

Willibald Maier, M.D.   Department of Cardiology, Cardiovascular Center, University Hospital Zurich, Zurich, Switzerland

Jonathan D. Marmur, M.D., F.R.C.P.(C.)   Assistant Professor, Department of Medicine, Mount Sinai School of Medicine, New York, New York

Bernhard Meier, M.D., FESC, FACC   Professor and Chairman, Swiss Cardiovascular Center Bern, University Hospital, Bern, Switzerland

Jason T. Motz   Research Assistant, George R. Harrison Spectroscopy Laboratory, Massachusetts Institute of Technology, Cambridge, Massachusetts

Jacqueline Müller-Nordhorn, M.D., D.P.H.   Research Assistant, Institute of Social Medicine and Epidemiology, Charité Hospital, Humboldt University of Berlin, Berlin, Germany

Piers Nash, B.Sc.   Department of Microbiology and Immunology, University of Western Ontario, London, Ontario, Canada

Kevin M. Rankin, M.D., F.A.C.C.   Assistant Professor, Cardiology Section, Department of Internal Medicine, Wake Forest University School of Medicine, Winston-Salem, North Carolina

Luis E. P. Rohde, M.D.   Cardiovascular Division, Department of Medicine, Brigham and Women's Hospital, and Harvard Medical School, Boston, Massachusetts

Nelson Ruiz-Opazo, Ph.D.   Professor of Medicine, Whitaker Cardiovascular Institute, Boston University School of Medicine, Boston, Massachusetts

Benjamin Scirica, M.D.   Clinical Fellow, Department of Medicine, Harvard Medical School, Boston, Massachusetts

Christodoulos Stefanadis, M.D.   Department of Cardiology, Athens University, Athens, Greece

Konstantinos Toutouzas, M.D.   Department of Cardiology, Athens University, Athens, Greece

Pavlos Toutouzas, M.D.   Department of Cardiology, Athens University, Athens, Greece

Russell P. Tracy, Ph.D.   Professor, Departments of Pathology and Biochemistry, University of Vermont, Colchester, Vermont

Eleftherios Tsiamis, M.D.   Department of Cardiology, Athens University, Athens, Greece

Babak A. Vakili, M.D.   Senior Fellow, Division of Cardiovascular Medicine, Department of Medicine, Albert Einstein College of Medicine and Montefiore Medical Center, Bronx, New York

Sweder W. E. van de Poll, M.D.   Department of Cardiology, Cleveland Clinic Foundation, Cleveland, Ohio, and Department of Cardiology, Leiden University Medical Center, Leiden, The Netherlands

Anton F. W. van der Steen, Ph.D.   Thoraxcentre, Rotterdam, The Netherlands

Allard C. van der Wal, M.D., Ph.D.   Department of Cardiovascular Pathology, Academic Medical Center, University of Amsterdam, Amsterdam, The Netherlands

Renu Virmani, M.D.   Chairperson, Department of Cardiovascular Pathology, Armed Forces Institute of Pathology, Washington, D.C.

Neil J. Weissman, M.D.   Director, Echocardiography and Ultrasound Laboratories, Cardiovascular Research Institute, Washington Hospital Center, Washington, D.C.

Stefan N. Willich, M.D., M.P.H.   Professor of Medicine, Institute of Social Medicine and Epidemiology, Charité Hospital, Humboldt University of Berlin, Berlin, Germany

Paul G. Yock, M.D.   Weiland Professor of Medicine, Center for Research in Cardiovascular Interventions, Stanford University School of Medicine, Stanford, California

Christian V. Zalai, B.Sc., M.Sc.   Department of Microbiology and Immunology, University of Western Ontario, London, Ontario, Canada

1
Development of the Atherosclerotic Plaque

Joan W. Berman, Marwan Kazimi, and Harry Ma
Albert Einstein College of Medicine, Bronx, New York

I. OVERVIEW OF ATHEROSCLEROSIS

Atherosclerosis is a pathological condition that is characterized by the development of plaques within arteries. There are numerous known risk factors for the development of atherosclerosis, including elevated plasma concentrations of cholesterol, in particular the low-density lipoprotein (LDL) fraction, hypertension, diabetes mellitus, smoking, and genetic predisposition (1–3). This disease is thought to be inflammatory in nature with lesions involving both lipid and cellular accumulation within the vessel wall and reactive intimal thickening of the artery (4). The onset of disease begins as early as childhood with the development of the fatty streak (5, 6), followed by lipid deposition and accumulation of both extracellular matrix and intimal smooth muscle cells (7). Once the characteristic plaque has formed, it may remain asymptomatic for many years. However, as the disease progresses, ischemia can occur with progressive occlusion of the vessel, or the plaque can suddenly rupture, resulting in thrombus formation. Rupture of a plaque frequently results in one of the acute coronary syndromes, which include sudden death, acute myocardial infarction, or unstable angina (8, 9).

The most important manifestation of atherosclerosis is cardiovascular disease, which accounts for 44% of mortality in the United States and is the nation's leading killer for both men and women (9, 10). The impact of this disease on health care costs is staggering. The American Heart Association estimated costs (combined direct costs and indirect costs) of treating cardiovascular disease (CVD), including strokes, for 1998 are $286.5 billion (11). Controlling risk factors and reducing the mortality and morbidity associated with CVD is an effective way of reducing costs associated with the disease (12).

A better understanding of the mechanisms of atherogenesis has emerged recently, revealing the multifactorial nature of both the pathogenesis and manifestations of this disease. Clinically, atherosclerotic CVD involves multiple vascular beds, such as coronary, cerebrovascular, and peripheral arteries. Moreover, the presence of one clinical manifestation increases the likelihood of additional manifestations of atherosclerosis developing (9, 10). The conversion of a stable atherosclerotic plaque to an unstable plaque, followed by rupture and thrombus formation, often precedes the development of an acute presentation of the disease. The prevention and treatment of atherosclerosis depends on understanding both the mechanisms of this disease process and that of plaque stability and instability.

II. PLAQUE MORPHOLOGY

Human atherosclerotic plaques have been classified by the American Heart Association (AHA) Committee on Vascular Lesions according to lesion morphological characteristics (13). Plaque progression, from fatty streak to the advanced complicated lesion, is divided into five phases (8). Figure 1 depicts this classification scheme and combines a clinical picture of each phase with the pathological description of the lesions.

Phase 1 consists of a small lesion of the type often found in those less than 35 years of age. These plaques can advance over time and are characterized as lesion types I, II, and III. Type I lesions consist of macrophage-derived foam cells that contain lipid. Type II lesions consist of both macrophages and smooth muscle cells surrounded by some extracellular fibrils and lipid droplets.

Phase 2 consists of plaques that may not exhibit stenosis but that may have high lipid content and, thus, may be susceptible to rupture. Such plaques are categorized morphologically as lesion types IV and Va. Type IV is characterized by confluent cellular content with an extensive amount of extracellular lipids, whereas type Va lesions contain extracellular lipid found in the core with an overlying fibrous cap.

Phase 2 may evolve into Phase 3 or Phase 4, and either of these can evolve into fibrotic Phase 5. Phase 3 is characterized by the acute "complicated" type VI lesion and usually results from rupture or fissure of a plaque of type IV or Va. This evolves into development of a mural thrombus that may not completely occlude the affected artery. Alterations in the shape of the disrupted plaque and organization of the thrombus by connective tissue can lead to the more stenotic and fibrotic type Vb or Vc lesions of Phase 5. Type Vb or Vc lesions may be manifested clinically by angina and evolve into occluding lesions. However, the final occlusion may be silent or subclinical (14). Unlike Phase 3, the severe com-

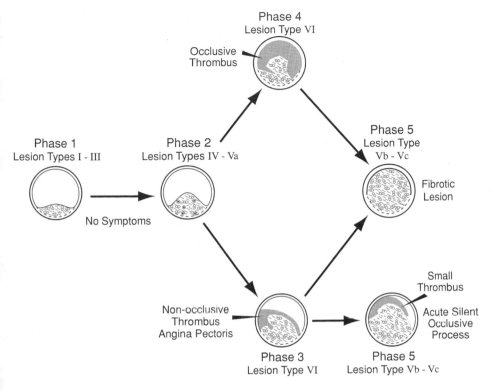

Figure 1 Illustrations of plaque morphology as defined by the American Heart Association Committee on Vascular Lesions (From Ref. 13.)

plicated type VI lesion of Phase 4 consists of an occluding thrombus with the development of an acute coronary episode. Such occluding thrombi may eventually progress to the Vb or Vc lesions of Phase 5. According to this scheme, the unstable plaque is considered as a Phase 2, type IV or type Va lesion.

III. RISK FACTORS

The incidence, severity, and progression of atherosclerosis vary to a large degree among individuals and groups, a finding that may contribute to an understanding of its pathogenesis. Although epidemiological data are expressed largely in terms of the incidence or the number of deaths attributable to ischemic heart disease, studies of material taken at surgery and at autopsy provide direct evidence of atherosclerotic lesions. Two of the most notable prospective studies performed on well-defined population groups, the Framingham Heart Study and the Multiple Risk Factor Intervention Trial (MRFIT), correlated atherosclerosis with increased age, male gender, certain genetic factors, and lifestyle (1–3). Of the various risk factors detected in such studies, the four considered most significant are diet/ hyperlipidemia, hypertension, cigarette smoking, and diabetes. More minor risk factors include obesity, physical inactivity, increasing age, stress, oral contraceptives, high carbohydrate intake, and homocysteinemia (15–17). Last, infection, specifically with *Chlamydia pneumonia*, herpes simplex virus type 1 (HSV-1), and cytomegalovirus (CMV), has been postulated to play a role in atherosclerosis, although studies on the subject have shown associations at times but have been inconclusive at others (18–20). It should be kept in mind that, as with most pathogenetic mechanisms and their related risk factors, genetics most likely plays both an overt (e.g., hypercholesteremia) and a subtle (e.g., basal levels of insulin and individual insulin sensitivity) role in atherogenesis.

The evidence linking hypercholesteremia and abnormalities in lipid metabolism to atherosclerosis is exhaustive. Atherosclerotic lesions are rich in cholesterol and cholesterol esters, and such lesions can be induced in animals, including subhuman primates, by feeding them diets high in cholesterol (21–24). Genetic diseases such as familial hypercholesteremia result in premature atherosclerosis that is often fatal at a young age, whereas acquired diseases that raise plasma cholesterol levels, such as the nephrotic syndrome and hypothyroidism, increase the risk of ischemic heart disease (IHD) (25–27). Treatment by altered diet and cholesterol-lowering drugs demonstrates some regression of coronary artery lesions in both men and women (28–30). Although no specific level of plasma cholesterol identifies individuals at risk for atherosclerosis, the risk is directly proportional to increasing concentrations of LDL, whereas risk is inversely proportional to levels of high-density lipoprotein (HDL) (31, 32). Risk of atherosclerosis rises more steeply with total cholesterol concentrations greater than 200 mg/dl (5.2 mmol/liter) (33).

On the basis of this association with cholesterol, diet plays a key role in atherosclerosis, although its effects may extend to other mechanisms discussed later. High dietary intake of cholesterol and saturated fats raises plasma cholesterol levels, whereas a diet low in cholesterol and low in the ratio of saturated/ polyunsaturated fats lowers plasma cholesterol levels (34, 35). Diets with a high content of omega-3 fatty acids are associated with low rates of IHD. Omega-3 fatty acids have been shown to lower plasma LDL, raise plasma HDL, and modify production by blood and vascular cells of prostaglandins and leukotrienes, mediators that affect platelet function and inflammation (36). Last, because overwhelming evidence indicates that increased vascular oxygen free radical levels constitute the central underlying mechanism for endothelial dysfunction (37), several studies have explored the link between the intake of antioxidants and atherosclerosis. Although not all the studies have been conclusive, and free radical scavengers such as vitamins C and E do not influence atherosclerosis to the same degree as plasma cholesterol levels, they are another potential component of diet that may modify the disease.

Elevated systolic or diastolic blood pressure influences atherogenesis and increases the incidence of IHD and cerebrovascular disease by mechanisms that have not yet been clarified (38). The MRFIT study demonstrated increased rates of death for those with systolic pressures greater than 110 mm Hg and diastolic pressures greater than 70 mm Hg. Interestingly, after the age of 45, hypertension shows a stronger correlation with the clinical manifestations of atherosclerosis than does hypercholesterolemia.

Cigarette smoking is also an established risk factor for coronary heart disease and peripheral vascular disease. It is associated with a greater severity of disease, but alone does not account for the twofold or greater risk of coronary heart disease among smokers (39). Smoking is specifically associated with a much greater risk of severe atherosclerosis of the abdominal aorta, consistent with a greater risk of peripheral vascular disease and aortic aneurysm among smokers. Cigarettes induce a variety of physiological responses that contribute to atherogenesis: increased plasma LDL and reduced plasma HDL concentrations, elevation in plasma fibrinogen concentration, and elevation in blood leukocyte count. Animal studies have demonstrated that the nicotine component of cigarettes may play a role in accelerating atherosclerosis through its activation of the sympathetic nervous system, the main effects of which are increased heart rate, blood pressure, and myocardial contractility. Although human studies have shown only the possibility that nicotine plays a role in the process, studies of individuals using transdermal nicotine patches support the idea that cigarette toxins other than nicotine are important causes of acute cardiovascular events (40).

Another factor implicated increasingly in atherosclerosis, specifically of the coronary arteries, is the insulin resistance syndrome, the precursor to non-insulin dependent, or type II, diabetes mellitus (NIDDM). Insulin resistance and hyperinsulinemia often cosegregate with factors that independently increase the risk for coronary artery disease. Studies demonstrate that atherosclerosis begins to appear in patients within a few years of onset of diabetes, and that fewer than 5% of nondiabetic patients but greater than 75% of diabetic patients show some evidence of atherosclerosis before the age of 45 (41, 42). Nevertheless, the classification of insulin resistance as an independent risk factor remains controversial (43).

Examples of the components of insulin resistance syndrome and NIDDM that correlate with heightened risk of atherosclerosis are low HDL cholesterol (44), obesity (45), oxidized LDL cholesterol (37), high triglycerides (46), and hypertension (55). Although several large prospective studies demonstrated a correlation between insulin resistance and coronary artery disease (CAD) using multivariate analysis (47–49), a review of several smaller studies found no significant link (47). To date, most studies on the subject have focused on the relationship between atherosclerosis and insulin levels, which are a marker for insulin resistance, but not a direct measure. The few patients so far tested by directly assessing the actions of insulin suggest that insulin resistance correlates more closely with atherosclerosis than does plasma insulin concentration (50, 51).

In MRFIT, fasting hyperinsulinemia was found not to be a risk factor for women but was a risk factor for those men with the apolipoprotein E 3/2 phenotype, rather than the more common E 3/3 phenotype. Furthermore, age may play a role as to whether insulin resistance is a risk, because insulin levels do not correlate with atherosclerosis in elderly populations, but do appear to contribute to CAD in Caucasian men 40 to 60 years old (52). The role of gender in negating the effect of insulin levels and/or resistance as a risk factor for atherosclerosis is supported by other studies (53).

Another aspect of insulin resistance, hyperglycemia, most likely contributes to atherogenesis. Chronic hyperglycemia alters tissue glycation, thus damaging vascular tissue and leading to oxidation of and delayed metabolism of LDL cholesterol (54). Nonenzymatic glycation of LDL makes it less able to bind to LDL receptors, inhibiting what is considered the most important mechanism for maintaining lower plasma cholesterol levels, whereas glycosylation of HDL renders it more susceptible to degradation (55).

Formation of early glycation end products is reversible, but further molecular alterations resulting in advanced glycation end products (AGEs) are often irreversible. The receptor for advanced glycation end products (RAGE) is a member of the immunoglobulin superfamily of cell surface molecules and has been hypothesized to play a central role in the accelerated atherosclerosis seen in diabetic patients (56). One pathway of RAGE-dependent intracellular signal transduction results in the nuclear translocation of transcription factor NF-κB. Expression of NF-κB–regulated genes has been observed with concurrent expression of RAGE and its ligands in pathological samples, together with increased expression of vascular cell adhesion molecule-1 (VCAM-1) (57, 58). In the AGE-enriched tissue and vessels of diabetic patients, the addition of a second stress, such as lipoprotein retention or oxidant formation typical of atherosclerosis, may result in exaggerated or accelerated inflammation and intimal formation (59).

Although various studies may conflict, and not all pathogenetic mechanisms behind epidemiological findings have been clarified, the overall picture indicates a contributory role for insulin resistance, if not hyperinsulinemia, in men. For women, insulin resistance itself does not appear to be a risk factor, but the components associated with NIDDM, as listed previously, certainly do.

Both obesity and sedentary lifestyle have been associated with an increased risk of atherosclerosis in human studies (17). Although each of these risk factors directly affects two major contributors to atherosclerosis, diabetes and hypertension, and a sedentary lifestyle may lead to higher LDL and lower HDL plasma levels (60), it remains difficult to control for all the associated variables. Thus, it can only be stated with certainty that "healthier" lifestyles, consisting of some degree of exercise and fitness, have positive effects on atherosclerosis.

Postmenopausal use of estrogen is associated with a decrease in cardiovascular disease and its risk factors in older women (61). There are many mechanistic explanations for the cardioprotective action of circulating estrogens. For example, they have been shown to reduce LDL, total cholesterol, and fibrinogen levels and to increase HDL cholesterol levels (62). Decreased neointimal hyperplasia and reduction of smooth muscle cell collagen synthesis have also been attributed to the actions of estrogen in animal studies (63). Some evidence also exists that estrogen may function as an antioxidant, inhibiting the oxidation of LDL (64). Thus, although precise reasons for the protective effects of estrogen with respect to atherosclerosis are not yet known, several possibilities have been demonstrated.

Studies have shown an association between the incidence of atherosclerosis and the presence of at least three types of infectious organisms—HSV-1, *Chlamydia pneumonia*, and CMV (65–67). All three organisms have been found in atheromatous lesions in coronary arteries and other organs obtained at autopsy (65, 67). However, there is no direct proof that infection with these organisms can cause the lesions of atherosclerosis in humans (68).

Elevated plasma homocysteine levels were first associated with advanced atherosclerosis on the basis of autopsy findings in patients with homozygous defects in enzymes necessary for homocysteine metabolism, such as cystathione β-synthase or methylene tetrahydrofolate reductase (16, 69–71). Patients with such defects have severe atherosclerosis develop in childhood and may have their first myocardial infarction before the age of 20 (71). Plasma homocysteine levels are slightly elevated in many patients who have no enzymatic defects in homocysteine metabolism, and such patients are at increased risk for symptomatic atherosclerosis (72). Treatment with folic acid can lower plasma homocysteine levels to normal, but it is still unknown whether such treatment can prevent the progression of atherosclerotic lesions in these patients (73). Potential mechanisms by which elevated plasma homocysteine may contribute to atherogenesis include its prothrombotic effects and its ability to increase collagen production and to decrease the availability of nitric oxide (NO) (74–76).

The relative contributions of the major and minor risk factors already noted to atherosclerosis initiation and progression are difficult to assess. Clearly, relationships between diet, physical activity, obesity, diabetes, and hypertension do exist, and the evidence discussed previously outlines their roles in the initiation and development of atherosclerosis. Genetics further complicates all such associations, because allelic distributions likely influence these risk factors in a multifactorial manner. Further research will continue to characterize the roles of the myriad risk factors both in their interactions with each other and in their direct contributions to atherosclerotic disease.

IV. INITIAL INJURY

A. Introduction

Many investigators believe that fatty infiltration of the arterial wall, while exhibiting different distributions in children than adults, represents the initial lesion of atherosclerosis, with other factors shaping the nature of the final, more clinically significant lesions (77, 78). The fatty streak is ubiquitous in children and was found by Stary to be present in early life at the same anatomical sites as predominantly smooth-muscle-rich fibrous plaques at older ages (5), confirming observations made by others. Although the work of Brown and Goldstein demonstrated the key role played by LDL in atherogenesis, atherosclerosis has been shown more recently to resemble a chronic inflammatory process, with histological evidence of inflammatory cells, cytokines, and adhesion molecules in human atherosclerotic lesions (79–81). The original response-to-injury hypothesis proposed that endothelial denudation initiated atherosclerosis (82). Although the hypothesis may hinge on a precise definition of endothelial injury, updated versions categorize injury as a spectrum of insults that may or may not morphologically alter the endothelium—from denudation or disjunction of endothelial cells, to alteration in permeability, to the subtler changes of growth factor secretion or cytokine expression. Thus, insults such as elevated levels of modified LDL, hypertension, diabetes mellitus, cigarette smoke, and other forms of oxidative damage may all contribute to atherosclerosis by causing endothelial dysfunction.

LDL, which may be modified by oxidation, glycation (as in diabetes), aggregation, association with proteoglycans, or incorporation into immune complexes, is a major cause of injury to the endothelium and smooth muscle (83, 84). Furthermore, the local inflammatory response can have a significant effect on lipoprotein movement within the artery. Specifically, mediators of inflammation such as tumor necrosis factor-alpha (TNF-α), interleukin-1 beta (IL-1β), and macrophage-colony stimulating factor (M-CSF) increase binding of LDL to endothelium and smooth muscle and increase the transcription of the LDL-receptor gene (85, 86). Thus, an autocrine loop is set in motion between LDL movement and modification within the arterial wall and the inflammatory reaction that characterizes atherosclerosis.

Hypertension elicits proinflammatory responses as well, by increasing smooth muscle lipoxygenase activity, which in turn can increase inflammation and the oxidation of LDL (55). Hypertension is characterized by increased levels of angiotensin II (Ang II) that can contribute to endothelial dysfunction and activation and alter smooth muscle cell viability (87). Hypertension may also be characterized by increased formation of H_2O_2, superoxide anion, and hydroxyl radicals in plasma, all of which can promote endothelial dysfunction by reducing the production of NO (88), promoting leukocyte adhesion (89), and increasing peripheral resistance (90). This last effect may contribute to initiation of atherosclerosis, because changes in flow alter the expression of certain genes that have shear stress responsive elements in their promoter regions, for instance intercellular adhesion molecule-1 (ICAM-1), platelet-derived growth factor-β (PDGF-β), and tissue factor (91, 92).

Endothelial dysfunction resulting from injury effects a compensatory response that contributes to the initiation of atherosclerosis by altering the normally nonthrombotic, nonadhesive endothelial surface. Vascular permeability and leukocyte infiltration may be increased, as well as secretion of vasoactive molecules, cytokines, and growth factors. The response may be viewed as inflammatory, and so far has been shown to be mediated by monocyte-derived macrophages and specific subtypes of T lymphocytes characteristic of a chronic inflammatory response (81).

B. Role of LDL

Chronically elevated levels of lipoproteins in the plasma, specifically very low-density lipoprotein (VLDL), and LDL, have been shown by numerous epidemiological studies to be associated with an increased incidence of atherosclerosis (93). The cellular and molecular bases for the regulation of plasma LDL levels were detailed by the work of Brown and Goldstein on the LDL receptor. That work led to the correlation of LDL binding by cells with the rate of cholesterol biosynthesis through the 3-hydroxy-3-methylglutaryl CoA (HMG CoA) reductase pathway. The normal homeostatic mechanism protects cells from excess cholesterol accumulation by decreasing the number of LDL receptors on the cell surface in response to elevated intracellular levels of LDL cholesterol. This protective mechanism, however, also leads to a decrease in the removal of LDL from the circulation and an increase in plasma LDL, establishing the noteworthy risk factor for atherosclerosis. Explanation of the pathway also established the basis for a new class of cholesterol-lowering drugs, which act through inhibition of the rate-limiting enzyme, HMG CoA reductase.

In the 1980s researchers began to notice that not all cholesterol accumulation within developing atherosclerotic lesions could be accounted for by the cellular uptake of LDL through the classic LDL receptor (94). Instead, a modified form of LDL (unknown at the time) appeared to be taken up by alternative receptors for LDL. This conclusion was based on two noteworthy observations. First, patients and animals with mutations rendering them completely devoid of the LDL receptor nevertheless accumulate lipid-laden foam cells in the same way as patients and animals with normal LDL receptors. Second, the two cell types found in atherosclerotic lesions that can take up cholesterol, and thus become foam cells (monocytes/macrophages and smooth muscle cells), do not accumulate cholesterol in vitro even in the presence of high concentrations of LDL.

Acetylation of LDL, originally performed with the aim of isolating the altered form of LDL that was responsible for the preceding observations, produces a modified LDL that can promote cholesterol accumulation in macrophages (95). This receptor, cloned and termed scavenger receptor A (SRA), is *not* down-regulated when the cholesterol content of a cell increases (96). Its expression is increased by the growth factor M-CSF, which is released by activated endothelial cells and smooth muscle cells (97). Although acetylated LDL could, in theory, contribute to foam cell formation, its true importance was in pointing the way to the discovery of another form of modified LDL. This form, which turned out to be oxidized LDL (oxLDL), appeared after overnight incubation of LDL with monolayers of human arterial endothelial or smooth muscle cells (98). Further research has shown that oxidation of LDL in the intimal space by free radicals or lipoxygenase causes alterations in the apolipoprotein B receptor binding domain (99). The oxidized LDL no longer expresses the native recognition site, and the particles can no longer undergo normal LDL uptake by the apolipoprotein B/E-sensitive LDL receptor (LDL-R). OxLDL then remains available for uptake by the macrophage SRA, resulting in the formation of the foam cells that are the hallmark of fatty streaks (98).

Although it remains to be proven that hypercholesteremia alone can induce changes characteristic of endothelial dysfunction and thus lead to the initiation of atherosclerotic plaques, recent investigations draw convincing connections between the in vitro effects of oxLDL on endothelial cells, smooth muscle cells, and macrophages (100–102). Aside from recognition by SRA and its subsequent role in foam cell formation, oxLDL exhibits several other pro-atherogenic effects. OxLDL is by itself a chemoattractant for monocytes (103, 104) and may inhibit the motility of tissue macrophages (105), thus contributing to macrophage accumulation in the intima. Furthermore, oxLDL is mitogenic for macrophages and smooth muscle cells (106) and can stimulate the release of the growth factor M-CSF from endothelial cells (107). OxLDL causes as many as 20 other biological effects in vitro, but very few have been evaluated in vivo (83). Several of these biological effects can be produced by minimally oxidized LDL (mmLDL), apparently attributable to partially oxidized phospholipids that might mimic the effects of platelet-activating factor or autocoids (108). The observation that minimal oxidation of LDL causes secretion of monocyte chemoattractant protein-1 (MCP-1) by human endothelial cells (109) suggests a mechanism whereby initial entry of LDL into the arterial intima, before the influx of leukocytes, may set the stage for the inflammatory reaction. It has been proposed that oxidation of the lipid-protein matrix of a plasma membrane is somewhat analogous to the oxidation of an LDL particle, and that the oxidation of the cell plasma membrane itself may exert a number of effects relevant to conditions of high oxidative stress, such as atherosclerosis (83).

Although most studies have focused on the role of oxLDL in atherogenesis, other oxidized lipoproteins might also contribute to the process. Oxidation products of both unesterified and esterified cholesterol have been demonstrated to be present in the arterial wall and to be highly toxic to a number of cell types in culture (110, 111), whereas oxidized fatty acids have been found in atherosclerotic lesions (112). Products of phospholipid oxidation have also been shown to regulate vascular function and to serve as indicators of oxidative stress. Isoprostane, one class of products formed by phospholipid oxidation, has been found in conditions of oxidant stress characteristic of atherosclerosis and its risk factors (113).

Although a growing body of evidence supports the important influence of oxLDL on endothelial cell activation and atherogenesis, much less is known about mechanisms by which LDL itself activates or injures endothelial cells. As alluded to previously with mmLDL, many investigators believe that some form of injury must be elicited by native LDL, or a just slightly modified form of LDL, because the monocytes responsible for the major modifications of LDL trapped in arterial endothelium are not present at the very start of fatty streak formation. When endothelial cells are incubated with native LDL, activation of the cells occurs, causing alterations in free radical formation and arachidonate metabolism, as well as a decrease in tissue plasminogen activator (114) and an increase in monocyte recruitment (115). Native LDL also up-regulates several genes involved in atherogenesis, including ICAM-1, VCAM-1, E-selectin, and the early growth response gene-1 (116–119).

Although the effects of native LDL on cultured endothelial cells appear similar to those of oxLDL, increasing evidence has shown that LDL perturbs endothelial cell function by mechanisms that differ from those attributed to oxLDL. At the level of transcription, it appears that oxLDL activates the transcription factor NF-κB, whereas LDL preferentially activates the transcription factor activator protein-1 (AP-1) (120, 121). Mechanisms of endothelial cell activation by native LDL involve calcium mobilization, activation of protein kinases, specifically JNK/SAPK, and an increase in the transcription factor c-Jun/AP-1 (122). In smooth muscle cells and macrophages, but not in human endothelial cells, both native and modified LDL have been shown to stimulate mitogen-activated protein (MAP) kinase and *c-fos* activation (106, 123, 124). Finally, recent work has shown that oxLDL is capable of activating the transcription factor peroxisome proliferator activator receptor-gamma (PPAR-γ), perhaps indicating another link between fat metabolism and the development of atherosclerosis (125).

C. Adhesion Molecules

A dominant factor in establishing the inflammatory aspect of the atherosclerotic lesion is the adhesion of leukocytes to the endothelial surface, with subsequent transmigration from the arterial lumen to the intima. The binding of leukocytes is mediated by specific adhesion molecules expressed on the luminal surface of the endothelium, as well as on leukocytes. The up-regulation of these proteins on endothelial cells is a process common to inflammation in many tissues and has been observed in such diverse conditions as transplant rejection, contact dermatitis, septic shock, and rheumatoid arthritis (126–128). Two families of endothelial cell adhesion molecules, the selectin family and the immunoglobulin (Ig) superfamily, play key roles in this interaction. Adhesion molecules believed to be involved in atherogenesis are outlined in Table 1.

Each member of the selectin family of adhesion molecules is composed of a lectin domain and an epithelial-like growth factor region. Two types of selectins, E-selectin and P-selectin, are thought to participate in atherogenesis. E-selectin, or endothelial leukocyte adhesion molecule-1 (ELAM-1), participates in the binding of monocytes and neutrophils to endothelial surfaces. The molecule is not expressed in normal arteries but is found in atherosclerotic lesions (129). E-selectin has been shown to mediate recruitment of leukocytes and a subset of T-lymphocytes to sites of inflammatory response (130, 131). P-selectin (GMP-140), originally identified on the surface of platelets, is released from intracellular endothelial stores on stimulation by cytokines or oxygen radicals and rapidly shuttled to the plasma membrane. P-selectin is also synthesized *de novo* after exposure to cytokines. The role of P-selectin in fatty streak formation has been demonstrated by experiments in mice susceptible to atherosclerosis (132). Another indication of the potential role that P-selectin may play in atherogenesis is the observation that oxLDL causes a redistribution of P-selectin to the surface of human aortic endothelial cells (133). Last, immunohistochemical staining of endothelial cells in human fatty streak lesions displays elevated levels of P-selectin compared with normal areas (134).

Although E-selectin and P-selectin allow the initial tethering and rolling of leukocytes or lymphocytes along a layer of endothelial cells, firm adhesion and subsequent transmigration in response to chemotactic factors are mediated by the immunoglobulin superfamily of endothelial cell adhesion molecules (ECAMs) (135). These adhesion molecules are characterized by immunoglobulin-like subunits. Two in particular, ICAM-1 and VCAM-1, have been demonstrated in human atherosclerotic lesions (79). ICAM-1 binds to beta-2 integrins such as LFA-1 (CD11a/CD18) and Mac-1 (CD11b/CD18) that are present on all leukocytes. VCAM-1 binds to the ligand VLA-4, present on lymphocytes, monocytes, and eosinophils.

VCAM-1 is absent or minimally expressed on normal endothelium, whereas ICAM-1 is present at a low constitutive level. On activation by alterations in shear stress, by exposure to lipopolysaccharide (LPS), or by exposure to the cytokines IL-1β, TNF-α, interferon-gamma (IFN-γ), and IL-4 (VCAM-1 only), expression is up-regulated. The regulatory cascades of both ICAM-1 and

Table 1 Endothelial Cell Adhesion Molecules Involved in Atherosclerosis

Molecule	Ligand	Binds with	Function
E-selectin/ELAM-1	SFLs	M, N, mT	Initial contact, rolling
P-selectin/GMP-140	SFLs, PSGL-1, L-selectin	Leukocytes	Tethering
ICAM-1	LFA-1 (CD11a/CD18), Mac-1 (CD11b/CD18), fibrinogen	Leukocytes	Firm adhesion
VCAM-1	VLA-4	Eos, Lymphocytes, M	Firm adhesion
PECAM/CD31	PECAM, GAGs	P, M, T	Transmit activation signals to monocytes, maintain endothelial monolayers
IG9	As yet unknown	M	As yet unknown
VMAP-1	As yet unknown	M	As yet unknown

Eos, eosinophils, M, monocytes/macrophages; N, neutrophils; P, platelets; T, T cells; mT, memory T cells; GAGs, glycosaminoglycons, PSGL-1, P-selectin glycoprotein ligand; SFLs, sialylated fucosylated lactosamines.

VCAM-1 have received much attention, as has the possibility of limiting atherosclerotic initiation and/or progression by limiting adhesion molecule expression (136, 137).

Platelet-endothelial cell adhesion molecule (PECAM/CD31) is a homotypic cell adhesion molecule present on endothelial cells, mainly at cell junctions, as well as on platelets, T cells, and monocytes (138). PECAM is thought to mediate signal delivery to monocytes and to maintain endothelial monolayers (139). It has been shown to activate T lymphocytes by increasing the affinity of the VLA-4 ligand for VCAM-1. It may also participate in immobilizing macrophages within the intima (79). Although PECAM can be found on both normal and atherosclerotic endothelium, its various effects on endothelial monolayers and on monocytes imply a role in atherosclerosis.

Another molecule, the monocyte binding protein identified by the antibody IG9, was shown by immunohistochemistry to be present in human and rabbit atherosclerotic coronary arteries on the surface of both endothelial cells and smooth muscle cells (140). Expression of this 105-kD protein on endothelial cells is increased by exposure to TNF-α, IL-1β, and LPS but not by IFN-γ. IG9 can be upregulated in vitro on human aortic and human umbilical vein endothelial cells treated with mmLDL for 24 hours, whereas levels of E-selectin, ICAM-1, and VCAM-1 are not up-regulated by mmLDL (140). This activation by mmLDL implicates IG9 as a key mediator in the recruitment of monocytes during the initial injury phase of atherosclerosis. Future studies in animal models of atherosclerosis will characterize the functional role of IG9 in vivo.

Another endothelial cell molecule shown to be up-regulated by mmLDL, the novel vascular adhesion associated protein (VMAP-1), has been shown to play a role in the adhesion of monocytes to activated endothelium (141). A monoclonal antibody specific for human VMAP-1 blocked binding of human monocytes to stimulated rabbit aortic endothelial cells in vitro.

The expression of endothelial cell adhesion molecules in general is strongly associated with certain risk factors for atherosclerosis, such as hypertension, hyperlipidemia, and oxidative stress (142). Because levels of ICAM-1, VCAM-1, and E-selectin are regulated in part by the pro-inflammatory transcription factors NF-κB, AP-1, and Egr-1, common pathways may exist for the induction of activated endothelium. NF-κB has been identified in situ in smooth muscle cells, macrophages, and endothelial cells of human atherosclerotic plaques and, in contrast, is absent in normal vessels (143). All three of the aforementioned transcription factors also function to drive expression of various cytokines and growth factors, further promoting the inflammatory environment that may cause the initiation and progression of atherosclerosis. The effects of atherosclerotic risk factors on the molecular mechanisms that promote leukocyte-endothelial interaction, including the expression of adhesion molecules, will continue to be defined.

D. Chemokines

The recruitment of mononuclear leukocytes to the vessel wall in atherogenesis depends on the presence of both cytokines, which affect adhesion molecule expression on endothelial cells, and chemokines (chemotactic cytokines), which induce complementary integrins on leukocytes (144, 145). Chemokines have been a focus of atherosclerosis research by virtue of their ability to induce directional migration and activation of leukocytes on establishing a chemokine gradient. Chemokines are members of a superfamily of more than 50 small, inducible, secreted polypeptides (146). The two chemokine subfamilies that have been implicated in the initial injury of atherosclerosis are designated as C-C and C-X-C, according to the spacing of the first two of four conserved cysteine residues (145, 147). Endothelial cells, fibroblasts, monocytes, and smooth muscle cells are capable of producing chemokines (Table 2).

MCP-1 was the first chemokine to be implicated in leukocyte-mediated inflammation of atherosclerosis. The expression and release of MCP-1 in macrophage-abundant arterial walls of patients has been detected by Northern blot analysis, in situ hybridization, and immunocytochemistry (148). Endothelial cells, monocytes, and smooth muscle cells secrete MCP-1 in vitro in response to mmLDL, oxLDL, IL-1β, TNF-α, PDGF, basic fibroblast growth factor (bFGF), or CD40/CD40L activation (149, 150). Recent studies have shown that activated NF-κB induces MCP-1 (151), TGF-β inhibits MCP-1 expression (152), and complement component membrane attack complex (MAC) induces release of MCP-1 from human smooth muscle cells (153, 154). In vitro, the chemotactic transmigration of monocytes in response to oxLDL is mediated by MCP-1, and MCP-1 also regulates the activation of leukocyte integrins containing beta family subunits, providing for higher affinity binding to integrin ligands (155, 156).

Although MCP-1 is the classic C-C chemokine believed to play a role in atherosclerosis, others have the potential to mediate atherogenesis. MCP-2 and MCP-3, which target a host of inflammatory cells but not smooth muscle cells (SMC), bind to several chemokine receptors other than CCR1 and CCR2. Their roles in atherogenesis have not yet been fully explored. MCP-4, which chemoattracts monocytes and T cells in addition to eosinophils, is 60% homologous to MCP-1, shares the ability to bind the MCP-1 receptor, CCR2B, and, like MCP-1, is expressed by endothelial cells and macrophages in atherosclerotic lesions (157). High levels of mRNA for MIP-1α, MIP-1β, and RANTES have been demonstrated in carotid plaques, coronary atherosclerotic lesions, and in atherosclerotic allogeneic heart transplants (158–160). In these instances, the C-C chemokine mRNAs were coexpressed and could only be detected in the macrophages migrating through the neointima. The differential expression of C-C chemokines by different cell types in atherosclerosis suggests that chemokines may help cre-

Table 2 Chemokines That May Be Involved in Atherosclerosis (145, 147)

Chemokine	Receptor	Cells able to produce the chemokine	Stimuli	Target cells
CXC				
ENA-78	CXCR1, CXCR2	EC, F, SMC	IL-1, LPS, TNF	EC, N
GRO (α,β,γ)	CXCR2, (CXCR1)	EC, F, M, T	IL-1, LPS, TNF	EC, F, N, SMC
IL-8	CXCR1, CXCR2	EC, F, M, N, SMC, T	IL-1, LPS, TNF, mitogens microorganisms	B, EC, N, NK, SMC, T
IP-10	CXCR3	EC, F, M, T	IFN, LPS, TNF	EC, M, NK, T
MIG	CXCR3	M	IFN—γ	EC, T
NAP-2	CXCR2, (CXCR1)	EC, F, SMC	Platelet activation	EC, N
PF4	Unknown	P	Platelet activation	EC, F
CC				
MCP-1	CCR2, CCR10	All types	IFN-γ, IL-1, TNF, growth factors, LPS, mitogens,	N, SMC, T
MCP-2	CCR1, CCR2, CCR5	F, M	IFN, IL-1, LPS, mitogens, virus	Bas, D, Eos, M, NK, T
MCP-3	CCR1, CCR2, CCR3, CCR10	F, M	IFN, mitogens, LPS	Bas, D, Eos, M, N, NK, T
MCP-4	CCR2, CCR3	M,	Inflammatory stimuli	Bas, Eos, M
MCP-5	CCR2	M, SMC	Inflammatory stimuli	N, SMC, T
MIP-1α	CCR1, CCR3, CCR5	F, M, T	Inflammatory stimuli, mitogens	M, N, NK, T
MIP-1β	CCR5	F, M, T	Inflammatory stimuli	M, NK, T
RANTES	CCR1, CCR3, CCR5	EC, P, T	Inflammatory stimuli, mitogens	M, NK, T
TARC (TECK)	CCR4	DC, EC	Inflammatory stimuli	M, T

Eos, eosinophils; M, monocytes/macrophages; N, neutrophils; P, platelets; mT, memory T cells; ESL-1, E-selectin ligand-1; GAGs, glycosaminoglycans; PSGL-1, P-selectin glycoprotein ligand-1; SFLs, sialylated fucosylated lactosamines; EC, endothelial cells; B, B cells; Bas, basophils; D, dendratic cells; F, fibroblasts; NK, natural killer cells; SMC, smooth muscle cells; T, T cells; IFN, interferon; IL-1, interleukin-1; LPS, lipopolysaccharide; TNF, tumor necrosis factor-α ate a network of signals at specific sites of the microenvironment to modulate inflammation.

The C-X-C chemokines generally target neutrophils and natural killer cells (161). Two members of this family, IL-8 and growth-regulated oncogene (GROα) can participate in chronic inflammation because of their ability to act as endothelial growth factors (162) and chemoattractants of subsets (mostly CD8+) of T lymphocytes (163). Physical arterial injury, certain intralesional cytokines, complement activation, thrombin, acetylated LDL, mmLDL, oxLDL, and *Chlamydia pneumonia* cultured from atheroma are examples of stimuli that induce the expression of IL-8 and/or GROα in monocyte-macrophages, endothelial cells, and/ or SMC (147). The observation that oxLDL-induced expression of IL-8 by monocytes involves activation of p50/p65 heterodimers of the NF-κB/rel transcription factor family (164) draws together the putative role of oxLDL with the potential role of NF-κB in atherosclerosis.

The potential atherogenic effects of IL-8, GROα, and other C-X-C chemokines have received relatively little attention until recently, mostly because of their major chemoattractant effects for neutrophils, which are not frequently detected in atherosclerotic lesions. In situ studies of atherosclerotic lesions in mice have shown abundant intimal GROα expression (165), whereas expression of IL-8 by macrophage-derived foam cells taken from human atherosclerotic lesions has also been seen (166). In advanced human atherosclerotic lesions, intimal macrophages have been shown to express the GROα and IL-8 receptor CXCR2 (165). A role for CXCR2 ligands in atherosclerosis was demonstrated by their ability to induce monocyte adhesion to mmLDL-stimulated endothelium (167). In addition, expression of IL-8, as well as other chemokines, is induced during the adhesion of monocytes to endothelial cells in vitro (168).

Although evidence now exists for the presence and potential mediating effects of CXC chemokines and their receptors in atherogenesis, the exact mechanisms are unknown. Possibilities include both the recruitment of circulating monocytes and the activation and/or growth of monocytes, endothelial cells, and SMC within lesions. IL-8 may play a role in the pathogenesis of atherosclerosis in diabetes mellitus, because elevated glucose concentrations have been shown to induce IL-8 expression by endothelial cells (169). Although atherosclerotic lesions themselves have not been shown to contain many neutrophils, they do exhibit expression of E-selectin and ICAM-1, major endothelial ligands for neutrophil adhesion molecules, as well as neutrophil chemotactic factors IL-8 and GROα. Finally, GROα and IL-8 are able to stimulate reduced nicotinamide adenine dinucleotide phosphate (NADPH) oxidase activity in peripheral blood monocytes (170), and may stimulate macrophages to perform pro-atherogenic activities, including oxidation of LDL and expression of other inflammatory mediators (84).

The possible mechanisms of chemokine involvement in atherosclerosis may be summarized as follows. The initial step is though to be entrapment of

LDL in the subendothelial space, isolated from plasma-borne antioxidants. Oxidation of LDL may occur by several pathways, and the initial product, mmLDL, can induce the production by overlying endothelium or underlying smooth muscle cells of MCP-1 with concomitant expression of adhesion molecules for monocytes. These molecules, in turn, induce monocyte and T lymphocyte adhesion and transendothelial migration. The release of reactive oxygen intermediates and aldehydes further modifies the mmLDL into a form of oxLDL that is avidly taken up by macrophages, resulting in foam cell formation.

V. INTIMAL THICKENING AND THE ROLE OF SMC

A central feature of atherosclerosis is the reactive intimal thickening that follows the lipid deposition and/or injury to the vascular wall during the progression of the disease or by interventions such as balloon angioplasty or endarterectomy. Intimal hyperplasia results from two distinct processes, the inappropriate migration and proliferation of vascular SMC into the intima and the accumulation of extracellular matrix deposited by the SMC. If this process continues, stenosis and occlusion of the artery can occur.

A normal artery wall is composed of three layers: intima, media, and adventitia. Under normal circumstances the intima is composed of a monolayer of endothelial cells resting on a basement membrane, which is separated from the media by the internal elastic lamina. SMC play a role in maintaining the extracellular matrix within the wall by secreting various types of collagen and elastin. In addition to this homeostatic function, SMC are essential for vasodilation and vasoconstriction in response to both physiological and pharmacological stimuli. The phenotype of SMC in the media of normal arteries can best be described as "contractile" (171). This is accompanied by the predominant expression of the α-smooth muscle actin isoform and expression of intermediate filaments such as vimentin and desmin (172, 173). This phenotype is altered during intimal hyperplasia, with the SMC adopting a dedifferentiated state that is characterized by a synthetic phenotype with a greater expression of β-nonmuscle actin and γ-smooth muscle actin (174, 175), as well as increased levels of vimentin and decreased levels of desmin (171). Studies from resected human lesions also correlate with findings of increased nonmuscle myosin heavy chain-β synthesis that may increase the risk of restenosis after atherectomy (176).

In a rat model of intimal hyperplasia, damage to the endothelium resulted in reactive intimal thickening. However, if the injury to the vessel wall included damage to the media, the result was greater intimal hyperplasia, suggesting that injury to the media is important in neointimal formation. Although the stimulus for intimal hyperplasia can vary, the one common factor is damage to the endothelium and media of the artery. This injury triggers a complex series of events that leads to a thickened intima. Endothelial dysfunction and denudation from the vessel wall has been implicated as the initial step in plaque formation (37, 82, 177). The result of this dysfunction or denuding is a compensatory response that alters the function of SMC and causes intimal thickening. In addition, the presence of modified LDL can stimulate an inflammatory response (105, 108). This response can be mediated by numerous cell types. SMC are capable of responding to and producing numerous cytokines and growth factors. Platelets are also important because they bind to the exposed basal lamina on endothelial denuding and also elaborate a variety of factors that contribute to intimal thickening. The endothelium is also capable of responding to such stimuli by altering its expression of cell surface proteins and by producing soluble mediators that are important for promoting intimal hyperplasia (178, 179).

Determining the mechanisms that regulate SMC growth is essential for a more complete understanding of the pathophysiology of intimal hyperplasia. Intimal thickening occurs after the initial injury to the vascular wall and formation of the fatty streak. During fatty streak formation there is infiltration of the intimal layer with lipoprotein particles, in particular LDL. In cases of hypercholesterolemia, where there are high levels of LDL in the serum, large amounts of LDL become trapped in arterial walls and undergo subsequent oxidation (108, 112). This oxLDL, which can no longer be recognized by its native receptor, serves as the active initiator of plaque formation, resulting in monocyte/macrophage recruitment. Internalization of oxLDL particles occurs by means of scavenger receptors, resulting in the formation of foam cells. Within the core of the developing plaque there is deposition of both soluble and crystalline cholesterol esters and formation of lipid peroxides (108, 112). As this process continues, the oxLDL can generate other free-radical molecules that can injure the endothelium and SMC, further perpetuating the inflammatory response by increasing soluble factors, such as MCP-1 and M-CSF, that recruit more monocytes (107, 109). Thus, LDL and its various modified forms serve not only to initiate the process of plaque formation but also to perpetuate and amplify the inflammatory process by stimulating the production of soluble factors that recruit inflammatory cells (108, 180).

The importance of lowering LDL levels in patients is important for prevention of atherosclerosis. The use of HMG-CoA reductase inhibitors has clearly been shown to reduce the progression of atherosclerosis (181, 182). However, several studies demonstrated that the effects of this class of drugs are due not only to lipid lowering but also to aiding in the decrease in migration and proliferation of SMC. The mechanism by which this occurs appears to be related to the ability of these drugs to prevent formation of mevalonic acid, the product of the HMG-CoA reductase activity (181). Studies in rabbit models indicate that lower lipid levels favor the mature SMC phenotype in plaques (182). Together these findings indicate the importance of lipids, in particular LDL and cholesterol, in the initiation and progression of the atheroma. Perhaps by lowering LDL levels, the number of inflammatory cells that are recruited to the site of injury can be reduced. The importance of these inflammatory cells is though to be their ability to modulate the activity of SMC through the production of various cytokines and growth factors (179). Interaction of SMC with the extracellular matrix and subsequent autocrine regulation by SMC can also be contributing factors (183).

PDGF has been shown to be a crucial regulator of SMC proliferation and migration. There are various isoforms of PDGF, PDGF-AA, PDGF-AB, and PDGF-BB, (caused by the two different polypeptide chains, A and B), along with different receptor types, PDGF-α-receptor and PDGF-β-receptor. SMC from injured arteries secrete only the PDGF-AA despite expressing the genes for both chains (184). Yet the receptor type that is expressed in these SMC is the β-receptor (185). It is uncertain why these cells would express one ligand and another type of receptor. The answer may be that different isoforms are generated for different functions with different target cells. Injury to the artery also exposes the underlying SMC to circulating platelets, which have been shown to adhere to the injured vessel, as well as being a source of PDGF-BB (186). In a rat model of vascular injury by balloon angioplasty, the resulting intimal hyperplasia could be blocked through the use of a specific inhibitor of PDGF-receptor tyrosine kinase (CGP53716) (187). This study indicated that PDGF-R activation was important in both SMC migration and proliferation; however, migration was shown to be affected to a greater extent. The various sources of PDGF in a plaque include endothelial cells, SMC, and platelets (188). On endothelial disruption or dysfunction, platelets can adhere to the basement membrane, resulting in release of PDGF-BB, or the endothelium can produce the PDGF-BB, which can then act as a chemotactic agent for SMC. The resulting migration of SMC from the media to the intima followed by subsequent stimuli leads to their proliferation and intima formation.

The heparin-binding growth factors, acidic fibroblast growth factor (aFGF) and basic fibroblast growth factor (bFGF), are also potentially important growth factors that can stimulate the proliferation of both SMC and endothelial cells (189, 190). They are normally bound to the extracellular matrix and can be released on mechanical injury such as that introduced by balloon angioplasty (191, 192). Once released from the matrix, FGF is free to bind its receptors on both SMC and endothelial cells, resulting in cellular proliferation. As in the case of PDGF, vascular injury serves not only to increase the availability of FGF to the cells but also to up-regulate the receptors for FGF (189). Animal models used to study the role of FGFs in intimal hyperplasia have shown that bFGF promotes intimal growth and its inhibition by an antibody can decrease intimal growth (193, 194). Studies conducted with aFGF produced mixed results. Infusion of aFGF decreases intimal hyperplasia (190), but the introduction of the aFGF gene within the cells lining the artery increases intimal growth and angiogenesis (195).

The effects of this growth factor are complicated by its interactions with other cytokines that are present within the plaque, such as transforming growth factor-β (TGF-β), which inhibits its actions on endothelial cells. Heparin, which is in the extracellular matrix, can also alter the action of the two types of FGFs in the plaque by altering the affinity of the receptors to the ligand (189).

Because hypertension is a risk factor for the development of atherosclerosis, researchers have investigated the role of the renin-angiotensin system in intimal proliferation, in particular the role of angiotensin II (AngII). There are two distinct receptors for AngII, AT1, expressed mainly on SMC, and AT2, expressed mainly on endothelial cells (196). As in the case of PDGF, vascular injury results in an up-regulation of only the AT2 receptor, and on binding AngII, SMC undergo both hypertrophy and proliferation (197). Studies with inhibitors of angiotensin-converting enzyme and AT1 receptor antagonist have demonstrated a reduction of intimal growth (198), but in studies with AT2 receptor inhibition has been demonstrated as well. The use of an AT2 receptor antagonist reduces intimal hyperplasia when administered directly into the region of vascular injury, whereas systemic administration of the inhibitor is ineffective (199).

Other factors that promote SMC proliferation and subsequent intimal thickening include α-thrombin, which is important in the clotting cascade, and insulin-like growth factor-1 (IGF-1). Both these substances appear to participate in the progression of the lesion and intimal thickening (200, 201). In the case of α-thrombin, which is associated within the matrix of the media, its activation depends on both its release from the matrix on injury and the up-regulation of its receptor by bFGF (202). In addition, the expression of its receptor is associated with SMC that produce PDGF (202). Use of inhibitors of thrombin such as hirudin has been reported to reduce restenosis after angioplasty (203, 204). Although IGF-1 can increase the ability of PDGF to induce SMC proliferation, it may play a more important role in remodeling the extracellular matrix by enhancing production of hydroxyproline and increasing the organization and maturation of collagen (205).

Despite the production of these growth-promoting cytokines and growth factors as a result of vascular injury, not all substances produced by these stimuli result in intimal hyperplasia. In particular, factors such as heparin, TGF-β, and NO can inhibit SMC proliferation. The role of heparin in intimal hyperplasia is rather complex and is still not fully understood. What is known is that SMC from regions of intimal thickening seem to be less sensitive to the actions of heparin than SMC from other regions (206). It is thought that heparin may mediate its effects through its ability to interact with the extracellular matrix, growth factors, such as FGF, and through its ability to alter matrix production by SMC (207, 208).

The negative effects of TGF-β on intimal growth can be attributed to its ability to inhibit SMC proliferation and migration (202). Other actions of TGF-β that can be important are its ability to modulate the production of extracellular matrix and the proteases that can be generated to destabilize the matrix (202). By decreasing SMC growth and increasing extracellular matrix production, TGF-β can stabilize the plaque and prevent the progression of the lesion.

Last, the production of NO provides a protective effect on intimal thickening and restenosis (209). In studies that increased NO production by supplying L-arginine there was a reduction in intimal thickening and an increase in endothelial function as measured by endothelium-dependent vasodilation (210). Activation of inducible NO synthase in SMC can occur with cytokines such as IL-1, which is also seen within the atheroma (211). Perhaps intimal thickening occurs when the balance of these growth-inhibiting factors is outweighed by growth-promoting factors. This possibility suggests targets for the control of intimal hyperplasia and warrants further studies.

These various growth promoters and inhibitors all have one thing in common, they all affect the activity of the SMC within the media causing the cell to undergo the changes necessary for migration and proliferation. Through the use of animal models of vascular injury, researchers have shown that SMC respond within 48 hours of injury, and there is synchronous entry of SMC into S phase (208). This response is also accompanied by changes in SMC phenotype from "contractile" to "synthetic" as the cells begin to proliferate (171). Factors that regulate this response generally activate either the G-protein coupled receptors or tyrosine kinase coupled receptors, which in turn leads to the activation of mitogen-activated protein kinases, resulting in induction of *c-Myc, c-Fos*, and *c-Jun*, followed by cell proliferation (212). Expression of the many growth factors mentioned previously is also up-regulated in this response, providing a positive feedback mechanism for SMC growth.

An atherosclerotic plaque consists of more than just lipids and the SMC that occupy most of the thickened intima. As mentioned earlier, athersclerosis can be described as an inflammatory disease involving monocytes, macrophages, and T cells (4). These inflammatory cells play an important role in reactive intimal hyperplasia through the production of cytokines and growth factors that can induce SMC migration and proliferation, as well as perpetuate the inflammatory process by recruiting more inflammatory cells (4, 180). Animal studies of vascular injury demonstrated that JE, the murine homolog of MCP-1, is expressed soon after injury to the vessel, resulting in recruitment of monocytes (213). The importance of MCP-1 has been demonstrated through antibody-blocking studies that result in a reduction of plaque size and intimal thickness (202). MCP-1 is present within human lesions, providing support for its role in both human and animal models of vascular injury (148).

The ability of leukocytes to infiltrate a lesion depends on the presence of the chemotactic agent and the expression of cell adhesion molecules on the surface of the endothelium. On injury of the vascular wall, there is an up-regulation of adhesion molecules on the endothelium (128, 214). This increase in cell adhesion proteins is an important step in the development of the plaque and the ensuing intimal reaction, as discussed previously. Inhibiting the interaction between leukocytes and these cell adhesion molecules can reduce infiltration of these inflammatory cells into the plaque, resulting in reduction in plaque size and intimal thickness (215).

Platelet binding to the exposed subendothelium on vascular injury results in the release of additional substances that can act as mitogens and chemotactic agents for SMC. Release of these factors, which include von Willebrand factor and thromboxane A_2, requires the activation and adhesion of platelets to the subendothelial matrix (216). Because platelet adhesion occurs early in the process of vascular injury, these factors may play an early role in intimal hyperplasia, but it is unlikely that they contribute to chronic intimal growth. In animals that are thrombocytopenic, there is no reduction in intimal size, illustrating the fact that platelets can provide the initial stimulus but are not necessary in this chronic process (217).

Development of intimal hyperplasia and the atheroma involves many cell types and is regulated by numerous factors. Proliferation of SMC is important as is migration of SMC from the media to the intima. Both PDGF and FGF can act as chemotactic agents for SMC, and there also appears to be a SMC-derived factor that acts as an autoregulatory agent that mediates SMC migration (218). During migration, SMC do not appear to proliferate, but on arrival in the intima, many of the SMC begin another phase of cell division (202). Thus, there are two stages of proliferation involved in neointimal formation, the initial dedifferentiation of SMC followed by proliferation within the media, and a second proliferative stage after migration into the intima has occurred. The migratory phase is regulated by interactions between the extracellular matrix and the integrin family of cell surface receptors (219, 220). One such interaction is the binding of vitronectin (a glycoprotein found in the matrix) by $\alpha V\beta 3$ and $\alpha V\beta 5$ integrins on SMC (220). Therefore, an additional regulatory step for SMC migration and proliferation can be through the modulation of extracellular matrix secreted by SMC.

The ultimate consequence of atherosclerosis is formation of a plaque that can lead to either occlusion of the artery or rupture of the plaque resulting in thrombus formation. Sudden rupture of the plaque results in acute symptoms such as a myocardial infarction or stroke (98). A major component of the plaque is the SMC population that has migrated and proliferated in the intima. Once located in the intima, the SMC interact with inflammatory cells and secrete extracellular matrix that adds to plaque size. This dynamic interaction between SMC and inflammatory cells contributes significantly to the phenotype of the plaque.

VI. DETERMINANTS OF PLAQUE STABILITY

Atherosclerosis results in the development of various symptoms, depending on the vascular bed that is affected (9). The most significant and potentially lethal manifestations of atherosclerosis are the development of unstable angina, myocardial infarction, or cerebral vascular ischemia, which can result from plaque rupture with thrombus formation (98). Understanding the determinants of plaque stability and factors that can lead to instability and rupture of a plaque is crucial in preventing these complications of atherosclerosis.

The structure of an atheroma can be divided into two regions, the lipid core, which is hypocellular and avascular, and the fibrous cap. Within the lipid core there is deposition of cholesterol ester crystals, modified lipoproteins, necrotic cellular debris, monocytes, macrophages, and foam cells (108, 180). Covering this lipid core is the fibrous cap that is predominantly occupied by SMC and the extracellular matrix they secrete (7). Disruption of the fibrous cap exposes the contents of the lipid core to platelets and other activators of the clotting cascade, resulting in thrombus. Pathological examination of human atheroma has identified several characteristics that contribute to plaque stability. Those that weaken the plaque make it more prone to rupture and thrombus formation. Plaques that have thin, eccentric fibrous caps and a large lipid core that is filled with lipids and necrotic debris tend to be relatively unstable. These morphological features are consistently seen with unstable atheroma, and many of these features are associated with plaque rupture in cases of sudden death (221). Plaques that contain a smaller lipid core and a thick fibrous cap tend to be more stable (222, 223).

One of the differences between stable and unstable plaques is the relative proportion of the lipid core. Plaques that have larger lipid cores tend to be more vulnerable to rupture than plaques that have smaller lipid cores (224, 225). Analysis of plaques has demonstrated that lesions with a lipid core occupying greater than 40% of the plaque size have a higher risk of rupture and thrombus formation (226). Plaques that contain large lipid cores tend to be softer than more fibrous plaques, and this softness can contribute to the instability of the lesion, because there is greater stress imposed on the fibrous cap of this type of plaque (222). In particular, the regions of high stress are located at the junction between the plaque and normal vessel, which corresponds to regions of rupture (222). Studies have shown that lipid-lowering agents have been successful in lowering the progression of atherosclerosis and the incidence of acute coronary events (227). One possible explanation for this effect is that lowering of serum cholesterol can alter the morphology of the plaque, increasing stability and decreasing the likelihood of rupture. Lowering lipid content in the plaque causes the plaque to be stiffer, reducing the strain on the fibrous cap (228). Although lipid-lowering drugs appear to provide more than one antiatherogenic mechanism, lowering lipid content within lesions may serve to prevent plaque rupture and the acute thrombotic events that follow.

The other feature of a plaque that plays an important role in determining the stability of an atheroma is the fibrous cap. Although the content and size of the lipid core can alter the level of stress that the fibrous cap receives, plaques with similar characteristics can have different clinical manifestations (228). This suggests that there are other factors that regulate the strength of the fibrous cap and thereby increase or decrease the stability of the plaque. Because the fibrous plaque is composed mainly of extracellular matrix components (particularly collagen, elastin, and proteoglycans), factors that regulate matrix production and degradation can affect the stability of a plaque. There is significant extracellular matrix in the plaque of lesions that are stable and produce chronic ischemia rather than frank thrombus formation, as opposed to the reduced matrix material present in unstable lesions (229). This combination of increased mechanical stress and insufficient extracellular matrix weakens the fibrous cap allowing rupture to occur.

In atherosclerosis, one of the central characteristics is increased extracellular matrix accumulation within the vessel wall. The major source of this material is the vascular smooth muscle cell. During intimal hyperplasia SMC proliferate and migrate into the intima where they also begin to produce extracellular matrix. The presence of cytokines and growth factors in the atheroma can regulate the production of matrix. For example, the presence of TGF-β results in increased collagen synthesis that provides tensile strength allowing the plaque to withstand greater amounts of stress (230). Once collagen and other matrix proteins have been elaborated, they can be reorganized in the presence of SMC. This process is mediated in part by β1-integrins on SMC (231).

The extracellular matrix can interact with more than the cell surface receptors; it also interacts with other molecules within the matrix such as cytokines and growth factors. An example of this type of interaction is the ability of FGF to bind to heparin sulfate in the matrix (232). In this regard, the extracellular matrix is regulating the presentation of FGF to its receptor. Although interactions between extracellular matrix, growth factors, and cells are important, their relevance in plaque stability is not fully understood.

Blood pressure changes have been proposed as a trigger for plaque rupture. For example, the cyclic pressure changes that an artery undergoes can lead to continuous stresses on a plaque (233). The correlation between blood pressure and tension is defined by LaPlace's law, which states that tension in the vessel wall increases with increasing blood pressure and intraluminal diameter. Thus, increases in blood pressure may be sufficient to raise the tension in the plaque to levels that exceed the ability of the plaque to compensate, resulting in rupture. It may be that normal cyclic changes in blood pressure do not overwhelm the plaque, but the repetitive stress of bending and compression weakens the plaque, making it susceptible to spontaneous rupture (233, 234). This is important in eccentric plaques that, when bent, do not have an equal distribution of stress (235).

In the normal artery wall, there is a microvascular network called the vasa vasorum that is located in the adventitia and media of the vessel. A second mechanism for increasing stress on the fibrous plaque is by increasing intraplaque pressure through intraplaque hemorrhage from the vaso vasorum. Although it has been documented that intraplaque hemorrhages occur with resulting increases in intraplaque pressure, this rise in pressure in most cases is not likely to exceed the intraluminal pressure of the artery, making it unlikely to cause rupture of the fibrous cap (228, 236). During vasospasm, the arterial diameter decreases, resulting in decreased tension in the vessel wall, but the physical action of vasospasm can alter the shape of the plaque, redistributing the tension to weaker points in the fibrous cap. Despite the overall decrease in tension, the plaque may still rupture (237). Although there are indications that plaque rupture and vasospasm colocalize, vasospasm is not the only factor that is involved in rupture (228). The different mechanisms of increasing intraplaque pressure are not sufficient to cause rupture alone but may play a role in conjunction with other determinants of plaque stability.

The third mechanism that may result in plaque rupture is weakening of the fibrous cap by degradation of the extracellular matrix, which provides the plaque with tensile strength. There are three main categories of proteases that can actively degrade the extracellular matrix proteins: serine proteases, cysteine proteases, and matrix metalloproteinases (MMPs). The serine family of proteases includes proteins such as urokinase-type plasminogen activator, plasmin, and other membrane-associated proteases. Although there is an increased expression of urokinase receptor in human lesions, serine protease activity is not augmented in unstable plaques (237). In general these proteases are involved in cell migration and digest laminin, fibronectin, and proteoglycans within the matrix (238).

The cysteine proteases, predominantly the cathepsin family of intracellular proteases, usually localize within the lysosomal compartment. Atherosclerotic plaques contain both macrophages and SMC that have expanded lysosomal compartments, suggesting a role for these cysteine proteases in matrix degradation (239). Although these cathepsins function optimally in acidic environments, cathepsin S has been shown to be active at neutral pH, and it is expressed in human lesions in regions of high susceptibility for rupture (237). The expression of cathepsin S can be modulated by cytokines that are found in atheromas, such as IL-β and IFN-γ, both of which result in secretion of active cathespin S from SMC in vitro (239). Cathespin K has also been identified as being present in the lesions, but the mechanism regulating its production is as yet unknown (240). Localization of these proteases to regions prone to rupture and their regulation by factors within the plaque provide a distinct mechanism that can lead to plaque instability.

The MMP family is composed of 16 zinc-dependent proteases. These proteases are defined by several characteristics: (a) they are able to degrade extracellular matrix; (b) they are secreted as a zymogen and require proteolytic cleavage before activation; (c) they can function at neutral pH; and (d) each protease binds zinc ions at the active site and also binds calcium ions for stability (241). These proteases often have a broad range of substrates with overlap among members of the family, but there are preferential substrates for specific MMPs. Stimulation of MMP production is regulated by various cytokines (242). Once secreted, the MMPs require proteolytic cleavage to be activated, and although this mechanism is unclear in humans, it is speculated that plasmin may be involved (237). Inhibition of MMP activity is regulated in part by the presence of tissue inhibitors of metalloproteinases (TIMPs) (243, 244).

MMPs may contribute to plaque rupture because of their ability to degrade matrix proteins in neutral pH. In human atherosclerotic plaque there is increased expression of MMPs in the shoulder region, where rupture of plaques commonly occurs (245). In situ hybridization studies of lesions demonstrated the presence of MMP-1, MMP-2, MMP-7, MMP-9, and MMP-12 that are expressed by macrophages within the lesion (246, 247). In situ zymography demonstrated that these MMPs are active enzymes (246). In comparison only MMP-2 was detected within the vessel wall of normal arteries (237, 246). Together these data suggest that MMP activity can participate in reducing the strength of the fibrous cap through degradation of extracellular matrix proteins, in particular collagen type I.

Other studies have shown that endothelial cells (EC), SMC, and monocytes are also capable of producing a variety of MMPs (247–249). Studies in vitro demonstrated that SMC stimulated by cytokines present in lesions increased their production of MMPs. For example, IL-1β and TNF-α can stimulate SMC to secrete MMP-1 and MMP-3 (248). One source of these cytokines is likely to be the monocytes or macrophages present in the lesion. MMP-1 and MMP-3 production is augmented by coculturing monocytes with SMC, which can be inhibited by antibodies to IL-1β (248).

Monocytes and macrophages can produce MMPs in addition to stimulating their production from SMC. In vitro studies of foam cells obtained from animal models of atherosclerosis revealed that these cells are constitutively active producers of MMPs (250). Separate studies done with human macrophages demonstrated their ability to degrade matrix in culture, providing a mechanism for plaque instability (251). However, these animal studies and culture models do not provide direct evidence for MMP activity in developing unstable plaques. Analysis of human lesions demonstrated a link between macrophages and plaque stability by identifying an increased density of macrophages infiltrating the fibrous plaque of unstable atheroma (252). Therefore, regulation of macrophage content in plaques may provide a way of stabilizing plaques.

It has been well documented that macrophage accumulation is stimulated by increased serum cholesterol levels, in particular the LDL fraction. An additional benefit to lipid-lowering therapies may be the reduction of MMP levels caused by a decrease in the number of macrophages within a plaque. This was illustrated in a rabbit model of atherosclerosis that demonstrated that lipid lowering resulted in a reduction of both macrophages and MMP-1 activity (253).

As discussed previously, the strength of the fibrous cap is due mainly to the presence of extracellular matrix proteins produced by SMC, which can be destabilized by factors including MMPs. Thus, a reduction in SMC and an increase in macrophages within a plaque would favor instability. It has been demonstrated in unstable plaques that numerous SMC are undergoing apoptosis (254). This process of programmed cell death is regulated by many factors, such as TNF-α and IL-1β, which can be present in the plaque (237, 255). Furthermore, IFN-γ secreted from activated T cells within the plaque can inhibit SMC growth (256). Interestingly, these T cells are located in the shoulder region of the plaque, supporting their presence as a mechanism for plaque instability. Indeed, a decrease in SMC and an increase in macrophages corresponds to a thin fibrous cap (229). Table 3 summarizes the various factors associated with plaque instability.

Rupture alone does not account for all clinical manifestations of atherosclerosis. When the fibrous cap is disrupted, the contents of the plaque are exposed to the bloodstream, triggering the clotting cascade, which results in thrombus formation. A key initiator of coagulation is tissue factor (TF), a membrane-bound glycoprotein that is located in abundance within the plaque (257). Activation of the clotting cascade by TF results in the conversion of fibrinogen to fibrin, a major component of thrombus formation. In addition to fibrin, the thrombus contains platelets, white blood cells, red blood cells, and circulating proteins that are trapped in the forming thrombus. The cellular components of the thrombus may

Table 3   Factors Involved in Plaque Instability

Eccentric and less stenotic lesions
Thin fibrous cap
Large lipid pool
Decreased collagen production
Decrease in smooth muscle cells
Increased amounts of free or esterfied cholesterol
Increase in macrophages and T cells
Increased protease production (MMPs, cathepsins, and others)

be involved in the progression of the lesion through the various factors that they are capable of secreting.

In normal arteries, TF mRNA and protein are found in the adventitia but are not expressed by the endothelium of normal arteries (257). In several studies of human lesions, TF mRNA and protein were found to be expressed by SMC, monocytes, and foam cells within the atherosclerotic lesions (258). The thrombogenicity of plaques after rupture has been attributed to the accumulation of TF within the core of the plaque and to a lesser extent within the endothelium. Regulation of TF production by SMC, EC, and monocytes is of importance to the development of many acute complications of atherosclerosis. In cell culture studies of SMC, MCP-1, PDGF, epidermal growth factor, α-thrombin, and AngII induced the expression of TF mRNA (258, 259). Many of these factors are present in lesions and are involved in the progression of atherosclerosis. Tissue factor mRNA is induced in endothelial cells by IL-1, TNF, thrombin, and shear stress (258). These findings suggest that many mediators of plaque development are also important in TF production and accumulation within lesions.

Another major stimulus for TF production is arterial injury. This is of particular importance in balloon angioplasty or atherectomy, where injury to the vessel wall contributes to plaque formation and restenosis. It has been demonstrated that SMC are responsible for the production of TF in response to arterial injury (260). Furthermore, in animal models of arterial injury, the location of TF accumulation corresponds to regions of intimal thickening, suggesting that TF may mediate intimal hyperplasia and thrombus formation. With increased TF production, the developing lesion is primed for thrombus formation after rupture of the plaque.

The correlation between plaque stability and TF is seen in patients with unstable angina. Lesions from these patients show a greater level of TF expression (261). In these lesions, the TF was located in a cellular region that contained both macrophages and SMC. However, in lesions from patients with stable angina, the TF was located predominantly in an acellular region. This association of TF with macrophages provides a link between plaque rupture and thrombus formation because macrophages play an important role in destabilizing the plaque, resulting in rupture and subsequent exposure of TF to the circulation.

VII. ANGIOGENESIS AND ATHEROSCLEROSIS

Development of the intimal hyperplasia associated with atherosclerosis is accompanied by neovascularization in the vaso vasorum of many plaques (262, 263). The role of these newly formed vessels is not fully understood nor is the mechanism of this neovascularization. Several theories have been proposed to explain their presence within atherosclerotic lesions, with researchers focusing on the role of neovascularization in the progression, instability, and rupture of lesions.

In studies of human and animal lesions there is evidence that neovascularization can promote the progression of the lesion. Histological analysis of human lesions indicates a higher prevalance of neovascularization within plaques that have signs of rupture, hemorrhage in the vessel wall, or unstable angina (264). In addition, a greater degree of neovascularization is seen in higher histological grades of plaque (using the American Heart Association classification system) (265, 266). Animal models of arterial injury have also demonstrated neovascularization within the adventitia that correlated with plaque development (267, 268). Furthermore, inhibiting angiogenesis by treatment with endostatin or TNP-470, an inhibitor of endothelial proliferation and migration, resulted in decreased plaque growth in apolipoprotein-E (apoE)-deficient mice (269). These findings support the concept that angiogenesis in plaques plays a role in the progression of the lesion, but it does not exclude the possibility that new vessels form in plaques to supply the thickened vessel wall with oxygen and nutrients.

Because many of these new vessels are located in the shoulder region of the plaque, which contains T-cell infiltrates and foam cells, neovascularization may be an important aspect of the inflammatory nature of atherogenesis (270). In human coronary plaques, the expression of cell adhesion molecules was detected in the vaso vasorum, suggesting a mechanism by which these newly formed vessels can facilitate entry of inflammatory cells into the plaque (270). Once located within the plaque, the inflammatory cells can then act to weaken the plaque by the mechanisms described previously. Thus, neovascularization of plaques can lead to disruption of the plaque, resulting in the development of acute coronary symptoms. In addition, angiogenesis within the plaque requires migration of endothelial cells through the extracellular matrix, which is accomplished by protease production that could also contribute to weakening of the fibrous cap, making a lesion prone to rupture (246).

The development of vessels within an atherosclerotic plaque involves many soluble factors, including chemokines. The family of C-X-C chemokines can be subdivided into chemokines that contain the conserved amino acid sequence Glu-Leu-Arg (the ELR motif) and those that lack this motif. C-X-C chemokines that contain the ELR motif include IL-8, GROα, NAP-2, GCP-2, and ENA-78 (145, 271) and have been shown to be potent angiogenic factors, inducing endothelial cell migration and proliferation in vitro, as well as corneal neovascularization in vivo (272). Thus, the presence of these chemokines within the lesion can serve a dual function, to recruit inflammatory cells and to promote neovascularization.

It is also important to note that C-X-C chemokines that do not have the ELR motif, such as IP-10, MIG, and PF4, are potent angiostatic factors (272). Thus, neovascularization in the plaque may depend on the balance between the various angiogenic and angiostatic factors present in the lesion.

Another angiogenic factor that may regulate this process is vascular endothelial growth factor (VEGF) (265). VEGF is an important angiogenic factor that is involved in vessel development and wound healing. It can induce endothelial cell migration, increase vascular permeability, increase integrin expression, and modulate coagulation-related proteins on endothelial cells by binding to its receptors, flt-1 and flk-1 (273). More recently, it has been shown that monocytes express the flt-1 receptor and that the expression of this receptor is responsible for the effects of VEGF on monocytes (274).

There are several cellular sources of VEGF in plaques: tissue culture systems, SMC, macrophages, and endothelial cells all secrete VEGF. Hypoxia, IL-1, TGF-β, Ang II, and bFGF can induce the production of VEGF (275, 276). These factors have all been found in lesions, providing a possible stimulus for VEGF secretion in vivo. The amount of VEGF seen in atherosclerotic lesions corresponds to the level of neovascularization that occurs in plaques (277). Plaques that contain the greatest amount of vessel formation also express the highest level of VEGF by SMC, activated macrophages, and endothelial cells within the newly formed vessels (265). The role of VEGF in progression of the lesion is strengthened by animal studies, where overexpression of VEGF induced angiogenesis and intimal formation (278, 279). There may be other factors, including ELR-containing C-X-C chemokines, that are important in this process, but it appears that VEGF plays an important role in neovascularization within atherosclerotic plaques.

VIII. CONCLUSION

Studies of the developmental stages of atherosclerosis have underscored the importance of the vascular endothelium as a modulator of atherogenesis and plaque stability. The working model of atherosclerosis as a chronic inflammatory reaction initiated by injury from a myriad of atherosclerotic risk factors, environmental factors, infectious agents, or genetic factors provides a framework for understanding contributors to plaque formation and disruption. Figure 2 illustrates the possible mechanisms involved in atherosclerosis. The following chapters of this text describe the components that may be involved in plaque rupture in an attempt to understand the process and suggest directions for future therapies.

A.

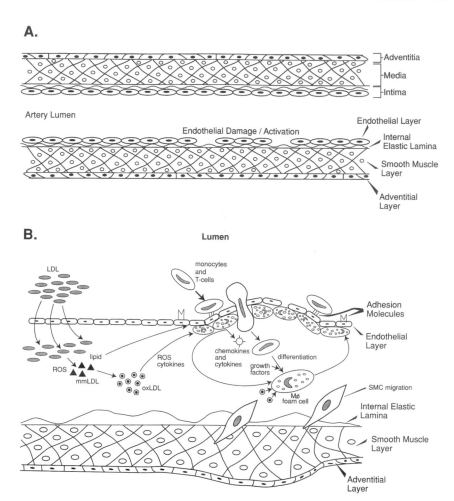

Figure 2 (A) The development of an atherosclerotic plaque. Endothelial activation fa-
vors the development of an atherosclerotic plaque. Various agents, such as elevated and
modified LDL, free radicals, cytokines, growth factors, and proteolytic enzymes, damage
and/or activate the vascular endothelium. Endothelial injury is manifest by increased permeability, a transition from anticoagulant to procoagulant properties, and increased adhesion of leukocytes and platelets. (B) In response to endothelial damage, an inflammatory
response is elicited. LDL, a necessary component in experimental induction of atherosclerosis, most likely contributes to early plaque formation. Oxidized and modified LDL promote atherogenesis by attracting monocytes, increasing the expression of monocyte adhesion molecules, inhibiting the mobility of smooth muscle cells that have migrated into
the plaque, stimulating the release of cytokines and growth factors, and acting as a direct
toxin and immunogen. Chemokines elaborated by cells within the plaque further promote
the chemotaxis of monocytes and T cells into the plaque, whereas cytokines increase adhesion molecule expression, and growth factors promote the differentiation of monocytes

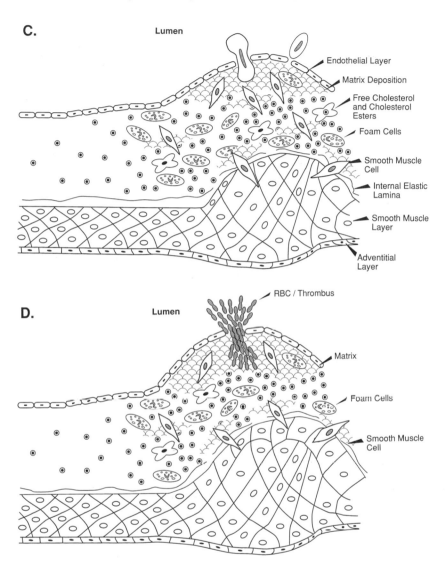

C.
Lumen

Endothelial Layer

Matrix Deposition

Free Cholesterol and Cholesterol Esters

Foam Cells

Smooth Muscle Cell

Internal Elastic Lamina

Smooth Muscle Layer

Adventitial Layer

RBC / Thrombus

D.
Lumen

Matrix

Foam Cells

Smooth Muscle Cell

into macrophages and foam cells. (C) Continued infiltration of monocytes and smooth muscle cells into the developing plaque amplifies the pathologic process. Deposition of matrix by smooth muscle cells causes the plaque size to increase, while the ratio of macrophages to fibrous tissue is thought to determine plaque stability. At this stage, the endothelium separating the plaque from the arterial lumen is also known as the fibrous cap. (D) Significant stress on the plaque or weakening of the fibrous covering can result in plaque rupture. This event is characterized by thrombus formation and platelet deposition in response to released plaque contents. Plaque rupture may be clinically significant in cases in which the thrombotic response causes complete or near-complete occlusion of the arterial lumen or in which an embolism results (refer to Figure 1).

REFERENCES

1. Cohen JD, Grimm RH Jr, Smith WM. Multiple risk factor intervention trial (MRFIT). Prev Med 1981; 10:501–518.
2. Dawber TR, Kannel WB. The Framingham study. An epidemiological approach to coronary heart disease. Circulation 1966; 34:553–555.
3. Kannel WB, McGee D, Gordon T. A general cardiovascular risk profile: the Framingham Study. Am J Cardiol 1976; 38:46–51.
4. Ross R. Atherosclerosis—an inflammatory disease. N Engl J Med 1999; 340:115–126.
5. Stary HC. Evolution and progression of atherosclerotic lesions in coronary arteries of children and young adults. Arteriosclerosis 1989; 9:I19–32.
6. Napoli C, D'Armiento FP, Mancini FP, et al. Fatty streak formation occurs in human fetal aortas and is greatly enhanced by maternal hypercholesterolemia. Intimal accumulation of low density lipoprotein and its oxidation precede monocyte recruitment into early atherosclerotic lesions. J Clin Invest 1997; 100:2680–2690.
7. Ross R. Mechanisms of atherosclerosis—a review. Adv Nephrol Necker Hosp 1990; 19:79–86.
8. Fuster V. Human lesion studies. Ann N Y Acad Sci 1997; 811:207–224; discussion 224–225.
9. Gonzalez ER, Kannewurf BS. Atherosclerosis: a unifying disorder with diverse manifestations. Am J Health Syst Pharm 1998; 55:S4–7.
10. Kannel WB. Overview of atherosclerosis. Clin Ther 1998; 20:B2–17.
11. 1999 Heart and Stroke Statistical Update. Dallas, TX: American Heart Association, 1998.
12. Stone NJ. The clinical and economic significance of atherosclerosis. Am J Med 1996; 101:4A6S–9S.
13. Stary HC, Chandler AB, Dinsmore RE, et al. A definition of advanced types of atherosclerotic lesions and a histological classification of atherosclerosis. A report from the Committee on Vascular Lesions of the Council on Arteriosclerosis, American Heart Association. Circulation 1995; 92:1355–1374.
14. Fuster V, Lewis A. Conner Memorial Lecture. Mechanisms leading to myocardial infarction: insights from studies of vascular biology [published erratum appears in Circulation 1995 Jan 1;91(1):256]. Circulation 1994; 90:2126–2146.
15. Denke MA. Diet and lifestyle modification and its relationship to atherosclerosis. Med Clin North Am 1994; 78:197–223.
16. Nehler MR, Taylor LM Jr, Porter JM. Homocysteinemia as a risk factor for atherosclerosis: a review. Cardiovasc Surg 1997; 5:559–567.
17. Kannel WB. New perspectives on cardiovascular risk factors. Am Heart J 1987; 114:213–219.
18. Chiu B, Viira E, Tucker W, Fong IW. Chlamydia pneumoniae, cytomegalovirus, and herpes simplex virus in atherosclerosis of the carotid artery. Circulation 1997; 96:2144–2148.
19. Ellis RW. Infection and coronary heart disease. J Med Microbiol 1997; 46:535–539.

20. Nieminen MS, Mattila K, Valtonen V. Infection and inflammation as risk factors for myocardial infarction. Eur Heart J 1993; 14(suppl K):12–16.
21. Experimental atherosclerosis in rabbits. Nutr Rev 1965; 23:329–330.
22. Reddick RL, Read MS, Brinkhous KM, Bellinger D, Nichols T, Griggs TR. Coronary atherosclerosis in the pig. Induced plaque injury and platelet response. Arteriosclerosis 1990; 10:541–550.
23. Mahley RW, Weisgraber KH, Innerarity T. Atherogenic hyperlipoproteinemia induced by cholesterol feeding the Patas monkey. Biochemistry 1976; 15:2979–2985.
24. Zhang SH, Reddick RL, Piedrahita JA, Maeda N. Spontaneous hypercholesterolemia and arterial lesions in mice lacking apolipoprotein E. Science 1992; 258:468–471.
25. Hopp L, Gilboa N, Kurland G, Weichler N, Orchard TJ. Acute myocardial infarction in a young boy with nephrotic syndrome: a case report and review of the literature. Pediatr Nephrol 1994; 8:290–294.
26. Stehbens WE. The epidemiological relationship of hypercholesterolemia, hypertension, diabetes mellitus and obesity to coronary heart disease and atherogenesis. J Clin Epidemiol 1990; 43:733–741.
27. Cullen P, Funke H, Schulte H, Assmann G. Lipoproteins and cardiovascular risk-from genetics to CHD prevention. J Atheroscler Thromb 1997; 4:51–58.
28. Wissler RW. Evidence for regression of advanced atherosclerotic plaques. Artery 1979; 5:398–408.
29. Nash DT, Gensini G, Esente P. Effect of lipid-lowering therapy on the progression of coronary atherosclerosis assessed by scheduled repetitive coronary arteriography. Int J Cardiol 1982; 2:43–55.
30. Olsson AG, Carlson LA, Erikson U, Hemius G, Hemmingsson A, Ruhn G. Regression of computer estimated femoral atherosclerosis after pronounced serum lipid lowering in patients with asymptomatic hyperlipidaemia [letter]. Lancet 1982; 1:1311.
31. Kannel WB, Castelli WP, Gordon T, McNamara PM. Serum cholesterol, lipoproteins, and the risk of coronary heart disease. The Framingham study. Ann Intern Med 1971; 74:1–12.
32. Brown MS, Goldstein JL. A receptor-mediated pathway for cholesterol homeostasis. Science 1986; 232:34–47.
33. Stamler J, Shekelle R. Dietary cholesterol and human coronary heart disease. The epidemiologic evidence. Arch Pathol Lab Med 1988; 112:1032–1040.
34. Brinton EA, Eisenberg S, Breslow JL. A low-fat diet decreases high density lipoprotein (HDL) cholesterol levels by decreasing HDL apolipoprotein transport rates. J Clin Invest 1990; 85:144–151.
35. Blankenhorn DH, Johnson RL, Mack WJ, el Zein HA, Vailas LI. The influence of diet on the appearance of new lesions in human coronary arteries [see comments]. Jama 1990; 263:1646–1652.
36. Knapp HR, Reilly IA, Alessandrini P, FitzGerald GA. In vivo indexes of platelet and vascular function during fish-oil administration in patients with atherosclerosis. N Engl J Med 1986;314:937–942.
37. Hennig B, Chow CK. Lipid peroxidation and endothelial cell injury: implications in atherosclerosis. Free Radic Biol Med 1988; 4:99–106.

38. Chobanian AV. The influence of hypertension and other hemodynamic factors in atherogenesis. Prog Cardiovasc Dis 1983; 26:177–196.

39. McGill HC, Jr. The cardiovascular pathology of smoking. Am Heart J 1988; 115: 250–257.

40. Benowitz NL. The role of nicotine in smoking-related cardiovascular disease. Prev Med 1997; 26:412–417.

41. Pyorala K. Diabetes and coronary heart disease. Acta Endocrinol Suppl 1985; 272: 11–19.

42. Stout RW. Diabetes and atherosclerosis. Biomed Pharmacother 1993; 47:1–2.

43. Howard G, O'Leary DH, Zaccaro D, et al. Insulin sensitivity and atherosclerosis. The Insulin Resistance Atherosclerosis Study (IRAS) Investigators [see comments]. Circulation 1996; 93:1809–1817.

44. Gordon DJ, Probstfield JL, Garrison RJ, et al. High-density lipoprotein cholesterol and cardiovascular disease. Four prospective American studies. Circulation 1989; 79:8–15.

45. Lew EA, Garfinkel L. Variations in mortality by weight among 750,000 men and women. J Chronic Dis 1979; 32:563–576.

46. Hulley SB, Rosenman RH, Bawol RD, Brand RJ. Epidemiology as a guide to clinical decisions. The association between triglyceride and coronary heart disease. N Engl J Med 1980; 302:1383–1389.

47. Elliott TG, Viberti G. Relationship between insulin resistance and coronary heart disease in diabetes mellitus and the general population: a critical appraisal. Baillieres Clin Endocrinol Metab 1993; 7:1079–1103.

48. Pyorala K. Relationship of glucose tolerance and plasma insulin to the incidence of coronary heart disease: results from two population studies in Finland. Diabetes Care 1979; 2:131–141.

49. Welborn TA, Wearne K. Coronary heart disease incidence and cardiovascular mortality in Busselton with reference to glucose and insulin concentrations. Diabetes Care 1979; 2:154–160.

50. Howard G, Bergman R, Wagenknecht LE, et al. Ability of alternative indices of insulin sensitivity to predict cardiovascular risk: comparison with the "minimal model." Insulin Resistance Atherosclerosis Study (IRAS) Investigators. Ann Epidemiol 1998; 8:358–369.

51. Wagenknecht LE, Mayer EJ, Rewers M, et al. The insulin resistance atherosclerosis study (IRAS) objectives, design, and recruitment results. Ann Epidemiol 1995; 5: 464–472.

52. Haffner SM, Miettinen H. Insulin resistance implications for type II diabetes mellitus and coronary heart disease. Am J Med 1997; 103:152–162.

53. Ferrara A, Barrett-Connor E, Wingard DL, Edelstein SL. Sex differences in insulin levels in older adults and the effect of body size, estrogen replacement therapy, and glucose tolerance status. The Rancho Bernardo Study, 1984–1987. Diabetes Care 1995; 18:220–225.

54. Reaven P, Merat S, Casanada F, Sutphin M, Palinski W. Effect of streptozotocin-induced hyperglycemia on lipid profiles, formation of advanced glycation endproducts in lesions, and extent of atherosclerosis in LDL receptor-deficient mice. Arterioscler Thromb Vasc Biol 1997; 17:2250–2256.

55. Hsueh WA, Law RE. Cardiovascular risk continuum: implications of insulin resistance and diabetes. Am J Med 1998; 105:4S–14S.
56. King GL, Brownlee M. The cellular and molecular mechanisms of diabetic complications. Endocrinol Metab Clin North Am 1996; 25:255–270.
57. Richardson M, Hadcock SJ, DeReske M, Cybulsky MI. Increased expression in vivo of VCAM-1 and E-selectin by the aortic endothelium of normolipemic and hyperlipemic diabetic rabbits. Arterioscler Thromb 1994; 14:760–769.
58. Nishio Y, Kashiwagi A, Taki H, et al. Altered activities of transcription factors and their related gene expression in cardiac tissues of diabetic rats. Diabetes 1998; 47:1318–1325.
59. Schmidt AM, Yan SD, Wautier JL, Stern D. Activation of receptor for advanced glycation end products: a mechanism for chronic vascular dysfunction in diabetic vasculopathy and atherosclerosis. Circ Res 1999; 84:489–497.
60. Miller TD, Balady GJ, Fletcher GF. Exercise and its role in the prevention and rehabilitation of cardiovascular disease. Ann Behav Med 1997; 19:220–229.
61. Manolio TA, Furberg CD, Shemanski L, et al. Associations of postmenopausal estrogen use with cardiovascular disease and its risk factors in older women. The CHS Collaborative Research Group. Circulation 1993; 88:2163–2171.
62. Effects of estrogen or estrogen/progestin regimens on heart disease risk factors in postmenopausal women. The Postmenopausal Estrogen/Progestin Interventions (PEPI) Trial. The Writing Group for the PEPI Trial [see comments] [published erratum appears in JAMA 1995 Dec 6;274(21):1676]. JAMA 1995; 273:199–208.
63. Celermajer DS, Sorensen KE, Gooch VM, et al. Non-invasive detection of endothelial dysfunction in children and adults at risk of atherosclerosis. Lancet 1992; 340: 1111–1115.
64. Rifici VA, Khachadurian AK. The inhibition of low-density lipoprotein oxidation by 17-beta estradiol. Metabolism 1992; 41:1110–1114.
65. Hendrix MG, Salimans MM, van Boven CP, Bruggeman CA. High prevalence of latently present cytomegalovirus in arterial walls of patients suffering from grade III atherosclerosis. Am J Pathol 1990; 136:23–28.
66. Melnick JL, Adam E, Debakey ME. Cytomegalovirus and atherosclerosis. Eur Heart J 1993; 14(suppl K):30–38.
67. Jackson LA, Campbell LA, Schmidt RA, et al. Specificity of detection of *Chlamydia pneumoniae* in cardiovascular atheroma: evaluation of the innocent bystander hypothesis. Am J Pathol 1997; 150:1785–1790.
68. Nicholson AC, Hajjar DP. Herpesvirus in atherosclerosis and thrombosis: etiologic agents or ubiquitous bystanders? Arterioscler Thromb Vasc Biol 1998; 18:339–348.
69. McCully KS. Vascular pathology of homocysteinemia: implications for the pathogenesis of arteriosclerosis. Am J Pathol 1969; 56:111–128.
70. Mudd SH, Skovby F, Levy HL, et al. The natural history of homocystinuria due to cystathionine beta-synthase deficiency. Am J Hum Genet 1985; 37:1–31.
71. Malinow MR. Plasma homocyst(e)ine and arterial occlusive diseases: a mini-review. Clin Chem 1995; 41:173–176.
72. Verhoef P, Stampfer MJ. Prospective studies of homocysteine and cardiovascular disease. Nutr Rev 1995; 53:283–288.

73. Omenn GS, Beresford SA, Motulsky AG. Preventing coronary heart disease: B vitamins and homocysteine [editorial; comment]. Circulation 1998; 97:421–424.
74. Hajjar KA. Homocysteine-induced modulation of tissue plasminogen activator binding to its endothelial cell membrane receptor. J Clin Invest 1993; 91:2873–2879.
75. Majors A, Ehrhart LA, Pezacka EH. Homocysteine as a risk factor for vascular disease. Enhanced collagen production and accumulation by smooth muscle cells. Arterioscler Thromb Vasc Biol 1997; 17:2074–2081.
76. Upchurch GR Jr, Welch GN, Fabian AJ, et al. Homocyst(e)ine decreases bioavailable nitric oxide by a mechanism involving glutathione peroxidase. J Biol Chem 1997; 272:17012–17017.
77. McGill HC Jr. George Lyman Duff memorial lecture. Persistent problems in the pathogenesis of atherosclerosis. Arteriosclerosis 1984; 4:443–451.
78. Wissler RW, Strong JP. Risk factors and progression of atherosclerosis in youth. PDAY Research Group. Pathological Determinants of Atherosclerosis in Youth. Am J Pathol 1998; 153:1023–1033.
79. Davies MJ, Gordon JL, Gearing AJ, et al. The expression of the adhesion molecules ICAM-1, VCAM-1, PECAM, and E-selectin in human atherosclerosis. J Pathol 1993; 171:223–229.
80. Watanabe T, Haraoka S, Shimokama T. Inflammatory and immunological nature of atherosclerosis. Int J Cardiol 1996; 54(suppl):S51–60.
81. Jonasson L, Holm J, Skalli O, Bondjers G, Hansson GK. Regional accumulations of T cells, macrophages, and smooth muscle cells in the human atherosclerotic plaque. Arteriosclerosis 1986; 6:131–138.
82. Ross R, Glomset J, Harker L. Response to injury and atherogenesis. Am J Pathol 1977; 86:675–684.
83. Steinberg D. Low density lipoprotein oxidation and its pathobiological significance. J Biol Chem 1997; 272:20963–20966.
84. Navab M, Berliner JA, Watson AD, et al. The Yin and Yang of oxidation in the development of the fatty streak. A review based on the 1994 George Lyman Duff Memorial Lecture. Arterioscler Thromb Vasc Biol 1996; 16:831–842.
85. Morel DW, Hessler JR, Chisolm GM. Low density lipoprotein cytotoxicity induced by free radical peroxidation of lipid. J Lipid Res 1983; 24:1070–1076.
86. Griendling KK, Alexander RW. Oxidative stress and cardiovascular disease [editorial; comment]. Circulation 1997; 96:3264–3265.
87. Kim JA, Gu JL, Natarajan R, Berliner JA, Nadler JL. A leukocyte type of 12-lipoxygenase is expressed in human vascular and mononuclear cells. Evidence for upregulation by angiotensin II. Arterioscler Thromb Vasc Biol 1995; 15:942–948.
88. Vanhoutte PM, Boulanger CM. Endothelium-dependent responses in hypertension. Hypertens Res 1995; 18:87–98.
89. Serrano CV Jr, Mikhail EA, Wang P, Noble B, Kuppusamy P, Zweier JL. Superoxide and hydrogen peroxide induce CD18-mediated adhesion in the postischemic heart. Biochim Biophys Acta 1996; 1316:191–202.
90. Lyons D. Impairment and restoration of nitric oxide-dependent vasodilation in cardiovascular disease. Int J Cardiol 1997; 62(Suppl 2):S101–109.
91. Resnick N, Collins T, Atkinson W, Bonthron DT, Dewey CF Jr, Gimbrone MA

Jr. Platelet-derived growth factor B chain promoter contains a cis-acting fluid shear-stress-responsive element [published erratum appears in Proc Natl Acad Sci USA 1993 Aug 15;90(16):7908]. Proc Natl Acad Sci USA 1993; 90:4591–4595.

92. Nagel T, Resnick N, Atkinson WJ, Dewey CF Jr, Gimbrone MA Jr. Shear stress selectively upregulates intercellular adhesion molecule-1 expression in cultured human vascular endothelial cells. J Clin Invest 1994; 94:885–891.

93. Steinberg D. Lipoproteins and the pathogenesis of atherosclerosis. Circulation 1987; 76:508–514.

94. Knight BL, Soutar AK. Degradation of normal and abnormal plasma lipoproteins by cultured macrophages. Agents Actions Suppl 1984; 16:129–143.

95. Ottnad E, Parthasarathy S, Sambrano GR, et al. A macrophage receptor for oxidized low density lipoprotein distinct from the receptor for acetyl low density lipoprotein: partial purification and role in recognition of oxidatively damaged cells. Proc Natl Acad Sci USA 1995; 92:1391–1395.

96. Sambrano GR, Steinberg D. Recognition of oxidatively damaged and apoptotic cells by an oxidized low density lipoprotein receptor on mouse peritoneal macrophages: role of membrane phosphatidylserine. Proc Natl Acad Sci USA 1995; 92: 1396–1400.

97. Clinton SK, Underwood R, Hayes L, Sherman ML, Kufe DW, Libby P. Macrophage colony-stimulating factor gene expression in vascular cells and in experimental and human atherosclerosis. Am J Pathol 1992; 140:301–316.

98. Henriksen T, Mahoney EM, Steinberg D. Enhanced macrophage degradation of low density lipoprotein previously incubated with cultured endothelial cells: recognition by receptors for acetylated low density lipoproteins. Proc Natl Acad Sci USA 1981; 78:6499–6503.

99. Steinbrecher UP. Oxidation of human low density lipoprotein results in derivatization of lysine residues of apolipoprotein B by lipid peroxide decomposition products. J Biol Chem 1987; 262:3603–3608.

100. Parthasarathy S, Quinn MT, Steinberg D. Is oxidized low density lipoprotein involved in the recruitment and retention of monocyte/macrophages in the artery wall during the initiation of atherosclerosis? Basic Life Sci 1988; 49:375–380.

101. Mougenot N, Lesnik P, Ramirez-Gil JF, et al. Effect of the oxidation state of LDL on the modulation of arterial vasomotor response in vitro. Atherosclerosis 1997; 133:183–192.

102. Thorne SA, Abbot SE, Winyard PG, Blake DR, Mills PG. Extent of oxidative modification of low density lipoprotein determines the degree of cytotoxicity to human coronary artery cells. Heart 1996; 75:11–16.

103. Quinn MT, Parthasarathy S, Fong LG, Steinberg D. Oxidatively modified low density lipoproteins: a potential role in recruitment and retention of monocyte/macrophages during atherogenesis. Proc Natl Acad Sci USA 1987; 84:2995–2998.

104. Quinn MT, Parthasarathy S, Steinberg D. Lysophosphatidylcholine: a chemotactic factor for human monocytes and its potential role in atherogenesis. Proc Natl Acad Sci USA 1988; 85:2805–2809.

105. Quinn MT, Parthasarathy S, Steinberg D. Endothelial cell-derived chemotactic activity for mouse peritoneal macrophages and the effects of modified forms of low density lipoprotein. Proc Natl Acad Sci USA 1985; 82:5949–5953.

106. Deigner HP, Claus R. Stimulation of mitogen activated protein kinase by LDL and oxLDL in human U-937 macrophage-like cells. FEBS Lett 1996; 385:149–153.
107. Rajavashisth TB, Andalibi A, Territo MC, et al. Induction of endothelial cell expression of granulocyte and macrophage colony-stimulating factors by modified low-density lipoproteins. Nature 1990; 344:254–257.
108. Berliner JA, Navab M, Fogelman AM, et al. Atherosclerosis: basic mechanisms. Oxidation, inflammation,and genetics. Circulation 1995; 91:2488–2496.
109. Cushing SD, Berliner JA, Valente AJ, et al. Minimally modified low density lipoprotein induces monocyte chemotactic protein 1 in human endothelial cells and smooth muscle cells. Proc Natl Acad Sci USA 1990; 87:5134–5138.
110. Rosenfeld ME, Khoo JC, Miller E, Parthasarathy S, Palinski W, Witztum JL. Macrophage-derived foam cells freshly isolated from rabbit atherosclerotic lesions degrade modified lipoproteins, promote oxidation of low-density lipoproteins, and contain oxidation-specific lipid-protein adducts. J Clin Invest 1991; 87: 90–99.
111. Zhang HF, Basra HJ, Steinbrecher UP. Effects of oxidatively modified LDL on cholesterol esterification in cultured macrophages. J Lipid Res 1990; 31:1361–1369.
112. Palinski W, Rosenfeld ME, Yla-Herttuala S, et al. Low density lipoprotein undergoes oxidative modification in vivo. Proc Natl Acad Sci USA 1989; 86:1372–1376.
113. Witztum JL, Berliner JA. Oxidized phospholipids and isoprostanes in atherosclerosis. Curr Opin Lipidol 1998; 9:441–448.
114. Levin EG, Miles LA, Fless GM, et al. Lipoproteins inhibit the secretion of tissue plasminogen activator from human endothelial cells. Arterioscler Thromb 1994; 14:438–442.
115. Pritchard KA Jr, Total RR, Lin JH, et al. Native low density lipoprotein. Endothelial cell recruitment of mononuclear cells. Arterioscler Thromb 1991; 11:1175–1181.
116. Smalley DM, Lin JH, Curtis ML, Kobari Y, Stemerman MB, Pritchard KA Jr. Native LDL increases endothelial cell adhesiveness by inducing intercellular adhesion molecule-1. Arterioscler Thromb Vasc Biol 1996; 16:585–590.
117. Allen S, Khan S, Al-Mohanna F, Batten P, Yacoub M. Native low density lipoprotein-induced calcium transients trigger VCAM-1 and E-selectin expression in cultured human vascular endothelial cells. J Clin Invest 1998; 101:1064–1075.
118. Lin JH, Zhu Y, Liao HL, Kobari Y, Groszek L, Stemerman MB. Induction of vascular cell adhesion molecule-1 by low-density lipoprotein. Atherosclerosis 1996; 127: 185–194.
119. Ko Y, Totzke G, Seewald S, et al. Native low-density lipoprotein (LDL) induces the expression of the early growth response gene-1 in human umbilical arterial endothelial cells. Eur J Cell Biol 1995; 68:306–312.
120. Cominacini L, Garbin U, Fratta Pasini A, et al. Lacidipine inhibits the activation of the transcription factor NF-kappaB and the expression of adhesion molecules induced by pro-oxidant signals on endothelial cells. J Hypertens 1997; 15:1633–1640.
121. Zhu Y, Lin JH, Liao HL, Verna L, Stemerman MB. Activation of ICAM-1 promoter by lysophosphatidylcholine: possible involvement of protein tyrosine kinases. Biochim Biophys Acta 1997; 1345:93–98.

122. Zhu Y, Lin JH, Liao HL, et al. LDL induces transcription factor activator protein-1 in human endothelial cells. Arterioscler Thromb Vasc Biol 1998; 18:473–480.

123. Yamakawa T, Eguchi S, Yamakawa Y, et al. Lysophosphatidylcholine stimulates MAP kinase activity in rat vascular smooth muscle cells. Hypertension 1998; 31: 248–253.

124. Chatterjee S, Bhunia AK, Snowden A, Han H. Oxidized low density lipoproteins stimulate galactosyltransferase activity, ras activation, p44 mitogen activated protein kinase and c- fos expression in aortic smooth muscle cells. Glycobiology 1997; 7:703–710.

125. Nagy L, Tontonoz P, Alvarez JG, Chen H, Evans RM. Oxidized LDL regulates macrophage gene expression through ligand activation of PPAR gamma. Cell 1998; 93:229–240.

126. Das PK, de Boer OJ, Visser A, Verhagen CE, Bos JD, Pals ST. Differential expression of ICAM-1, E-selectin and VCAM-1 by endothelial cells in psoriasis and contact dermatitis. Acta Derm Venereol Suppl 1994; 186:21–22.

127. Ferro CJ, Webb DJ. Endothelial dysfunction and hypertension. Drugs 1997; 53: 30–41.

128. Cotran RS, Mayadas-Norton T. Endothelial adhesion molecules in health and disease. Pathol Biol (Paris) 1998; 46:164–170.

129. Tenaglia AN, Buda AJ, Wilkins RG, et al. Levels of expression of P-selectin, E-selectin, and intercellular adhesion molecule-1 in coronary atherectomy specimens from patients with stable and unstable angina pectoris. Am J Cardiol 1997; 79: 742–747.

130. Frenette PS, Wagner DD. Insights into selectin function from knockout mice. Thromb Haemost 1997; 78:60–64.

131. Austrup F, Vestweber D, Borges E, et al. P- and E-selectin mediate recruitment of T-helper-1 but not T-helper-2 cells into inflamed tissues. Nature 1997; 385:81–83.

132. Johnson RC, Chapman SM, Dong ZM, et al. Absence of P-selectin delays fatty streak formation in mice. J Clin Invest 1997; 99:1037–1043.

133. Vora DK, Fang ZT, Liva SM, et al. Induction of P-selectin by oxidized lipoproteins. Separate effects on synthesis and surface expression. Circ Res 1997; 80:810–818.

134. Johnson-Tidey RR, McGregor JL, Taylor PR, Poston RN. Increase in the adhesion molecule P-selectin in endothelium overlying atherosclerotic plaques. Coexpression with intercellular adhesion molecule-1. Am J Pathol 1994; 144:952–961.

135. Gonzalez-Amaro R, Diaz-Gonzalez F, Sanchez-Madrid F. Adhesion molecules in inflammatory diseases. Drugs 1998; 56:977–988.

136. Nageh MF, Sandberg ET, Marotti KR, et al. Deficiency of inflammatory cell adhesion molecules protects against atherosclerosis in mice. Arterioscler Thromb Vasc Biol 1997; 17:1517–1520.

137. Ruffolo RR, Jr., Feuerstein GZ. Pharmacology of carvedilol: rationale for use in hypertension, coronary artery disease, and congestive heart failure. Cardiovasc Drugs Ther 1997; 11(Suppl 1):247–256.

138. Cotran RS, Gimbrone MA Jr, Bevilacqua MP, Mendrick DL, Pober JS. Induction and detection of a human endothelial activation antigen in vivo. J Exp Med 1986; 164:661–666.

139. Tanaka Y, Albelda SM, Horgan KJ, et al. CD31 expressed on distinctive T cell subsets is a preferential amplifier of beta 1 integrin-mediated adhesion. J Exp Med 1992; 176:245–253.

140. Calderon TM, Factor SM, Hatcher VB, Berliner JA, Berman JW. An endothelial cell adhesion protein for monocytes recognized by monoclonal antibody IG9. Expression in vivo in inflamed human vessels and atherosclerotic human and Watanabe rabbit vessels. Lab Invest 1994; 70:836–849.

141. McEvoy LM, Sun H, Tsao PS, Cooke JP, Berliner JA, Butcher EC. Novel vascular molecule involved in monocyte adhesion to aortic endothelium in models of atherogenesis. J Exp Med 1997; 185:2069–2077.

142. Ridker PM. Inflammation, atherosclerosis, and cardiovascular risk: an epidemiologic view. Blood Coagul Fibrinolysis 1999; 10(Suppl 1):S9–12.

143. Brand K, Page S, Rogler G, et al. Activated transcription factor nuclear factor-kappa B is present in the atherosclerotic lesion. J Clin Invest 1996; 97:1715–1722.

144. Zlotnik A, Morales J, Hedrick JA. Recent advances in chemokines and chemokine receptors. Crit Rev Immunol 1999; 19:1–47.

145. Wang JM, Su S, Gong W, Oppenheim JJ. Chemokines, receptors, and their role in cardiovascular pathology. Int J Clin Lab Res 1998; 28:83–90.

146. Adams DH, Lloyd AR. Chemokines: leucocyte recruitment and activation cytokines. Lancet 1997; 349:490–495.

147. Terkeltaub R, Boisvert WA, Curtiss LK. Chemokines and atherosclerosis. Curr Opin Lipidol 1998; 9:397–405.

148. Yla-Herttuala S, Lipton BA, Rosenfeld ME, et al. Expression of monocyte chemoattractant protein 1 in macrophage-rich areas of human and rabbit atherosclerotic lesions. Proc Natl Acad Sci USA 1991; 88:5252–5256.

149. Wempe F, Lindner V, Augustin HG. Basic fibroblast growth factor (bFGF) regulates the expression of the CC chemokine monocyte chemoattractant protein-1 (MCP-1) in autocrine-activated endothelial cells. Arterioscler Thromb Vasc Biol 1997; 17:2471–2478.

150. Lei XF, Ohkawara Y, Stampfli MR, et al. Disruption of antigen-induced inflammatory responses in CD40 ligand knockout mice. J Clin Invest 1998; 101:1342–1353.

151. Landry DB, Couper LL, Bryant SR, Lindner V. Activation of the NF-kappa B and I kappa B system in smooth muscle cells after rat arterial injury. Induction of vascular cell adhesion molecule-1 and monocyte chemoattractant protein-1. Am J Pathol 1997; 151:1085–1095.

152. Kitamura M. Identification of an inhibitor targeting macrophage production of monocyte chemoattractant protein-1 as TGF-beta 1. J Immunol 1997; 159:1404–1411.

153. Torzewski J, Oldroyd R, Lachmann P, Fitzsimmons C, Proudfoot D, Bowyer D. Complement-induced release of monocyte chemotactic protein-1 from human smooth muscle cells. A possible initiating event in atherosclerotic lesion formation. Arterioscler Thromb Vasc Biol 1996; 16:673–677.

154. Torzewski M, Torzewski J, Bowyer DE, et al. Immunohistochemical colocalization of the terminal complex of human complement and smooth muscle cell alpha-actin in early atherosclerotic lesions. Arterioscler Thromb Vasc Biol 1997; 17:2448–2452.

155. Gyetko MR, Todd RF 3rd, Wilkinson CC, Sitrin RG. The urokinase receptor is required for human monocyte chemotaxis in vitro. J Clin Invest 1994; 93:1380–1387.

156. Faull RJ, Ginsberg MH. Inside-out signaling through integrins. J Am Soc Nephrol 1996; 7:1091–1097.

157. Berkhout TA, Sarau HM, Moores K, et al. Cloning, in vitro expression, and functional characterization of a novel human CC chemokine of the monocyte chemotactic protein (MCP) family (MCP-4) that binds and signals through the CC chemokine receptor 2B. J Biol Chem 1997; 272:16404–16413.

158. Wilcox JN, Nelken NA, Coughlin SR, Gordon D, Schall TJ. Local expression of inflammatory cytokines in human atherosclerotic plaques. J Atheroscler Thromb 1994; 1:S10–13.

159. Pattison JM, Nelson PJ, Huie P, Sibley RK, Krensky AM. RANTES chemokine expression in transplant-associated accelerated atherosclerosis. J Heart Lung Transplant 1996; 15:1194–1199.

160. Fairchild RL, VanBuskirk AM, Kondo T, Wakely ME, Orosz CG. Expression of chemokine genes during rejection and long-term acceptance of cardiac allografts. Transplantation 1997; 63:1807–1812.

161. Hoch RC, Schraufstatter IU, Cochrane CG. In vivo, in vitro, and molecular aspects of interleukin-8 and the interleukin-8 receptors. J Lab Clin Med 1996; 128:134–145.

162. Koch AE, Polverini PJ, Kunkel SL, et al. Interleukin-8 as a macrophage-derived mediator of angiogenesis [see comments]. Science 1992; 258:1798–1801.

163. Qin S, LaRosa G, Campbell JJ, et al. Expression of monocyte chemoattractant protein-1 and interleukin-8 receptors on subsets of T cells: correlation with transendothelial chemotactic potential. Eur J Immunol 1996; 26:640–647.

164. Brand K, Eisele T, Kreusel U, et al. Dysregulation of monocytic nuclear factor-kappa B by oxidized low-density lipoprotein. Arterioscler Thromb Vasc Biol 1997; 17:1901–1909.

165. Boisvert WA, Santiago R, Curtiss LK, Terkeltaub RA. A leukocyte homologue of the IL-8 receptor CXCR-2 mediates the accumulation of macrophages in atherosclerotic lesions of LDL receptor-deficient mice. J Clin Invest 1998; 101:353–363.

166. Wang N, Tabas I, Winchester R, Ravalli S, Rabbani LE, Tall A. Interleukin 8 is induced by cholesterol loading of macrophages and expressed by macrophage foam cells in human atheroma. J Biol Chem 1996; 271:8837–8842.

167. Schwartz D, Andalibi A, Chaverri-Almada L, et al. Role of the GRO family of chemokines in monocyte adhesion to MM-LDL-stimulated endothelium. J Clin Invest 1994; 94:1968–1973.

168. Lukacs NW, Strieter RM, Elner V, Evanoff HL, Burdick MD, Kunkel SL. Production of chemokines, interleukin-8 and monocyte chemoattractant protein-1, during monocyte: endothelial cell interactions. Blood 1995; 86:2767–2773.

169. Urakaze M, Temaru R, Satou A, Yamazaki K, Hamazaki T, Kobayashi M. The IL-8 production in endothelial cells is stimulated by high glucose. Horm Metab Res 1996; 28:400–401.

170. Walz A, Meloni F, Clark-Lewis I, von Tscharner V, Baggiolini M. [Ca2+]i changes

and respiratory burst in human neutrophils and monocytes induced by NAP-1/interleukin-8, NAP-2, and gro/MGSA. J Leukoc Biol 1991; 50:279–286.

171.   Kocher O, Gabbiani F, Gabbiani G, et al. Phenotypic features of smooth muscle cells during the evolution of experimental carotid artery intimal thickening. Biochemical and morphologic studies. Lab Invest 1991; 65:459–470.

172.   Kocher O, Skalli O, Bloom WS, Gabbiani G. Cytoskeleton of rat aortic smooth muscle cells. Normal conditions and experimental intimal thickening. Lab Invest 1984; 50:645–652.

173.   Gabbiani G, Rungger-Brandle E, de Chastonay C, Franke WW. Vimentin-containing smooth muscle cells in aortic intimal thickening after endothelial injury. Lab Invest 1982; 47:265–269.

174.   Owens GK, Loeb A, Gordon D, Thompson MM. Expression of smooth muscle-specific alpha-isoactin in cultured vascular smooth muscle cells: relationship between growth and cytodifferentiation. J Cell Biol 1986; 102:343–352.

175.   Okamoto E, Suzuki T, Aikawa M, et al. Diversity of the synthetic-state smooth-muscle cells proliferating in mechanically and hemodynamically injured rabbit arteries. Lab Invest 1996; 74:120–128.

176.   Simons M, Leclerc G, Safian RD, Isner JM, Weir L, Baim DS. Relation between activated smooth-muscle cells in coronary-artery lesions and restenosis after atherectomy. N Engl J Med 1993; 328:608–613.

177.   Reidy MA, Fingerle J, Lindner V. Factors controlling the development of arterial lesions after injury. Circulation 1992; 86:III43–46.

178.   Davies PF, Tripathi SC. Mechanical stress mechanisms and the cell. An endothelial paradigm. Circ Res 1993; 72:239–245.

179.   Ross R. Growth factors in the pathogenesis of atherosclerosis. Acta Med Scand Suppl 1987; 715:33–38.

180.   Ross R. The pathogenesis of atherosclerosis: a perspective for the 1990s. Nature 1993; 362:801–809.

181.   Bellosta S, Bernini F, Ferri N, et al. Direct vascular effects of HMG-CoA reductase inhibitors. Atherosclerosis 1998; 137(suppl):S101–109.

182.   Bustos C, Hernandez-Presa MA, Ortego M, et al. HMG-CoA reductase inhibition by atorvastatin reduces neointimal inflammation in a rabbit model of atherosclerosis. J Am Coll Cardiol 1998; 32:2057–2064.

183.   Casscells W. Smooth muscle cell growth factors. Prog Growth Factor Res 1991; 3:177–206.

184.   Consigny PM, Bilder GM. Expression and release of smooth muscle cell mitogens in the arterial wall after balloon angioplasty. J Vas Med Biol 1993; 4:1–8.

185.   Majesky MW, Reidy MA, Bowen-Pope DF, Hart CE, Wilcox JN, Schwartz SM. PDGF ligand and receptor gene expression during repair of arterial injury. J Cell Biol 1990; 111:2149–2158.

186.   Bowen-Pope DF, Hart CE, Seifert RA. Sera and conditioned media contain different isoforms of platelet-derived growth factor (PDGF) which bind to different classes of PDGF receptor. J Biol Chem 1989; 264:2502–2508.

187.   Major TC, Keiser JA. Inhibition of cell growth: effects of the tyrosine kinase inhibitor CGP 53716. J Pharmacol Exp Ther 1997; 283:402–410.

188.   Ross R. Platelet-derived growth factor. Lancet 1989; 1:1179–1182.

189. Klagsbrun M, Edelman ER. Biological and biochemical properties of fibroblast growth factors. Implications for the pathogenesis of atherosclerosis. Arteriosclerosis 1989; 9:269–278.

190. Bjornsson TD, Dryjski M, Tluczek J, et al. Acidic fibroblast growth factor promotes vascular repair. Proc Natl Acad Sci USA 1991; 88:8651–8655.

191. Edelman ER, Nugent MA, Smith LT, Karnovsky MJ. Basic fibroblast growth factor enhances the coupling of intimal hyperplasia and proliferation of vasa vasorum in injured rat arteries. J Clin Invest 1992; 89:465–473.

192. Edelman ER, Nugent MA, Karnovsky MJ. Perivascular and intravenous administration of basic fibroblast growth factor: vascular and solid organ deposition. Proc Natl Acad Sci USA 1993; 90:1513–1517.

193. Lindner V, Majack RA, Reidy MA. Basic fibroblast growth factor stimulates endothelial regrowth and proliferation in denuded arteries. J Clin Invest 1990; 85:2004–2008.

194. Lindner V, Reidy MA. Proliferation of smooth muscle cells after vascular injury is inhibited by an antibody against basic fibroblast growth factor. Proc Natl Acad Sci USA 1991; 88:3739–3743.

195. Nabel EG, Yang ZY, Plautz G, et al. Recombinant fibroblast growth factor-1 promotes intimal hyperplasia and angiogenesis in arteries in vivo. Nature 1993; 362:844–846.

196. Griendling KK, Murphy TJ, Alexander RW. Molecular biology of the renin-angiotensin system. Circulation 1993; 87:1816–1828.

197. Itoh H, Mukoyama M, Pratt RE, Gibbons GH, Dzau VJ. Multiple autocrine growth factors modulate vascular smooth muscle cell growth response to angiotensin II. J Clin Invest 1993; 91:2268–2274.

198. Kauffman RF, Bean JS, Zimmerman KM, Brown RF, Steinberg MI. Losartan, a nonpeptide angiotensin II (Ang II) receptor antagonist, inhibits neointima formation following balloon injury to rat carotid arteries. Life Sci 1991; 49:L223–228.

199. Bilazarian SD, Currier JW, Kakuta T, Haudenschild CC, Faxon DP. Angiotensin II antagonism does not prevent restenosis after rabbit iliac angioplasty (abstr). Circulation 1992; 86:I187.

200. Sara VR, Hall K. Insulin-like growth factors and their binding proteins. Physiol Rev 1990; 70:591–614.

201. Okazaki H, Majesky MW, Harker LA, Schwartz SM. Regulation of platelet-derived growth factor ligand and receptor gene expression by alpha-thrombin in vascular smooth muscle cells. Circ Res 1992; 71:1285–1293.

202. Davies MG, Hagen PO. Pathobiology of intimal hyperplasia. Br J Surg 1994; 81:1254–1269.

203. Gertz SD, Fallon JT, Gallo R, et al. Hirudin reduces tissue factor expression in neointima after balloon injury in rabbit femoral and porcine coronary arteries. Circulation 1998; 98:580–587.

204. Heras M, Chesebro JH, Webster MW, et al. Hirudin, heparin, and placebo during deep arterial injury in the pig. The in vivo role of thrombin in platelet-mediated thrombosis. Circulation 1990; 82:1476–1484.

205. Lynch SE, Colvin RB, Antoniades HN. Growth factors in wound healing. Single

and synergistic effects on partial thickness porcine skin wounds. J Clin Invest 1989; 84:640–646.

206. Chan P, Munro E, Patel M, et al. Cellular biology of human intimal hyperplastic stenosis. Eur J Vasc Surg 1993; 7:129–135.

207. Majack RA, Clowes AW. Inhibition of vascular smooth muscle cell migration by heparin-like glycosaminoglycans. J Cell Physiol 1984; 118:253–256.

208. Majesky MW, Schwartz SM, Clowes MM, Clowes AW. Heparin regulates smooth muscle S phase entry in the injured rat carotid artery. Circ Res 1987; 61:296–300.

209. Garg UC, Hassid A. Nitric oxide-generating vasodilators and 8-bromo-cyclic guanosine monophosphate inhibit mitogenesis and proliferation of cultured rat vascular smooth muscle cells. J Clin Invest 1989; 83:1774–1777.

210. Tarry WC, Makhoul RG. L-arginine improves endothelium-dependent vasorelaxation and reduces intimal hyperplasia after balloon angioplasty. Arterioscler Thromb 1994; 14:938–943.

211. Busse R, Mulsch A. Induction of nitric oxide synthase by cytokines in vascular smooth muscle cells. FEBS Lett 1990; 275:87–90.

212. Rao GN, Berk BC. Active oxygen species stimulate vascular smooth muscle cell growth and proto-oncogene expression. Circ Res 1992; 70:593–599.

213. Taubman MB, Rollins BJ, Poon M, et al. JE mRNA accumulates rapidly in aortic injury and in platelet-derived growth factor-stimulated vascular smooth muscle cells. Circ Res 1992; 70:314–325.

214. Tanaka H, Sukhova GK, Swanson SJ, et al. Sustained activation of vascular cells and leukocytes in the rabbit aorta after balloon injury. Circulation 1993; 88:1788–1803.

215. Rogers C, Edelman ER, Simon DI. A mAb to the beta2-leukocyte integrin Mac-1 (CD11b/CD18) reduces intimal thickening after angioplasty or stent implantation in rabbits. Proc Natl Acad Sci USA 1998; 95:10134–10139.

216. Marmur JD, Taubman MB, Fuster V. Pathophysiology of restenosis: the role of platelets and thrombin. Journal of Vascular Medicine and Biology 1993; 4:55–63.

217. Fingerle J, Johnson R, Clowes AW, Majesky MW, Reidy MA. Role of platelets in smooth muscle cell proliferation and migration after vascular injury in rat carotid artery. Proc Natl Acad Sci USA 1989; 86:8412–8416.

218. Koyama N, Harada K, Yamamoto A, Morisaki N, Saito Y, Yoshida S. Purification and characterization of an autocrine migration factor for vascular smooth muscle cells (SMC), SMC-derived migration factor. J Biol Chem 1993; 268:13301–13308.

219. Jones JI, Doerr ME, Clemmons DR. Cell migration: interactions among integrins, IGFs and IGFBPs. Prog Growth Factor Res 1995; 6:319–327.

220. Slepian MJ, Massia SP, Dehdashti B, Fritz A, Whitesell L. Beta3-integrins rather than beta1-integrins dominate integrin-matrix interactions involved in postinjury smooth muscle cell migration. Circulation 1998; 97:1818–1827.

221. Davies MJ, Bland JM, Hangartner JR, Angelini A, Thomas AC. Factors influencing the presence or absence of acute coronary artery thrombi in sudden ischaemic death. Eur Heart J 1989; 10:203–208.

222. Loree HM, Kamm RD, Stringfellow RG, Lee RT. Effects of fibrous cap thickness on peak circumferential stress in model atherosclerotic vessels. Circ Res 1992; 71:850–858.

223. Richardson PD, Davies MJ, Born GV. Influence of plaque configuration and stress distribution on fissuring of coronary atherosclerotic plaques [see comments]. Lancet 1989; 2:941–944.

224. Lundberg B. Chemical composition and physical state of lipid deposits in atherosclerosis. Atherosclerosis 1985; 56:93–110.

225. Gertz SD, Roberts WC. Hemodynamic shear force in rupture of coronary arterial atherosclerotic plaques [editorial]. Am J Cardiol 1990; 66:1368–1372.

226. Davies MJ, Richardson PD, Woolf N, Katz DR, Mann J. Risk of thrombosis in human atherosclerotic plaques: role of extracellular lipid, macrophage, and smooth muscle cell content. Br Heart J 1993; 69:377–381.

227. Randomised trial of cholesterol lowering in 4444 patients with coronary heart disease: the Scandinavian Simvastatin Survival Study (4S) [see comments]. Lancet 1994; 344:1383–1389.

228. Gronholdt ML, Dalager-Pedersen S, Falk E. Coronary atherosclerosis: determinants of plaque rupture. Eur Heart J 1998; 19 Suppl C:C24–29.

229. Arroyo LH, Lee RT. The unstable atheromatous plaque. Can J Cardiol 1998; 14(Suppl B):11B–13B.

230. Amento EP, Ehsani N, Palmer H, Libby P. Cytokines and growth factors positively and negatively regulate interstitial collagen gene expression in human vascular smooth muscle cells. Arterioscler Thromb 1991; 11:1223–1230.

231. Lee RT, Berditchevski F, Cheng GC, Hemler ME. Integrin-mediated collagen matrix reorganization by cultured human vascular smooth muscle cells. Circ Res 1995; 76:209–214.

232. Yayon A, Klagsbrun M, Esko JD, Leder P, Ornitz DM. Cell surface, heparin-like molecules are required for binding of basic fibroblast growth factor to its high affinity receptor. Cell 1991; 64:841–848.

233. Lee RT, Kamm RD. Vascular mechanics for the cardiologist. J Am Coll Cardiol 1994; 23:1289–1295.

234. Shah PK. Pathophysiology of plaque rupture and the concept of plaque stabilization. Cardiol Clin 1996; 14:17–29.

235. MacIsaac AI, Thomas JD, Topol EJ. Toward the quiescent coronary plaque. J Am Coll Cardiol 1993; 22:1228–1241.

236. Barger AC, Beeuwkes Rd. Rupture of coronary vasa vasorum as a trigger of acute myocardial infarction. Am J Cardiol 1990; 66:41G–43G.

237. Lee RT, Libby P. The unstable atheroma. Arterioscler Thromb Vasc Biol 1997; 17:1859–1867.

238. Fazioli F, Blasi F. Urokinase-type plasminogen activator and its receptor: new targets for anti-metastatic therapy? Trends Pharmacol Sci 1994; 15:25–29.

239. Sukhova GK, Shi GP, Simon DI, Chapman HA, Libby P. Expression of the elastolytic cathepsins S and K in human atheroma and regulation of their production in smooth muscle cells. J Clin Invest 1998; 102:576–583.

240. Bossard MJ, Tomaszek TA, Thompson SK, et al. Proteolytic activity of human osteoclast cathepsin K. Expression, purification, activation, and substrate identification. J Biol Chem 1996; 271:12517–12524.

241. Matrisian LM. Metalloproteinases and their inhibitors in matrix remodeling. Trends Genet 1990; 6:121–125.

242. Galis ZS, Muszynski M, Sukhova GK, et al. Cytokine-stimulated human vascular smooth muscle cells synthesize a complement of enzymes required for extracellular matrix digestion. Circ Res 1994; 75:181–189.

243. Fabunmi RP, Sukhova GK, Sugiyama S, Libby P. Expression of tissue inhibitor of metalloproteinases-3 in human atheroma and regulation in lesion-associated cells: a potential protective mechanism in plaque stability. Circ Res 1998; 83:270–278.

244. Willenbrock F, Murphy G. Structure-function relationships in the tissue inhibitors of metalloproteinases [published erratum appears in Am J Respir Crit Care Med 1995 Mar; 151(3 Pt 1):926]. Am J Respir Crit Care Med 1994; 150:S165–170.

245. Nikkari ST, O'Brien KD, Ferguson M, et al. Interstitial collagenase (MMP-1) expression in human carotid atherosclerosis. Circulation 1995; 92:1393–1398.

246. Galis ZS, Sukhova GK, Lark MW, Libby P. Increased expression of matrix metalloproteinases and matrix degrading activity in vulnerable regions of human atherosclerotic plaques. J Clin Invest 1994; 94:2493–2503.

247. Ye S, Humphries S, Henney A. Matrix metalloproteinases: implication in vascular matrix remodelling during atherogenesis. Clin Sci (Colch) 1998; 94:103–110.

248. Lee E, Grodzinsky AJ, Libby P, Clinton SK, Lark MW, Lee RT. Human vascular smooth muscle cell-monocyte interactions and metalloproteinase secretion in culture. Arterioscler Thromb Vasc Biol 1995; 15:2284–2289.

249. Welgus HG, Campbell EJ, Cury JD, et al. Neutral metalloproteinases produced by human mononuclear phagocytes. Enzyme profile, regulation, and expression during cellular development. J Clin Invest 1990; 86:1496–1502.

250. Galis ZS, Sukhova GK, Kranzhofer R, Clark S, Libby P. Macrophage foam cells from experimental atheroma constitutively produce matrix-degrading proteinases. Proc Natl Acad Sci USA 1995; 92:402–406.

251. Shah PK, Falk E, Badimon JJ, et al. Human monocyte-derived macrophages induce collagen breakdown in fibrous caps of atherosclerotic plaques. Potential role of matrix-degrading metalloproteinases and implications for plaque rupture. Circulation 1995; 92:1565–1569.

252. Moreno PR, Falk E, Palacios IF, Newell JB, Fuster V, Fallon JT. Macrophage infiltration in acute coronary syndromes. Implications for plaque rupture. Circulation 1994; 90:775–778.

253. Aikawa M, Rabkin E, Okada Y, et al. Lipid lowering by diet reduces matrix metalloproteinase activity and increases collagen content of rabbit atheroma: a potential mechanism of lesion stabilization [see comments]. Circulation 1998; 97:2433–2444.

254. Kockx MM, Herman AG. Apoptosis in atherogenesis: implications for plaque destabilization. Eur Heart J 1998; 19(Suppl G):G23–28.

255. Geng YJ, Libby P. Evidence for apoptosis in advanced human atheroma. Colocalization with interleukin-1 beta-converting enzyme [see comments]. Am J Pathol 1995; 147:251–266.

256. Geng YJ, Wu Q, Muszynski M, Hansson GK, Libby P. Apoptosis of vascular smooth muscle cells induced by in vitro stimulation with interferon-gamma, tumor necrosis factor-alpha, and interleukin-1 beta. Arterioscler Thromb Vasc Biol 1996; 16:19–27.

257. Wilcox JN, Smith KM, Schwartz SM, Gordon D. Localization of tissue factor in

the normal vessel wall and in the atherosclerotic plaque. Proc Natl Acad Sci USA 1989; 86:2839–2843.

258. Taubman MB, Fallon JT, Schecter AD, et al. Tissue factor in the pathogenesis of atherosclerosis. Thromb Haemost 1997; 78:200–204.

259. Schecter AD, Rollins BJ, Zhang YJ, et al. Tissue factor is induced by monocyte chemoattractant protein-1 in human aortic smooth muscle and THP-1 cells. J Biol Chem 1997; 272:28568–28573.

260. Marmur JD, Rossikhina M, Guha A, et al. Tissue factor is rapidly induced in arterial smooth muscle after balloon injury. J Clin Invest 1993; 91:2253–2259.

261. Marmur JD, Thiruvikraman SV, Fyfe BS, et al. Identification of active tissue factor in human coronary atheroma. Circulation 1996; 94:1226–1232.

262. O'Brien ER, Garvin MR, Dev R, et al. Angiogenesis in human coronary atherosclerotic plaques. Am J Pathol 1994; 145:883–894.

263. Barger AC, Beeuwkes Rd, Lainey LL, Silverman KJ. Hypothesis: vasa vasorum and neovascularization of human coronary arteries. A possible role in the pathophysiology of atherosclerosis. N Engl J Med 1984; 310:175–177.

264. Tenaglia AN, Peters KG, Sketch MH Jr, Annex BH. Neovascularization in atherectomy specimens from patients with unstable angina: implications for pathogenesis of unstable angina. Am Heart J 1998; 135:10–14.

265. Chen YX, Nakashima Y, Tanaka K, Shiraishi S, Nakagawa K, Sueishi K. Immunohistochemical expression of vascular endothelial growth factor/vascular permeability factor in atherosclerotic intimas of human coronary arteries. Arterioscler Thromb Vasc Biol 1999; 19:131–139.

266. Kumamoto M, Nakashima Y, Sueishi K. Intimal neovascularization in human coronary atherosclerosis: its origin and pathophysiological significance. Hum Pathol 1995; 26:450–456.

267. Gertz SD, Gimple LW, Ragosta M, et al. Response of femoral arteries of cholesterol-fed rabbits to balloon angioplasty with or without laser: emphasis on the distribution of foam cells. Exp Mol Pathol 1993; 59:225–243.

268. Kwon HM, Sangiorgi G, Ritman EL, et al. Enhanced coronary vasa vasorum neovascularization in experimental hypercholesterolemia. J Clin Invest 1998; 101:1551–1556.

269. Moulton KS, Heller E, Konerding MA, Flynn E, Palinski W, Folkman J. Angiogenesis inhibitors endostatin or TNP-470 reduce intimal neovascularization and plaque growth in apolipoprotein E-deficient mice [see comments]. Circulation 1999; 99:1726–1732.

270. O'Brien KD, McDonald TO, Chait A, Allen MD, Alpers CE. Neovascular expression of E-selectin, intercellular adhesion molecule-1, and vascular cell adhesion molecule-1 in human atherosclerosis and their relation to intimal leukocyte content. Circulation 1996; 93:672–682.

271. Baggiolini M, Dewald B, Moser B. Interleukin-8 and related chemotactic cytokines-CXC and CC chemokines. Adv Immunol 1994; 55:97–179.

272. Strieter RM, Polverini PJ, Kunkel SL, et al. The functional role of the ELR motif in CXC chemokine-mediated angiogenesis. J Biol Chem 1995; 270:27348–27357.

273. Klagsbrun M, D'Amore PA. Vascular endothelial growth factor and its receptors. Cytokine Growth Factor Rev 1996; 7:259–270.

274. Barleon B, Sozzani S, Zhou D, Weich HA, Mantovani A, Marme D. Migration of human monocytes in response to vascular endothelial growth factor (VEGF) is mediated via the VEGF receptor flt-1. Blood 1996; 87:3336–3343.

275. Ferrara N, Bunting S. Vascular endothelial growth factor, a specific regulator of angiogenesis. Curr Opin Nephrol Hypertens 1996; 5:35–44.

276. Williams B, Baker AQ, Gallacher B, Lodwick D. Angiotensin II increases vascular permeability factor gene expression by human vascular smooth muscle cells. Hypertension 1995; 25:913–917.

277. Inoue M, Itoh H, Ueda M, et al. Vascular endothelial growth factor (VEGF) expression in human coronary atherosclerotic lesions: possible pathophysiological significance of VEGF in progression of atherosclerosis. Circulation 1998; 98:2108–2116.

278. Lazarous DF, Shou M, Scheinowitz M, et al. Comparative effects of basic fibroblast growth factor and vascular endothelial growth factor on coronary collateral development and the arterial response to injury. Circulation 1996; 94:1074–1082.

279. Yonemitsu Y, Kaneda Y, Morishita R, Nakagawa K, Nakashima Y, Sueishi K. Characterization of in vivo gene transfer into the arterial wall mediated by the Sendai virus (hemagglutinating virus of Japan) liposomes: an effective tool for the in vivo study of arterial diseases. Lab Invest 1996; 75:313–323.

2
Clinical and Pathological Correlates

Renu Virmani, Allen P. Burke, Andrew Farb, and Frank D. Kolodgie
Armed Forces Institute of Pathology, Washington, D.C.

I. INTRODUCTION

The incidence of atherosclerotic sudden coronary death has not changed in the last few decades despite a significant drop in hospital-based coronary death rates. Much has been learned about plaque morphology and the role of inflammation in plaque rupture and luminal thrombosis. Most studies have emphasized plaque rupture as a mechanism of coronary thrombosis (1–5), with little attention devoted to other causes of thrombosis (6). We have recently shown that thrombosis occurs from two main causes, plaque rupture and plaque erosion. We have demonstrated that risk factors may predict, to a degree, the type of plaque morphology that underlies luminal thrombus.

II. MORPHOLOGICAL CHARACTERISTICS OF PLAQUE RUPTURE

Atherosclerotic plaque rupture is characterized by exposure of the necrotic core beneath a thin fibrous cap that has torn, allowing contact between the lipid-rich plaque and blood flow in the arterial lumen (Figure 1). The necrotic core is rich in free cholesterol (cholesterol crystals). The fibrous cap is infiltrated by foamy macrophages and monocytes and, to a lesser degree, lymphocytes, and measures

---

The opinions or assertions contained herein are the private views of the authors and are not to be construed as official or reflecting the views of the Department of the Army, the Department of the Air Force, or the Department of Defense.

51

near the site of rupture about 25-μm thick [mean, 23 ± 19 μm, with 95% of the caps measuring less than 64 μm (7)]. The fibrous cap is made up of collagen with few scattered smooth muscle cells. A most intriguing question is, what are the constituents of the plaque that make the plaque rupture? We have reported that patients with plaque rupture have other sites within their coronary tree that have similar characteristics (vulnerable plaque) as those stated previously but do not have a disrupted fibrous cap or an overlying luminal thrombus (7). We have analyzed quantitatively the following characteristics of plaque rupture and compared them with plaque erosion, vulnerable plaque, and stable plaque: the percent area occupied by the necrotic core, the percentage of macrophages within the fibrous cap, the number of cholesterol clefts within the necrotic core, the number of vasa vasorum, and the number of hemosiderin-laden macrophages (Table 1 and 2). The necrotic core is largest in plaque rupture and therefore must be an important component of plaque rupture. The number of cholesterol clefts in the plaque, reflecting the presence of free cholesterol, is significantly greater in plaque rupture compared with erosion and stable plaque and therefore is likely to contribute to rupture. Similarly, macrophage content was also highest in the fibrous cap of ruptured plaques compared with other plaque types. Therefore, these characteristics of the plaque are likely important in the causation of rupture.

Preliminary studies in our laboratory show that in hearts with acute plaque rupture, plaque hemorrhages are more frequent in other coronary segments, suggesting that plaque hemorrhage may be a precursor to plaque rupture. The mean

Table 1 Comparison of the Size of the Necrotic Core, Number of Cholesterol Clefts, and Macrophage Infiltration in Ruptured Plaques, Vulnerable Plaque, Plaque Erosion, and Stable Plaque Among Men Dying of Sudden Coronary Death.

Plaque type	% Necrotic core, plaque area	No. Cholesterol clefts, cross section of necrotic core	% Macrophage infiltration, fibrous cap
Rupture	34 ± 17[a,b]	169 ± 218[c,d]	26 ± 20[e,f]
Vulnerable	25 ± 17	96 ± 104	15 ± 14
Erosion	14 ± 14[a]	9.6 ± 36[c]	10 ± 12[e]
Stable	12 ± 25[b]	0 ± 0[d]	3 ± 0.7[f]

[a] $p = 0.002$.
[b] $p = 0.05$.
[c] $p = 0.03$.
[d] $p = 0.02$.
[e] $p < 0.0001$.
[f] $p = 0.0001$.

Table 2 Comparison of the Number of Vasa Vasorum Within Atherosclerotic Plaque and Hemosiderin-Laden Macrophages in Rupture, Vulnerable Plaque, Erosion, and Stable Plaque

Plaque type	Mean vasa vasorum, atherosclerotic plaque	Hemosiderin laden macrophages	p vs. rupture
Rupture	44 ± 22	18.9 ± 11	—
Vulnerable	26 ± 23	4.4 ± 3.6	0.07/0.001
Erosion	28 ± 18	4.3 ± 4.7	0.02/<0.0001
Stable	13 ± 9	5.0 ± 9.3	0.01/0.03

number of hemorrhages in the coronary tree of patients with plaque rupture was 2.5 ± 1.3, vs none in erosion ($p = 0.0001$) and 0.05 ± 0.6 in stable plaques ($p = 0.04$). Intraplaque hemorrhage probably occurs through rupture of vasa vasorum, which has been shown to be highest in ruptured compared with other types of plaque (Table 2). These results indicate that (Table 2) intraplaque hemorrhage may contribute to the plaque's vulnerability to rupture.

Recent work by Felton et al (8) in the human aorta corroborates our morphological findings in the coronary arteries. They showed that the lipid concentration was highest at the site of disrupted plaque compared with plaques away from the disrupted plaque and in nondisrupted plaques (85.3, 52.0, and 28.9 mg/g w/w, respectively). Likewise, the concentrations of esterified and free cholesterol were higher in disrupted than nondisrupted plaque or plaque away from the site of disrupted plaque and were approximately double in the plaques away from the site of disrupted plaques compared with nondisrupted plaques. In disrupted plaque, the concentration of free cholesterol was increased a further twofold compared with plaque away from the disrupted plaque. Esterified cholesterol was highest at the center of plaque, away from the disrupted plaque, and free cholesterol was higher in the center of the disrupted plaque. There was a good correlation between cholesterol ester concentration with macrophage area at the center and edge of all plaque types. Free cholesterol was negatively associated with minimum fibrous cap thinness in the center and edges of the plaques that were away from the rupture site and in the disrupted plaques.

Therefore, the combination of a thin fibrous cap, which is infiltrated by macrophages and an underlying necrotic core, with a high cholesterol cleft content are the essential elements of a plaque that is likely to rupture. These morphological characteristics of a plaque rupture may help in the future to identify plaques by noninvasive means such as magnetic resonance invaging or by antibody tagging to an element of the plaque that is present at sites of rupture and not in sites away from the disrupted plaque.

III. SITE OF PLAQUE RUPTURE, SHOULDER VS. CENTRAL REGION OF THE FIBROUS CAP

Work by Richardson et al. in 1989 (9) investigated the site of plaque rupture. They classified the lesions with a lipid pool or a necrotic core as either eccentric (86%) or concentric (14%). They found that the rupture site was the shoulder region (lateral tear) in 49%, central region of the necrotic core in 29%, and in 21% the rupture site was seen in concentric plaques. Of these 21%, a necrotic core was present in 9%. By computer modeling, the regions of high circumferential stress correlated well with the site of intimal tear. Loree et al (10, 11) showed by finite element analysis that by reducing the thickness of the fibrous cap there was a dramatic increase in peak circumferential stress in the plaque. The same group further showed that maximal circumferential stress in plaques that rupture was significantly higher than maximal stress in stable plaques and that there are often multiple sites of high stress (pressure of more than 2250 mmHg).

As predicted by mechanical models, the rupture often, but not always, occurs at the site of maximum circumferential stress, which has been predicted to be the shoulder region (12). We evaluated the site of plaque rupture in cases of sudden coronary death. The most frequent site of rupture was located in the central region of the necrotic core (42%), followed by the shoulder region of the necrotic core (36%), and circumferentially (4%) (Figure 1). In 18% of ruptures it was not possible to determine the exact location because of extensive destruc-

---

Figure 1 Patterns of acute plaque rupture, coronary arteries. (A) A 54-year-old African-American man experienced chest pain and had a cardiac affect while driving to the hospital. He had no prior medical history. At autopsy, the left anterior descending coronary artery was 80% narrowed (shown in figure). (B) A higher magnification demonstrates the centrally thinned necrotic cap in the left anterior descending coronary artery with the rupture site (arrow). (C) A 38-year-old white man had a fever develop, and went to bed. His wife was alerted by labored respirations and witnessed his cardiac arrest. At autopsy, the left anterior descending coronary artery demonstrated a plaque rupture. (D) A higher magnification shows the central rupture site (arrows). (E) A 69-year-old white man was found dead at home. At autopsy, the coronary arteries showed a 70% narrowing of the left anterior descending artery, 70% narrowing, of the left circumflex artery, a 75% lesion in the right coronary artery with thrombus (shown), and a transmural acute myocardial infarct of the posterior right and left ventricle. (F) A higher magnification of the rupture site demonstrates the tear at the shoulder region (arrow). (G) A 56-year-old man arrested while eating supper. He had a history of cigarette smoking and vague chest pains that had not been evaluated by a physician. At autopsy, his heart weight was 760 g. He had severe three-vessel coronary artery disease with an acute thrombus in the proximal right coronary artery (shown). (H) A higher magnification demonstrates a circumferential necrotic core, with the rupture site shown by arrows.

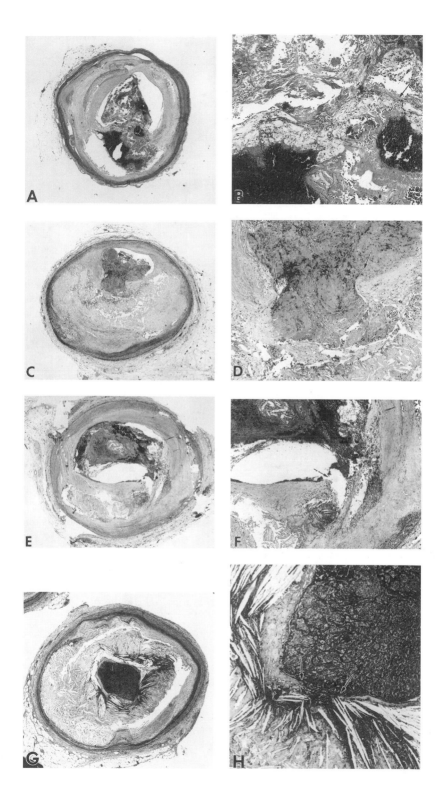

tion of the rupture site. Furthermore, we have discovered that rupture sites differ between exercise-related deaths and deaths at rest. The central region is the commonest site of plaque rupture in exercise-related death, whereas at rest the rupture site is usually in the shoulder region. These results suggest that there are several factors that influence the site of plaque rupture.

IV. RISK FACTORS ASSOCIATED WITH PLAQUE RUPTURE IN MEN AND WOMEN

We examined hearts from 113 men who died of sudden coronary death (SCD) (7). SCD was defined as death having occurred within 6 hours of onset of symptoms or within 24 hours of the time that the victim was last seen alive in a normal state of health. Death from coronary cause was defined as luminal narrowing of a major coronary artery by at least 75% by an atherosclerotic plaque or by the presence of luminal thrombus all other causes of death had to be ruled out by a complete autopsy including toxicological screen. All patients had blood analyzed post-mortem for serum total cholesterol (TC), high-density lipoprotein (HDL) cholesterol, serum thiocyanate level to identify smokers (>90 μmol/liter), and glycohemoglobin. Hypertension was determined on the basis of history and microscopic analysis of renal vasculature. Hypercholesterolemia was defined as TC >210 mg/dl or a ratio (TC/HDL-C) greater than 5.0. The hearts were studied after perfusion fixation of the coronary arteries and then cut at 3-mm intervals and when necessary decalcified before cutting. All arteries with $>50\%$ luminal narrowing were submitted for histological examination. Of 113 patients, 59 patients had acute coronary thrombi. Thrombi were further classified into those with plaque rupture as defined previously and plaque erosion, which was defined as an acute luminal thrombus in direct contact with intimal plaque that is rich in smooth muscle cells within a proteoglycan matrix (Figure 2). In plaque erosion, either the necrotic core was absent or small and on serial sectioning did not communicate with the luminal thrombus. Lesions that did not have luminal thrombi were further classified into vulnerable plaque, if there was a thin fibrous cap (<65 mm thick) infiltrated by macrophages with an underlying necrotic core. A stable plaque was defined as cross-sectional luminal narrowing of at least 75% in the absence of luminal thrombus.

We observed that men with thrombi were younger and more often smokers than men with stable plaques (75% vs. 41%, Table 3). Men with thrombi were more frequently normotensive (43%) than hypertensive (19%). No other risk factor was associated with thrombosis. However, when the thrombi were further classified as plaque rupture and plaque erosion, there were significant differences in the presence of risk factors. Plaque rupture was associated with high TC, lower HDL cholesterol, and a higher TC/HDL ratio than men with plaque erosion (Table 4). Hy-

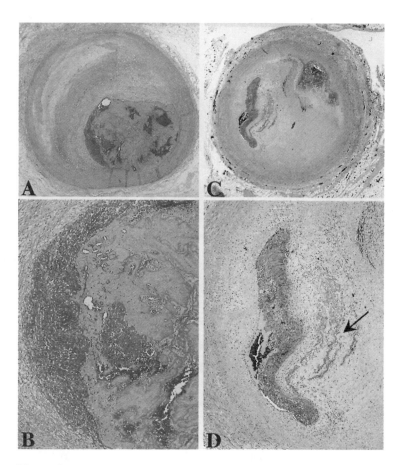

Figure 2 Plaque erosion. (A) A 23-year-old African-American man had a 2-year history of epigastric and chest pain. His father had died at the age of 27 with a myocardial infarction. At autopsy, the left anterior descending coronary artery showed a 60% lesion with an occlusive thrombus (shown). The other epicardial vessels were open. The thrombus propagated to the left circumflex artery. (B) A higher magnification of the thrombus in the left anterior descending artery shows the inflamed cap with overlying thrombus. (C) A 28-year-old woman complained of chest pain and dizziness, progressing to cardiac arrest. At autopsy, the 430-g heart demonstrated severe narrowing of the left circumflex artery, left obtuse marginal artery, and left anterior descending artery. The left anterior descending artery showed acute thrombus (shown), and the right coronary artery was free of disease. (D) A higher magnification of the thrombus showed layering (arrow) of the plaque, suggestive of repeated episodes of thrombosis.

Table 3   Risk Factors and Presence of Acute Coronary Thrombus, 113 Men Dying Suddenly with Severe Coronary Artery Disease

Risk factor	Acute thrombus ($n = 59$)	Stable plaque ($n = 54$)	p Value (univariate)	p Value (multivariate)[a]
Cigarette smokers (n, %)	44 (75)	22 (41)	<0.001	0.004
Age, mean (yr)	47.3 ± 8.9	52.7 ± 11.0	0.005	0.24
Hypertension (n, %)	11 (19)	23 (43)	0.008	0.22
Total cholesterol, mg/dl[b]	249 ± 62	222 ± 100	0.08	>0.4[c]
High-density lipoprotein cholesterol, mg/dl	39 ± 15	45 ± 18	0.10	0.16
Black: white	11:48	16:38	0.19	0.38
Glycosylated hemoglobin, percent	7.6 ± 2.1	7.5 ± 2.5	0.90	>0.4[c]

[a] By logistic stepwise regression, p value to remove.
[b] Conversion factor to SI: 0.026.
[c] Dropped from analysis.
Source: Ref. 7.

pertension, cigarette smoking, and glycosylated hemoglobin were not predictive of the type of thrombosis. The number of vulnerable plaques were associated with serum cholesterol concentration ($r^2 = 0.08$, $p = 0.003$), the HDL cholesterol concentration ($r^2 = 0.04$, $p = 0.03$), the ratio of TC/HDL cholesterol ($r^2 = 0.11$, $p < 0.001$), and with white race ($p = 0.02$). There was no association between glycosylated hemoglobin, hypertension, and the number of vulnerable plaques.

Table 4   Risk Factors and the Type of Coronary Thrombus, 59 Men Studied Who Died Suddenly and Had Acute Thrombus

Risk factor	Plaque rupture ($n = 41$)	Eroded plaque ($n = 18$)	p Value (univariate)	p Value (multivariate)[a]
HDL-C, mg/dl[b]	35.8 ± 13.5	46.9 ± 16.1	0.008	0.003
TC, mg/dl[b]	262 ± 58	220 ± 61	0.014	0.003
TC/HDL-C	8.5 ± 4.0	5.0 ± 1.8	0.001	0.003
Age, yr	48.4 ± 8.8	44.8 ± 9.0	0.16	0.30
Cigarette smoking (n, %)	29 (71)	15 (83)	0.35	0.16
Hypertension (n, %)	9 (22)	2 (11)	0.48	0.09
Glycosylated Hgb, %	7.9 ± 2.2	6.9 ± 1.7	0.11	>0.4[c]

[a] By logistic stepwise regression, p value to remove.
[b] Conversion factor to SI: 0.026.
[c] Dropped from analysis.
Source: Ref. 7.

Table 5 Risk Factors and Mechanism of Death, 51 Women with Severe Coronary Atherosclerosis

Risk factor	Plaque rupture (n = 8)	Plaque erosion (n = 18)	Stable plaque, healed MI (n = 18)	Stable plaque, no MI (n = 7)	p Values (if < 0.05)
Age, yr mean ± SD	58 ± 12[a]	45 ± 8[a]	54 ± 13	43 ± 9	[a]0.01 vs. erosion, 0.02 vs. stable, no MI;[b] 0.04 vs. stable plaque, healed MI
Age > 50 years, n (%)	7 (87)[a]	3 (17)	9 (50)	2 (29)	[a]0.001 vs. plaque erosion; 0.03 vs. stable plaque, no infarct
TC, mg/dl, mean ± SD	270 ± 55[a]	188 ± 48	203 ± 71	201 ± 57	[a]0.007 vs. erosion; 0.007 vs. stable plaque, healed MI; 0.02 vs. stable plaque
HDL-C, mg/dl, mean ± SD	46 ± 12	39 ± 21	40 ± 23	48 ± 32	—
TC/HDL-C, mean ± SD	6.2 ± 1.8	6.0 ± 3.7	6.6 ± 3.9	5.2 ± 2.7	—
BMI, kg/m², mean ± SD	31 ± 4[a]	27 ± 4	28 ± 9	30 ± 11	[a]0.02 vs. erosion
GlycoHgb, %, mean ± SD	8.8 ± 4.4	6.7 ± 0.7	10.2 ± 5.0[a]	8.0 ± 4.5	[a]0.006 vs. erosion
Ht wt, g, mean ± SD	483 ± 108	372 ± 87[a]	460 ± 105	375 ± 129	[a]0.01 vs. rupture and stable plaque, healed MI
Htwt/BMI, mean ± SD	1.6 ± 0.5	1.4 ± 0.4	1.7 ± 0.4[a]	1.3 ± 0.2	[a]0.02 vs. stable plaque; 0.04 vs. erosion
Smokers, n (%)	4 (50)	14 (78)	9 (50)	2 (29)	—
Htn, n (%)	3 (38)	4 (22)	9 (50)	2 (29)	—

MI, myocardial infarct; TC, total cholesterol; HDL-C, high-density lipoprotein cholesterol; Ht wt, heart weight; BMI, body mass index; Htn, hypertension.
[a] Statistically significant differences between values within the same row.
Source: Ref. 13.

We examined 51 women who died of sudden coronary death and compared these with 15 women who died to trauma (13). The culprit plaques were similarly classified as in men into plaque rupture with thrombus ($n = 8$), plaque erosion with thrombus ($n = 18$), stable plaque with healed myocardial infarction ($n = 18$), and stable plaque without myocardial infarction ($n = 7$). Women with plaque rupture were older (58 ± 12 vs. 45 ± 8 years), had higher TC (270 ± 55 vs. 188 ± 48 mg/dl) and higher BMI (31 ± 4 vs. 27 ± 4) than women with erosion (Table 5). Of all plaque ruptures, 87% occurred in women older than 50 years; in contrast, of all plaque erosions, only 17% occurred in women older than 50 years. Higher levels of glycosylated hemoglobin and hypertension were associated with healed myocardial infarction and stable plaque (Table 5). Compared with controls, women with plaque rupture had elevated TC (270 ± 55 vs. 194 ± 44 mg/dl, $p = 0.002$), and those with erosion were more likely to be smokers (78% vs. 33%, $p = 0.01$). Vulnerable plaques were associated with age >50 years and hypercholesterolemia. Thus, although the effects of risk factors on plaque morphology seem similar in women as in men who die of sudden coronary death, they appear significantly altered by menopausal status.

REFERENCES

1. Falk E. Coronary thrombosis: pathogenesis and clinical manifestations. Am J Cardiol 1991; 68:28B–35B.
2. Falk E. Morphologic features of unstable atherothrombotic plaques underlying acute coronary syndromes. Am J Cardiol 1989; 63:114E–120E.
3. Falk E. Why do plaques rupture? Circulation 1992; 86:III30–42.
4. Davies MJ. Anatomic features in victims of sudden coronary death. Coronary artery pathology. Circulation 1992; 85:I19–24.
5. Davies MJ, Thomas AC. Plaque fissuring-the cause of acute myocardial infarction, sudden ischaemic death, and crescendo angina. Br Heart J 1985; 53:363–373.
6. van der Wal AC, Becker A, van der Loos CM, Das PK. Site of intimal rupture or erosion of thrombosed coronary atherosclerotic plaques is characterized by an inflammatory process irrespective of the dominant plaque morphology. Circulation 1994; 89:36–44.
7. Burke AP, Farb A, Malcom GT, Liang Y-H, Smialek J, Virmani R. Coronary risk factors and plaque morphology in patients with coronary disease dying suddenly. N Engl J Med 1997; 336:1276–1282.
8. Felton CV, Crook D, Davies MJ, Oliver MF. Relation of plaque lipid composition and morphology to the stability of human aortic plaques. Arterioscler Thromb Vasc Biol 1997; 17:1337–1345.
9. Richardson PD, Davies MJ, Born GV. Influence of plaque configuration and stress distribution on fissuring of coronary atherosclerotic plaques. Lancet 1989; 2:941–944.
10. Loree HM, Kamm RD, Stringfellow RG, Lee RT. Effects of fibrous cap thickness

on peak circumferential stress in model atherosclerotic vessels. Circ Res 1992; 71: 850–858.

11. Loree HM, Tobias BJ, Gibson LJ, Kamm RD, Small DM, Lee RT. Mechanical properties of model atherosclerotic lesion lipid pools. Arterioscler Thromb 1994; 14:230–234.

12. Hayashi K, Imai Y. Tensile property of atheromatous plaque and an analysis of stress in atherosclerotic wall. J Biomech 1997; 30:573–579.

13. Burke AP, Farb A, Malcom GT, Liang Y-H, Smialek J, Virmani R. Effect of risk factors on the mechanism of acute thrombosis and sudden coronary death in women. Circulation 1998; 97:2110–2116.

3

The Role of Inflammation in Plaque Rupture

Anton E. Becker and Allard C. van der Wal
Academic Medical Center, University of Amsterdam, Amsterdam, The Netherlands

I. INTRODUCTION

Inflammation is defined as the reponse of tissue to injury. A principal and early feature is accumulation at the site of injury of leukocytes, cells that are specialized to destroy injurious agents. In the early stages of tissue damage, therefore, leukocytes serve in host defense and have a protective function; but in the long term, once the inflammation turns into a more chronic stage, secretory products may damage preexisting tissue components and, hence, may induce additional tissue injury. Inflammation, moreover, initiates a series of events that should lead to the reconstitution of the injured tissue, either by regeneration of damaged preexistent cells or by replacement of irreversibly injured tissue by fibrous tissue (fibrosis or scar formation). In other words, tissue injury will evoke inflammation that will set into motion a process of repair.

Both inflammation and repair are key events in the natural course of atherosclerosis (1, 2). Moreover, intraplaque inflammation appears to be closely related to the onset of plaque rupture (3, 4). In this chapter we describe the cellular basis of intraplaque inflammation and, in particular, its relationship with plaque rupture.

II. RECRUITMENT OF INFLAMMATORY CELLS

Adhesion and migration of inflammatory cells through an apparently intact endothelial cell layer is the first recognizable morphological phenomenon of lesion

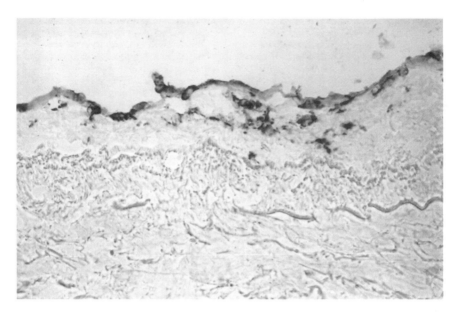

Figure 1 Section through a human coronary artery with diffuse intimal thickening, showing subendothelial accumulation of macrophages. F8RA/HLA-DR double stain. (See also color insert.)

formation (Figure 1). It starts early in life and initially shows preference for so-called lesion-prone areas, such as flow dividers and branching points (5). Recently it has been shown that atherosclerotic lesions in coronary arteries develop preferentially in regions exposed to low mean shear stress (6). Later in life, and in particular under atherogenic conditions, such as hypercholesterolemia, other arterial sites become involved as well.

To this end it is important to reiterate that recruitment of inflammatory cells is not a feature of plaque initiation only but occurs throughout the long-lasting period of lesion formation. It can be observed in precursor lesions (fatty streaks) and in fully developed atherosclerotic plaques.

A.   Adhesion Molecules and Atherogenesis

The adhesion of leukocytes requires induction or up-regulation of specific adhesion molecules at the outer membrane of both endothelial and inflammatory cells. Several adhesion proteins appear to be involved, including vascular cell adhesion molecule (VCAM), E-selectin, intracellular adhesion molecule-1 (ICAM-1), and CD40 (7–10). These phenotypic changes probably reflect the first response to injury of the vessel wall. It not only promotes adherence of leukocytes to the surface endothelial cell layer, but it is also associated with increased procoagulant activity and increased permeability of the endothelium. In hypercholesterolemic rabbits, the formation of fatty streaklike lesions is preceded by *de novo* expression of a newly recognized adhesion protein, initially named athero-ELAM, which appears to be a rabbit homologue of the human VCAM-1 molecule (10).

There are several candidates for induction of leukocyte recruitment in atherosclerosis. Of particular interest are oxidized low-density lipoprotein (ox-LDL) derivatives, such as lysophosphatidylcholine, which exerts proinflammatory effects through the induction of VCAM-1 expression on endothelial cells (11). In fact, plasma of hypercholesterolemic patients contains increased levels of phosphatidylcholines, providing clinical evidence for the potential atherogenic effects of ox-LDL. Shear stress is another stimulator of adhesion proteins as observed in vitro using monolayers of endothelial cells cultured under controlled flow conditions (12–14). Moreover in vivo up-regulation of ICAM-1 and VCAM on endothelial cells has been observed on the surface lining of atherosclerotic lesions in the ascending aorta at sites of altered stress, a phenomenon even more pronounced under hypercholesterolemic conditions. Once monocytes have migrated into the intima, they differentiate into tissue macrophages. The inflammatory reaction so induced may lead to the secretion of cytokines, such as interleukin-1 (IL-1), tumor necrosis factor-α (TNF-α), and the macrophage chemotactic protein (MCP-1), which may facilitate further recruitment of mononuclear cells.

B. Neovascularization in the Plaque

It is an old observation that advanced atherosclerotic plaques contain newly formed capillary vessels derived from the underlying vasa vasorum that occupy the base of the atheroma and the shoulder parts of plaques (15). The latter areas are of interest because they represent the vulnerable sites of plaques where most ruptures take place. Recent studies have demonstrated abundant expression of the adhesion molecules VCAM, E-selectin, ICAM-1, and CD40 on the microvascular endothelium, as well as their counter structures (ligands) on bordering T cells and macrophages (Figure 2) (16, 17). These vessels may provide an alternative pathway for leukocyte recruitment in the so-called rupture prone sites of advanced plaques (17).

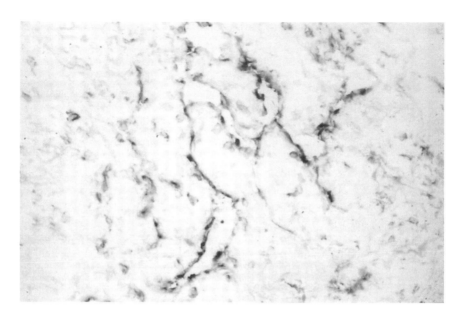

Figure 2   Neovascularization of an advanced atherosclerotic plaque. The microvascular endothelium shows UEA expression. There is perivascular infiltration of CD40-positive inflammatory cells. UEA/CD40 immunodouble stain. (See also color insert.)

III.   INFLAMMATORY CELLS IN THE PLAQUE

Immunohistochemical studies of human atherosclerotic plaques have shown that macrophages, T lymphocytes, and, to a lesser extent, mast cells are the most prominent cells, whereas B lymphocytes and neutrophils are rarely encountered (18–20). Subpopulations of these inflammatory cells express certain activation markers indicating their functional capacity to produce cytokines and other inflammatory mediators (18, 19, 21–25). It thus appears that regulatory networks of cellular communication are operative in plaques, albeit precise understanding of these complex interactions remains to be explained. Indeed, most factors considered to play a role act on different cell types and, moreover, induce multiple and sometimes divergent functions. Nevertheless, present insights into the molecular biology of intraplaque inflammatory processes could provide the background for understanding the pathological features considered characteristic of atherosclerotic plaques, such as cell proliferation and differentiation, vasoreactivity and lipid metabolism, and complicating aspects, such as plaque rupture.

A. Macrophages

Once monocytes have entered the arterial intima, they undergo transformation into tissue macrophages capable of phagocytosis. Indeed, phagocytosis of lipids has long been considered the principal function of macrophages in the plaque. LDL is endocytosed by specific LDL receptors, equipped with an internal feedback control mechanism; the more LDL internalized the less surface receptors expressed and vice versa. The scavenger pathway, on the other hand, allows unlimited uptake of ox-LDL and, hence, may lead to the formation of lipid-laden foam cells (26–28). In addition, macrophages within arterial plaque become activated, which causes an increase in cell size and phagocytic capacity and also induces the potential to produce and secrete a wide variety of biologically active substances. Such activation stimuli, relevant in the setting of atherosclerosis, includes cytokines derived from sensitized T lymphocytes, mast cells and other macrophages, various chemical mediators, extracellular matrix proteins, and probably endotoxins. A variety of inflammatory mediators, often with opposing functional capacities, can be produced by macrophages. Some may induce or promote further tissue injury, such as proteolytic enzymes (metalloproteinases), toxic oxygen metabolites, coagulation factors (tissue factor), arachidonic acid metabolites, and nitric oxide. Other factors, however, play a role in repair and promote fibrosis in plaques, such as growth factors, angiogenesis factors, and remodeling collagenases (14, 28). It is likely that local circumstances, such as the presence or absence of inflammatory stimuli, determine which of these effects is predominant. The complexity of these biological effects may be illustrated by the observation that macrophages within one and the same plaque express a variety of function-associated surface antigens and secretory products in part depending on their location in relation to the lipid core (Figure 3) (24, 29, 30). It appears, therefore, that local variations in macrophage functional status can occur, resulting in local variations within the same plaque.

B. T Lymphocytes

T cell responses are initiated through a process of antigen presentation. An antigen-presenting cell presents a processed antigen, bound to a major histocompatibility complex (MHC) molecule, HLA-DR, to the T cell that results in sensitization of the T cell. This is followed by clonal proliferation, expression of various activation antigens, and the production of cytokines, of which interferon-γ (IFN-γ) appears to be the most specific. T cells are regularly found in atherosclerotic plaques and often in close association with macrophages (Figure 4). Several studies have documented the presence of activation markers on T cells in human atherosclerotic plaques. A large proportion of T cells within randomly sampled

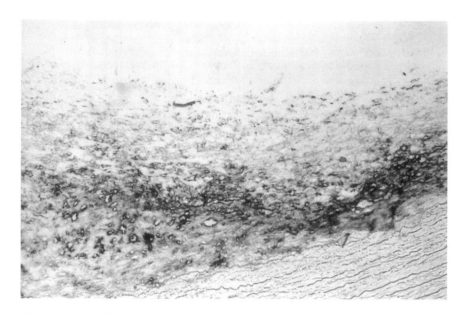

Figure 3 Shoulder part of an atherosclerotic plaque in a human carotid artery. Two distinct subpopulations of macrophages are visualized using a double immunostaining technique with CD14/CD36. The macrophages bordering on the lipid core stain positive with CD36; the more superficial macrophages stain positive with CD14. (See also color insert.)

plaques present the very late activation antigen VLA-1 and HLA-DR molecules, whereas relatively low numbers express interleukin-2 receptors (IL-2R) (19, 23). This suggests on the average a state of long-term low-level activation in atherosclerosis.

The expression of IL-2R on T cells is of particular interest, because it indicates a state of recent activation of these cells in a cell-mediated immune response. IL-2R activity appears on the cell surface of T cells shortly (within 2–24 hours) after cytokine stimulation by macrophages and persists for only a few days once the stimulating agents diminish. During this period a wide variety of inflammatory mediators can be produced, particularly by cytokine-activated macrophages and the T cells themselves (31, 32). The immunocytochemical detection of IL-2R on T lymphocytes is considered a strong indication that recent antigenic stimulation has taken place. Indeed, the microenvironment of atherosclerotic plaques contains additional components necessary for antigenic stimulation, such as HLA-DR-positive macrophages (which may serve as antigen presenting cells), and sets of co-stimulatory molecules and their ligands on both macrophages and T cells (24). Moreover, in situ studies of human plaque tissues

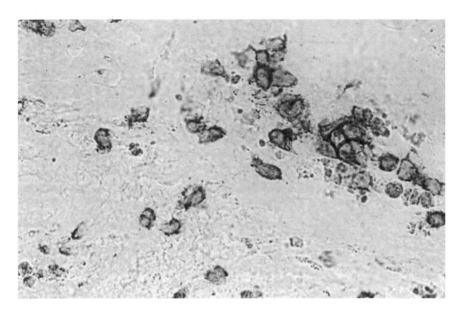

Figure 4 Detail of an atherosclerotic plaque showing a cluster of CD3-positive T lymphocytes clustered around ceroid granules. (See also color insert.)

have shown that the panel of cytokines produced by the inflammatory cells includes IFN-γ and IL-12, but virtually lacks IL-4 (24, 33, 34). This indicates a preference for a proinflammatory (Th1) response in atherosclerotic plaques. Thus far, studies on T cell activation were carried out on randomly selected mostly uncomplicated plaques, but recently we demonstrated that the percentage of IL-2R–positive T cells is markedly increased in culprit lesions of patients with severe forms of unstable angina and patients with acute myocardial infarction (35), thus suggesting that the crescendo course of the acute coronary syndromes relates to some, as yet unknown, agent causing recent activation of T cells within the plaques.

C. Mast Cells

A relationship between mast cells and atherosclerosis was first suggested by Constantinides in 1953 (36). Initially, the mast cell attracted attention only as an endogenous source of heparin in the plaque, but presently there is a renewed interest for these cells because of the studies of Kovanen and Kaartinen (20, 37).

Mast cells are characterized by secretory granules within the cytoplasm, which contain inflammatory mediators such as histamine and the neutral proteases, tryptase and chymase. On activation, the granules are released in the surrounding microenvironment. In addition to the classic IgE-mediated stimulation of mast cells, degranulation can be provoked also by T cells, macrophages, and complement fragments. And, indeed, fatty streaks and the shoulder region of advanced atherosclerotic plaques contain many degranulated mast cells, which reflects recent activation of these cells (Figure 5) (20). Although the number of mast cells in plaques is relatively low compared with the abundant presence of macrophages, their secretory products may serve unique functions in atherogenesis. For instance, heparin, proteoglycans, and chymase released by exocytosed granules promote foam cell production (37, 38), but at the same time exhibit antioxidative effects, so that activated mast cells may provide both proatherogenic and antiatherogenic stimuli (38). Tryptase and chymase, albeit themselves proteolytic enzymes, appear to have a limited direct potential regarding breakdown of the extracellular matrix of plaques. However, they effectively activate the proenzyme forms of metalloproteinases (MMPs), and thus provide a plasmin-independent pathway of MMP activation in plaques (39). In addition, several mast cell products, including histamine, heparin, and the neutral proteases, are angiogenic factors that could stimulate the formation of neovascular sprouts in

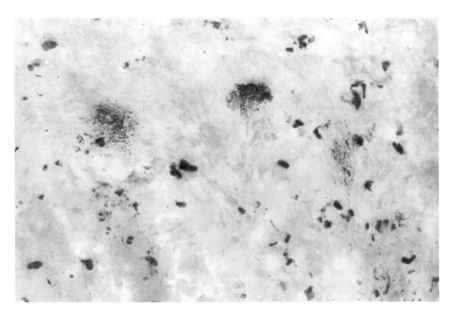

Figure 5   Mast cells in a coronary atherectomy specimen of a patient with unstable angina. The mast cells are degranulated, indicating activation of the cells. Antitriptase stain. (See also color insert.)

advanced plaques (38). It appears, therefore, that mast cells in atherosclerotic plaques may be much more important than initially thought.

IV. INFLAMMATION AND PLAQUE RUPTURE

The various inflammatory mediators that have been detected in atherosclerotic plaque tissue are not unique for atherosclerosis. They are active also in other immune-mediated inflammatory diseases, such as rheumatoid arthritis, in which tissue lysis and fibrosis are the key features. The analogy with those disease processes strongly suggests that a number of inflammatory mediators may have profound effects on the integrity of the connective tissue meshwork of plaques. From a theoretical point of view these processes may work in two ways: they may either stimulate the synthesis of extracellular matrix components and, hence, fibrosis, which may stabilize plaques, or they may lead to degradation of the matrix components, thus inducing plaque instability.

A. Stimulation of Fibrosis in the Plaque

Smooth muscle cells (SMCs) produce all the extracellular matrix components of a plaque, including collagens, elastin, and various types of proteoglycans. Transforming growth factor-β (TFG-β) is one of the most potent stimulators of connective tissue production by SMCs. Large amounts of this growth factor are detected in restenosis lesions after angioplasty (40), and TGF-β also participates in the repair process after natural plaque disruption. TGF-β and other growth factors, including platelet-derived growth factor (PDGF), collagen growth factor (CTGF), and basic fibroblast growth factor (bFGF) play important roles in wound healing and the reparative stage of many chronic inflammatory diseases. Thus, one may anticipate that in atherosclerosis they have a stabilizing effect on plaque structure (41).

B. Inhibition of Collagen Production in the Fibrous Cap

The T-cell cytokine, IFN-γ, produced by activated T lymphocytes and macrophages in plaques, plays an important role in the process of plaque destabilization (41). It inhibits the proliferation of SMCs and selectively decreases their synthesis of collagens by inhibiting the expression of the interstitial collagen-1 gene, even when SMCs previously have been stimulated with the anti-inflammatory cytokine TGF-β (41). Another exclusive effect of IFN-γ is the induction of HLA-DR expression on SMCs (42). Although the functional significance of this phenomenon is still speculative, it may serve as a marker for the activity of IFN-γ in plaques, because HLA-DR–positive SMCs can indeed be observed in plaques at sites of inflammation (3).

At present, there is increasing interest in the induction of apoptosis in plaques. Apoptosis is an intrinsically programmed form of cell death, which can be activated by the cytokines TNF-α and IL-1. Apoptosis is recognized as a mechanism of foam cell death, which results in the spillage of lipids and, hence, the enlargement of the soft core of extracellular lipids. The CD36 scavenging receptor, which is up-regulated in these cells, plays a role in this process. Apoptosis of SMCs has been observed in atherosclerotic plaques in humans and in rabbit models of vascular disease (43–45). The increased rates of SMC apoptosis in intimal lesions might be explained by a combination of proapoptotic signals (cytokines and growth factors) and a decreased expression of the antiapoptotic Bcl-xL gene, which has recently been documented (45). In early lesions, SMC apoptosis could have beneficial effects in promoting regression of the volume of SMCs, but in the fibrous cap of advanced lesions it introduces an additional potential of plaque destabilization because of the loss of the repair functions of these cells.

C.   Matrix Degrading Effects of Metalloproteinases

Apart from the inhibiting effects on extracellular matrix production, plaque inflammation may initiate an even more powerful pathway of plaque degradation by the secretion of extracellular matrix degrading MMPs (Figure 6). MMPs are proteolytic enzymes, which are normally involved in the physiological process of connective tissue turnover. In pathological states such as chronic inflammation, however, their synthesis and activation can be markedly up-regulated (46). Several types of MMPs have been identified in human plaques, including collagenase (MMP1), gelatinases A and B (MMP2 and 9), stromelysin-1 (MMP3), and matrilysin (MMP8) (47, 48). The secretion of these enzymes is stimulated by the cytokines TNF and IL-1, and in the extracellular space of the plaque they are activated by plasmin or, alternatively, by mast cell products. In the activated state, MMPs initiate a cascade of proteolytic activities with a very broad substrate specificity, which basically includes all extracellular matrix components of the fibrous cap.

Tissue inhibitors of metalloproteinases (TIMPs) are able to control the strong proteolytic activities of MMPs under normal conditions, but in contrast to MMPs the secretion of TIMPs is only marginally up-regulated by inflammatory cytokines. This phenomenon thus creates a situation in favor of the degrading activities of MMPs (46). In fact, the net effect of matrix lysis has been demonstrated with in situ zymographic studies, which revealed that the vulnerable (macrophage-rich) regions of plaques contained high proteolytic enzyme activity (49). Another observation of particular interest is that synthesis and lytic activity of these enzymes is most abundant in the lipid-laden macrophages and in the extra-

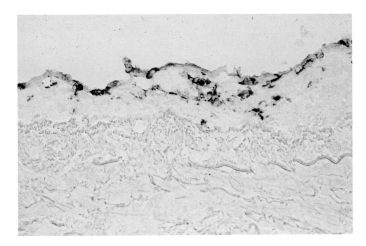

Figure 3.1 Section through a human coronary artery with diffuse intimal thickening, showing subendothelial accumulation of macrophages. F8RA/HLA-DR double stain. Endothelial cells (F8RA) in blue, macrophages (HLA/DR) in brown.

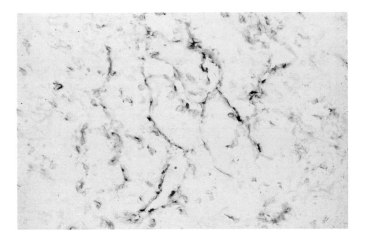

Figure 3.2 Neovascularization of an advanced atherosclerotic plaque. The microvascular endothelium shows UEA expression (blue). There is perivascular infiltration of CD40-positive inflammatory cells (brown). UEA/CD40 immunodouble stain.

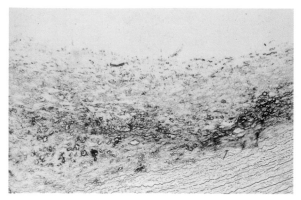

Figure 3.3 Shoulder part of an atherosclerotic plaque in a human carotid artery. Two distinct subpopulations of macrophages are visualized using a double immunostaining technique with CD14/CD36. The macrophages bordering on the lipid core stain positive with CD36 (blue); the more superficial macrophages stain positive with CD14 (brown).

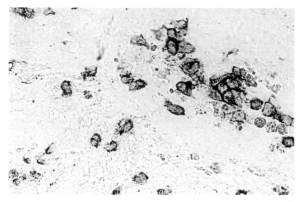

Figure 3.4 Detail of an atherosclerotic plaque showing a cluster of CD3-positive T lymphocytes (brown) clustered around ceroid granules.

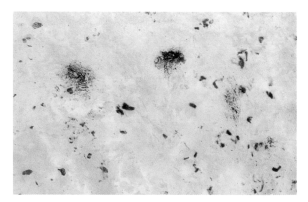

Figure 3.5 Mast cells in a coronary atherectomy specimen of a patient with unstable angina. The mast cells are degranulated, indicating activation of the cells. Antitriptase stain (brick red).

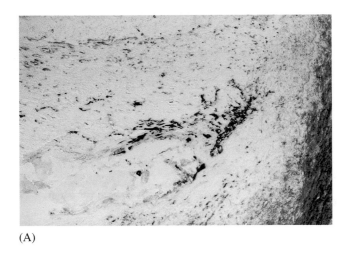

(A)

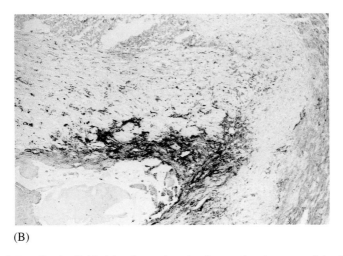

(B)

Figure 3.6 Detail of a lipid-rich atherosclerotic plaque, showing part of the lipid core together with the shoulder part and fibrous cap. (A) Double immunostain, anti-CD68/anti-α actin, showing foam cell macrophages (red) bordering on the lipid core and smooth muscle cells (blue) in the fibrous cap and the adjacent media. (B) Adjacent section shows abundant MMP3 staining of foam cell macrophages around the lipid core and to a lesser extent some smooth muscle cells in the fibrous cap (anti-MMP immunostain). (From Ref. 4.)

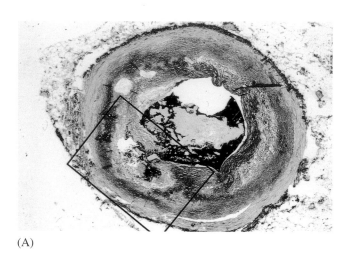

(A)

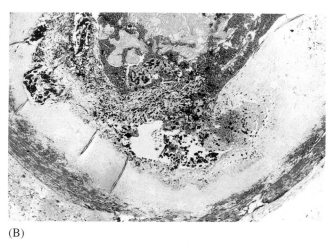

(B)

Figure 3.7 Atherosclerotic plaque in a coronary artery of a 67-year-old man, showing an eccentric mildly stenotic plaque with complete disruption of the fibrous cap (boxed area), mural thrombus, and hemorrhage into the lipid core. (A) Picrosirius red stain (collagen stains red). (B) Detail of the boxed area in A. An adjacent tissue section shows accumulation of macrophages (red) at the rupture site. Smooth muscle cells in the media stain blue (anti-CD68/anti-α actin immunodouble stain). (From Ref. 4.)

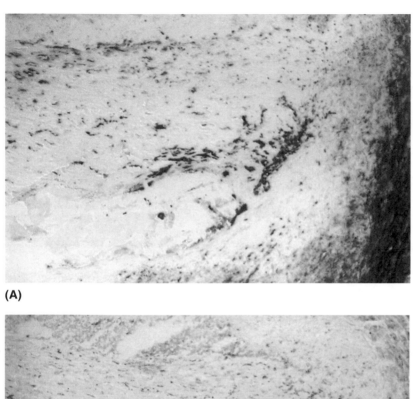

(A)

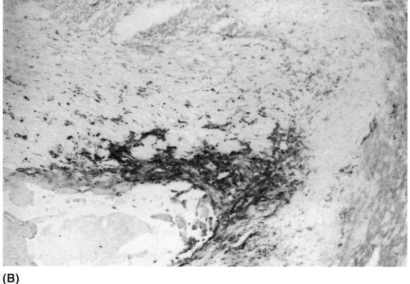

(B)

Figure 6   Detail of a lipid-rich atherosclerotic plaque, showing part of the lipid core together with the shoulder part and fibrous cap. (A) Double immunostain, anti-CD68/anti-α actin, showing foam cell macrophages bordering on the lipid core and smooth muscle cells in the fibrous cap and the adjacent media. (B) adjacent section shows abundant MMP3 staining of foam cell macrophages around the lipid core and to a lesser extent some smooth muscle cells in the fibrous cap (anti-MMP immunostain). (See also color insert.) (From Ref. 4.)

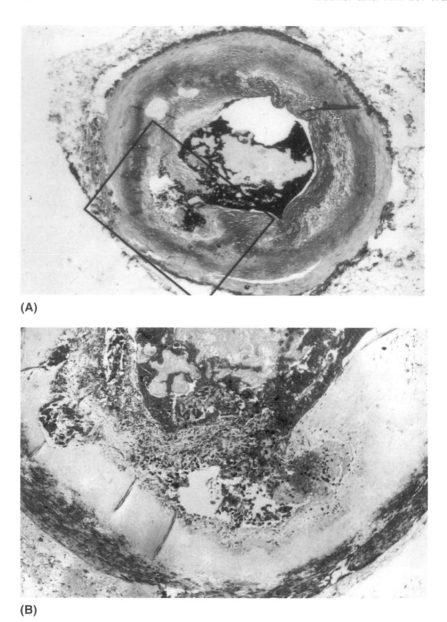

(A)

(B)

Figure 7 Atherosclerotic plaque in a coronary artery of a 67-year-old man, showing an eccentric mildly stenotic plaque with complete disruption of the fibrous cap (boxed area), mural thrombus, and hemorrhage into the lipid core. (A) Picrosirius red stain. (B) Detail of the boxed area in A. An adjacent tissue section shows accumulation of macrophages at the rupture site. Smooth muscle cells in the media stain positive for α-actin (anti-CD68/anti-α actin immunodouble stain). (See also color insert.)(From Ref. 4.)

cellular space around lipid cores of plaques. Studies on experimental atheromas have endorsed these observations: lipid loading of isolated macrophages augments the production of collagenases (49). These observations provide a link between lipids and inflammation and, furthermore, might explain why the degradative effects of inflammation are most prominent in lipid-rich plaques.

V. CONCLUSIONS

As alluded to previously, there is accumulating evidence that a relationship exists between intraplaque inflammation and plaque complications, of which, in general terms, plaque rupture is the most common condition underlying acute myocardial infarction (Figure 7). The study of athertectomy specimens obtained from patients with coronary syndromes have shown unequivocally that a direct link exists between the amount of inflammatory cells present and the severity of the underlying clinical syndrome. In addition, these studies have explained that recent onset activation, IL-2R expression on T lymphocytes, correlates directly with the most severe forms of unstable angina pectoris and acute myocardial infarction.

The observation that the inflammatory process present in atherosclerotic plaques is an immune-mediated disease with secretion of cytokines and growth factors introduces the potential for inflammation-mediated effects on the matrix components of the plaque. Indeed, one may hypothesize that once the antigenic stimuli have been removed, for instance, through lipid-lowering therapy, the balance of the inflammatory secretory products may well veer toward repair with accumulation of extracellular matrix components and eventually fibrous tissue. However, in the setting of augmented antigenic stimulation, one may conceptualize a situation in which breakdown of extracellular matrix prevails. As indicated previously much evidence supports this particular phenomenon in human atherosclerotic plaques that are at risk.

This is not to say that other factors cannot play a role, such as shear stress, vascular wall reactivity, and tissue stress factors; each of these in their own right may contribute to the eventual rupture. In our views, however, the degrading effects of the inflammatory products on the extracellular matrix most often provide the setting for disruption of the integrity of the plaque.

REFERENCES

1. Munro JM, Cotran RS. The pathogenesis of atherosclerosis: atherogenesis and inflammation. Lab Invest 1988; 58:249–261.
2. Ross R. The pathogenesis of atherosclerosis: a perspective for the 1990s. Nature 1993; 362:801–809.

3. van der Wal AC, Becker AE, van der Loos CM, Das PK. Site of intimal rupture
    or erosion of thrombosed coronary atherosclerotic plaques is characterized by an
    inflammatory process irrespective of the dominant plaque morphology. Circulation
    1994; 89:36–44.
4. van der Wal AC, Becker AE. Atherosclerotic plaque rupture—pathologic basis of
    plaque instability and instability. Cardiovasc Res 1999; 41:334–444.
5. Stary HC. Evolution and progression of atherosclerotic lesions in coronary arteries
    of children and young adults. Arteriosclerosis 1989; 9(suppl 1):19–32.
6. Krams R, Wentzel JJ, Oomen JAF, Vinke R, Schuurbiers JCH, de Feyter PJ, Serruys,
    PW, Slager CJ. Evaluation of endothelial shear stress and 3D geometry as factors
    determining the development of atherosclerosis and remodeling in human coronary
    arteries in vivo: combining 3D reconstruction from angiography and IVUS (AN-
    GUS) with computational fluid dynamics. Atheroscler Thromb Vasc Biol 1997; 17:
    2061–2065.
7. Poston RN, Haskard DO, Coucher JR, Gall NP, Johnson-Tidey RR. Expression of
    intercellular adhesion molecule-1 in atherosclerotic plaques. Am J Pathol 1992; 140:
    665–673.
8. van der Wal AC, Das PK, Tigges AJ, Becker AE. Adhesion molecules on the endo-
    thelium and mononuclear cells in human atherosclerotic lesions. Am J Pathol 1992;
    141:1427–1433.
9. Duplaa C, Coufinhall T, Labat L, Moreau C, Petit-Jean ME, Doutre MS, Lamaziere JM,
    Bonnet J. Monocyte/macrophage recruitment and expression of endothelial adhesion
    proteins in human atherosclerotic lesions. Atherosclerosis 1996; 121:253–266.
10. Cybulsky MI, Gimbrone MA, Jr. Endothelial expression of a monocyte leukocyte
    adhesion molecule during atherogenesis. Science 1991; 251:788–791.
11. Kume N, Cybulsky MI, Gimbrone MA, Jr. Lysophosphatidylcholine, a component
    of atherogenic lipoproteins, induces mononuclear leukocyte adhesion in cultured
    human rabbit arterial endothelial cells. J Clin Invest 1992; 90:1138–1144.
12. Gimbrone MA Jr, Cybulsky MI, Kume N, Collins T, Resnick N. Vascular endothe-
    lium: an integrator of pathophysiological stimuli in atherogenesis. Ann N Y Acad
    Sci 1995; 748:122–132.
13. Walpola PL, Gotlieb AI, Cybulsky MI, Langille BL. Expression of ICAM-1 and
    VCAM-1 and monocyte adherence in arteries exposed to altered shear stress. Arte-
    rioscler Thromb Vasc Biol 1995; 15:2–10.
14. Tropea BI, Huie P, Cooke JP, Tsao PS, Sibley RK, Zarins CK. Hypertension-
    enhanced monocyte adhesion in experimental atherosclerosis. J Vasc Surg 1996; 23:
    596–605.
15. Geiringer E. Intimal vascularization and atherosclerosis. J Pathol Bacteriol 1951;
    63:201–211.
16. O'Brien KD, McDonald TO, Chait A, Allen MD, Alpers CE. Neovascular expres-
    sion of E-selection, intercellular adhesion molecule-1, and vascular adhesion mole-
    cule-1 in human atherosclerosis and their relation to intimal leukocyte content. Cir-
    culation 1996; 93:672–682.
17. de Boer OJ, van der Wal AC, Teeling P, Becker AE. Leucocyte recruitment in rup-
    ture prone regions of lipid-rich plaques: a prominent role for neovascularization.
    Cardiovasc Res 1999; 41:443–449.

18. Jonasson L, Holm J, Skalli O, Bondjers G, Hansson GK. Regional accumulation of T-cells, macrophages, and smooth muscle cells in the human atherosclerotic plaque. Atherosclerosis 1986; 6:131–138.

19. van der Wal AC, Das PK, Bentz van de Berg DB, van der Loos CM, Becker AE. Atherosclerotic lesions in humans. In situ immunophenotypic analysis suggesting an immune mediated response. Lab Invest 1989; 61:166–170.

20. Kaartinen M, Penttila A, Kovanen PT. Accumulation of activated mast cells in the shoulder region of human coronary atheroma, the predilection site of atheromatous rupture. Circulation 1994; 90:1669–1678.

21. van der Wal AC, de Boer OJ, Becker AE. Immune and inflammatory responses in the atherosclerotic plaque. In: Schultheiss HP, Schwimmbeck P, eds. The Role of Immune Mechanisms in Cardiovascular Disease. Berlin: Springer Verlag, 1997: 205–212.

22. Hansson GK, Holm J, Jonasson L. Detection of activated T lymphocytes in the human atherosclerotic plaque. Am J Pathol 1989; 135:169–175.

23. Stemme S, Holm J, Hansson GK. T lymphocytes in human atherosclerotic plaques are memory cells expressing CD45RO and the integrin VLA-1. Arterioscler Thromb 1991; 12:206–211.

24. de Boer OJ, Hirsch F, van der Wal AC, van der Loos CM, Das PK, Becker AE. Costimulatory molecules in human atherosclerotic plaques: an indication of antigen specific T lymphocyte activation. Atherosclerosis 1997; 133:227–234.

25. Hansson GK. Cell-mediated immunity in atherosclerosis. Curr Opin Lipidol 1997; 8:301–311.

26. Steinberg D, Witztum JL. Lipoproteins and atherogenesis: current concepts. JAMA 1990; 264:3047–3052.

27. Brown MS, Goldstein JL. Atherosclerosis. Scavenging for receptors. Nature 1990; 343:508–509.

28. Mitchinson MJ, Ball RY. Macrophages and atherogenesis. Lancet 1987; 2:146–148.

29. van der Wal AC, Das PK, Tigges AJ, Becker AE. Macrophage differentiation in atherosclerosis. An in situ immunohistochemical analysis in humans. Am J Pathol 1992; 141:161–168.

30. Nagornev VA, Maltseva SV. The phenotype of macrophages which are not transformed into foam cells in atherogenesis. Atherosclerosis 1996; 121:245–251.

31. Waldmann TA. The structure,function, and expression of interleukin-2 receptors on normal and malignant lymphocytes. Science 1986; 232:727–732.

32. Poulton TA Gallagher A, Potts RC, Beck JS. Changes in activation markers and cell membrane receptors on human peripheral blood T lymphocytes during cell cycle progression after PHA stimulation. Immunology 1988; 64:419–425.

33. Uyemura K, Demer LL, Castle SC, Julien D, Berliner JA, Gately MK, Warrier RR, Pham N, Fogelman AM, Modlin RL. Cross regulatory roles of interleukin (IL)-12 and IL-10 in atherosclerosis. J Clin Invest 1996; 97:2130–2138.

34. de Boer OJ, van der Wal AC, Verhagen CE, Becker AE. Cytokine secretion profiles of cloned T cells from human aortic atherosclerotic plaques. J Pathol 1999; 188: 174–179.

35. van der Wal AC, Piek JJ, de Boer OJ, Koch KT, Teeling P, van der Loos CM,

Becker AE. Recent activation of the plaque immune response in coronary lesions underlying acute coronary syndromes. Heart 1998; 80:14–18.

36. Constantinides P. Mast cells and susceptibility to experimental atherosclerosis. Science 1953; 117:505–506.

37. Kokkonen JO, Kovanen PT. Stimulation of mast cells leads to cholesterol accumulation in macrophages in vitro by a mast cell granule mediated uptake of low density lipoprotein. Proc Natl Acad Sci USA 1987; 84:2287–2291.

38. Kaartinen M. Mast cells in human arterial intima. Implications for atherosclerosis and its complications. Academic dissertation, University of Helsinki, 1996.

39. Kaartinen M, van der Wal AC, van der Loos CM, Piek JJ, Koch KT, Becker AE, Kovanen PT. Mast cell infiltration in acute coronary syndromes. Implications for plaque rupture. J Am Coll Cardiol 1998; 32:606–612.

40. Nikol S, Isner JM, Pickering JG, Kearney M, Leclerc G, Weir L. Expression of transforming growth factor-beta 1 is increased in human vascular restenosis lesons. J Clin Invest 1992; 90:1582–1592.

41. Libby P. Molecular bases of the acute coronary syndromes. Circulation 1995; 91: 2844–2850.

42. Warner SJ, Friedman GB, Libby P. Regulation of major histocompatibility gene expression in human vascular smooth muscle cells. Arteriosclerosis 1989; 9:279–288.

43. Geng YJ, Libby P. Evidence for apoptosis in advanced human atheroma; colocalization with interleukin-1 beta-converting enzyme. Am J Pathol 1995; 147:251–266.

44. Isner JM, Kearney M, Bortman S, Passeri J. Apoptosis in human atherosclerosis and restenosis. Circulation 1995; 91:2703–2711.

45. Pollman MJ, Hall JL, Mann MJ, Zhang L, Gibbons GH. Inhibition of neointimal bcl-x expression induces apoptosis and regression of vascular disease. Nature Medicine 1998; 4:222–227.

46. Lee RT, Libby P. Metalloproteinases and atherosclerotic plaque rupture. In: Schultheiss HP, Schwimmbeck P, eds. The Role of Immune Mechanisms in Cardiovascular Disease. Berlin: Springer Verlag, 1997:238–245.

47. Henney AM, Wakeley PR, Davies MJ, Foster K, Hembry R, Murphy G, Humphries S. Localization of stromclysin gene expression in atherosclerotic plaques by in situ hybridization. Proc Natl Acad Sci USA 1991; 88:8154–8158.

48. Galis ZS, Sukhova GK, Lark MW, Libby P. Increased expression of matrix metalloproteinases and matrix degrading activity in vulnerable regions of human atherosclerotic plaques. J Clin Invest. 1994; 94:2493–2503.

49. Galis ZS, Sukhova GK, Kranzhofer R, Clark S, Libby P. Macrophage foam cells from experimental atheroma constitutively produce matrix degrading proteinases. Proc Natl Acad Sci USA 1995; 92:402–406.

4
Molecular Mechanisms of Plaque Weakening and Disruption

Zorina S. Galis
Emory University School of Medicine, Atlanta, Georgia

I. PLAQUE STABILITY AND TISSUE WEAKENING

Wisdom achieved during the last few years, mainly through careful pathological analysis of fatally occluded vessels (1–4), has led to the final realization that such fatal cardiovascular events are more likely due to artery occlusion by thrombi rather than to the simple obliteration of arterial lumen by atheroma. During the natural history of atherosclerosis, the affected arteries undergo a continuous process of remodeling (Figure 1), during which they initially adapt, compensating for the development of intimal atherosclerotic lesions with an overall increase in their diameter (5, 6). The demise of the lesion occurs through destabilization. Thrombi develop in places where the continuity of a plaque's fibrous cap is disrupted by fissures (4) or in places where the endothelial lining is eroded (7). The recently recognized clinical importance of plaque disruption initiated a quest for factors that may contribute to plaque weakening and destabilization. Observation of ruptured plaques has also shown that the wall structure fails in predictable spots, called the ''shoulders'', where the plaque meets the normal wall. A combination of passive and active factors is currently suspected as being responsible for weakening of tissue in these vulnerable areas (8). Pathological determinants associated with instability include a high lipid content and an increased number of macrophage-derived foam cells (9). The composition of individual atheroma is related to tissue strength, and, together with the geometrical parameters, determines the intensity of the mechanical forces that develop in the plaque (10). Mathematical modeling has revealed that the typically asymmetrical geometry of atherosclerotic vessels imposes an increased mechanical stress at the plaque

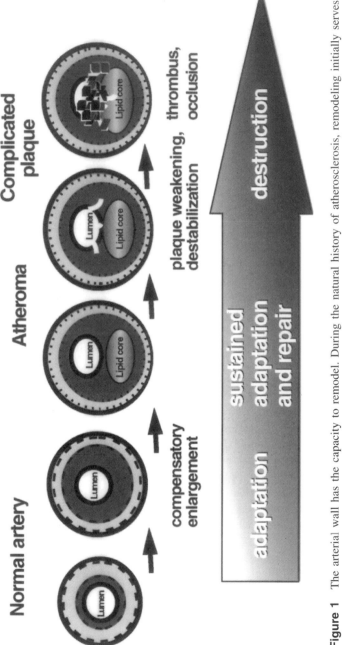

Figure 1 The arterial wall has the capacity to remodel. During the natural history of atherosclerosis, remodeling initially serves a beneficial adaptive function, but later may progress toward destructive stages in which the tissue weakens and the plaque structure is compromised. Loss of the nonthrombogenic endothelial layer and further exposure of the thrombogenic material through plaque erosion, fissuring, and rupture triggers the development of superimposed thrombosis and can lead to lumen occlusion, a main cause of acute cardiovascular syndromes.

shoulders (11). In addition to these previously recognized features, which will be discussed in detail in other chapters, we have investigated the hypothesis that a dynamic process of weakening contributes to plaque failure. Specifically, we suspected that active destruction of the extracellular matrix, the plaque's scaffold, occurs in advanced plaques, and we set out to identify and characterize potential matrix-degrading enzymes. The action of enzymes specialized in matrix degradation, called matrix metalloproteinases (MMPs), had been previously recognized and investigated in relation to tissue invasion, remodeling, and inflammation (12). We hypothesized that the cells of large blood vessels might also be able to produce MMPs, which would participate in vascular remodeling in general and would be specifically associated with the development and complications of human atherosclerotic plaques. Since then, numerous reports have enhanced our understanding of MMP biology, and many pieces of evidence have accumulated to support a major role of MMPs in vascular pathological conditions. This chapter will focus on regulation of vascular MMPs and the evidence for their likely role in plaque destabilization and disruption.

II. MATRIX METALLOPROTEINASES (MMPs)

A. General Characteristics

More than 20 members of the MMP family of enzymes have been identified and described so far. Each enzyme degrades at least one and sometimes several components of the extracellular matrix (13). Because matrix degradation is a necessary component of tissue shaping and remodeling, the action of MMPs has been studied in connection with many physiological and pathological processes, including embryonic development, wound healing, inflammation, and cancer (12, 14–16). The MMPs have fairly homologous amino acid domains and share several important features that account for their collective grouping. All cell-secreted MMPs described so far are produced as latent proenzymes (or zymogens). Thus, an essential common regulatory feature of MMP action is related to a necessary posttranslational conversion to the active forms (17). The mechanism of activation, known as the ''cysteine switch'' mechanism (18), can be initiated either through conformational modifications of the proenzyme molecule or through the proteolytic removal of its prodomain. Either pathway must result in breaking the coordination between essential cysteine residues in the prodomain and the zinc atom in the enzyme's catalytic center, which otherwise keeps the proenzyme folded on itself. This first event leads to generation of a partially activated enzyme. Even in this stage, the MMP can bind and digest the substrate; it can also initiate the autocatalysis of the partially activated enzyme. Through a consecutive series of autolytic steps, the MMP molecules are then progressively shortened, going through a fully activated stage, and later with more processing, lose the catalytic domain and thus lose the enzymatic activity. This molecular processing is characteristic of MMPs, whose enzymatic activity is absent in tissues under normal conditions because the stored zymogens are inactive and subsequent initiation of activation results in a limited life span for the enzyme. Cells also secrete natural MMP inhibitors, called tissue inhibitors of metalloproteinases, or TIMPs (19), which can interfere with zymogen activation and with substrate degradation by activated MMPs (20).

B. MMP Classes

MMPs have been classified into several classes, each class including members with a high degree of amino acid sequence homology and similar substrate specificity. Substrate specificity can be fairly restricted, as in the case of the interstitial collagenase (MMP-1) (21), which is thought to be dedicated to digestion of interstitial collagens. Worth noting is that the triple helical structure of these fibrillar collagens is resistant to most other known proteases. In contrast, other MMPs, such as the members of the stromelysin-1 (MMP-3) class, have broad proteolytic activities. Among main extracellular matrix (ECM) components, stromelysin substrates include proteoglycans, fibronectin, and laminin (22). The zymogens of other MMPs are also an important class of substrates (23, 24) for MMP-3, placing the stromelysins at the top of the MMP activation cascade (25).

Yet another class of MMPs is the gelatinases, MMP-2 and MMP-9. These enzymes were initially described as specialized for degradation of collagens IV and V, the nonfibrillar collagens abundant in the cellular basal lamina. Gelatinases are also thought to complete the degradation of interstitial collagen, hydrolyzing the two characteristic fragments generated by MMP-1, although subsequent studies suggest that, under inhibitor-free conditions, gelatinases may even cleave intact interstitial collagen (26). MMP-2 and MMP-9 were also found to be efficient elastases (27–29). A recent study investigating glomerular mesangial cells suggested the interesting possibility that besides its widely recognized function of digesting matrix components, active MMP-2 may also regulate cell proliferation and differentiation (30).

Until the last few years, it was believed that all MMPs were secreted proteins. With the discovery of the membrane type (MT)1-MMP (31), the first cell membrane–associated MMP, a new, and rapidly growing class was added to the list of MMPs (32). MT1-MMP was initially identified as the cell-associated activator of secreted pro-MMP-2. As for the other MMPs, the MT-MMPs also turned out to have broader substrate degrading capacity (33).

The number of identified members of the MMP family is still growing, as is the array of substrates susceptible to the action of the various MMPs. Interestingly, many of the more recently described MMP substrates: cytokines (34), growth factors and their receptors (35), plasminogen, and plasminogen activator

(36, 37), are not structural components of the matrix. Proteolytic processing of these biologically active factors leads either to activation or inhibition of their biological action, resulting in regulation of the multitude of processes controlled by such mediators. Thus, most likely, the role of MMPs within tissues reaches beyond direct degradation of ECM components, as originally thought, and might still be underestimated.

III. MMPs IN THE NORMAL AND DISEASED ARTERIAL WALL

Obvious primary questions are: do cells of normal or atherosclerotic arteries produce MMPs and are there any differences associated with vascular pathological conditions? If so, what are the factors that may regulate MMP expression and activation in the context of atherosclerosis?

A. MMP Expression

Henney and colleagues (38) showed by in situ hybridization that mRNA transcripts for MMP-3 can be selectively detected in atherosclerotic plaques. Positive signals were associated with macrophage-derived foam cells and the smooth muscle cells (SMC) of the fibrous cap. We used immunocytochemistry and biochemical analysis to examine the presence of several MMPs and TIMPs 1 and 2, in normal or atherosclerotic human coronary and carotid arteries (39). In normal human arteries, we found that MMP-2 and TIMPs are homogeneously distributed across the wall. Other MMPs, such as MMP-1, MMP-3, and MMP-9, were not detectable by immunocytochemistry. In contrast, strong immunostaining, suggesting focal overexpression of all investigated MMPs, (i.e., MMP-1, MMP-2, MMP-3, and MMP-9) was detected in the plaque's shoulders, which are believed to be "vulnerable" because of their tendency to rupture (1). Further immunocytochemical characterization of specimens using cell typing also indicated the cellular sources of MMPs and provided us with hints regarding the factors that might modulate their expression and activation in the atherosclerotic vessel wall. A major source of MMPs were the foam cells, macrophages, or SMC containing intracellular lipid accumulations. Cells expressing MMPs also included the endothelium covering plaques, or lining the vasa plaquorum, as well as SMC forming the fibrous cap, or localized between breaks in the internal elastic lamina. Interestingly, coexpression of TIMPs was detected in these areas, thus confounding the essential question regarding the capacity of MMPs to degrade matrix in these sites. Expression of two other broad-acting MMPs, matrilysin and macrophage metalloelastase (40), was also detected exclusively in atherosclerotic plaques of human carotid arteries compared with normal arteries. The distribution of MMPs was restricted to the macrophage-derived foam cells in the area between the acellular lipid core and the overlying fibrous cap (41), further supporting a role of macrophage MMPs in the detachment of the fibrous cap. Interestingly, immunodetection of versican, a preferred proteoglycan substrate of matrilysin, showed a specific distribution around the matrilysin-expressing foam cells. Although histological examination does not provide the time sequence, and thus the cause-effect relation is not certain, these observations support the view that macrophages may tailor their expression of matrix-degrading enzymes in accordance with the matrix environment.

B. MMP Activity

Because the local enzymatic activity of MMPs is a balance between the amount of active enzyme generated and the inhibitors present, this issue cannot be settled by use of either immunocytochemical analysis, which does not distinguish active enzymes or give quantitative information, or by the biochemical characterization of whole tissue homogenates, which may inadvertently mix enzymes and inhibitors confined initially to different locations. We therefore developed a method that preserves the tissue structure while allowing detection of MMP enzymatic activity in situ (42). Investigation of freshly excised human carotid endarterectomy specimens using "in situ zymography" showed that active MMPs prevail in the vulnerable shoulders of atheroma (Figure 2). However, no MMP activity

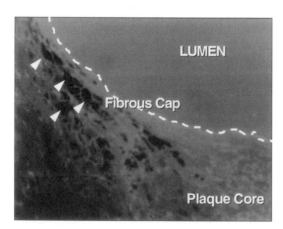

Figure 2 Detection of matrix-degrading activity in the fibrous cap of a human atherosclerotic plaque (coronary artery) by in situ zymography. The tissue specimens were laid on a film of substrate coupled to a fluorescent reporter molecule (casein-resorufin) to reveal the holes drilled by the active enzymes (arrowheads). Such activity weakens the matrix and is likely responsible for destabilization of the fibrous cap at the vulnerable shoulders.

was detected in normal human or rabbit arteries (39, 42). These observations thus furnished strong support for a role of MMP activity in the weakening of atherosclerotic plaques leading to plaque destabilization. These studies also allowed identification of the macrophage-derived foam cells as the main producers of MMP activity in atheroma. The role of macrophage-derived MMPs was elegantly confirmed in subsequent studies demonstrating their capacity to induce breakdown of collagen in the fibrous cap of human atherosclerotic lesions (43). Recent evidence has added mast cells as potential sources of active MMPs in the plaque shoulders (44).

Increased expression of MMPs seems to be a consistent feature of atherosclerotic lesions regardless of the artery type. Li et al. (45) reported that human aortic atherosclerotic lesions have increased levels of latent and active MMP-2 compared with normal aortas. An increase in arterial MMP expression and activity, especially of MMP-9, was found to be associated with unstable and degenerative vascular syndromes: unstable angina (46), ruptured aortic aneurysms (47–49), or temporal arteritis (50).

IV. REGULATION OF VASCULAR MMP EXPRESSION AND ACTIVATION IN VITRO

A. Vascular MMP Expression

Examination in situ of MMP expression and activity implied correlations with pathological features of human arteries. No matter how suggestive, observations made on tissue specimens can only offer a still picture of the situation. To validate insights gained from the morphological analysis, one needs to turn to studies using vascular cells in culture in conditions that allow testing of potential regulatory factors. Some features of MMP expression by the main cellular constituents of blood vessels, the endothelial and the smooth muscle cells, in vitro and in situ are summarized in Table 1.

1. Endothelial MMPs

Endothelial cells (EC) form the innermost layer of blood vessels. In culture they synthesize several MMPs and their natural inhibitors (51, 52, 56). The spectrum of MMPs secreted in vitro reportedly varies according to the source of EC and depends on cell culture conditions (52). All cultured EC seem to constitutively secrete the zymogen form of MMP-2, thought to be necessary for the normal turnover of all cellular basement membranes. Expression of MMP-1 and MMP-3 by EC is induced or enhanced, depending on the vascular source of EC, by exposure to cytokines or phorbol esters (52, 56). Cytokines also stimulate in vitro expression of MT1-MMP in human saphenous vein EC (Figure 3) and in SMC (65).

Table 1 Main Human Vascular MMPs and TIMPs

Enzyme	Major substrate(s)	Expression	Known stimuli
MMP-1 (interstitial collagenase)	Fibrillar collagen	Constitutive/inducible in EC in vitro (51, 52); Inducible in SMC in vitro; In situ atherosclerotic coronary artery: EC (39, 53, 54), SMC (39); macrophages (39, 43, 55)	Phorbol Esters, IL-1β, TNF-α (52, 56, 57), linoleic acid hydroperoxide (58), FGF-2 (59), CD-40 ligand (60)
MMP-2 (the 72-kD gelatinase, gelatinase A)	Degraded collagen, Collagen IV, V, Elastin	Constitutive in EC in vitro (52, 58); Constitutive in SMC in vitro (57); In situ: normal coronary artery EC, SMC (39); In situ atherosclerotic coronary artery: EC, SMC, macrophages (39)	
MMP-3 (stromelysin 1)	Proteoglycans, Fibronectin, Laminin, Pro-MMP-1/-9	Constitutive/inducible in EC in vitro (51, 52); Inducible in SMC in vitro (57); In situ atherosclerotic coronary artery EC, SMC, macrophages (38, 39)	Phorbol Esters, IL-1β, TNF-α (52, 56, 57), linoleic acid hydroperoxide (58), thrombin (61), CD-40 ligand (60)
MMP-9 (the 92-kD gelatinase, gelatinase B)	Degraded collagen, Collagen IV, V, Elastin	Inducible in EC in vitro (52); Inducible in SMC in vitro (57); Constitutive monocyte/monocytic cells; In situ atherosclerotic coronary artery: SMC, macrophages (39, 46); In situ aneurysmal aorta (48); In situ saphenous vein SMC (62)	IL-1β, TNF-α (52, 57, 63), interaction with EC (64), CD-40 ligand (60)
Matrilysin (MMP-7)	Proteoglycans (versican)	In situ atherosclerotic coronary artery (41)	
MT1-MMP	Pro-MMP-2	Constitutive/inducible in EC in vitro (65)	H_2O_2 (66), collagen I lattice (67), IL-1β, TNF-α, oxidized LDL (65)
TIMP-1	MMP-1, MMP-3, MMP-9	Constitutive/inducible in SMC in vitro (57); Normal arteries (39); Atheroma (39, 54)	PMA (52), PDGF, TGF-β
TIMP-2	Pro-/MMP-2	Constitutive in SMC in vitro (57); Normal coronary artery EC, SMC (39); In situ atherosclerotic coronary artery (39)	
TIMP-3 (68)		Constitutive/inducible in SMC in vitro (69); In situ atherosclerotic carotid artery, aorta (69)	PDGF, TGF-β (69)

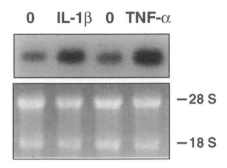

Figure 3 Cytokines increase the constitutive levels of mRNA of MT1-MMP in cultured endothelial cells (EC). Total RNA was extracted from cultured unstimulated (0) human saphenous vein endothelial cells (EC), or EC stimulated with interleukin (IL)-1 or tumor necrosis factor (TNF)-α, and probed using Northern blotting. Increased expression of MT1-MMP is seen in lanes 2 & 4. Loading of the lanes is illustrated in the lower panel by ethidium bromide staining of ribosomal RNA.

2. Smooth Muscle MMPs

Vascular SMC constitute most of the cells in the blood vessel wall and thus are likely the main contributors to protein synthesis in general, and vascular matrix specifically. In vitro, SMC isolated from various vascular sources of different species have been shown to produce several members of the MMP family (57, 70–74). Experiments using synthetic and natural MMP inhibitors, in vitro (74, 75) and in vivo (76, 77), helped highlight the role of different MMPs in SMC migration and proliferation. For example, unstimulated confluent human SMC produce and secrete, in vitro, the proform of MMP-2 (57, 71). We found pro-MMP-2 to be a major in vitro protein product of SMC, thus likely to be abundant in the wall of arteries, and it may well be the main vascular MMP under physiological conditions. The idea that MMP-2 is continuously produced by SMC in situ and deposited in the extracellular space was also suggested by the immunocytochemical and biochemical analysis of normal human arteries (39). Interestingly, most of the pro-MMP-2 secreted in vitro by human SMC was found in a complex with its natural inhibitor, TIMP-2 (57). Presence of TIMP-2 acts as an efficient regulator of pro-MMP-2 activation (78), a feature that could be important because large quantities of pro-MMP-2 might be available for activation in arteries under normal conditions. Expression of additional MMP zymogens, pro-MMP-9, pro-MMP-1 (57, 71), and pro-MMP-3 (57), by human SMC is induced in vitro by growth factors or cytokines, which are preferentially expressed in atherosclerotic vessels in areas infiltrated with inflammatory cells (79). In our experiments in vitro, stimulation with cytokines did not significantly affect the level of MMP inhibitors secreted by cultured human SMC. Furthermore, we noticed that cytokine stimulation also increased the level of activated MMP-2 (57). Finding the stimulatory effect of cytokines on expression of the membrane-associated activator MT1-MMP in subsequent studies (65) provides a plausible explanation. Thus, stimulated SMC produce a combination of MMPs that have the capacity to degrade all major components of the vascular matrix (57). Taken together, the comparison of in situ expression in atherosclerotic vs. nondiseased arteries and the results from these in vitro studies support the notion that locally produced cytokines enhance MMP expression and matrix degradation in areas of inflammatory cell infiltrates of atheroma (57, 80).

Other mechanisms that could regulate the expression of MMPs in SMC of atheroma were recently explored. Previously, Lee et al. (55) combined mathematical modeling with morphological analysis of plaques to reveal coincidence of highest tensile stress and overexpression of MMP-1 in the rupture-prone shoulders of human atherosclerotic plaques. The importance of this finding for plaque destabilization is obvious: the weakest spots might be subjected to the highest mechanical stress. Beyond being a mere, indeed unfortunate, coincidence, this occurrence might point to a causal relation. On the basis of this lead, the same group recently studied the effect of cyclical stretch on MMP production in vitro (81) but unexpectedly found that cyclic stretch actually down-regulated the expression of MMP-1. We have also investigated the possibility that stretch modulates the expression and function of SMC-derived MMPs (82) and have found that the in vitro response of SMC depends on the type of stretch. We confirmed that, compared with the conventional static cell culture conditions, cyclic stretch decreases the expression of MMP-2 in human SMC. In contrast, stationary stretch highly significantly increased not only the level of MMP-2 mRNA but also the levels of secreted latent and active MMP-2 (Figure 4). Similar modulatory effects were detected also for MMP-9 protein.

Detection of active MMP-2 in the culture media of SMC after stationary stretch has important functional implications and suggested novel MMP activation pathways. One possible pathway is through up-regulation of MT1-MMP, the cell-associated activator of MMP-2 (31), which is expressed by SMC and levels of which are enhanced by cytokines and oxidized LDL (65). Another potential mechanism of MMP-2 activation under conditions of imposed mechanical strain could involve the generation of reactive oxygen species (ROS). In vitro, ROS can activate latent forms of gelatinases secreted by cultured human SMC (83). Production of ROS known to be present in atheroma is commonly attributed to inflammatory cells; however, ROS can also be produced by vascular SMC, especially on stimulation (84). The concept that mechanical stretch may stimulate vascular cell ROS production is also supported by recent evidence that stretched EC release hydrogen peroxide (85).

Our results support the notion that cyclic stretch down-regulates production of MMPs. This fits with the view that the matrix-degrading activity in healthy

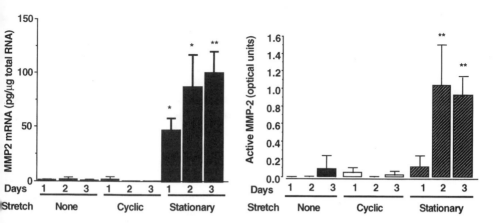

Figure 4 Effect of mechanical uniaxial stretch on expression and activity of MMP-2 by human smooth muscle cells (SMC) cultured for up to 3 days on silicone membranes maintained at resting length (Stretch: ''None''), or stretched either by imposing cyclic (1 Hz), or stationary stretch. Left panel, Stationary stretch increases the level of mRNA severalfold over nonstretch or cyclic stretch conditions. Total cellular RNA was extracted from confluent human saphenous vein SMC. Level of MMP-2 mRNA was determined with quantitative competitive reverse transcriptase–polymerase chain reaction. Bars represent mean values ±S.D. (*$p < 0.05$, ** $p < 0.01$, compared with similar time points from both other groups). Right panel, The level of secreted active MMP-2 is significantly increased after stationary stretch of SMC (** $p < 0.01$ compared with similar time points from both other groups).

arteries, constantly undergoing cyclic stretching, is low. However, the wall of atherosclerotic arteries is subjected to increased circumferential tensile stress (86), whereas the normal cyclic expansion and recoil of arteries is structurally and functionally impaired (87) by many factors, including increased stiffening associated with the development of advanced calcified lesions and poor vasodilation caused by the increased oxidative stress (88). Under these conditions, increased continuous stretch may act as a stimulus to enhance production of matrix-degrading enzymes by the SMC of the diseased artery, possibly as a mechanism to allow compensatory expansion of the arterial wall. Thus, our in vitro results provide a likely mechanistic explanation for the observations made by in situ analysis of human atheroma (55) showing increased MMP expression in plaque areas where stress is maximal (i.e., the shoulders) (11). The sustained increased degradation of matrix would thus weaken and ultimately promote rupture at the plaque shoulders.

Similar reactions of SMC to increased tensile stretch, allowing remodeling and adaptation of vessels through matrix degradation, may take place chronically in hypertension or may occur as an acute reaction to the stretch experienced by arteries expanded with balloon catheters during vascular interventions. Both conditions are associated with an enhancement of the atherosclerotic process.

3. Macrophage MMPs

Blood-borne cells are not a common component of the normal vessel, but inflammatory cells, probably recruited as part of the tissue's intention to heal (89), become a prominent feature of the diseased human arterial wall (90). The monocyte-derived macrophage seems to be prevalent among the several types of inflammatory cells, including macrophages, T lymphocytes, and mast cells, detected in human atherosclerotic lesions. As described earlier in the text, analysis of atherosclerotic plaques showed intense MMP immunopositive staining of resident macrophages (39). This finding suggested high levels of MMP expression, but was also compatible with the mere ingestion of MMPs by macrophages. We will next summarize studies in which we investigated the capacity of macrophage-derived foam cells of atheroma to synthesize, secrete, and activate MMPs.

By nature, activated inflammatory cells have the ability to penetrate tissues, a capacity largely attributed to the matrix-degrading action of MMPs (91). After recruitment from blood by molecules expressed on the luminal surface of the activated endothelium (92), inflammatory cells first attach to and then move through this endothelial monolayer and its supporting basement membrane. Direct interaction with a monolayer of human EC was shown to increase the production of MMP-9 secreted by monocytic cells several fold (64). Data regarding the mechanism are not available yet but are suggested by an earlier article by Romanic and Madri (93), who studied in vitro the interaction between T cells, another type of inflammatory cells, and EC monolayers. In those experiments, the direct cellular interaction triggered T-cell secretion of MMP-2, the other basement membrane–degrading MMP, and was dependent on the expression of the vascular cell adhesion molecule (VCAM)-1 by the EC. Once inside the arterial wall, the MMP action is, no doubt, further necessary for macrophages to penetrate the interstitial space tightly webbed with ECM components. In vitro investigation of factors that may up-regulate MMP expression in monocytes and monocytic cell lines indicates that their repertoire and levels of MMPs depend on the stage of cellular differentiation (94). These studies have shown that the binding of bacterial antigens, which enhances monocyte differentiation, also up-regulates the production of MMPs (95). Although pathogens might play a role in atherogenesis, a hypothesis gaining increasing support [reviewed in (96)], the likely modulator of MMP production by monocytes within arteries is the interaction with common plaque components: other cells (97, 98) or their soluble products (99) and with matrix (100, 101). We found in vitro that interaction of human monocytes with a substrate of collagen I, the major component of atherosclerotic plaque matrix, enhances their differentiation, expression of MMP-9, and intracellular accumulation of lipid (101).

Because the typical phenotype of macrophage resident in atheroma is the foam cell, we chose to develop a model foam cell in vivo to allow detailed in vitro investigation of MMP synthesis and secretion. Although culturing cells on a collagen I substrate also increased intracellular lipid accumulation (101), neither this nor any other maneuver previously used in vitro had been able to produce a genuine in vitro counterpart for the foam cell of atheroma. This phenotype was sought in many experimental studies because it is thought to be closely associated with the characteristic behavior of macrophages in plaque. Therefore, we induced formation of these cells in vivo under hypercholesterolemic conditions. The tissue macrophages accumulated lipid in atherosclerotic lesions and in subcutaneous granulomas induced in rabbits, acquiring the foam cell phenotype found in human atheroma (102). The production of MMPs by macrophages and macrophage-derived foam cells isolated from normal and hypercholesterolemic rabbit tissue was studied in vitro (103, 104). The aortic lipid-laden macrophages of hypercholesterolemic rabbits maintained their capacity to produce MMP-1 and MMP-3 for days after isolation from the experimental atherosclerotic lesions (Figure 5). In contrast, the nonlipid-laden macrophages isolated by bronchoalveolar lavage from the same rabbits did not produce these MMPs (103). When we compared production of MMPs by macrophages isolated from the subcutaneous granulomas of normocholesterolemic and hypercholester-

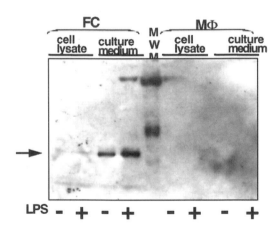

Figure 5 Detection of stromelysin (MMP-3) produced in vitro by aortic macrophage-derived foam cells (FC) or by alveolar macrophages (Mφ) isolated from hypercholesterolemic rabbits (Western blot). Culture medium of FC, but not their cell lysates, contains MMP-3 (arrow) indicating that MMP-3 is produced and released by FC but not by Mφ isolated from the same rabbits. MMP-3 was detectable without additional exogenous stimulation in FC, but in vitro stimulation with lipopolysaccharide (LPS) increased levels of MMP-3. (Molecular weight markers, MWM, were loaded on one lane. Apparent molecular weights, upper band, 110, lower, 68 kD.)

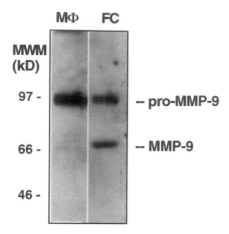

Figure 6 Detection of MMP-9 released in culture by macrophages (MΦ) or macrophage-derived foam cells (FC) isolated from subcutaneous granulomas of normocholesterolemic or hypercholesterolemic rabbits, respectively (Western blot). The latent form (pro-MMP-9) was identified as secreted by both macrophage populations. Culture media harvested from FC also contain active MMP-9. Migration of molecular weight markers (MWM) is indicated on the left in kiloDaltons (kD).

olemic rabbits (104), we found that both macrophages and macrophage-derived foam cells secreted pro-MMP-9 (Figure 6). This was not surprising, because MMP-9 was previously shown to be constitutively produced by circulating monocytes and most macrophages and was implicated in a variety of other pathological situations with an inflammatory component, such as rheumatoid arthritis, as well as in metastasis (105). A distinctive finding in our experiments was that the culture medium harvested from foam cells contained, in addition to the zymogen, the active form of MMP-9, showing that the foam cells had the capacity to activate the zymogen.

When we did these experiments, macrophage MMP activation in an isolated in vitro system was not reported. This observation permitted detailed studies investigating the hypothesis that ROS contribute to the activation of latent MMPs. Thus, besides producing cytokines, the mediators of inflammation that stimulate MMP expression in vascular cells (80), macrophages of atheroma also actively produce MMPs themselves. Monocyte-derived lipid-laden macrophages secrete a larger spectrum of matrix-degrading enzymes compared with either the nontissue alveolar macrophages or the nonlipid-laden tissue macrophages, and they possess a mechanism by which they can activate latent MMPs. Again, these results are in accord with in situ detection of MMP protein and activity in plaque areas rich in inflammatory infiltrates (39, 42).

B. Vascular TIMPs

The scenarios presented previously are complicated, however, by the presence of the aforementioned MMP inhibitors. Both normal and diseased human arteries contain immunoreactive TIMPs (39). The biological action of MMPs in the tissue thus depends on the local balance between levels of active MMPs and TIMPs. As mentioned earlier, TIMPs inhibit activation of MMP zymogens (106) and limit binding of substrates by active MMPs. Less consistent data are available regarding regulation of TIMP expression by vascular cells compared with MMPs. In cell culture, human vascular cells constitutively produce the MMP inhibitors, TIMP-1, TIMP-2 (52, 57), and TIMP-3 (69). Levels of TIMP-1 were enhanced by phorbol myristate acetate (PMA) in human EC (52), whereas we found that neither TIMP-1 nor TIMP-2 levels were affected by exposure of SMC to interleukin (IL)-1α or tumor necrosis factor (TNF)-α (57).

Explanations at the level of RNA transcription have been sought. Partial identification of regions of the human TIMP-1 promoter (107) confirmed the presence of several transcription factor activator protein 1 (AP-1) binding sites (108). Similar promoter analysis showed that the human TIMP-2 promoter was unresponsive to PMA stimulation despite the presence of a complete AP-1 binding site (109) and showed that TIMP-2 gene has several features observed in housekeeping genes. For TIMP-3, expression may be connected to cell cycle progression: with information available only for the murine promoter, both AP-1 binding sites and a putative p53 site (110) appear to be important controlling elements. In human SMC, TIMP-3 expression is increased by platelet-derived growth factor (PDGF) and transforming growth factor (TGF)-β (69). Recent experiments also examined effects of overexpression of the three different TIMPs in rat SMC (111). This study found similar inhibitory effects on the capacity of SMC to migrate in vitro though a reconstituted basement membrane, a process that depends on the action of MMPs, but revealed quite divergent effects of TIMPs on cell proliferation and survival. Although overexpression of TIMP-1 did not affect cell proliferation, that of TIMP-2 caused a dose-dependent reduction in proliferation, whereas TIMP-3 overexpression induced DNA synthesis and promoted SMC death by apoptosis. These latter effects could not be reproduced by using synthetic inhibitors of MMPs, suggesting the possibility that TIMPs may have important functions that are independent of their MMP inhibitory activity or the possibility that synthetic inhibitors lack the access to the necessary compartments.

C. Factors That May Activate MMPs in Atheroma

Because of their characteristic secretion as zymogens, the MMPs can exert their enzymatic action only after activation. Thus, the activation step is crucial for their biological function, and aside from its basic scientific interest, the understanding of the pathways that work in different settings could lead to development of therapeutic approaches. Traditional studies of proteolytic activation of MMPs have examined, almost exclusively, the plasmin/plasminogen pathway (112). This pathway initiates in vitro a metalloprotease cascade leading to activation of some members of the MMP family (113, 114). However, the participation of the plasminogen pathway cannot be accounted for in many cases in which MMP activity leads to matrix degradation, and furthermore, pro-MMP-2, the major vascular MMP, is not activatable through this mechanism. Thus, what activation mechanisms are likely to trigger MMP-dependent degradation of matrix in atheroma? By combining knowledge of MMP biochemical properties and characteristic features of atheroma, one can seek to find pathways biologically relevant in the context of atherosclerosis. We examined the possibility that one such pathway is a consequence of redox stress in the environment of atheroma, and another is related to thrombosis. Results of these investigations will be discussed in the next two sections. Previous studies suggested that activated neutrophils may also be capable of autoactivating latent collagenase (115). Although no direct evidence was presented, the authors proposed the hypothesis that activation might occur through pro-MMP reaction with hypochlorous acid generated by the action of myeloperoxidase, which has been detected in atherosclerotic vessels (116). Thus, hypochlorous acid may also contribute to the activation of MMPs in atheroma. More recent evidence suggests that yet another mechanism of MMP zymogen activation in atheroma relies on lytic processing by other proteases secreted by mast cells in the plaque (44). Johnson et al. found that, in addition to the mast cell neutral proteases, trypase and chymase, mast cells also express MMP-1 and -3. Use of in situ zymography revealed that such sites were also characterized by the presence of active MMPs. The contribution of mast cell proteases was further supported by in vitro experiments. Chemical induction of mast cell degranulation, known to result in the release of trypase and chymase, also increased the activity of MMPs released by plaque specimens. Conversely, in vitro addition of specific inhibitors of mast cell proteases reduced activation of MMPs, confirming a relation between the two types of proteases.

1. The Redox Environment of the Atherosclerotic Plaque and Matrix Degradation

The increased redox stress to which the vessel wall is subjected in a number of pathological situations, such as atherosclerosis (117), certain forms of hypertension (118), and diabetes mellitus (119), has been discovered during the past several years. Reactive oxygen species (ROS) is a collective name for highly chemically active derivatives of oxygen, including both free radicals [e.g., superoxide ($\cdot O_2^-$), hydroxyl (OH$\cdot$), nitric oxide (NO$\cdot$), and peroxynitrite (ONOO$^-$)], and nonradical oxygen derivatives such as hydrogen peroxide (H_2O_2). The capacity for producing ROS is not uniquely restricted to macrophages (120) as originally thought. Production of ROS occurs as a result of normal cellular metabolism (121) through the action of several enzyme systems, including components of mitochondrial electron transport, xanthine oxidase, cyclooxygenase, lipoxygenase, NO⁺ synthase, reduced nicotinamide adenine dinucleotide phosphate (NADPH), and reduced nicotinamide adenine dinucleotide (NADH) oxidases. Vascular cells also possess the necessary cellular machinery, thus both the smooth muscle (84) and the endothelial cell (122, 123) produce ROS. Vascular cells, as most mammalian cells, have numerous antioxidant defense mechanisms including enzymes such as superoxide dismutase (SOD), catalase, glutathione peroxidase, and reduced sulfhydryl groups that normally prevent ROS accumulation. Interestingly, such systems could sometimes work against the cells. For example, the antioxidant mechanism by which SOD inactivates •O_2^- produces H_2O_2, which has a longer lifetime and thus could be potentially more harmful than the initial ROS. For example, we believe that the atherosclerotic process is exacerbated by the peroxidase activity of a novel form of extracellular SOD expressed by macrophage-derived foam cells (124). An increased production or inefficient inactivation of ROS in biological systems results in redox stress (125).

Cell-derived ROS participate in secondary reactions that result in formation of derivative ROS, such as hydroxyl radical (OH•), which results from reduction of H_2O_2 in the presence of transition metals by the Fenton reaction (125). Another radical that results from the interaction between superoxide and nitric oxide (126) is peroxynitrite ($ONOO^-$). Unscavenged ROS react with various intracellular or extracellular biological targets, leading to chemical modification of protein, lipid, or DNA molecules. Many of these interactions have important biological consequences, such as inactivation of enzymes (127), lipid peroxidation (128–130), and cell signaling (131). Escalating redox stress in tissues can lead to deleterious effects that may range from DNA strand breakage to cell death and rampant tissue destruction. Implications of the oxidative modification of lipoproteins accumulated in the atherosclerotic plaque, considered to be a major pathway for the development of lesions, have been extensively studied and reviewed (132, 133). More recently, we proposed activation of MMP zymogens to mediate some of the ROS effects in the tissue.

MMP zymogens are prime candidates for modification by ROS, because ROS easily undergo reactions with thiol groups. Thiols are involved in preserving MMP latency, and their reduction could serve as a common mechanism of activation for several different MMPs. Thus, the biochemical compatibility and availability of reactants, together with our in situ observations indicating MMP activity in areas of atheroma rich in macrophage-derived foam cells (39, 42), suggested to us the hypothesis that zymogen activation may occur through interaction with ROS released by foam cells.

First, we confirmed the capacity of lipid-laden macrophages to produce ROS and defined the nature of these ROS (83). Macrophage-derived foam cells, whether isolated from aortic atheroma or subcutaneous granuloma of hypercholesterolemic animals, produce substantial amounts of $O_2^{\cdot -}$ compared with non-lipid-laden macrophages obtained from the same animals (83). Production of peroxides was detected exclusively in foam cells. Lipid-laden macrophages also express varying amounts of NO synthase activity. In contrast, NO synthase activity was undetectable in alveolar macrophages. We also tested the effects of these ROS, $O_2^{\cdot -}$, H_2O_2, $\cdot NO$, and $ONOO^-$, generated in vitro by donors or added exogenously, on activation of gelatinases produced by cultured SMC or macrophages. ROS generated by the xanthine/xanthine oxidase system activated the affinity-purified zymogens of human SMC-derived MMP-2 and MMP-9 (Figure 7). Direct addition of H_2O_2 causes modulation of gelatinase activity produced by human SMC (83) and by rabbit macrophages (Figure 8). Pro-MMP-9 zymogen, the only form secreted constitutively by alveolar macrophages, was converted to the active

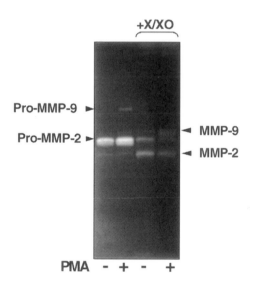

Figure 7   Reactive oxygen species generated by xanthine and xanthine oxidase (X/XO; 100 μM:0.0025 U) activate affinity-purified zymogens of MMP-2 and MMP-9 gelatinases (sodium dodecyl sulfate–polyacrylamide gel electrophoresis [SDS-PAGE] zymography). Proteins are analyzed in SDS-PAGE gels containing gelatin. Presence of gelatinases is indicated by lysed bands in stained gels. Pro-MMPs were isolated from the culture medium of unstimulated (−) or phorbol myristate acetate (PMA)-stimulated (+) human smooth muscle cells. Conversion of the zymogens to the active forms is indicated by the drop in the apparent molecular weight in the X/XO treated samples.

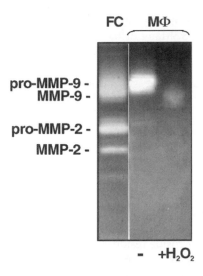

Figure 8 Gelatinolytic activity released in culture by macrophage foam cells (FC) isolated from rabbit atherosclerotic intima or by alveolar macrophages of same rabbit (Mφ) sodium dodecyl sulfate–polyacrylamide gel electrophoresis [SDS-PAGE] gelatin zymography). Culture medium conditioned by FC, loaded on the first lane, contains both zymogens, pro-MMP-2 and pro-MMP-9, and their activated forms. Medium harvested from Mφ (second lane) contains only pro-MMP-9. Incubation of this culture media with 4 μM hydrogen peroxide (''+ H_2O_2'') triggers activation of pro-MMP-9 to MMP-9, as indicated by the shift of the gelatinolytic band to a lower molecular weight associated with the active form.

form after in vitro incubation with H_2O_2. Of note, the culture medium of macrophage-derived foam cells already contains active MMP-9. We found a biphasic effect of H_2O_2 on MMP-2 activity. Low doses of H_2O_2 (4 μM) produced MMP-2 activation, whereas higher doses (10–50 μM) produced inactivation (83). High concentrations of H_2O_2 may inhibit MMP-2 enzymatic activity through either mobilization of the zinc atom at the catalytic site (134) or through extensive protein modification leading to degradation and could act as a regulatory mechanism for MMP activity. Thus, we found a direct activating effect of H_2O_2 on MMP-2 zymogen in cell-free conditions. In addition, subsequent studies showed that H_2O_2 treatment of EC in culture also increased expression of MT1-MMP (66), the cell-associated activator of pro-MMP-2. Therefore, it seems that the action of H_2O_2 can lead to activation of both interstitial and cell-bound MMP-2 zymogen. In such in vitro experiments, one cannot, however, exclude the possibility of formation of the OH^- radical by means of the H_2O_2-dependent Fenton reaction, which could be supported by free metals in the culture medium.

As mentioned earlier, macrophages and macrophage-derived foam cells also produce ˙NO, another major vascular ROS. Many of the known effects of ˙NO, including vasodilatation, lead to the general view that ˙NO is a "good" ROS. However, it is important to understand that ˙NO can interact with other ROS present within tissues (135), thus influencing the general balance of ROS and effects in vivo (129). We also tested the effects of several ˙NO donors upon MMP activation. In our in vitro experiments, generation of ˙NO under these conditions did not affect pro-MMP-2 produced by human SMC. However, a more recent study suggested that ˙NO can activate the pro-MMP-2 zymogen (136). In this latter study, rat mesangial cells were simultaneously incubated with cytokines, lipopolysaccharide, and ˙NO donors. Under such conditions, both ˙NO and $O_2^{˙-}$ may have been generated, leading to formation of $ONOO^-$, another ROS with strong oxidizing properties (137). $ONOO^-$ may be responsible for free-radical–dependent toxicity in atherosclerosis (138) and other pathological conditions (139). $ONOO^-$ has the ability to nitrate tyrosine residues of proteins (140, 141). When using an antinitrotyrosine antibody to investigate the distribution of such modified residues in atherosclerotic lesions, Beckman et al. (140) found an intense immunopositive reaction, but the functional consequences of these modifications were unclear. Thus, it is possible that the MMP-2 activating effect observed by Trachtman et al. (136) was due to $ONOO^-$, whose reaction with pro-MMP-2 leads to production of active MMP-2 (83) rather than to a direct effect of •NO. Another recent report re-examined the issue of direct vs. indirect effects of •NO on MMP-2 activity (142) and also found that •NO by itself had no effect.

We investigated the possibility that $ONOO^-$ reacts with MMP zymogens to modulate their activity (83). Our results showed that $ONOO^-$ triggered proteolytic conversion of pro-MMP-2. Assays with radiolabeled collagen substrate confirmed that conversion is associated with the acquisition of enzymatic activity. Incubation with inactivated $ONOO^-$, containing its decomposition products NO_3^- and NO_2^-, had no effect on pro-MMP-2. This was, to our knowledge, the first demonstration of a protein being activated by $ONOO^-$. Using consecutive immunoblotting with antinitrotyrosine, followed by anti-MPP-2 antibodies, we found almost exclusive modification of proteins migrating at ~70 kD and concomitant loss of reactivity to anti-MMP-2 antibodies. This suggested that activation of pro-MMP-2 occurred as a result of direct interaction with $ONOO^-$ and protein modification. Although the exact residues have not yet been identified, the putative nitration of tyrosine residues present in the hinge region between the folded propeptide and the active part may assist in unfolding of the zymogen. We found that, like H_2O_2, $ONOO^-$ also had a biphasic effect: increasing its concentration led to inactivation of the MMP-2 zymogen (83).

An interesting twist of the ROS contribution to matrix degradation, which would potentiate the metalloproteinase-mediated tissue weakening even further, is the reported inactivation of TIMPs. Frears et al. (143) found a dose-dependent inactivation of TIMP-1 by $ONOO^-$, which reduced the inhibitory activity of TIMP-1 toward MMP-2. At very high concentrations (500 µM), but still within the range found in pathophysiological states (144), $ONOO^-$ produced fragmentation of TIMP-1 (143). Thus, the local concentration of ROS may specifically modulate the action of MMPs. We suggest that the intense nitrotyrosine immunostaining pattern described in atheroma (140) is partially due to nitration of MMPs and TIMPs. Importantly, interaction with $ONOO^-$, as well as the other ROS released around activated macrophages, provides a likely mechanism that unleashes the MMP activity previously detected in vulnerable areas of the atherosclerotic plaque (39, 42).

2. Plaque Rupture and Thrombosis—The MMP-Thrombin Plaque Destabilizing Loop

What happens after the plaque's structure is compromised? It is known that plaque disruption entails superimposed thrombosis (1–4). The content of the atheromatous lipid core of the plaque and the interstitial collagen-rich matrix enhance formation of thrombus (145, 146). Thrombotic complications associated with plaque rupture might be exacerbated by the increased availability of plasminogen activator inhibitor type-1 (PAI-1), the principal inhibitor of the fibrinolytic system. Lupu et al. (147) reported increased PAI-1 synthesis by SMC within the fibrous cap and macrophages located at the periphery of the necrotic core, with extracellular accumulation of PAI-1 in the atherosclerotic lesions. Availability of tissue factor (TF), produced especially by the resident macrophages (148), is also considered essential.

In places where the structurally compromised wall is covered by thrombus, MMPs released by vascular cells are likely to come in direct contact with thrombin. We investigated in vitro the possibility that thrombin might be a proteolytic activator of pro-MMP-2 (149), the most widely expressed vascular MMP. This gelatinase zymogen had been previously shown to be refractory to activation by the plasmin system (150) or by an array of studied proteases (16), which are effective activators of other pro-MMPs. As mentioned, MT1-MMP, a plasma membrane–associated protease, can produce a localized, pericellular activation of pro-MMP-2 (31). Using cultured human SMC, we found that activation of the MMP-2 zymogen by thrombin was cell independent (151), because it also occurred on addition of active thrombin directly to culture media after harvesting it from SMC. The thrombin cleavage sites in the pro-MMP-2 zymogen have not been determined. It is also not known whether proteolytic processing is mediated by thrombin or whether it involves only initiation by thrombin followed by autolysis. This action of thrombin is particularly interesting, because it seems to overcome the inhibition imposed by the TIMP-2 molecule found to be typically bound to SMC-derived pro-MMP-2 (149) and that reportedly blocks its proteolytic conversion (16, 106). A possible activation scenario may involve cleavage of TIMP-2 by thrombin, which would remove its inhibitory capacity and thus allow autoactivation of the TIMP-2-free proenzyme. The latter possibility is supported by our experimental observations, and it is consistent with the presence of potential thrombin cleavage sites in the TIMP-2 amino acid sequence. At present, the activating action of thrombin appears to be specific for pro-MMP-2, because it was previously reported that thrombin does not directly activate the other gelatinase zymogen, pro-MMP-9 (152, 153). We also were unable to activate in vitro the recombinant pro-MMP-3 using thrombin (149). It is important to note, however, that it has been reported that active MMP-2 can initiate activation of other MMPs [e.g., latent interstitial collagenase, or pro-MMP-1 (154), and pro-MMP-9 (155)], and it enhances generation of active MMP-3 (156). Thus, after its proteolytic activation, MMP-2 could potentially propagate an in vivo MMP enzymatic cascade initiated by thrombin.

An important corollary is that the thrombin-mediated extracellular activation of pro-MMP-2 would not be spatially restricted to the cell plasma membrane. Instead, active MMP-2 might then catalyze widespread activation of any zymogen constitutively stored in the extracellular space of the arterial wall (39). A recent report by Sawicki et al. (157) provides exciting insight into the flip side of the MMP-2-thrombin interaction. They reported a positive correlation between the release of pro-MMP-2 during platelet aggregation induced by thrombin or collagen and the process of platelet aggregation, as well as a positive correlation between inhibition of pro-MMP-2 release and decreased platelet aggregation. On the basis of these results the authors suggested that active MMP-2 mediates a new pathway for platelet aggregation. Thus, at sites of tissue injury, generation of thrombin may lead to release and activation of latent MMP-2, which in turn can induce more platelet aggregation and further generation of thrombin. If mutual activation resulting in cyclic production of active matrix-degrading enzymes, platelet aggregation, and thrombin generation suggested by in vitro experiments occurs in vivo, it may contribute to augment and sustain the instability of weak spots in atherosclerotic plaques (Figure 9) and might therefore play an important role in perpetuating plaque instability and, thus, the acute vascular syndromes.

New evidence suggests that MMPs and thrombin potentially regulate each other's action in other indirect ways. For example, degradation of fibrinogen by MMP-3 renders it thrombin-unclottable (158). Also, MMP-3 can degrade cross-linked fibrin, suggesting that MMPs may interfere with coagulation/fibrinolysis. Thus, although MMP and thrombin actions might be parallel, as in degradation of matrix (159), or opposed, as suggested by the latter study showing fibrinolytic actions of MMPs, they still promote plaque instability.

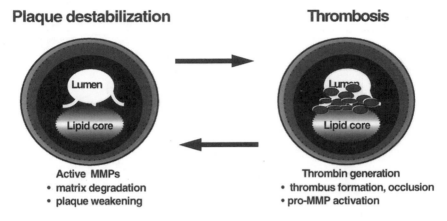

Plaque destabilization

Lumen

Lipid core

Thrombosis

Lumen

Lipid core

Active MMPs
* matrix degradation
* plaque weakening

Thrombin generation
* thrombus formation, occlusion
* pro-MMP activation

Figure 9 The MMP-thrombin positive feedback loop may contribute to, exacerbate, and sustain plaque instability. The matrix-degrading action of MMPs leads to tissue weakening and plaque destabilization triggering thrombosis. Recent evidence indicates that, besides causing the exposure of the thrombogenic content of the ruptured plaque, MMP activity directly contributes to platelet aggregation and thrombus formation. Thrombin activates conversion of MMP zymogens through cell-dependent and independent pathways, creating more plaque instability.

V. MACROPHAGES AND PLAQUE INSTABILITY

Although several aspects of macrophage involvement have been already discussed in the text, the potential role of resident macrophages in weakening plaque tissue certainly deserves a special note. Macrophage-rich infiltrates characterize sites of plaque disruption (160) and are associated with sites of thrombus formation in all ruptured plaques and in half of eroded plaques (7). The manifestly inflammatory nature of ruptured atherosclerotic plaques endorses the important role of macrophage-derived foam cells in plaque destabilization, as well as in thrombus formation, the disastrous combination that underlies most acute coronary syndromes (8). The procoagulant role of plaque macrophages is demonstrated by the capacity of stimulated macrophages to produce in vitro tissue factor (99, 161), essential for thrombus formation (162). Tissue factor production occurs in macrophages resident in atheroma (148) and is specifically associated with unstable coronary syndromes (163). The arsenal of activated macrophages is supplemented with cytokines, proteases, and ROS. Studies described previously have provided us with many pieces of information regarding the multiple involvement of resident macrophages in the process of matrix degradation by MMPs. These include (a) induction of MMP expression in other cells (by secretion of cyto-

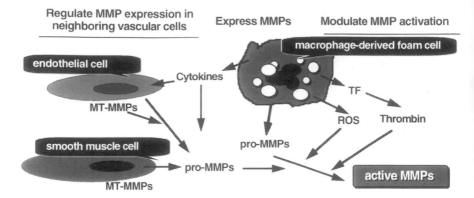

Figure 10 Macrophages regulate MMP-dependent matrix degradation at all levels. Cytokines, the active mediators secreted by macrophages, induce MMP genes in neighboring cells. Macrophages express their own MMPs. Macrophages also provide ways for conversion of MMP zymogens (pro-MMPs) into active enzymes. Activation of MMP zymogens by macrophages may occur directly, through interaction with macrophage-released reactive oxygen species (ROS), or indirectly, through stimulated expression of cellular MT-MMP by macrophage cytokines, or by macrophage tissue factor (TF)-mediated generation of thrombin.

kines), (b) production of their own MMPs, and (c) activation of MMP zymogens (by production of ROS). All these activities come together to support a major role for macrophages in weakening atherosclerotic tissue (Figure 10) and provide a likely explanation for their reported association with plaque instability.

VI. OTHER FORMS OF PLAQUE DESTABILIZATION AND MMPs

The two major presentations of compromised plaques are fissure/rupture of the fibrous cap and erosion of the superficial endothelial layer. In both of these the structural defect allows circulating blood from the lumen of the artery to come in contact with subendothelial components of the plaque. Extravasation of blood can also occur from within the plaque, leading to intraplaque hemorrhage. Intraplaque hemorrhage occurs through leakage of the vasa plaquorum, capillaries that develop within the intima of atherosclerotic vessels and supply the atheroma with blood. The extent of plaque neovascularization correlates with the extent of luminal stenosis and inflammation (164), indicating an essential role for neovascularization in plaque growth (4). Furthermore, neovascularization may be related to unstable syndromes, as suggested by a recent investigation by Tenaglia et al. (165), who showed that plaque neovascularization was correlated with unstable angina in a group of 28 patients.

The action of MMPs is known to be crucial for angiogenesis from recent genetic models of MMP deficiency (166) and many studies of cancer (167). A similar function is expected to be necessary for the process of neovascularization of atheroma. Supporting evidence comes from detection of MMP-1 in the capillary endothelial cells of vasa plaquorum (39). MMP-1 action may be essential for the sprouting of new vessels in the collagen-rich matrix of atheroma. However, sustained activity of this matrix-degrading enzyme might ultimately lead to leaky vessels, and, possibly, to hemorrhage in the plaque, as suggested by Nikkari et al. (53), who examined human carotid specimens. In their study, they found that, although undetectable in nonatherosclerotic carotid arteries, MMP-1 was strongly expressed by a subset of plaque macrophages located at the borders of the lipid core. Quantification of MMP-1 expression and extent of hemorrhage within plaques showed a strong correlation, supporting a role for this MMP in plaque destabilization through intraplaque hemorrhage.

The weakening action of MMPs has long been suspected in the pathogenesis of aneurysms, especially the aneurysmal dilatation of the abdominal aorta. The extensive destruction of the arterial wall tissue with infiltration of blood between the wall layers, which results in longitudinal dissection of the aorta, may be considered the ultimate destabilization of the atherosclerotic artery, and it is a cause of acute vascular syndromes and sudden death (168). Although in certain conditions such occurrence can be traced back to systemic defects in synthesis or assembly of matrix components, most commonly, aneurysms occur in advanced atherosclerotic disease. In such cases, extensive degradation of matrix components can be demonstrated, and it is associated with the presence of inflammatory cells. At variance with the importance traditionally attributed to the intimal layer in atherogenesis, most reports indicate that it is the adventitial layer that may play a particularly significant role in the pathogenesis of atherosclerotic aneurysms. Of note, an older theory of atherogenesis, which supports the notion that the seeds of atheroma must be sought in the adventitial layer, is gaining increasing support (169), and recent experimental evidence connects hypercholesterolemia, adventitial inflammation, atherosclerotic lesion development (170), and formation of aortic aneurysms (171). Tissue of aortic aneurysms (172, 173) and cerebral aneurysms (174) contains increased levels of MMPs, likely released by inflammatory infiltrates (47, 175). The type of MMPs expressed might be related to the severity of the aneurysmal dilatation, as suggested by McMillan et al. (176), who showed that MMP-9 may account for the AAA propensity to continue to expand. However, it is also possible that expression of MMP-9 depends on the phase at which the aneurysms are removed for study, as suggested by Schneiderman et al. (177), who showed MMP-9 level to be maximal in the acute phase. The study also showed colocalization with t-PA and u-PA, which suggests, again, cooperation of the fibrinolytic systems and MMP activity. Also supporting the role of MMPs in aneurysm formation, as well as the previously proposed mechanism of MMP zymogen activation by plasmin (178), Carmeliet et al. (179) showed that genetic deficiency of u-PA in mouse models protects against destruction of the medial layer and aneurysm formation.

VII. OTHER MECHANISMS THAT MAY LOWER THE STRENGTH OF ATHEROSCLEROTIC TISSUE

A. Other Proteases

The components of the ECM scaffold of late-stage atheroma may also be degraded by proteases other than MMPs. For example, thrombin digests proteoglycans (159), and the cathepsins (macrophage-derived cysteine proteases) have elastin and basement membrane–degrading activity (180, 181). Expression of cathepsins K and S was detected by immunocytochemistry in macrophages and intimal SMC in atheroma and was induced in vitro in SMC stimulated with IL-1β or interferon gamma (IFNγ) (182).

Different proteolytic pathways may intersect, and the various proteases can modulate each other's actions. For example, activation of MMP zymogens by proteases such as plasmin, thrombin, and mast cell proteases has been demonstrated, as discussed earlier. In turn, MMPs may also increase the enzymatic activity of other proteases. For example, the serine protease inhibitors (serpins), alpha$_1$-proteinase inhibitor, alpha$_1$-antitrypsin, and alpha$_1$-antichymotrypsin are among the nonmatrix substrates susceptible to the digestion of MMPs such as MMP-1 (183) and macrophage metalloelastase (40). Degradation of these inhibitors may lead to escalation of proteolytic activity at sites that contain active MMPs.

B. Decreased Production of Matrix

A decline in matrix-dependent tissue strength can occur not only through increased matrix degradation but also through decreased matrix synthesis. The main producers of ECM components in the intimal layer of arteries are the SMC. Matrix synthesis by SMC is finely tuned by the environment, being modulated by neighboring cells through soluble mediators, such as growth factors (184), cytokines (185), nitric oxide (186), and by the surrounding matrix itself (187). Factors such as the T cell–derived IFNγ, found in vitro to down-regulate SMC proliferation and synthesis of fibrillar collagen (185), the main provider of mechanical strength, are suspected to contribute to overall weakening of matrix in the plaques (80, 188). Naturally, the extreme situation of SMC loss, reported to occur frequently in human atheroma through apoptosis (189, 190), will result in decreased matrix synthesis and thus have an impact on the overall strength of matrix.

C. Cell Death

As mentioned earlier, loss of vascular cells, either by necrosis or apoptosis, decreases the tissue capacity to replenish the matrix of the atherosclerotic vessel wall. Furthermore, the death of cells in the plaque, especially of either SMC- or macrophage-derived foam cells, also contributes to plaque instability through the accrual of cellular remains that form the soft core characteristic of unstable plaques. Extensive apoptotic cell death is now a common finding in atherosclerotic lesions (189, 190). Although the mechanisms are still under investigation, cell apoptosis appears to be correlated with the inflammatory infiltrates (190), perhaps in relation to factors previously known to be associated with apoptosis: cytokines (191), Fas ligand (192), and increase in oxidative stress (193). Interestingly, it was reported that in human T cells, surface expression of Fas, which when released induces apoptosis in target cells, is regulated by Zn^{2+}-dependent metalloproteases (194). MMPs might also be related indirectly to apoptosis of vascular cells in the atherosclerotic plaque through degradation of the matrix necessary for survival of many cells (195), including the EC (196).

VIII. THERAPEUTIC INCREASE OF ATHEROSCLEROTIC PLAQUE STABILITY

The ultimate purpose of the effort to understand the cause of acute vascular syndromes is to intervene with new therapies to curb their dramatic consequences. Major advances have been made in the last few years, one of which is the identification of the fundamental importance of plaque stability. We are currently looking for culprits inside, rather than outside the atheroma. Several practical issues still impede our capacity to provide therapy. These include the continued inability to detect and monitor unstable plaques and the lack of adequate animal models for plaque destabilization. However, several promising therapeutic modalities have emerged. In some cases, we have identified new targets for ''not-so-new'' interventions. Nevertheless, the detailed comprehension of molecular targets is expected to help to better tune and direct our therapeutic efforts. Some of these efforts are expected to improve plaque stability.

A. Reduction of Oxidative Stress

Antioxidants have been reported to have beneficial cardiovascular effects in atherosclerosis and restenosis, both in patients (197) and in experimental models

(198–200), but the exact mechanism of action remains poorly understood. Treatment of animal models of atherosclerosis with probucol and vitamins E and C reduced lesions through a decrease in lipid and monocyte-macrophage content (201). In vivo use of agents targeting ROS (antioxidants and ROS scavengers) should oppose transcriptional and posttranslational events known to be mediated in vitro by ROS (e.g., intracellular activation of redox-sensitive genes and oxidative modification of lipoproteins, activation of latent MMPs, potential direct degradation of matrix components) (202). On the basis of our results showing the MMP-activating capacity of ROS, we tested the effect of N-acetyl-L-cysteine (NAC), an ROS scavenger, on the MMPs produced by macrophage-derived foam cells (104) induced in a hypercholesterolemic rabbit model (83). We found that treatment with 1 to 10 mmol/L NAC decreased not only the gelatinolytic activity released in vitro by foam cells but also the expression of the main macrophage MMP, MMP-9, in vitro and in situ, in the experimental atherosclerotic lesions. Although we did not perform experiments to test it, the exciting possibility exists now that such effect on MMPs may be used in advanced plaques to restrict the weakening of vascular matrix thought to be a major factor precipitating plaque destabilization. Complementary actions of antioxidants might also limit the extent of inflammation in general and its host of consequences. For instance, NAC inhibited the expression of the endothelial vascular adhesion molecule (VCAM)-1, the molecule recruiting the inflammatory cells into the vessel wall in vitro (203) and in vivo (204). The dietary supplementation with alpha-tocopherol in healthy human volunteers has been shown to reduce the production of soluble mediators of inflammation, ROS and cytokines, released by the monocytes isolated from their peripheral blood (205). In vitro, these monocytes were also found to be less prone to sticking to EC monolayers after activation, suggesting resistance to inflammatory stimuli. Such effects would reduce the infiltration of inflammatory cells, which no doubt occurs in the early stages of lesion development and possibly continues throughout the natural history of the lesion.

B.   Lipid Lowering

Lipid-lowering treatment has long been recognized in experimental models of atherosclerosis as an effective way to reduce the size of the lipid core and increase the percentage of connective tissue. Lipid regression studies done in primates (206) showed regression of atherosclerotic plaques, with enlargement of the artery lumen and improved endothelial function. More recently, using the hypercholesterolemic rabbit model, Aikawa et al. (207) showed that dietary reduction of lipid decreases MMP activity and increases the collagen content of rabbit atheroma. Furthermore, statins, developed as pharmacological agents for lipid-lowering therapy, provide another example of an intervention that unexpectedly turns out to directly modulate MMP expression. Fluvastatin has been shown in in vitro experiments to inhibit basal and phorbol ester-stimulated secretion of MMP-9 by human and mouse macrophages (208).

Thus, such therapies may work in vivo through a combination of pathways. The decrease in extracellular and intracellular lipid accumulation and oxidation decreases inflammation in atheroma, with subsequent reduction of monocyte recruitment and cellular activation and decreased production of mediators of inflammation: chemokines, ROS, and proteases. Another observed beneficial effect of lipid lowering and reduction of redox stress is improved endothelial function (209), which limits vasospasm, a possible trigger for plaque disruption. As the chemical and cellular composition of the plaque returns toward normal, the decreased lipid core and restored matrix improve the strength and stability of the atherosclerotic plaque.

ACKNOWLEDGMENTS

The author's research activities that generated results described in this manuscript have been supported through grants from the American Heart Association, the Whitaker Foundation, the National Institutes of Health, the Emory-Georgia Tech Biomedical Alliance, and the Emory University Research Committee. The author wishes to thank the many collaborators from the Emory University School of Medicine, Georgia Institute of Technology, and Brigham & Women's Hospital, with whom she had the good fortune to interact through the years, for their support and inspiration.

REFERENCES

1. Fuster V, Stein B, Ambrose JA, Badimon L, Badimon JJ, Chesebro JH. Atherosclerotic plaque rupture and thrombosis. Circulation 1990; 82(suppl II):II-47–II-59.
2. Falk E. Dynamics in thrombus formation. Ann NY Acad Sci 1992; 667:204–223.
3. Lendon CL, Born GV, Davies MJ, Richardson PD. Plaque fissure: the link between atherosclerosis and thrombosis. Nouv Rev Fr Hematol 1992; 34:27–29.
4. Constantinides P. Plaque hemorrhages, their genesis and their role in supra-plaque thrombosis and atherogenesis. In: Glagov S, Newman WPI, Schaffer SA, eds. Pathobiology of the Human Atherosclerotic Plaque. New York: Springer-Verlag, 1989:393–412.
5. Glagov S, Weisenberg E, Zarins CK, Stankunavicius R, Kolettis GJ. Compensatory enlargement of human atherosclerotic coronary arteries. N Engl J Med 1987; 316:1371–1375.

6. Clarkson TB, Prichard RW, Morgan TM, Petrick GS, Klein KP. Remodeling of coronary arteries in human and nonhuman primates [see comments]. JAMA 1994; 271:289–94.
7. Farb A, Burke AP, Tang AL, Liang TY, Mannan P, Smialek J, Virmani R. Coronary plaque erosion without rupture into a lipid core. A frequent cause of coronary thrombosis in sudden coronary death. Circulation 1996; 93:1354–1363.
8. Fuster V. Elucidation of the role of plaque instability and rupture in acute coronary events. Am J Cardiol 1995; 76:24C–33C.
9. Lendon CL, Davies MJ, Born GV, Richardson PD. Atherosclerotic plaque caps are locally weakened when macrophages density is increased. Atherosclerosis 1991; 87:87–90.
10. Davies MJ, Richardson PD, Woolf N, Katz DR, Mann J. Risk of thrombosis in human atherosclerotic plaques: role of extracellular lipid, macrophage, and smooth muscle cell content. Br Heart J 1993; 69:377–381.
11. Cheng GC, Loree HM, Kamm RD, Fishbein MC, Lee RT. Distribution of circumferential stress in ruptured and stable atherosclerotic lesions: a structural analysis with histopathologic correlation. Circulation 1993; 87:1179–1187.
12. Woessner JF Jr. Matrix metalloproteinases and their inhibitors in connective tissue remodeling. FASEB J 1991; 5:2145–2154.
13. Woessner JF Jr. The family of matrix metalloproteinases. Ann N Y Acad Sci 1994; 732:11–21.
14. Murphy G, Hembry RM, Hughes CE, Fosang AJ, Hardingham TE. Role and regulation of metalloproteinases in connective tissue turnover. Biochem Soc Trans 1990; 18:812–815.
15. Liotta LA, Steeg PS, Stetler-Stevenson WG. Cancer metastasis and angiogenesis: An imbalance of positive and negative regulation. Cell 1991; 64:327–336.
16. Stetler-Stevenson WG, Liotta LA, Kleiner DE. Extracellular matrix 6: Role of matrix metalloproteinases in tumor invasion and metastasis. FASEB J 1993; 7:1434–1441.
17. Nagase H. Activation mechanisms of matrix metalloproteinases. J Biol Chem 1997; 378:151–160.
18. Van Wart HE, Birkedal-Hansen H. The cysteine switch: a principle of regulation of metalloproteinase activity with potential applicability to the entire matrix metalloproteinase gene family. Proc Natl Acad Sci USA 1990; 87:5578–5582.
19. Gomez DE, Alonso DF, Yoshiji H, Thorgeirsson UP. Tissue inhibitors of metalloproteinases: structure, regulation and biological functions. Eur J Cell Biol 1997; 74:111–122.
20. Murphy G. Matrix metalloproteinases and their inhibitors. Acta Orthop Scand 1995; 266(Suppl):55–60.
21. Wilhelm SM, Eisen AZ, Teter M, Clark SD, Kronberger A, Goldberg G. Human fibroblast collagenase: glycosylation and tissue-specific levels of enzyme synthesis. Proc Natl Acad Sci USA 1986; 83:3756–3760.
22. Chin JR, Murphy G, Werb Z. Stromelysin, a connective tissue-degrading metalloendopeptidase secreted by stimulated rabbit synovial fibroblasts in parallel with collagenase. Biosynthesis, isolation, characterization, and substrates. J Biol Chem 1985; 260:12367–12376.

23. Murphy G, Cockett MI, Stephens P, Smith BJ, Docherty AJP. Stromelysin is an activator of procollagenase. Biochem J 1987; 248:265–268.

24. Ogata Y, Enghild JJ, Nagase H. Matrix metalloproteinase 3 (stromelysin) activates the precursor for the human matrix metalloproteinase 9. J Biol Chem 1992; 267: 3581–3584.

25. He C, Wilhelm SM, Pentland AP, Marmer BL, Grant GA, Eisen AZ, Goldberg GI. Tissue cooperation in a proteolytic cascade activating human interstitial collagenase. Proc Natl Acad Sci USA 1989; 86:2632–2636.

26. Aimes RT, Quigley JP. Matrix metalloproteinase-2 is an interstitial collagenase. Inhibitor-free enzyme catalyzes the cleavage of collagen fibrils and soluble native type I collagen generating the specific 3/4- and 1/4-length fragments. J Biol Chem 1995; 270:5872–5876.

27. Murphy G, Cockett MI, Ward RV, Docherty AJ. Matrix metalloproteinase degradation of elastin, type IV collagen and proteoglycan. A quantitative comparison of the activities of 95 kDa and 72 kDa gelatinases, stromelysins-1 and -2 and punctuated metalloproteinase (PUMP). Biochem J 1991; 277:277–279.

28. Senior RM, Griffin GL, Fliszar CJ, Shapiro SD, Goldberg GI, Welgus HG. Human 92- and 72-kilodalton type IV collagenases are elastases. J Biol Chem 1991; 266: 7870–7875.

29. Katsuda S, Okada Y, Okada Y, Imai K, Nakanishi I. Matrix metalloproteinase-9 (92-kd gelatinase/type IV collagenase equals gelatinase B) can degrade arterial elastin. Am J Pathol 1994; 145:1208–1218.

30. Turck J, Pollock AS, Lee LK, Marti HP, Lovett DH. Matrix metalloproteinase 2 (gelatinase A) regulates glomerular mesangial cell proliferation and differentiation. J Biol Chem 1996; 271:15074–15083.

31. Sato H, Takino T, Okada Y, Cao J, Shinagawa A, Yamamoto E, Seiki M. A matrix metalloproteinase expressed on the surface of invasive tumor cells. Nature 1994; 370:61–65.

32. Sato H, Okada Y, Seiki M. Membrane-type matrix metalloproteinases (MT-MMPs) in cell invasion. Thromb Haemost 1997; 78:497–500.

33. d'Ortho MP, Will H, Atkinson S, Butler G, Messent A, Gavrilovic J, Smith B, Timpl R, Zardi L, Murphy G. Membrane-type matrix metalloproteinases 1 and 2 exhibit broad-spectrum proteolytic capacities comparable to many matrix metalloproteinases. Eur J Biochem 1997; 250:751–757.

34. Gearing AJ, Beckett P, Christodoulou M, Churchill M, Clements J, Davidson AH, Drummond AH, Galloway WA, Gilbert R, Gordon JL, et al. Processing of tumor necrosis factor-alpha precursor by metalloproteinases. Nature 1994; 370:555–557.

35. Levi E, Fridman R, Miao HQ, Ma YS, Yayon A, Vlodavsky I. Matrix metalloproteinase 2 releases active soluble ectodomain of fibroblast growth factor receptor 1. Proc Natl Acad Sci USA 1996; 93:7069–7074.

36. Ugwu F, Van Hoef B, Bini A, Collen D, Lijnen HR. Proteolytic cleavage of urokinase-type plasminogen activator by stromelysin-1 (MMP-3). Biochemistry 1998; 37:7231–7236.

37. Lijnen HR, Ugwu F, Bini A, Collen D. Generation of an angiostatin-like fragment from plasminogen by stromelysin-1 (MMP-3). Biochemistry 1998; 37:4699–4702.

38. Henney AM, Wakeley PR, Davies MJ, Foster K, Hembry R, Murphy G, Humphries
     S. Localization of stromelysin gene expression in atherosclerotic plaques by in situ
     hybridization. Proc Natl Acad Sci USA 1991; 88:8154–8158.
39. Galis ZS, Sukhova GK, Lark MW, Libby P. Increased expression of matrix metallo-
     proteinases and matrix degrading activity in vulnerable regions of human athero-
     sclerotic plaques. J Clin Invest 1994; 94:2493–2503.
40. Gronski TJ Jr, Martin RL, Kobayashi DK, Walsh BC, Holman MC, Huber M, Van
     Wart HE, Shapiro SD. Hydrolysis of a broad spectrum of extracellular matrix pro-
     teins by human macrophage elastase. J Biol Chem 1997; 272:12189–12194.
41. Halpert I, Sires UI, Roby JD, Potter-Perigo S, Wight TN, Shapiro SD, Welgus HG,
     Wickline SA, Parks WC. Matrilysin is expressed by lipid-laden macrophages at
     sites of potential rupture in atherosclerotic lesions and localizes to areas of versican
     deposition, a proteoglycan substrate for the enzyme. Proc Natl Acad Sci USA 1996;
     93:9748–9753.
42. Galis Z, Sukhova G, Libby P. Microscopic localization of active proteases by in
     situ zymography: detection of matrix metalloproteinase activity in vascular tissue.
     FASEB J 1995; 9:974–980.
43. Shah PK, Falk E, Badimon JJ, Fernandez-Ortiz A, Mailhac A, Villareal-Levy G,
     Fallon JT, Regnstrom J, Fuster V. Human monocyte-derived macrophages induce
     collagen breakdown in fibrous caps of atherosclerotic plaques. Potential role of
     matrix-degrading metalloproteinases and implications for plaque rupture. Circula-
     tion 1995; 92:1565–1569.
44. Johnson JL, Jackson CL, Angelini GD, George SJ. Activation of matrix-degrading
     metalloproteinases by mast cell proteases in atherosclerotic plaques. Arterioscler
     Thromb Vasc Biol 1998; 18:1707–1715.
45. Li Z, Li L, Zielke HR, Cheng L, Xiao R, Crow MT, Stetler-Stevenson WG, Froeh-
     lich J, Lakatta EG. Increased expression of 72-kd type IV collagenase (MMP-2)
     in human aortic atherosclerotic lesions. Am J Pathol 1996; 148:121–128.
46. Brown DL, Hibbs MS, Kearney M, Loushin C, Isner JM. Identification of 92-kD
     gelatinase in human coronary atherosclerotic lesions. Association of active enzyme
     synthesis with unstable angina. Circulation 1995; 91:2125–2131.
47. Freestone T, Turner RJ, Coady A, Higman DJ, Greenhalgh RM, Powell JT. In-
     flammation and matrix metalloproteinases in the enlarging abdominal aortic aneu-
     rysm. Arterioscler Thromb Vasc Biol 1995; 15:1145–1151.
48. McMillan WD, Patterson BK, Keen RR, Shively VP, Cipollone M, Pearce WH.
     In situ localization and quantification of mRNA for 92-kD type IV collagenase and
     its inhibitor in aneurysmal, occlusive, and normal aorta. Arterioscler Thromb Vasc
     Biol 1995; 15:1139–1144.
49. Thompson RW, Holmes DR, Mertens RA, Liao S, Botney MD, Mecham RP, Wel-
     gus HG, Parks WC. Production and localization of 92-kilodalton gelatinase in ab-
     dominal aortic aneurysms. An elastolytic metalloproteinase expressed by aneu-
     rysm-infiltrating macrophages. J Clin Invest 1995; 96:318–326.
50. Nikkari ST, Hoyhtya M, Isola J, Nikkari T. Macrophages contain 92-kd gelatinase
     (MMP-9) at the site of degenerated internal elastic lamina in temporal arteritis. Am
     J Pathol 1996; 149:1427–1433.
51. Herron GS, Banda MJ, Clark EJ, Gavrilovic J, Werb Z. Secretion of metalloprotei-

nases by stimulated capillary endothelial cells. II. Expression of collagenase and stromelysin activities is regulated by endogenous inhibitors. J Biol Chem 1986; 261:2814–2818.

52. Hanemaaijer R, Koolwijk P, le Clercq L, de Vree WJ, van Hinsbergh VW. Regulation of matrix metalloproteinase expression in human vein and microvascular endothelial cells. Effects of tumour necrosis factor alpha, interleukin 1 and phorbol ester. Biochem J 1993; 296:803–809.

53. Nikkari ST, O'Brien KD, Ferguson M, Hatsukami T, Welgus HG, Alpers CE, Clowes AW. Interstitial collagenase (MMP-1) expression in human carotid atherosclerosis. Circulation 1995; 92:1393–1398.

54. Nikkari ST, Geary RL, Hatsukami T, Ferguson M, Forough R, Alpers CE, Clowes AW. Expression of collagen, interstitial collagenase, and tissue inhibitor of metalloproteinases-1 in restenosis after carotid endarterectomy. Am J Pathol 1996; 148: 777–783.

55. Lee RT, Schoen FJ, Loree HM, Lark MW, Libby P. Circumferential stress and matrix metalloproteinase 1 in human coronary atherosclerosis. Implications for plaque rupture. Arterioscler Thromb Vasc Biol 1996; 16:1070–1073.

56. Herron GS, Werb Z, Dwyer K, Banda MJ. Secretion of metalloproteinases by stimulated capillary endothelial cells. I. Production of procollagenase and prostromelysin exceeds expression of proteolytic activity. J Biol Chem 1986; 261:2810–2813.

57. Galis ZS, Muszynski M, Sukhova GK, Simon-Morrissey E, Unemori EN, Lark MW, Amento E, Libby P. Cytokine-stimulated human vascular smooth muscle cells synthesize a complement of enzymes required for extracellular matrix digestion. Circ Res 1994; 75:181–189.

58. Sasaguri Y, Kakita N, Murahashi N, Kato S, Hiraoka K, Morimatsu M, Yagi K. Effect of linoleic acid hydroperoxide on production of matrix metalloproteinases by human aortic endothelial and smooth muscle cells. Athcrosclcrosis 1993; 100: 189–196.

59. Pickering JG, Ford CM, Tang B, Chow LH. Coordinated effects of fibroblast growth factor-2 on expression of fibrillar collagens, matrix metalloproteinases, and tissue inhibitors of matrix metalloproteinases by human vascular smooth muscle cells. Evidence for repressed collagen production and activated degradative capacity. Arterioscler Thromb Vasc Biol 1997; 17:475–482.

60. Schonbeck U, Mach F, Sukhova GK, Murphy C, Bonnefoy JY, Fabunmi RP, Libby P. Regulation of matrix metalloproteinase expression in human vascular smooth muscle cells by T lymphocytes: a role for CD40 signaling in plaque rupture? Circ Res 1997; 81:448–454.

61. Duhamel-Clerin E, Orvain C, Lanza F, Cazenave JP, Klein-Soyer C. Thrombin receptor-mediated increase of two matrix metalloproteinases, MMP-1 and MMP-3 in human endothelial cells. Arterioscler Thromb Vasc Biol 1997; 17:1931–1938.

62. George SJ, Zaltsman AB, Newby AC. Surgical preparative injury and neointima formation increase MMP-9 expression and MMP-2 activation in human saphenous vein. Cardiovasc Res 1997; 33:447–459.

63. Partridge CA, Jeffrey JJ, Malik AB. A 96-kDa gelatinase induced by TNF-alpha contributes to increased microvascular endothelial permeability. Am J Physiol 1993; 265:L438–L447.

64. Amorino GP, Hoover RL. Interactions of monocytic cells with human endothelial cells stimulate monocytic metalloproteinase production. Am J Pathol 1998; 152: 199–207.

65. Rajavashisth TB, Galis ZS, Liao JK, Libby P. Cytokines increase the expression of membrane type-matrix metalloproteinase in cultured human vascular cells. Circulation 1995; 92:A0180.

66. Belkhiri A, Richards C, Whaley M, McQueen SA, Orr FW. Increased expression of activated matrix metalloproteinase-2 by human endothelial cells after sublethal H_2O_2 exposure. Lab Invest 1997; 77:533–539.

67. Haas TL, Davis SJ, Madri JA. Three-dimensional type I collagen lattices induce coordinate expression of matrix metalloproteinases MT1-MMP and MMP-2 in microvascular endothelial cells. J Biol Chem 1998; 273:3604–3610.

68. Apte SS, Olsen BR, Murphy G. The gene structure of tissue inhibitor of metalloproteinases (TIMP)-3 and its inhibitory activities define the distinct TIMP gene family. J Biol Chem 1995; 270:14313–14318.

69. Fabunmi RP, Sukhova GK, Sugiyama S, Libby P. Expression of tissue inhibitor of metalloproteinases-3 in human atheroma and regulation in lesion-associated cells: a potential protective mechanism in plaque stability. Circ Res 1998; 83:270–278.

70. Evans CH, Georgescu HI, Lin CW, Mendelow D, Steel DL, Webster MW. Inducible synthesis of collagenase and other neutral metalloproteinases by cells of aortic origin. J Surg Res 1991; 51:399–404.

71. Yanagi H, Sasaguri Y, Sugama K, Morimatsu M, Nagase H. Production of tissue collagenase (matrix metalloproteinase 1) by human aortic smooth muscle cells in response to platelet-derived growth factor. Atherosclerosis 1991; 91:207–216.

72. Southgate KM, Davies M, Booth RF, Newby AC. Involvement of extracellular-matrix-degrading metalloproteinases in rabbit aortic smooth-muscle cell proliferation. Biochem J 1992; 288:93–99.

73. Au YP, Montgomery KF, Clowes AW. Heparin inhibits collagenase gene expression mediated by phorbol ester-responsive element in primate arterial smooth muscle cells. Circ Res 1992; 70:1062–1069.

74. Pauly RR, Passaniti A, Bilato C, Monticone R, Cheng L, Papadopoulos N, Gluzband YA, Smith I., Weinstein C, Lakatta EG, Crow MT. Migration of cultured vascular smooth muscle cells through a basement membrane barrier requires type IV collagenase activity and is inhibited by cellular differentiation. Circ Res 1994; 75:41–54.

75. Newby AC, Southgate KM, Davies M. Extracellular matrix degrading metalloproteinases in the pathogenesis of arteriosclerosis. Basic Res Cardiol 1994; 89:59–70.

76. Zempo N, Kenagy RD, Au YPT, Bendeck M, Clowes MM, Reidy MA, Clowes AW. Matrix metalloproteinases of vascular wall cells are increased in balloon-injured rat carotid artery. J Vasc Surg 1994; 20:209–217.

77. Bendeck MP, Zempo N, Clowes AW, Galardy RE, Reidy MA. Smooth muscle cell migration and matrix metalloproteinase expression after arterial injury in the rat. Circ Res 1994; 75:539–545.

78. Fridman R, Bird RE, Hoyhtya M, Oelkuct M, Komarek D, Liang CM, Berman ML, Liotta LA, Stetler-Stevenson WG, Fuerst TR. Expression of human recombinant 72

kDa gelatinase and tissue inhibitor of metalloproteinase-2 (TIMP-2): characterization of complex and free enzyme. Biochem J 1993; 289:411–416.

79. Libby P, Hansson GK. Involvement of the immune system in human atherogenesis: Current knowledge and unanswered questions. Lab Invest 1991; 64:5–15.

80. Libby P, Galis ZS. Cytokines regulate genes involved in atherosclerosis. In: Numano F, Wissler RW, eds. Atherosclerosis III: Recent Advances in Atherosclerosis Research. New York: The New York Academy of Sciences, 1995:158–170.

81. Yang JH, Briggs WH, Libby P, Lee RT. Small mechanical strains selectively suppress matrix metalloproteinase-1 expression by human vascular smooth muscle cells. J Biol Chem 1998; 273:6550–6555.

82. Asanuma K, Meng X, Nerem RM, Galis ZS. Stationary stretch increases expression and activity of matrix metalloproteinases (MMPs) produced by human vascular SMC in vitro. Circulation 1998; 98:2420.

83. Rajagopalan S, Meng XP, Ramasamy S, Harrison DG, Galis ZS. Reactive oxygen species produced by macrophage-derived foam cells regulate the activity of vascular matrix metalloproteinases in vitro. Implications for atherosclerotic plaque stability. J Clin Invest 1996; 98:2572–2579.

84. Griendling KK, Minieri CA, Ollerenshaw JD, Alexander RW. Angiotensin II stimulates NADH and NADPH oxidase activity in cultured vascular smooth muscle cells. Circ Res 1994; 74:1141–1148.

85. Howard AB, Alexander RW, Nerem RM, Griendling KK, Taylor WR. Cyclic strain induces an oxidative stress in endothelial cells. Am J Physiol 1997; 272:C421–C427.

86. Richardson PD, Davies MJ, Born GV. Influence of plaque configuration and stress distribution on fissuring of coronary atherosclerotic plaques. Lancet 1989; 2:941–944.

87. Hickler RB. Aortic and large artery stiffness: current methodology and clinical correlations. Clin Cardiol 1990; 13:317–322.

88. Harrison DG, Ohara Y. Physiologic consequences of increased vascular oxidant stresses in hypercholesterolemia and atherosclerosis: implications for impaired vasomotion [see comments]. Am J Cardiol 1995; 75:75B–81B.

89. Ross R. Rous-Whipple Award Lecture. Atherosclerosis: a defense mechanism gone awry. Am J Pathol 1993; 143:987–1002.

90. Stary HC, Chandler AB, Glagov S, Guyton JR, Insull WJ, Rosenfeld ME, Schaffer SA, Schwartz CJ, Wagner WD, Wissler RW. A definition of initial, fatty streak, and intermediate lesions of atherosclerosis. A report from the Committee on Vascular Lesions of the Council on Atherosclerosis, American Heart Association. Circulation 1994; 89:2462–2478.

91. Goetzl EJ, Banda MJ, Leppert D. Matrix metalloproteinases in immunity. J Immunol 1996; 156:1–4.

92. Gimbrone MAJ, Bevilacqua MP, Cybulsky MI. Endothelial-dependent mechanisms of leukocyte adhesion in inflammation and atherosclerosis. Ann N Y Acad Sci 1990; 598:77–85.

93. Romanic AM, Madri JA. The induction of 72-kD gelatinase in T-cells upon adhesion to endothelial cells is VCAM-1 dependent. J Cell Biol 1994; 125:1165–1178.

94. Campbell EJ, Cury JD, Shapiro SD, Goldberg GI, Welgus HG. Neutral proteinases

of human mononuclear phagocytes. Cellular differentiation markedly alters cell phenotype for serine proteinases, metalloproteinases, and tissue inhibitor of metalloproteinases. J Immunol 1991; 146:1286–1293.

95. Pierce RA, Sandefur S, Doyle GA, Welgus HG. Monocytic cell type-specific transcriptional induction of collagenase. J Clin Invest 1996; 97:1890–1899.

96. Libby P, Egan D, Skarlatos S. Roles of infectious agents in atherosclerosis and restenosis: an assessment of the evidence and need for future research. Circulation 1997; 96:4095–4103.

97. Lacraz S, IsIer P, Vey E, Welgus HG, Dayer JM. Direct contact between T lymphocytes and monocytes is a major pathway for induction of metalloproteinase expression. J Biol Chem 1994; 269:22027–22033.

98. Malik N, Greenfield BW, Wahl AF, Kiener PA. Activation of human monocytes through CD40 induces matrix metalloproteinases. J Immunol 1996; 156:3952–3960.

99. Mach F, Schonbeck U, Bonnefoy JY, Pober JS, Libby P. Activation of monocyte/macrophage functions related to acute atheroma complication by ligation of CD40: induction of collagenase, stromelysin, and tissue factor. Circulation 1997; 96:396–399.

100. Shapiro SD, Kobayashi DK, Pentland AP, Welgus HG. Induction of macrophage metalloproteinases by extracellular matrix. Evidence for enzyme- and substrate-specific responses involving prostaglandin-dependent mechanisms. J Biol Chem 1993; 268:8170–8175.

101. Wesley RI, Meng X, Godin D, Galis Z. Extracellular matrix modulates macrophage functions characteristic to atheroma: collagen I enhances acquisition of resident macrophage traits by human peripheral blood monocytes in vitro. Arterioscl Thromb Vasc Biol 1998; 18:432–440.

102. Rosenfeld ME, Khoo JC, Miller E, Parthasarathy S, Palinski W, Witztum JL. Macrophage-derived foam cells freshly isolated from rabbit atherosclerotic lesions degrade modified lipoproteins, promote oxidation of low-density lipoproteins, and contain oxidation-specific lipid-protein adducts. J Clin Invest 1991; 87:90–99.

103. Galis ZS, Sukhova GK, Kranzhöfer R, Clark S, Libby P. Macrophage foam cells from experimental atheroma constitutively produce matrix-degrading proteinases. Proc Natl Acad Sci USA 1995; 92:402–406.

104. Galis Z, Asanuma K, Godin D, Meng X. N-acetyl-cysteine decreases the matrix-degrading capacity of macrophage-derived foam cells: new target for antioxidant therapy? Circulation 1998; 97:2445–2454.

105. Ueda Y, Imai K, Tsuchiya H, Fujimoto N, Nakanishi I, Katsuda S, Seiki M, Okada Y. Matrix metalloproteinase 9 (gelatinase B) is expressed in multinucleated giant cells of human giant cell tumor of bone and is associated with vascular invasion. Am J Pathol 1996; 148:611–622.

106. Ward RV, Atkinson SJ, Slocombe PM, Docherty AJ, Reynolds JJ, Murphy G. Tissue inhibitor of metalloproteinases-2 inhibits the activation of 72 kDa progelatinase by fibroblast membranes. Biochim Biophys Acta 1991; 1079:242–246.

107. Clark IM, Rowan AD, Edwards DR, Bech-Hansen T, Mann DA, Bahr MJ, Cawston TE. Transcriptional activity of the human tissue inhibitor of metalloproteinases 1

(TIMP-1) gene in fibroblasts involves elements in the promoter, exon 1 and intron 1. Biochem J 1997; 324:611–617.

108.   Karin M, Liu Z, Zandi E. AP-1 function and regulation. Curr Opin Cell Biol 1997; 9:240–246.

109.   Hammani K, Blakis A, Morsette D, Bowcock AM, Schmutte C, Henriet P, De-Clerck YA. Structure and characterization of the human tissue inhibitor of metallo-proteinases-2 gene. J Biol Chem 1996; 271:25498–25505.

110.   Bian J, Jacobs C, Wang Y, Sun Y. Characterization of a putative p53 binding site in the promoter of the mouse tissue inhibitor of metalloproteinases-3 (TIMP-3) gene: TIMP-3 is not a p53 target gene. Carcinogenesis 1996; 17:2559–2562.

111.   Baker AH, Zaltsman AB, George SJ, Newby AC. Divergent effects of tissue inhibitor of metalloproteinase-1, -2, or -3 overexpression on rat vascular smooth muscle cell invasion, proliferation, and death in vitro. TIMP-3 promotes apoptosis. J Clin Invest 1998; 101:1478–1487.

112.   Vassalli J-D, Sappino A-P, Belin D. The plasminogen activator/plasmin system. J Clin Invest 1991; 88:1067–1072.

113.   Murphy G, Atkinson S, Ward R, Gavrilovic J, Reynolds JJ. The role of plasminogen activators in the regulation of connective tissue metalloproteinase. Ann NY Acad Sci 1992; 667:1–12.

114.   Kleiner DE Jr, Stetler-Stevenson WG. Structural biochemistry and activation of matrix metalloproteases. Curr Opin Cell Biol 1993; 5:891–897.

115.   Weiss SJ, Peppin G, Ortiz X, Ragsdale C, Test ST. Oxidative autoactivation of latent collagenase by human neutrophils. Science 1985; 227:747–749.

116.   Daugherty A, Dunn JL, Rateri DL, Heinecke JW. Myeloperoxidase, a catalyst for lipoprotein oxidation, is expressed in human atherosclerotic lesions. J Clin Invest 1994; 94:437–444.

117.   Ohara Y, Peterson TE, Harrison DG. Hypercholesterolemia increases endothelial superoxide anion production. J Clin Invest 1993; 91:2546–2551.

118.   Rajagopalan S, Kurz S, Münzel T, Tarpey M, Freeman B, Griendling K, Harrison D. Angiotensin II-mediated hypertension in the rat increases vascular superoxide production via membrane NADH/NADPH oxidase activation: Contribution to alterations of vasomotor tone. J Clin Invest 1996; 97:1916–1923.

119.   Giugliano D, Ceriello A, Paolisso G. Diabetes mellitus, hypertension, and cardiovascular disease: which role for oxidative stress? Metabolism 1995; 44:363–368.

120.   Segal AW, Abo A. The biochemical basis of the NADPH oxidase of phagocytes. Trends Biochem Sci 1993; 18:43–47.

121.   Nohl H. Generation of superoxide radicals as byproduct of cellular respiration. Ann Biol Clin (Paris) 1994; 52:199–204.

122.   Matsubara T, Ziff M. Increased superoxide anion release from human endothelial cells in response to cytokines. J Immunol 1986; 137:3295–3302.

123.   Mohazzab KM, Kaminski PM, Wolin MS. NADH oxidoreductase is a major source of superoxide anion in bovine coronary artery endothelium. Am J Physiol 1994; 266:H2568–H2572.

124.   Fukai T, Galis ZS, Meng XP, Parthasarathy S, Harrison DG. Vascular expression of extracellular superoxide dismutase in atherosclerosis. J Clin Invest 1998; 101: 2101–2111.

125. McCord JM. Human disease, free radicals, and the oxidant/antioxidant balance. Clin Biochem 1993; 26:351–357.

126. Pryor WA, Squadrito GL. The chemistry of peroxynitrite: a product from the reaction of nitric oxide with superoxide [see comments]. Am J Physiol 1995; 268: L699–722.

127. Crow JP, Beckman JS, McCord JM. Sensitivity of the essential zinc-thiolate moiety of yeast alcohol dehydrogenase to hypochlorite and peroxynitrite. Biochemistry 1995; 34:3544–3552.

128. Radi R, Beckman JS, Bush KM, Freeman BA. Peroxynitrite-induced membrane lipid peroxidation: the cytotoxic potential of superoxide and nitric oxide. Arch Biochem Biophys 1991; 288:481–487.

129. Darley-Usmar V, Wiseman H, Halliwell B. Nitric oxide and oxygen radicals: a question of balance. FEBS Lett 1995; 369:131–135.

130. Gutteridge JM. Lipid peroxidation and antioxidants as biomarkers of tissue damage. Clin Chem 1995; 41:1819–1828.

131. Wang X, Martindale JL, Liu Y, Holbrook NJ. The cellular response to oxidative stress: influences of mitogen-activated protein kinase signalling pathways on cell survival. Biochem J 1998; 333:291–300.

132. Berliner JA, Heinecke JW. The role of oxidized lipoproteins in atherogenesis. Free Radic Biol Med 1996; 20:707–727.

133. Steinberg D. Oxidative modification of LDL and atherogenesis. Circulation 1997; 95:1062–1071.

134. Fliss H, Menard M. Oxidant-induced mobilization of zinc from metallothionein. Arch Biochem Biophys 1992; 293:195–199.

135. Freeman BA, White CR, Gutierrez H, Paler-Martinez A, Tarpey MM, Rubbo H. Oxygen radical-nitric oxide reactions in vascular diseases. Adv Pharmacol 1995; 34:45–69.

136. Trachtman H, Futterweit S, Garg P, Reddy K, Singhal PC. Nitric oxide stimulates the activity of a 72-kDa neutral matrix metalloproteinase in cultured rat mesangial cells. Biochem Biophys Res Commun 1996; 218:704–708.

137. Huie RE, Padmaja S. The reaction of NO with superoxide. Free Radic Res Commun 1993; 18:195–199.

138. Beckman JS, Beckman W, Chen J, Marshall PA, Freeman BA. Apparent hydroxyl radical production by peroxynitrite: implications for endothelial injury from nitric oxide and superoxide. Proc Natl Acad Sci USA 1990; 87:1620–1624.

139. Radi R, Beckman JS, Bush KM, Freeman BA. Peroxynitrite oxidation of sulfhydryls. The cytotoxic potential of superoxide and nitric oxide. J Biol Chem 1991; 266:4244–4250.

140. Beckmann JS, Ye YZ, Anderson PG, Chen J, Accavitti MA, Tarpey MM, White CR. Extensive nitration of protein tyrosines in human atherosclerosis detected by immunohistochemistry. Biol Chem Hoppe Seyler 1994; 375:81–88.

141. Ischiropoulos H, al-Mehdi AB. Peroxynitrite-mediated oxidative protein modifications. FEBS Lett 1995; 364:279–282.

142. Owens MW, Milligan SA, Jourd'heuil D, Grisham MB. Effects of reactive metabolites of oxygen and nitrogen on gelatinase A activity. Am J Physiol 1997; 273: L445–450.

143. Frears ER, Zhang Z, Blake DR, O'Connell JP, Winyard PG. Inactivation of tissue inhibitor of metalloproteinase-1 by peroxynitrite. FEBS Lett 1996; 381:21–24.
144. Ischiropoulos H, Zhu L, Beckman JS. Peroxynitrite formation from macrophage-derived nitric oxide. Arch Biochem Biophys 1992; 298:446–451.
145. Fernandez-Ortiz A, Badimon JJ, Falk E, Fuster V, Meyer B, Mailhac A, Weng D, Shah PK, Badimon L. Characterization of the relative thrombogenicity of atherosclerotic plaque components: implications for consequences of plaque rupture. J Am Coll Cardiol 1994; 23:1562–1569.
146. Holvoet P, Collen D. Thrombosis and atherosclerosis. Curr Opin Lipidol 1997; 8: 320–328.
147. Lupu F, Bergonzelli GE, Heim DA, Cousin E, Genton CY, Bachmann F, Kruithof EK. Localization and production of plasminogen activator inhibitor-1 in human healthy and atherosclerotic arteries. Arterioscler Thromb 1993; 13:1090–1100.
148. Wilcox JN, Smith KM, Schwartz SM, Gordon D. Localization of tissue factor in the normal vessel wall and in the atherosclerotic plaque. Proc Natl Acad Sci USA 1989; 86:2839–2843.
149. Galis ZS, Kranzhöfer R, Fenton II J, Libby P. Thrombin promotes activation of matrix metalloproteinase-2 (MMP-2) produced by cultured smooth muscle cells. Arterioscl Thromb Vasc Biol 1997; 17:483–489.
150. Tryggvason K, Huhtala P, Hoyhtya M, Hujanen E, Hurskainen T. 70 KD type IV collagenase (gelatinase). Matrix Suppl 1992; 1:45–50.
151. Galis ZS, Kranzhöfer R, Libby P. Thrombin promotes activation of matrix metalloproteinase-2 (MMP-2) produced by cultured smooth muscle cells. FASEB J 1995; 9:A413.
152. Okada Y, Gonoji Y, Naka K, Tomita K, Nakanishi I, Iwata K, Yamashita K, Hayakawa T. Matrix metalloproteinase 9 (92-kDa gelatinase/type IV collagenase) from HT 1080 human fibrosarcoma cells. Purification and activation of the precursor and enzymic properties. J Biol Chem 1992; 267:21712–21719.
153. Morodomi T, Ogata Y, Sasaguri Y, Morimatsu M, Nagase H. Purification and characterization of matrix metalloproteinase 9 from U937 monocytic leukaemia and HT1080 fibrosarcoma cells. Biochem J 1992; 285:603–611.
154. Crabbe T, O'Connell JP, Smith BJ, Docherty AJ. Reciprocated matrix metalloproteinase activation: a process performed by interstitial collagenase and progelatinase A. Biochemistry 1994; 33:14419–14425.
155. Fridman R, Toth M, Pena D, Mobashery S. Activation of progelatinase B (MMP-9) by gelatinase A (MMP-2). Cancer Res 1995; 55:2548–2555.
156. Knauper V, Will H, Lopez-Otin C, Smith B, Atkinson SJ, Stanton H, Hembry RM, Murphy G. Cellular mechanisms for human procollagenase-3 (MMP-13) activation. Evidence that MT1-MMP (MMP-14) and gelatinase a (MMP-2) are able to generate active enzyme. J Biol Chem 1996; 271:17124–17131.
157. Sawicki G, Salas E, Murat J, Miszta-Lane H, Radomski MW. Release of gelatinase A during platelet activation mediates aggregation. Nature 1997; 386:616–619.
158. Bini A, Itoh Y, Kudryk BJ, Nagase H. Degradation of cross-linked fibrin by matrix metalloproteinase 3 (stromelysin 1): hydrolysis of the gamma Gly 404-Ala 405 peptide bond. Biochemistry 1996; 35:13056–13063.
159. Benezra M, Vlodavsky I, Bar-Shavit R. Thrombin enhances degradation of heparan

sulfate in the extracellular matrix by tumor cell heparanase. Exp Cell Res 1992; 201:208–215.

160. van der Wal AC, Becker AE, van der Loos CM, Das PK. Site of intimal rupture or erosion of thrombosed coronary atherosclerotic plaques is characterized by an inflammatory process irrespective of the dominant plaque morphology. Circulation 1994; 89:36–44.

161. Edgington TS, Mackman N, Fan ST, Ruf W. Cellular immune and cytokine pathways resulting in tissue factor expression and relevance to septic shock. Nouv Rev Fr Hematol 1992; 34:S15–27.

162. Barstad RM, Hamers MJ, Kierulf P, Westvik AB, Sakariassen KS. Procoagulant human monocytes mediate tissue factor/factor VIIa-dependent platelet-thrombus formation when exposed to flowing nonanticoagulated human blood. Arterioscler Thromb 1995; 15:11–16.

163. Annex BH, Denning SM, Channon KM, Sketch MH Jr, Stack RS, Morrissey JH, Peters KG. Differential expression of tissue factor protein in directional atherectomy specimens from patients with stable and unstable coronary syndromes. Circulation 1995; 91:619–622.

164. Kumamoto M, Nakashima Y, Sueishi K. Intimal neovascularization in human coronary atherosclerosis: its origin and pathophysiological significance. Hum Pathol 1995; 26:450–456.

165. Tenaglia AN, Peters KG, Sketch MH Jr, Annex BH. Neovascularization in atherectomy specimens from patients with unstable angina: implications for pathogenesis of unstable angina. Am Heart J 1998; 135:10–14.

166. Vu TH, Shipley JM, Bergers G, Berger JE, Helms JA, Hanahan D, Shapiro SD, Senior RM, Werb Z. MMP-9/gelatinase B is a key regulator of growth plate angiogenesis and apoptosis of hypertrophic chondrocytes. Cell 1998; 93:411–422.

167. Moses MA. The regulation of neovascularization of matrix metalloproteinases and their inhibitors. Stem Cells 1997; 15:180–189.

168. Basso C, Morgagni GL, Thiene G. Spontaneous coronary artery dissection: a neglected cause of acute myocardial ischaemia and sudden death. Heart 1996; 75: 451–454.

169. Wilcox JN, Scott NA. Potential role of the adventitia in arteritis and atherosclerosis. Int J Cardiol 1996; 54:S21–35.

170. Seo HS, Lombardi DM, Polinsky P, Powell-Braxton L, Bunting S, Schwartz SM, Rosenfeld ME. Peripheral vascular stenosis in apolipoprotein E-deficient mice. Potential roles of lipid deposition, medial atrophy, and adventitial inflammation. Arterioscler Thromb Vasc Biol 1997; 17:3593–3601.

171. Freestone T, Turner RJ, Higman DJ, Lever MJ, Powell JT. Influence of hypercholesterolemia and adventitial inflammation on the development of aortic aneurysm in rabbits. Arterioscler Thromb Vasc Biol 1997; 17:10–17.

172. Herron GS, Unemori E, Wong M, Rapp JH, Hibbs MH, Stoney RJ. Connective tissue proteinases and inhibitors in abdominal aortic aneurysms. Involvement of the vasa vasorum in the pathogenesis of aortic aneurysms. Arterioscler Thromb 1991; 11:1667–1677.

173. Vine N, Powell JT. Metalloproteinases in degenerative aortic disease. Clin Sci (Colch) 1991; 81:233–239.

174. Kim SC, Singh M, Huang J, Prestigiacomo CJ, Winfree CJ, Solomon RA, Connolly ES Jr. Matrix metalloproteinase-9 in cerebral aneurysms. Neurosurgery 1997; 41: 642–666; discussion 646–647.

175. Newman KM, Jean-Claude J, Li H, Scholes JV, Ogata Y, Nagase H, Tilson MD. Cellular localization of matrix metalloproteinases in the abdominal aortic aneurysm wall. J Vasc Surg 1994; 20:814–820.

176. McMillan WD, Tamarina NA, Cipollone M, Johnson DA, Parker MA, Pearce WH. Size matters: the relationship between MMP-9 expression and aortic diameter [see comments]. Circulation 1997; 96:2228–2232.

177. Schneiderman J, Bordin GM, Adar R, Smolinsky A, Seiffert D, Engelberg I, Dilley RB, Thinnes T, Loskutoff DJ. Patterns of expression of fibrinolytic genes and matrix metalloproteinase-9 in dissecting aortic aneurysms. Am J Pathol 1998; 152: 703–710.

178. Jean-Claude J, Newman KM, Li H, Gregory AK, Tilson MD. Possible key role for plasmin in the pathogenesis of abdominal aortic aneurysms. Surgery 1994; 116: 472–478.

179. Carmeliet P, Moons L, Lijnen R, Baes M, Lemaitre V, Tipping P, Drew A, Eeckhout Y, Shapiro S, Lupu F, Collen D. Urokinase-generated plasmin activates matrix metalloproteinases during aneurysm formation. Nat Genet 1997; 17:439–444.

180. Werb Z, Banda MJ, Jones PA. Degradation of connective tissue matrices by macrophages. I. Proteolysis of elastin, glycoproteins, and collagen by proteinases isolated from macrophages. J Exp Med 1980; 152:1340–1357.

181. Reddy VY, Zhang QY, Weiss SJ. Pericellular mobilization of the tissue-destructive cysteine proteinases, cathepsins B, L, and S, by human monocyte-derived macrophages. Proc Natl Acad Sci USA 1995; 92:3849–3853.

182. Sukhova GK, Shi GP, Simon DI, Chapman HA, Libby P. Expression of the elastolytic cathepsins S and K in human atheroma and regulation of their production in smooth muscle cells. J Clin Invest 1998; 102:576–583.

183. Desrochers PE, Jeffrey JJ, Weiss SJ. Interstitial collagenase (matrix metalloproteinase-1) expresses serpinase activity. J Clin Invest 1991; 87:2258–2265.

184. Liau G, Chan LM. Regulation of extracellular matrix RNA levels in cultured smooth muscle cells. Relationship to cellular quiescence. J Biol Chem 1989; 264: 10315–10320.

185. Amento EP, Ehsani N, Palmer H, Libby P. Cytokines positively and negatively regulate interstitial collagen gene expression in human vascular smooth muscle cells. Arterioscler Thromb 1991; 11:1223–1230.

186. Myers PR, Tanner MA. Vascular endothelial cell regulation of extracellular matrix collagen: role of nitric oxide. Arterioscler Thromb Vasc Biol 1998; 18:717–722.

187. Thie M, Harrach B, Schonherr E, Kresse H, Robenek H, Rauterberg J. Responsiveness of aortic smooth muscle cells to soluble growth mediators is influenced by cell-matrix contact. Arterioscler Thromb 1993; 13:994–1004.

188. Libby P. Molecular bases of the acute coronary syndromes. Circulation 1995; 91: 2844–2850.

189. Geng YJ, Libby P. Evidence for apoptosis in advanced human atheroma. Colocalization with interleukin-1 beta-converting enzyme [see comments]. Am J Pathol 1995; 147:251–266.

190. Bjorkerud S, Bjorkerud B. Apoptosis is abundant in human atherosclerotic lesions, especially in inflammatory cells (macrophages and T cells), and may contribute to the accumulation of gruel and plaque instability. Am J Pathol 1996; 149:367–380.

191. Hansson GK. Cell-mediated immunity in atherosclerosis. Curr Opin Lipidol 1997; 8:301–311.

192. Liles WC, Kiener PA, Ledbetter JA, Aruffo A, Klebanoff SJ. Differential expression of Fas (CD95) and Fas ligand on normal human phagocytes: implications for the regulation of apoptosis in neutrophils. J Exp Med 1996; 184:429–440.

193. Buttke TM, Sandstrom PA. Redox regulation of programmed cell death in lymphocytes. Free Radic Res 1995; 22:389–397.

194. Mariani SM, Matiba B, Baumler C, Krammer PH. Regulation of cell surface APO-1/Fas (CD95) ligand expression by metalloproteases. Eur J Immunol 1995; 25: 2303–2307.

195. Frish SM, Francis H. Disruption of epithelial cell-matrix interactions induces apoptosis. J Cell Biol 1994; 124:619–626.

196. Meredith JE Jr, Fazeli B, Schwartz MA. The extracellular matrix as a cell survival factor. Mol Biol Cell 1993; 4:953–961.

197. Gaziano JM. Antioxidant vitamins and coronary artery disease risk. Am J Med 1994; 97:18S–21S; discussion 22S–28S.

198. Ferns GA, Forster L, Stewart-Lee A, Konneh M, Nourooz-Zadeh J, Anggard EE. Probucol inhibits neointimal thickening and macrophage accumulation after balloon injury in the cholesterolfed rabbit. Proc Natl Acad Sci USA 1992; 89:11312–11316.

199. Lafont AM, Chai YC, Cornhill JF, Whitlow PL, Howe PH, Chisolm GM. Effect of alpha-tocopherol on restenosis after angioplasty in a model of experimental atherosclerosis. J Clin Invest 1995; 95:1018–1025.

200. Nunes GL, Sgoutas DS, Redden RA, Sigman SR, Gravanis MB, King SBr, Berk BC. Combination of vitamins C and E alters the response to coronary balloon injury in the pig. Arterioscler Thromb Vasc Biol 1995; 15:156–165.

201. Baumann DS, Doblas M, Schonfeld G, Sicard GA, Daugherty A. Probucol reduces the cellularity of aortic intimal thickening at anastomotic regions adjacent to prosthetic grafts in cholesterol-fed rabbits. Arterioscler Thromb 1994; 14:162–167.

202. Hawkins CL, Davies MJ. Oxidative damage to collagen and related substrates by metal ion/hydrogen peroxide systems: random attack or site-specific damage? Biochim Biophys Acta 1997; 1360:84–96.

203. Marui N, Offermann MK, Swerlick R, Kunsch C, Rosen CA, Ahmad M, Alexander RW, Medford RM. Vascular cell adhesion molecule-1 (VCAM-1) gene transcription and expression are regulated through an antioxidant-sensitive mechanism in human vascular endothelial cells. J Clin Invest 1993; 92:1866–1874.

204. Fruebis J, Gonzalez V, Silvestre M, Palinski W. Effect of probucol treatment on gene expression of VCAM-1, MCP-1, and M-CSF in the aortic wall of LDL receptor-deficient rabbits during early atherogenesis. Arterioscler Thromb Vasc Biol 1997; 17:1289–1302.

205. Devaraj S, Li D, Jialal I. The effects of alpha tocopherol supplementation on monocyte function. Decreased lipid oxidation, interleukin 1 beta secretion, and monocyte adhesion to endothelium. J Clin Invest 1996; 98:756–763.

206. Williams JK, Anthony MS, Honore EK, Herrington DM, Morgan TM, Register TC, Clarkson TB. Regression of atherosclerosis in female monkeys. Arterioscler Thromb Vasc Biol 1995; 15:827–836.
207. Aikawa M, Rabkin E, Okada Y, Voglic SJ, Clinton SK, Brinckerhoff CE, Sukhova GK, Libby P. Lipid lowering by diet reduces matrix metalloproteinase activity and increases collagen content of rabbit atheroma: a potential mechanism of lesion stabilization [see comments]. Circulation 1998; 97:2433–2444.
208. Bellosta S, Via D, Canavesi M, Pfister P, Fumagalli R, Paoletti R, Bernini F. HMG-CoA reductase inhibitors reduce MMP-9 secretion by macrophages. Arterioscler Thromb Vasc Biol 1998; 18:1671–1678.
209. Ohara Y, Peterson TE, Sayegh HS, Subramanian RR, Wilcox JN, Harrison DG. Dietary correction of hypercholesterolemia in the rabbit normalizes endothelial superoxide anion production. Circulation 1995; 92:898–903.

5
Epidemiological Evidence for Inflammation in Plaque Rupture

Russell P. Tracy
University of Vermont, Colchester, Vermont

I. INTRODUCTION

The concept of inflammation as an integral part of atherothrombotic disease is not a new one. Early pioneers such as Virchow, Rokitansky, and Duguid wrote about inflammation and thrombosis as key components of cardiovascular disease (1–3), and recent developments have demonstrated how prescient these views were (4). Our modern views, however, are considerably more complex because they exist within the current molecular framework. Many details at the gene, protein, and cell biology levels are being developed, and it will take some time to meld all this detail into a comprehensive scheme.

Epidemiology has played a role in bringing us to our current position, by clearly showing that markers of inflammation are related to underlying atherothrombotic disease, on one hand, and the occurrence of future atherothrombotic events on the other. For example, as shown in Figure 1, in a cross-sectional study of older people, fibrinogen is strongly related to the degree of carotid artery stenosis as revealed by ultrasonography (5), whereas in the same population fibrinogen predicts future myocardial infarction, even after adjustment for the presence of subclinical cardiovascular disease (6).

From a pathophysiological standpoint, we are beginning to understand that the atherothrombotic process, which begins at an early age (7) and progresses through several phases (8–10), probably involves inflammation in different ways at different stages. As a corollary, an emerging epidemiological concept is that the nature of the association of inflammation with future atherothrombotic disease

Association of Fibrinogen with Stenosis

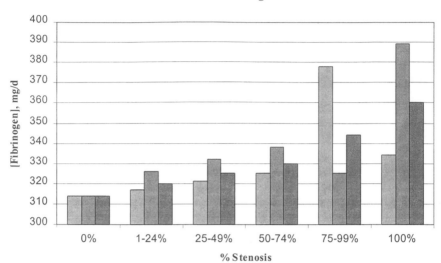

Association of Fibrinogen with Future CVD Events

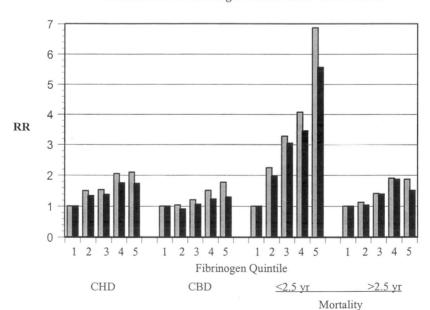

likely changes with age (11, 12). It is probably the degree of underlying atherothrombotic disease that is the true determinant, but age is an easily identifiable surrogate, at least in men. Evidence for this concept comes from genetic studies (13) and studies of molecular phenotypes such as fibrinogen and C-reactive protein (CRP). Besides age, other important modulators of the association of inflammation with disease outcome include sex (14) (Cushman M et al., manuscript submitted), adiposity (15, 16), smoking (17–19), and components of the metabolic syndrome (insulin resistance syndrome, or syndrome X) (20).

For each of the measurements being made epidemiologically that reflect some aspect of inflammation, it is an open question whether the marker reflects underlying pathophysiological processes, participates in those processes, or both (21). Again, fibrinogen is a good example, as shown in Figure 2. It is unlikely that epidemiology will yield the answers to these questions, because cause and effect are difficult to tease apart when the disease process is essentially lifelong and involves at least some aspects of inflammation at every stage. Animal models and controlled clinical studies and trials will be needed. As discussed later, the available data suggest that in fact inflammation is both a reflection of, and a participant in, atherothrombosis.

II. WHAT IS "INFLAMMATION"?

This is an important question that has an ever more complex answer as the scientific community uncovers more and more of the molecular factors and events

---

Figure 1 Association of plasma fibrinogen with the presence of subclinical atherothrombotic disease and the risk of future cardiovascular events. Both panels use data from the Cardiovascular Health Study, a longitudinal epidemiological study of healthy people (*n* = 5,201) >64 years at baseline (127). In the upper panel, modified from Ref. 5, the mean plasma fibrinogen values are expressed by the maximum degree of stenosis found in either the left or right, common or internal carotid artery by ultrasonography. The bars, progressing from light to dark gray, represent a subgroup free of clinical CVD at baseline; the group with clinical CVD at baseline; and the entire cohort. All data are adjusted for age, sex, height, weight, smoking status, LDL and HDL cholesterol, fasting glucose, and systolic and diastolic blood pressure. In the lower panel, modified from Ref. 6, the relative risk of a CVD event (from Cox proportional hazards models) is expressed against the quintile of baseline plasma fibrinogen level. The first quintile is used as the reference group and set to 1.0. The events were coronary heart disease (CHD); stroke or transient ischemic attack (CBD); or mortality from any cause occurring either within 2.5 years of baseline or after. The gray bars represent unadjusted data, whereas the black bars represent data adjusted for CVD risk factors and the presence or absence of significant subclinical atherothrombotic disease.

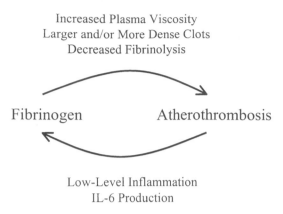

Increased Plasma Viscosity
Larger and/or More Dense Clots
Decreased Fibrinolysis

Fibrinogen   Atherothrombosis

Low-Level Inflammation
IL-6 Production

Figure 2 The association of fibrinogen with atherothrombotic disease. Fibrinogen levels predict future CVD events. This may be because, as an inflammation-sensitive protein, fibrinogen reflects the degree of underlying disease through low-level inflammatory changes. However, there are many studies describing mechanisms, whereby fibrinogen may cause atherothrombotic disease, such as by increasing viscosity or by increasing the likelihood of a larger, more dense blood clot. Because data exist to support both hypotheses, both may be true, with increasing disease causing elevations in fibrinogen, which in turn may exacerbate the disease process (21).

associated with what we have come to think of as "inflammation." This has led to the emergence of four new concepts with respect to the epidemiological application of markers of inflammation.

First, the traditional definition of inflammation is a ". . . complex of . . . reactions that occur in the affected blood vessels and adjacent tissues . . . in response to an injury or abnormal stimulation . . .", with the so-called cardinal signs of redness, swelling, heat, pain, and loss of function (22). However, in the modern context, when we speak of inflammation, it is likely that none of the cardinal signs will be evident, at least at the macroscopic level. For example, the high levels of CRP that predict future cardiovascular events are *far below* the values that have traditionally been used to detect inflammation and represent what one might think of as values in the upper part of the "normal range" (23). The same is true for the other markers of inflammation that have been examined epidemiologically, causing us to redefine "inflammation" as a chronic and extremely mild version of the traditional definition.

A second new concept is that, from an epidemiological viewpoint, we suggest considering "inflammation" as representative of a "supersystem," including either the entirety or elements of coagulation, fibrinolysis, complement activation, immune response, insulin, and glucose metabolism and the more generalized concept of inflammation comprising tissue damage and proinflammatory cytokine production. This is based on the consistent, strong associations we and others have observed between markers of inflammation and components of these "other" systems (18), as illustrated in Figure 3. As mentioned in the beginning of this review, we are still in the early stages of developing a more complete scheme that links all the relevant metabolic processes. The set mentioned previously are key in an epidemiological sense, because we have markers we can measure in populations. The synthetic work of Ross, Libby, Fuster, and others, representing research they and many others have done, has played and continues to play a critical role in this synthesis from the standpoint of molecular pathophysiology (4, 24, 25). In this review we will focus on factors more directly related to coagulation, fibrinolysis, and classic inflammation, but it is important to keep in mind the possible roles played by the components of these other "supersystem" members, and some mention of each will be made in the following.

Epidemiological work in this area started in earnest with thrombosis risk factors, specifically fibrinogen (26–28). This work was spurred on by clear evidence, which placed thrombosis in the causal pathway instead of in the group of postevent epiphenomena (29). As work has progressed, a third important concept has evolved: for most key factors, there are both positive and negative effects associated with changed levels of that factor, as dictated by the basic biological precept of feedback regulation (30). Thrombin, the ultimate enzyme in the coagulation cascade, is an excellent example. Although thrombin is clearly a major procoagulant factor at the site of exposed subendothelium and activated platelets and monocytes (31), thrombin is also an anticoagulant, responsible for the activation of protein C, the major plasma anticoagulant protein, when bound to thrombomodulin (32). In fact, this scheme becomes even more complex, because new evidence shows that thrombin-thrombomodulin is also antifibrinolytic, through the activation of TAFI [Thrombin-Activated Fibrinolysis Inhibitor (33)], and the competition of protein C and TAFI for the thrombin-thrombomodulin sites is likely to help regulate the speed and extent of both coagulation and fibrinolysis. Therefore, another complicating factor in interpreting epidemiological studies is that molecular measurements are likely to yield conflicting results, depending on the nature of the underlying pathological condition.

Finally, the fourth new concept regarding inflammation markers is that they appear to predict the occurrence of a number of chronic diseases of the elderly, not just cardiovascular disease. For example, fibrinogen is associated with not only cardiovascular disease mortality but all-cause mortality as well (6). Other examples, that use nonfatal outcomes include type 2 diabetes (34) and cancer (Andreescu et al, manuscript submitted). This should not be surprising because most of the chronic diseases of older age are associated with some degree of tissue damage or injury even in the very early stages. However, just as in atherothrombotic disease, a proinflammatory environment might also contribute to the development of such outcomes. As an example, the early stages of diabetes, characterized by the metabolic syndrome, are known to be associated with increased levels of inflammation

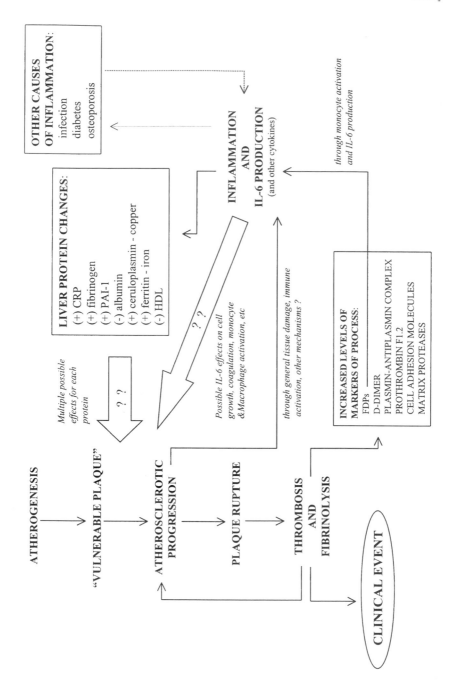

(20), so one might expect to be able to predict the future development of diabetes by markers of inflammation. In addition,increased levels of proinflammatory cytokines such as tumor necrosis factor-α (TNF-α) have recently been shown in in vitro studies to cause insulin resistance (35), and it has been proposed that a proinflammatory environment may lead to the development of type 2 diabetes (36).

III. FIBRINOGEN AND OTHER COMPONENTS OF COAGULATION AND FIBRINOLYSIS

Although many have contributed to our knowledge in this area, the work of Meade and colleagues has been key (37). Their work, along with the work of many others, has shown that fibrinogen is associated with both subclinical atherothrombotic disease (5, 38) and the risk of future cardiovascular outcomes (6, 39). This is true in both middle-aged and older adults and in both men and women. In younger adults and children, fibrinogen is associated with many cardiovascular risk factors (40), particularly adiposity (41).

We have observed a distinct time-to-event effect with fibrinogen in older people. In the Cardiovascular Health Study, fibrinogen predicted both total mortality (6) and cardiovascular mortality (Tracy RP, et al. manuscript in preparation) much more effectively when the event occurred within 2.5 years from the time of blood collection than when the event occurred after this time. This is in contrast with prediction by inflammation markers in younger individuals, which commonly are associated with little if any time-to-event effect (see section on CRP, later). On the basis of these epidemiological findings, we have suggested that the

---

Figure 3 An overview of the atherothrombotic process that includes elements of coagulation, fibrinolysis, oxidative damage, inflammation, and immunity. Disease progression from fatty streak to vulnerable plaque to more complex plaque with thrombosis results in the elaboration of products of cell damage, immune activation, and increases in markers of coagulation, fibrinolysis, and other aspects of atherothrombosis. These in turn cause generalized increases in inflammation mediators such as IL-6, through a number of mechanisms (e.g., the activation of monocytes by fibrin degradation products) (128). IL-6 and other proinflammatory mediators may have direct effects on the disease process through cell proliferation, immune activation, creating a hypercoagulable state, or other pathways. In addition, as pluripotent effector molecules, proinflammatory cytokines often cause dramatic changes in the production of a number of liver proteins such as fibrinogen, C-reactive protein, the fibrinolysis inhibitor PAI-1, and others. These changes may, over time, worsen the atherothrombotic process. In this model, other causes of inflammation would be expected to increase rates of CVD through changes invoked in these same intermediate factors. The figure is modified from Ref. 12.

increased short-term prediction of cardiovascular events seen in older people is due to the ''proximate pathophysiology'' of the atherothrombotic process in the setting of more complex, extensive pathophysiology (11, 12). This is also supported by results we have observed with markers of coagulation activation, which also vary between middle-aged and older people in their association with future events (see later). Because the nature of the culprit lesion may change with the subject's age (10), there may be an anatomical correlate to this hypothesis.

Factor VII has been proposed as a prospective risk factor on the basis of the original results from the Northwick Park Heart Study (42). However, more recent findings from the ARIC, CHS, and PROCAM studies (6, 43, 44) have not reproduced these findings. In addition, we and others have failed to find significant associations of factor VII with the extent of existing subclinical atherothrombotic disease (5, 38). Because factor VII along with all the vitamin K–dependent coagulation factors are known to be related to plasma lipid levels (45), this may have confounded identifying the true relationship of factor VII to cardiovascular events. It should be noted that a recent report concerning a common factor VII genetic polymorphism that is associated strongly with factor VII levels suggests that this polymorphism may be associated with the risk of future myocardial infarction in middle-aged men (46). Although at this time it seems unlikely that factor VII levels will prove useful in the prediction of future cardiovascular events, further work is needed to definitively answer this issue. Little is known about the other vitamin K–dependent procoagulation factors, factor IX, X, and prothrombin, from a prospective standpoint.

In general, one might expect that low levels of anticoagulants might be associated with an increased risk of thrombosis, and considering venous disease, they are. Deficiencies in protein C, protein S, and antithrombin are all associated with venous thrombosis (47). However, in general, they are not associated with arterial thrombosis. Because these anticoagulants require interaction with endothelial cells, this may be because arterial clot formation, unlike venous clotting, occurs in rapidly moving blood yielding little opportunity for endothelial cell–mediated anticoagulation events to occur other than downstream from the lesion. In fact, protein C levels are higher in those experiencing myocardial infarction than in controls (48), probably as a homeostatic response to increased coagulant activity in people prone to having a thrombotic episode. In the general population, as in the large prospective ARIC study, protein C and antithrombin were not associated with future events (44). We have demonstrated an association of tissue factor pathway inhibitor (TFPI) with the extent of subclinical atherothrombotic disease (49), but this association was relatively weak and this factor has not been explored prospectively.

These findings based on protein levels have been supported by recent results in the area of genetics. Factor V_{Leiden} is a mutation in the structural portion of the factor V gene, which makes the activated cofactor, factor Va, less susceptible to activated protein C–mediated inactivation (50). In essence, factor V_{Leiden}

should have the same consequences as protein C deficiency. In fact, factor V_{Leiden} is a major risk factor for venous events (51), but is not strongly associated with arterial thrombosis (52). If it plays any role at all, it appears to be in relatively small, specific subsets of individuals (53). A similar story is emerging for a recently uncovered genetic polymorphism in the prothrombin gene, called prothrombin$_{20210}$ (54). This genotype is in the 3'-flanking region of the gene and is associated with increased prothrombin levels. Again, although associated with venous disease, it does not appear to carry significant increased risk for arterial events (55), except possibly in specific subsets of people (56).

The major coagulation and anticoagulation cofactors are factor V (prothrombin activation), factor VIII (factor X activation), tissue factor (factor VIIa complex), and thrombomodulin (protein C activation). Of these, only factor VIII has been studied in any detail to date. Factor VIII levels are associated with the extent of subclinical disease (5, 38) and predict future coronary events. However, factor VIII is also known as an acute phase reactant, and it is not clear whether higher factor VIII levels predispose toward arterial thrombosis or if they reflect the extent of underlying disease.

Von Willebrand factor is produced in the liver and is a circulating protein that is polymorphic in structure (highly polymeric) and binds factor VIII, preventing factor VIII degradation; it is also an acute phase reactant (57). Endothelial cell–produced von Willebrand factor, when exposed, is capable of binding specific platelet proteins and participating in platelet adherence. In this sense it is a marker of endothelial cell function (58). Plasma levels of von Willebrand factor have been associated with future cardiovascular events, but whether this is due to an inflammatory response or endothelial cell damage is unclear (44).

The contact system (intrinsic system) of blood coagulation is not believed to play a major role in the initiation of arterial coagulation, a role currently ascribed to tissue factor/factor VIIa–mediated factor IX, and factor X activation (59). However, data support a role for the contact system in the extension of the coagulation reaction, in complement activation, and in the regulation of fibrinolysis (60, 61). Unfortunately, little is known about how the plasma levels of the contact system components may function as risk factors.

Although markers of recent coagulant and/or fibrinolytic activity [e.g., prothrombin fragment 1 + 2 (F1 + 2), thrombin-antithrombin, fibrinopeptide A (FPA), fibrin fragment D-dimer and plasmin-antiplasmin complex] do reflect the hypercoagulable state from the standpoint of deep vein thrombosis or disseminated intravascular coagulation (DIC), they have not proven to be important indicators of future cardiovascular risk in middle-aged subjects. In the Physician's Health Study, D-dimer levels were only associated with future cardiovascular events when in the upper 10% of values (62). In the elderly, we have observed that F1 + 2 and FPA do reflect, to a certain degree, the extent of underlying atherothrombotic disease (63), consistent with evidence for a relatively weak activation state in high-risk men (64). This is likely due to the extent of atherothrombotic disease burden, because D-dimer is also strongly related to cardiovascular events in men with peripheral vascular disease (65).

Several studies, but not all, have suggested that levels of fibrinolytic factors may have important roles in arterial atherothrombosis. Lower tissue plasminogen activator (t-PA) levels and higher plasminogen activator inhibitor-1 (PAI-1) levels characterize male myocardial infarction survivors and predict second myocardial infarction in that group (66, 67). In one study of middle-aged men, higher t-PA levels predicted future events (68), but this is most likely due to the assay used in that study, which reflected PAI-1 levels caused by circulating t-PA–PA-1 complexes. However, others have failed to observe an important independent role for PAI-1, even when underlying disease appears to contribute to increased coagulant activity (69).

Any true association of fibrinolytic factors with atherothrombotic disease is difficult to determine, because PAI-1 is the key determinant of such activity, and PAI-1 exhibits extensive correlation with other cardiovascular disease risk factors such as adiposity, triglyceride levels, and insulin levels (70). In addition, PAI-1 is a weak acute-phase reactant (71), suggesting it may, like fibrinogen etc., reflect subclinical disease. We have performed factor analysis to determine the strength of the various PAI-1 correlations when all are assessed together, and PAI-1 appears most closely related to insulin and body mass variables rather than fibrinolytic factors, triglyceride, or markers of fibrin formation (71a). The most extensively studied genetic polymorphism related to fibrinolytic function is the 4G/5G insertion polymorphism in the promoter region of the PAI-1 gene, which is associated with PAI-1 levels and responsiveness of the PAI-1 gene to inflammatory stimuli (72–74). This polymorphism has been shown to be related to atherothrombotic disease in some studies and not others, as recently reviewed (75). Taking all the evidence together, if PAI-1 levels play a role, it appears to be a minor one.

IV. C-REACTIVE PROTEIN AND OTHER MARKERS OF PROINFLAMMATORY CYTOKINE ACTIVITY

After the extensive work done by a wide variety of investigators with fibrinogen, a number of other markers of inflammation have been examined as risk factors for atherothrombotic events. Some of the work in this area has recently been reviewed (76). In addition, a number of other new cardiovascular risk factors might also be considered markers of inflammation. Table 1 is a partial listing of these markers. The most work has been done with CRP.

CRP is homopentamer (a so-called pentraxin) synthesized in the liver in response to levels of the proinflammatory cytokine interleukin-6 (IL-6) (77, 78). In fact, IL-6 is the only regulatory factor currently identified for CRP, which distinguishes it from other acute-phase reactants such as fibrinogen (79) and

Table 1 New CVD Risk Factors Related to Inflammation

Variable	Comment
C-reactive protein	An acute-phase protein, which reflects low-level inflammation (18, 83, 127, 128) and predict future CVD events (90, 92, 93)
Albumin	A negative acute-phase protein and low levels predict future CVD events (76, 129, 130)
Fibrinogen	An acute-phase protein (128), which predicts future CVD events (37)
Serum amyloid A	An acute-phase protein (128), which predicts future CVD events in those with pre-existing CVD (90)
Ceruloplasmin	An acute-phase protein (128), whose levels influence the assessment of copper, and predict future CVD events (131)
Bilirubin	Associates strongly with albumin and reflects albumin level under normal conditions (132); low levels predict future CVD events (133)
PAI-1	PAI-1 levels go up with inflammation (71), although levels also sensitive to obesity and insulin (15); may predict future CVD events (66, 75)
HDL	Levels go down with inflammation and low levels predict future events (134)
Ferritin	Influences the assessment of iron and goes up with inflammation (132); levels may predict future CVD events (135–137)

PAI-1 (80, 81). Although its function is not known for certain, various suggestions, based on limited data, have been put forward. CRP may act as a regulator of the immune system through either complement activation (82) or opsoninization (83). Alternatively, CRP has been shown to cause monocytes to elaborate tissue factor in vitro (84) and may affect cell-cell interaction (85).

The cross section correlates of CRP (17, 18) appear to reflect those characteristics and environments that are most closely related to increased levels of proinflammatory cytokines (86, 87). Although not all studies are completely consistent, taking the data together, CRP appears relatively strongly associated with adiposity, smoking, variables of the metabolic syndrome and/or the presence of diabetes, and markers of increased coagulation and fibrinolysis. CRP is more weakly associated with the degree of underlying atherothrombotic disease (18, 20). (Folsom A, et al. manuscripts submitted). As expected, CRP is usually associated with other inflammation markers such as increased fibrinogen, decreased HDL-cholesterol level, etc., presumably through common regulation by means of IL-6 and other proinflammatory mediators.

The association with adiposity is believed to reflect the prominent cytokine production by visceral adipocytes (16). Smoking is thought to increase CRP by producing endothelial damage. We have shown that the relationship of CRP to lifetime exposure to cigarette smoke is independent of smoking cessation, suggesting the damage is permanent (18). This is consistent with the finding that carotid wall thickness as revealed by ultrasonography is related to lifetime exposure to passive cigarette smoke and is also independent of cessation (19). The association with variables of the metabolic syndrome other than adiposity may reflect the possible role of proinflammatory cytokines in insulin resistance or may represent endothelial damage associated with the syndrome or with associated atherosclerotic disease. This most likely represents an association independent of adiposity, because in the IRAS study, insulin sensitivity was independently and strongly related to CRP levels (20). Finally, a relatively recent finding is that CRP levels are profoundly affected by pharmacological estrogen (88, 89). Whether this finding extends to physiological estrogen levels remains to be demonstrated.

Concerning prediction of future atherothrombotic events, CRP was first identified as a prospective risk factor in subjects with existing cardiovascular disease (90, 91). These results were soon followed by data showing that CRP predicted future events in men and women of middle age and older (92–95). As with fibrinogen, in older people CRP appeared associated with the time-to-event, consistent with the concept of proximate pathophysiology as discussed earlier (92). There has been remarkable consistency in the values of CRP across a variety of studies (23), once assays were developed that could accurately measure CRP in the healthy reference range (90, 96, 97). It has been suggested that a measure of inflammation may prove useful in the clinical assessment of cardiovascular risk (21, 98, 99) and that CRP, as such a measure, has several attributes that may make it a good candidate (21).

V. IL-6 AND OTHER PROINFLAMMATORY CYTOKINES

Pathophysiologically, it is clear that there is potential for proinflammatory cytokines themselves to participate in the atherothrombotic process, separate from any possible participation on the part of factors whose levels are affected by the cytokines. Sepsis has been studied extensively (100) and might be considered a "worst-case" model for the low-level, chronic inflammation considered important in atherothrombotic disease (101). IL-6 is a major proinflammatory cytokine in the sepsis model (102, 103), with powerful effects on cellular activation events, coagulation, and fibrinolysis (104), suggesting the possibility of an important role in atherothrombosis a well.

Concerning early lesion development, we have recently shown that, in mice, weekly injections of IL-6, sufficient to produce a mild inflammatory response, cause a twofold to fivefold increase in fatty lesion size (105) (Figure 4). Some evidence exists that IL-6 in this setting may function through immune activation (Huber et al., manuscript submitted).

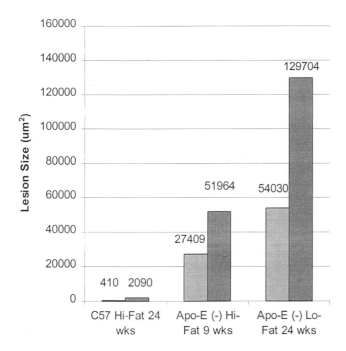

Figure 4 The introduction of IL-6 increases fatty lesion size in the C57B1/6 mouse model of atherosclerosis. In either C57B1/6 mice on high-fat diets for 24 weeks, or C57B1/6 apo-E knock-out mouse (either on a high-fat diet for 9 weeks or a low-fat diet for 24 weeks), weekly injections of IL-6 (darker bars) vs. vehicle (lighter bars) caused a twofold to fivefold increase in fatty lesion size, suggesting that in humans the elaborated IL-6 found in atherothrombotic disease may not be simply a passive marker of the disease process but may participate in some way, causing increased disease. Figure drawn from data presented in Table 1 of Ref. 105.

Recent advances in the immunoassays used to measure plasma cytokines have allowed the use of cytokine measures in epidemiological studies, and IL-6 has recently been studied as a prospective risk factor. In the setting of pre-existing cardiovascular disease, IL-6 levels, similar to CRP levels, predict the future outcome of patients with angina (106). In addition, in healthy elderly individuals, IL-6 levels are independent predictors of all-cause and cardiovascular mortality (87). Although important from the perspective of the underlying molecular pathology, it remains unclear whether direct cytokine measurements will prove superior to assays for cytokine-responsive proteins as clinical measures. Various factors will prove important, including the sensitivity and specificity of the assay and the biological variation in the protein.

VI. OTHER ISSUES

The preceding discussion raises an important question: are all measures of inflammation-sensitive markers equivalent with respect to risk prediction? It is tempting to conclude "yes" because several different markers have been associated with disease, as recently reviewed (76). However, the regulatory elements in these genes are not identical, suggesting they may reflect the inflammatory damage differently. Also, in several studies in which statistical models have been used to predict risk, adjustment for one marker has not removed the significance of the other (69). In addition, the proposed mechanistic contributions of these proteins are markedly different (e.g., fibrinogen and clot formation vs. CRP and complement activation). Finally, the degree of association with covariates also varies considerably when different measures are directly compared; a recent example looking at the association of five different markers with activity status illustrates this point (107). Therefore, at this time, we cannot conclude equivalency, with further work needed to definitively answer this question.

Recent work has implicated infections as a risk factor for atherothrombotic disease, and a recent review by Nieto has covered this area (108). Several infectious organisms have been implicated in different studies, including *Chlamydia*, herpes simplex virus-1, and cytomegalovirus. However, the results of different epidemiological studies have not been consistent (109–113). These organisms have been identified within the vasculature (114), suggesting a causal role possibly through damage and/or injury caused by the infection or by the local elaboration of cytokines during the localized inflammatory response. However, it is likely that these infections also cause a mild, chronic, systemic inflammatory response, and such a response may be associated with persistent increased risk of atherothrombotic progression remote from the site of actual infection.

Considering genetic analyses as a whole, several relatively frequent genotypes have been identified in inflammation-sensitive proteins that affect their levels; examples include fibrinogen (115) and PAI-1 (73). Also, polymorphisms have been identified in the genes for several inflammation-related cytokines including IL-6 (116) and TNF-α (117). The usefulness of these polymorphisms has been, and continues to be, studied actively. In general, results have been inconsistent across studies. A good example includes several polymorphisms in the fibrinogen gene, many of which are in linkage disequilibrium (118). In some studies, the presence of a specific genotype has been associated with disease, whereas in others it has not (119–123). In the case of PAI-1, a recent meta-analysis has concluded that it is likely there is an association, but the effect is small (75). Many of the studies are relatively small case-control studies that may lead to either type 2 error or type 1 error (124, 125). In addition, variations in outcome phenotype may complicate these results. For example, recent autopsy-based studies have shown that thrombosis is not present in all cases of myocardial infarction and may be related to the type of precipitating lesion, rupture, or erosion (10). Using myocardial infarction as an outcome phenotype in studies of thrombosis-related genotypes, therefore, might be expected to yield conflicting results, especially if the studies were small, with the possibility of disproportionate representation of the fraction of events involving thrombosis across the different studies.

It appears likely that individual genotypes associated with quantitative traits will exert an effect in specific settings (i.e., in gene-gene or gene-environment interactions) (126). As an example, this has been suggested by Rosendaal and colleagues (52) with respect to the factor V_{Leiden} mutation, which appears to exert an effect on atherothrombotic risk in young women with other thrombosis risk factors (53) but not in the general population. Taken together with the potential error involved when studying small groups, significantly larger studies are required to determine for genetic associations with disease.

VII. CONCLUSIONS

Inflammation, coagulation, and several other systems need to be considered as a single "super-system." A number of intermediate components of this system, which can be measured in blood-based samples, reflect the degree of underlying disease and the risk of future atherothrombotic events. Many questions exist, however, about the nature of these associations. It is unknown whether the various measures are equivalent. And, in particular, it remains unclear for a number of these assays whether the component in question either reflects the degree of underlying disease or participates in the pathophysiology or both. This has important implications for possible interventions. This point is complicated by the complexity of the pathways. Important components often have both "positive" and "negative" effects within these pathways, and under different conditions one or the other may predominate.

The degree of "inflammation" that is involved with atherothrombotic risk is relatively mild compared with the traditional interpretation of the term "inflammation." For example, the predictive risk for CRP is encompassed almost exclusively within what is generally considered the "normal range" of CRP. Also, the relationship between these markers and future risk appears to change over time, based on the evolving atherothrombotic lesion ("proximate pathophysiology"). In particular, inflammation markers predicting atherothrombotic events in younger individuals do so over long periods of time, whereas in older individuals, they appear to predict events occurring soon after blood collection, thus opening new possibilities for the use of inflammation markers in risk prediction.

ACKNOWLEDGMENTS

I wish to thank Drs. Lew Kuller and Mary Cushman for many helpful conversations. The writing of this review was supported by NIH RO1 Awards HL46696 and HL58329.

REFERENCES

1. Virchow R. Die Cellularpathologie in ihrer Begründung auf physiologische und pathologische Gewebelehre. Berlin, 1858.
2. Rokitansky C. A Manual of Pathological Anatomy. Philadelphia: Blanchard and Lee, 1855.
3. Duguid J. Thrombosis as a factor in the pathogenesis of coronary atherosclerosis. J Pathol Bacterial 1946; 58:207–212.
4. Ross R. Atherosclerosis—an inflammatory disease. N Engl J Med 1999; 340:115–126.
5. Tracy R, Bovill E, Yanez D, Psaty B, Fried L, Heiss G, Lee M, Polak J, Savage P, for the CHS Investigators. Fibrinogen and factor VIII, but not factor VII, are associated with measures of subclinical cardiovascular disease in the elderly: results from the Cardiovascular Health Study. Arterioscler Thromb Vasc Biol 1995; 15: 1269–1279.
6. Tracy RP, Arnold AM, Ettinger W, Fried L, Meilahn E, Savage P. The relationship of fibrinogen and factors VII and VIII to incident cardiovascular disease and death in the elderly: results from the Cardiovascular Health Study. Arterioscler Thromb Vasc Biol 1999; 19:1776–1783.
7. Strong JP, Malcom GT, McMahan CA, Tracy RE, Newman WP, 3rd, Herderick EE, Cornhill JF. Prevalence and extent of atherosclerosis in adolescents and young adults: implications for prevention from the Pathobiological Determinants of Atherosclerosis in Youth Study. JAMA 1999; 281:727–735.
8. Stary H, Chandler A, Glagov S, Guyton J, Insull W, Rosenfield M, Schaffer S, Schwartz C, Wagner W, Wissler R. A definition of initial, fatty streak, and intermediate lesions of atherosclerosis. Circulation 1994; 89:2462–2478.
9. Stary H, Chandler A, Dinsmore R, Fuster V, Glalov S, Insull W, Rosenfield M, Schwartz C, Wagner W, Wissler R. A definition of advanced types of atherosclerotic lesions and a histological classification of atherosclerotic lesions and a histological classification of atherosclerosis. Circulation 1995; 92:1355–1374.
10. Burke AP, Farb A, Malcom GT, Liang YH, Smialek J, Virmani R. Coronary risk factors and plaque morphology in men with coronary disease who died suddenly [see comments]. N Engl J Med 1997; 336:1276–1282.
11. Tracy RP. Inflammation markers and coronary heart disease. Curr Opin Lipidol 1999; 10:435–441.
12. Tracy R. Epidemiological evidence for inflammation in cardiovascular disease. Thromb Haemost 1999; 82:826–831.
13. Bray P. Integrin polymorphisms as risk factors for thrombosis. Thromb Haemost 1999; 82:337–344.

14. Cushman M, Arnold A, Kuller L, Psaty B, Manolio T, Burke G, Polak J, Tracy R. C-reactive protein and risks of myocardial infarction, stroke and death in an elderly cohort (abstrt). Circulation 1999; 98:1108.

15. Loskutoff DJ, Samad F. The adipocyte and hemostatic balance in obesity: studies of PAI-1. Arterioscler Thromb Vasc Biol 1998; 18:1–6.

16. Yudkin JS, Stehouwer CD, Emesis JJ, Coppack SW. C-reactive protein in healthy subjects: associations with obesity, insulin resistance, and endothelial dysfunction: a potential role for cytokines originating from adipose tissue? Arterioscler Thromb Vasc Biol 1999; 19:972–978.

17. Mendall MA, Patel P, Ballam L, Strachan D, Northfield TC. C reactive protein and its relation to cardiovascular risk factors: a population based cross sectional study. BMJ 1996; 312:1061–1065.

18. Tracy R, Macy E, Bovill E, Cushman M, Psaty B, Cornell E, Kuller L. Lifetime smoking exposure affects the association of C-reactive protein with cardiovascular disease risk factors and subclinical disease in healthy elderly subjects. Arterioscler Thromb Vasc Biol 1997; 17:2167–2176.

19. Howard G, Wagenknecht L, Burke G, Diez-Roux A, Evans G, McGovern P, Nieto F, Tell G, for the ARIC Investigators. Cigarette smoking and progression of atherosclerosis: The Atherosclerosis Risk in Communities (ARIC) study. JAMA 1998; 279:119–124.

20. Festa A, D'Agostino R Jr, Howard G, Mykkanen L, Tracy RP, Haffner SM. Chronic subclinical inflammation as part of the insulin resistance syndrome: The insulin resistance atherosclerosis study (IRAS). Circulation 2000; 102:42–47.

21. Tracy RP. Inflammation in cardiovascular disease: cart, horse, or both? Circulation 1998; 97:2000–2002.

22. Stedman's Medical Dictionary. Baltimore, MD: The Williams & Wilkins Co., 1976:1678.

23. de Maat M, Haverkate F, Kluft C. C-reactive protein: a cardiovascular risk factor. Report on the CRP hot-topic workshop of October 1, 1997. Fibrinolysis Proteolysis 1998; 12:323–327.

24. Fuster V. Elucidation of the role of plaque instability and rupture in acute coronary events. Am J Cardiol 1995; 76:24C–33C.

25. Libby P. Molecular bases of the acute coronary syndromes. Circulation 1995; 91: 2844–2850.

26. Meade T, Chakrabarti R, Haines A, North W, Stirling Y, Thompson S. Haemostatic function and cardiovascular death: early results of a prospective study. Lancet 1980; i:1050–1054.

27. Wilhelmsen L, Svardsudd K, Korsan-Bengtsen K, Larsson B, Welin L, Tibblin G. Fibrinogen as a risk factor for stroke and myocardial infarction. N Eng J Med 1984; 311:501–505.

28. Stone M, Thorp J. Plasma fibrinogen—a major coronary risk factor. J R Coll Gen Pract 1985; 35:565–569.

29. DeWood M, Spores J, Notske R, Mouser L, Burroughs R, Goldens M, Lang H. Prevalence of total coronary occlusion during the early hours of transmural myocardial infarction. N Engl J Med 1980; 303:897–902.

30. Alberts B, Bray D, Lewis J, Raff M, Roberts K, Watson J. Molecular Biology of the Cell. New York: Garland Publishing, 1989:1219.

31. Mann K. Prothrombin and thrombin. In: Colman R, Hirsh J, Marder V, Salzman
     E, eds. Hemostasis and Thrombosis: Basic Principles and Clinical Practice. Phila-
     delphia: J. B. Lippincott, 1994:184–199.
32. Esmon C. The protein C anticoagulant pathway. Arterioscler Thromb 1992; 12:
     135–145.
33. Nesheim M, Wang W, Boffa M, Nagashima M, Morser J, Bajzar L. Thrombin,
     thrombomodulin and TAFI in the molecular link between coagulation and fibrinol-
     ysis. Thromb Haemost 1997; 78:386–391.
34. Schmidt MI, Duncan BB, Sharrett AR, Lindberg G, Savage PJ, Offenbacher S,
     Azambuja MI, Tracy RP, Heiss G. Markers of inflammation and prediction of dia-
     betes mellitus in adults (Atherosclerosis Risk in Communities study): a cohort
     study. Lancet 1999; 353:1649–1652.
35. Cheung AT, Ree D, Kolls JK, Fuselier J, Coy DH, Bryer-Ash M. An in vivo model
     for elucidation of the mechanism of tumor necrosis factor-alpha (TNF-alpha)-
     induced insulin resistance: evidence for differential regulation of insulin signaling
     by TNF-alpha. Endocrinology 1998; 139:4928–4935.
36. Peraldi P, Spiegelman B. TNF-alpha and insulin resistance: summary and future
     prospects. Mol Cell Biochem 1998; 182:169–175.
37. Meade T. The epidemiology of haemostatic and other variables in coronary artery
     disease. In: Verstraete M, Vermylen J, Lijnen H, Arnout J, eds. Thromb. and Hae-
     mostasis 1987. Leuven: International Society on Thrombosis and Haemostasis and
     Leuven University Press, 1987:37–59.
38. Folsom A, Wu K, Shahar E, Davis C. Association of hemostatic variables with
     prevalent cardiovascular disease and asymptomatic carotid artery atherosclerosis.
     The Atherosclerosis Risk in Communities (ARIC) study. Aretioscler Thromb 1993;
     13:1829–1836.
39. Folsom A, Wu K, Rosamond W, Sharrett A, Chambless L. Hemostatic factors and
     incidence of coronary heart disease in the Atherosclerosis Risk in Communities
     (ARIC) study (abstrt). Circulation 1996; 93:622.
40. Folsom AR, Qamhieh HT, Flack JM, Hilner JE, Liu K, Howard BV, Tracy RP.
     Plasma fibrinogen: levels and correlates in young adults. The Coronary Artery Risk
     Development in Young Adults (CARDIA) study. Am J Epidemiol 1993; 138:1023–
     1036.
41. Shea S, Isasi CR, Couch S, Starc TJ, Tracy RP, Deckelbaum R, Talmud P, Berglund
     L, Humphries SE. Relations of plasma fibrinogen level in children to measures of
     obesity, the (G-455 → A) mutation in the beta-fibrinogen promoter gene, and family
     history of ischemic heart disease: the Columbia University BioMarkers Study. Am
     J Epidemiol 1999; 150:737–746.
42. Meade T, Brozovic M, Chakrabarti R, Haines A, Imeson J, Mellows S, Miller G,
     North W, Stirling Y, Thompson S. Haemostatic function and ischaemic heart disease:
     principal results of the Northwick Park Heart Study. Lancet 1986; ii:533–537.
43. Heinrich J, Balleisen L, Schulte H, Assmann G, van de Loo J. Fibrinogen and factor
     VII in the prediction of coronary risk: Results from the PROCAM study in healthy
     men. Arterioscler Thromb 1994; 14:54–59.
44. Folsom AR, Wu KK, Rosamond WD, Sharrett AR, Chambless LE. Prospective
     study of hemostatic factors and incidence of coronary heart disease: the Atheroscle-
     rosis Risk in Communities (ARIC) study. Circulation 1997; 96:1102–1108.

45. Tracy R, Losito R, Howard P, Cushman M, Bovill E. The association of plasma lipids and vitamin K-dependent coagulation factors. In: Bray G, Ryan D, eds. Nutrition, Genetics and Heart Disease. Vol. 6. Baton Rouge: LSU Press, 1996:29–49.

46. Iacoviello L, Di Castelnuovo A, De Knijff P, D'Orazio A, Amore C, Arboretti R, Kluft C, Benedetta Donati M. Polymorphisms in the coagulation factor VII gene and the risk of myocardial infarction. N Engl J Med 1998; 338:79–85.

47. Comp P. Overview of the hypercoagulablae states. Semin Thromb Hemost 1990; 16:158–161.

48. Callas P, Tracy R, Bovill E, Cannon C, Thompson B, Mann K. The association of anticoagulant protein concentrations with acute myocardial infarction in the Thrombolysis in Myocardial Infarction Phase II (TIMI II) trial. J Thromb Thrombol 1998; 5:53–60.

49. Sakkinen PA, Cushman M, Psaty BM, Kuller LH, Bajaj SP, Sabharwal AK, Boineau R, Macy E, Tracy RP. Correlates of antithrombin, protein C, protein S, and TFPI in a healthy elderly cohort. Thromb Haemost 1998; 80:134–139.

50. Bertina R, Koeleman B, Koster T, Rosendaal F, Dirven R, deRonde H, van der Velden P, Reitsma P. Mutation in blood coagulation factor V associated with resistance to activated protein C. Nature 1994; 369:64–67.

51. Bertina R. Factor V leiden and other coagulation factor mutations affecting thrombotic risk. Clin Chem 1997; 43:1678–1682.

52. Cushman M, Rosendaal FR, Psaty BM, Cook EF, Valliere J, Kuller LH, Tracy RP. Factor V Leiden is not a risk factor for arterial vascular disease in the elderly: results from the Cardiovascular Health Study. Thromb Haemost 1998; 79:912–915.

53. Rosendaal FR, Siscovick DS, Schwartz SM, Beverly RK, Psaty BM, Longstreth WT, Jr., Raghunathan TE, Koepsell TD, Reitsma PH. Factor V Leiden (resistance to activated protein C) increases the risk of myocardial infarction in young women. Blood 1997; 89:2817–2821.

54. Bertina R. The prothrombin 20210 G to A variant and thrombosis. Curr Opin Hematol 1998; 5:339–342.

55. Ridker P, Hennekens C, Miletich J. G20210A mutation in prothrombin gene and risk of myocardial infarction, stroke, and venous thrombosis in a large cohort of US men. Circulation 1999; 99:999–1004.

56. Rosendaal F, Siscivick D, Schwartz S, Psaty B, Raghunathan T, Vos H. A common prothrombin variant (20210 G to A) increases the risk of myocardial infarction in young women. Blood 1997; 90:1747–1750.

57. de Groot P, Sixma J. Role of von Willebrand factor in the vessel wall. Semin Thromb Hemost 1987; 13:416–424.

58. Blann A, Dobrotova M, Kubisz P, McCollum C. von Willebrand factor, soluble P-selectin, tissue plasminogen activator and plasminogen activator inhibitor in atherosclerosis. Thromb Haemost 1995; 74:626–630.

59. Mann K, Krishnaswamy S, Lawson J. Surface dependent hemostasis. Blood 1992; 29:213–226.

60. Naito K, Fujikawa K. Activation of human blood coagulation factor XI independent of factor XII. Factor XI is activated by thrombin and factor XIa in the presence of negatively charged surfaces. J Biol Chem 1991; 266:7353–7358.

61. Jansen P, Pixley R, Brouwer M, deJong I, Chang A, Hack C, Taylor F, Colman R. Inhibition of factor XII in septic baboons attenuates the activation of complement

and fibrinolytic systems and reduces the release of interleukin-6 and neutrophil elastase. Blood 1996; 87:2337–2344.

62. Ridker P, Hennekens C, Cerskus A, Stampfer M. Plasma concentration of cross-linked fibrin degradation product (D-Dimer) and the risk of future myocardial infarction among apparently healthy men. Circulation 1994; 90:2236–2240.

63. Cushman M, Psaty B, Macy E, Bovill E, Cornell E, Kuller L, Tracy R. Correlates of thrombin markers in an elderly cohort free of clinical cardiovascular disease. Arterioscler Thromb Vasc Biol 1996; 16:1163–1169.

64. Miller G, Bauer K, Barzegar S, Cooper J, Rosenberg R. Increased activation of the haemostatic system in men at high risk of fatal coronary heart disease. Thromb Haemost 1996; 75:767–771.

65. Fowkes F, Lowe G, Housley E, Rattray A, Rumley A, Elton R, MacGregor I, Dawes J. Cross-linked fibrin degradation products, progression of peripheral arterial disease, and risk of coronary heart disease. Lancet 1993; 342:84–86.

66. Hamsten A, de Faire U, Walldius G, Dahlen G, Szamosi A, Landou C, Blomback M, Wiman B. Plasminogen activator inhibitor in plasma: risk factor for recurrent myocardial infarction. Lancet 1987; ii:3–9.

67. Hamsten A, Wiman B, de Faire U, Blomback M. Increased plasma levels of a rapid inhibitor of tissue plasminogen activator in young survivors of myocardial infarction. N Engl J Med 1985; 313:1557–1563.

68. Ridker P, Vaughan D, Stampfer M, Manson J, Hennekens C. Endogenous tissue-type plasminogen activator and risk of myocardial infarction. Lancet 1993; 341:1165–1168.

69. Cushman M, Lemaitre R, Kuller L, Psaty B, Macy E, Sharrett A, Tracy R. Fibrinolytic Activation Markers Predict Myocardial Infarction in the Elderly: The Cardiovascular Health Study. Arterioscler Thromb Vasc Biol 1999; 19:493–498.

70. Juhan-Vague I, Alessi M, Vague P. Increased plasma plasminogen activator inhibitor 1 levels: a possible link between insulin resistance and atherothrombosis. Diabetologia 1991; 34:457–462.

71. Kluft C, Verheijen J, Jie A, Rijken D, Preston F, Sue-Ling H, Jespersen J, Aasen A. The post-operative fibrinolytic shutdown: a rapidly reverting acute phase pattern for the fast acting inhibitor of tissue-type plasminogen activator after trauma. Scand J Clin Lab Invest 1985; 45:605–610.

71a. Sakkinen PA, Wahl P, Cushman M, Lewis MR, Tracy RP. Clustering of procoagulation, inflammation, and fibrinolysis variables with metabolic factors in insulin resistance syndrome. Am. J Epidemiol 2000; 152:897–907.

72. Panahloo A, Mohamed-Ali V, Lane A, Humphries S, Yudkin J. Determinants of plasminogen activator inhibitor 1 activity in treated NIDDM and its relation to a polymorphism in the plasminogen activator inhibitor 1 gene. Diabetes 1995; 44:37–42.

73. Dawson S, Hamsten A, Wiman B, Henney A, Humphries S. Genetic variation at the plasminogen activator inhibitor-1 locus is associated with altered levels of plasminogen activator inhibitor-1 activity. Arterioscler Thromb 1991; 11:183–190.

74. Humphries S, Lane A, Dawson S, Green F. The study of gene-environment interactions that influence thrombosis and fibrinolysis: genetic variation at the loci for factor VII and plasminogen activator inhibitor-1. Arch Pathol Lab Med 1992; 116:1322–1329.

75. Iacoviello L, Burzotta F, Di Castelnuovo A, Zito F, Marchioli R, Donati MB. The 4G/5G polymorphism of PAI-1 promoter gene and the risk of myocardial infarction: a meta-analysis. Thromb Haemost 1998; 80:1029–1030.
76. Danesh J, Collins R, Appleby P, Peto R. Association of fibrinogen, C-reactive protein, albumin, or leukocyte count with coronary heart disease: meta-analyses of prospective studies. JAMA 1998; 279:1477–1482.
77. Pepys M, Baltz M. Acute phase proteins with special reference to C-reactive protein and related proteins and serum amyloid A protein. Adv Immunol 1983; 34:141–212.
78. Bataille R, Klein B. C-reactive protein levels as a direct indicator of interleukin-6 levels in humans in vivo. Arth Rheum 1992; 35:982–984.
79. Amrani D. Regulation of fibrinogen biosynthesis: glucocorticoid and interleukin-6 control. Blood Coagulation Fibrinolysis 1990; 1:443–446.
80. Alessi M, Juhan-Vague I, Kooistra T, Declerck P, Collen D. Insulin stimulates the synthesis of plasminogen activator inhibitor 1 by the human hepatocellular cell line HepG2. Thromb Haemost 1988; 60:491–494.
81. Schneider D, Sobel B. Augmentation of synthesis of plasminogen activator inhibitor type 1 by insulin and insulin-like growth factor type I: implications for vascular disease in hyperinsulinemic states. Proc Natl Acad Sci USA 1991; 88:9959–9963.
82. Lagrand WK, Visser CA, Hermens WT, Niessen HW, Verheugt FW, Wolbink GJ, Hack CE. C-reactive protein as a cardiovascular risk factor: more than an epiphenomenon? Circulation 1999; 100:96–102.
83. Pepys M. C-reactive protein fifty years on. Lancet 1981; i:653–656.
84. Cermak J, Key N, Bach R, Balla J, Jacob H, Vercellotti G. C-reactive protein induces human peripheral blood monocytes to synthesize tissue factor. Blood 1993; 82:513–520.
85. Zouki C, Beauchamp M, Baron C, Filep JG. Prevention of In vitro neutrophil adhesion to endothelial cells through shedding of L-selectin by C-reactive protein and peptides derived from C-reactive protein. J Clin Invest 1997; 100:522–529.
86. Mendall MA, Patel P, Asante M, Ballam L, Morris J, Strachan DP, Camm AJ, Northfield TC. Relation of serum cytokine concentrations to cardiovascular risk factors and coronary heart disease. Heart 1997; 78:273–277.
87. Harris TB, Ferrucci L, Tracy RP, Corti MC, Wacholder S, Ettinger WH, Jr., Heimovitz H, Cohen HJ, Wallace R. Associations of elevated interleukin-6 and C-reactive protein levels with mortality in the elderly. Am J Med 1999; 106:506–512.
88. Cushman M, Legault C, Barrett-Connor E, Stefanick ML, Kessler C, Judd HL, Sakkinen PA, Tracy RP. Effect of postmenopausal hormones on inflammation-sensitive proteins: the Postmenopausal Estrogen/Progestin Interventions (PEPI) study. Circulation 1999; 100:717–722.
89. Cushman M, Meilahn EN, Psaty BM, Kuller LH, Dobs AS, Tracy RP. Hormone replacement therapy, inflammation, and hemostasis in elderly women. Arterioscler Thromb Vasc Biol 1999; 19:893–899.
90. Liuzzo G, Biasicci LM, Gallimore JR, Grillo R, Rebuzzi A, Pepys M, Maseri A. The prognostic value of C-reactive protein and serum amyloid A protein in severe unstable angina. New Engl J Med 1994; 331:417–424.
91. Haverkate F, Thompson S, Pyke S, Gallimore J, Pepys M. Production of C-reactive protein and risk of coronary events in stable and unstable angina. Lancet 1997; 349:462–466.

92. Tracy R, Lemaitre R, Psaty B, Ives D, Evans R, Cushman M, Meilahn E, Kuller L. Relationship of C-reactive protein to risk of cardiovascular disease in the elderly: results from the Cardiovascular Health Study and Rural Health Promotion Project. Arterioscler Thromb Vasc Biol 1997; 17:1121–1127.

93. Ridker P, Cushman M, Stampfer M, Tracy R, Hennekens C. Inflammation, aspirin, and the risk of cardiovascular disease in apparently healthy men. N Engl J Med 1997; 336:973–979.

94. Koenig W, Sund M, Frohlich M, Fischer H-G, Lowel H, Doring A, Hutchinson W, Pepys M. C-reactive protein, a sensitive marker of inflammation, predicts future risk of coronary heart disease in initially healthy middle-aged men. Circulation 1999; 99:237–242.

95. Sakkinen P, Abbott R, Curb J, Rodriguez B, Yano K, Tracy R. C-reactive protein and incident myocardial infarction in Japanese American men (abstr). Circulation 1999; 99:1121.

96. Macy E, Hayes T, Tracy R. Variability in the measurement of C-reactive protein in healthy subjects: implications for reference interval and epidemiological applications. Clin Chem 1997; 43:52–58.

97. Rifai N, Tracy RP, Ridker PM. Clinical efficacy of an automated high-sensitivity C-reactive protein assay. Clin Chem 1999; 45:2136–2141.

98. Ridker PM, Glynn RJ, Hennekens CH. C-reactive protein adds to the predictive value of total and HDL cholesterol in determining risk of first myocardial infarction. Circulation 1998; 97:2007–2011.

99. Ernst E, Resch K. Fibrinogen as a cardiovascular risk factor: A meta-analysis and review of the literature. Ann Intern Med 1993; 118:956–963.

100. Esmon C, Taylor F, Snow T. Inflammation and coagulation: linked processes potentially regulated through a common pathway mediated by protein C. Thromb Haemost 1991; 66:160–165.

101. Clinton S, Libby P. Cytokines and growth factors on atherogenesis. Arch Pathol Lab Med 1992; 116:1292–1300.

102. Le J, Vilcek J. Biology of disease. Interleukin 6: a multifunctional cytokine regulating immune reactions and the acute phase protein response. Lab Invest 1989; 61: 588–602.

103. Waage A, Brandtzaeg P, Halstennsen A, Kierulf P, Espevik T. The complex pattern of cytokines in serum from patients with meningococcal septic shock. J Exp Med 1989; 169:333–338.

104. van der Poll T, Levi M, Hack E, ten Cate H, van Deventer S, Eerenberg A, de Groot E, Jansen J, Gallati H, Buller H, ten Cate J, Aarden L. Elimination of interleukin 6 attenuates coagulation activation in experimental endotoxemia in chimpanzees. J Exp Med 1994; 179:1253–1259.

105. Huber SA, Sakkinen P, Conze D, Hardin N, Tracy R. Interleukin-6 exacerbates early atherosclerosis in mice. Arterioscler Thromb Vasc Biol 1999; 19:2364–2367.

106. Biasucci L, Vitelli A, Liuzzo G, Altamura S, Caligiuri G, Monaco C, Rebuzzi A, Ciliberto G, Maseri A. Elevated levels of interleukin-6 in unstable angina. Circulation 1996; 94:874–877.

107. Geffken DF, Cushman M, Burke GL, Polak JF, Sakkinen PA, Tracy RP. Association between physical activity and markers of inflammation in a healthy elderly population. Am J Epidemiol 2000; 153:242–250.

108. Nieto F. Infections and atherosclerosis: new clues from an old hypothesis? Am J Epidemiol 1998; 148:937–948.

109. Patel P, Mendall M, Carrington D, Strachan D, Leatham E, Molineaux N, Levy J, Blakeston C, Seymour C, Camm A. Association of helicobactor pylori and chlamydia pneumoniae infections with coronary heart disease and cardiovascular risk factors. BMJ 1995; 311:711–714.

110. Davidson M, Kuo CC, Middaugh JP, Campbell LA, Wang SP, Newman WP 3rd, Finley JC, Grayston JT. Confirmed previous infection with *Chlamydia pneumoniae* (TWAR) and its presence in early coronary atherosclerosis. Circulation 1998; 98:628–633.

111. Ridker P, Hennekens C, Stampfer M, Wang F. Prospective study of herpes simplex virus, cytomegalovirus, and the risk of future myocardial infarction and stroke. Circulation 1998; 98:2796–2799.

112. Melnick S, Shahar E, Folsom A, Grayson J, Sorlie P, Wang S, Szklo M. Past infection by *Chlamydia* pneumonia strain TWAR and asymptomatic carotid atherosclerosis. The Atherosclerosis Risk in Communities (ARIC) study Investigators. Am J Med 1993; 95:499–504.

113. Saikku P, Leinonen M, Tenkanen L, Manninen V, Huttunen J. Chronic chlamydia pneumoniae infection as a risk factor for coronary heart disease (CHD) in the Helsinki Heart Study (HHS). Ann Intern Med 1992; 116:273–278.

114. Fryert R, Schwobe E, Woods M, Rodgers G. Chlamydia species infect human vascular endothelial cells and induce procoagulant activity. J Invest Med 1997; 45:168–174.

115. Humphries S, Cook M, Dubowitz M, Stirling Y, Meade T. Role of genetic variation at the fibrinogen locus in determination of plasma fibrinogen concentrations. Lancet 1987; i:1452–1455.

116. Fugger L, Morling N, Bendtzen K, Ryder L, Andersen V, Heilman C, Karup Pedersen F, Friis J, Halbert P, Svejgaard A. IL-6 gene polymorphism in rheumatoid arthritis, pauciarticular juvenile rheumatoid arthritis, systemic lupus erythematosus, and in healthy Danes. J Immunogenet 1989; 16:461–465.

117. Brinkman B, Zuijdgeest D, Kaijzel E, Breedveld F, Verweij C. Relevance of the tumor necrosis factor alpha (TNFa)-308 promoter polymorphism in TNFa gene regulation. J Inflammation 1996; 46:32–41.

118. Thomas A, Lamlum H, Humphries S, Green F. Linkage disequilibrium across the fibrinogen locus as shown by five genetic polymorphisms, G/A-455 (*HaeIII*), C/T-148 (*HindIII*/A1uI), T/G + 1689 (*AvaII*), and BclI (B-Fibrinogen) and *TaqI* (a-Fibrinogen), and their detection by PCR. Human Mutation 1994; 3:79–81.

119. Schmidt H, Schmidt R, Niederkorn K, Horner S, Becsagh P, Reinhart B, Schumacher M, Weinrauch V, Kostner GM. Beta-fibrinogen gene polymorphism (C148 → T) is associated with carotid atherosclerosis: results of the Austrian Stroke Prevention Study. Arterioscler Thromb Vasc Biol 1998; 18:487–492.

120. Gardemann A, Schwartz O, Haberbosch W, Katz N, WeiB T, Tillmanns H, Hehrlein F, Waas W, Eberbach A. Positive association of the B fibrinogen H1/H2 gene variation to basal fibrinogen levels and to the increase in fibrinogen concentration during acute phase reaction but not to coronary artery disease and myocardial infarction. Thromb Haemost 1997; 77:1120–1126.

121. de Maat MP, Kastelein JJ, Jukema JW, Zwinderman AH, Jansen H, Groenemeier B, Bruschke AV, Kluft C. −455G/A polymorphism of the beta-fibrinogen gene is associated with the progression of coronary atherosclerosis in symptomatic men:

proposed role for an acute-phase reaction pattern of fibrinogen. REGRESS group. Arterioscler Thromb Vasc Biol 1998; 18:265–271.

122. Humphries SE, Ye S, Talmud P, Bara L, Wilhelmsen L, Tiret L. European Athero-sclerosis Research Study: genotype at the fibrinogen locus (G-455-A beta-gene) is associated with differences in plasma fibrinogen levels in young men and women from different regions in Europe. Evidence for gender-genotype-environment inter-action. Arterioscler Thromb Vasc Biol 1995; 15:96–104.

123. Wang XL, Wang J, McCredie RM, Wilcken DE. Polymorphisms of factor V, factor VII, and fibrinogen genes. Relevance to severity of coronary artery disease. Arte-rioscler Thromb Vasc Biol 1997; 17:246–251.

124. Lander ES, Schork NJ. Genetic dissection of complex traits [published erratum appears in Science 1994 Oct 21; 266(5184):353]. Science 1994; 265:2037–2048.

125. Lander ES. The new genomics: global views of biology. Science 1996; 274:536–539.

126. Boerwinkle E, Ellsworth D, Hallman D, Biddinger A. Genetic analysis of athero-sclerosis: a research paradigm for the common chronic disease. Hum Mol Genet 1996; 5 Review: 1405–1410.

127. Fried L, Borhani N, Enright P, Furberg C, Gardin J, Kronmal R, Kuller L, Manolio T, Mittelmark M, Newman A, O'Leary D, Psaty B, Rautaharju P, Tracy R, Weiler P, for the CHS Research Group. The Cardiovascular Health Study: design and ratio-nale. Ann Epidemiol 1991; 1:263–276.

128. Ritchie D, Levy B, Adams M, Fuller G. Regulation of fibrinogen synthesis by plasmin-derived fragments of fibrinogen and fibrin: an indirect feedback pathway. Proc Natl Acad Sci USA 1982; 79:1530–1534.

129. Phillips A, Shaper A, Whincup P. Association between serum albumin and mortality from cardiovascular disease, cancer, and other causes. Lancet 1989; i:1434–1436.

130. Kuller L, Eichner J, Orchard T, Grandits G, McCallum, L, Tracy R, and the MRFIT Research Group. The relation between serum albumin levels and risk of coronary heart disease in the Multiple Risk Factor Intervention Trial. Am J Epidemiol 1991; 134:1266–1277.

131. Reunanen A, Knekt P, Aaran RK. Serum ceruloplasmin level and the risk of myo-cardial infarction and stroke. Am J Epidemiol 1992; 136:1082–1090.

132. Tietz N, ed. Clinical Guide to Laboratory Tests. Philadelphia: W.B. Saunders Co, 1990.

133. Schwertner H, Jackson W, Tolan G. Association of low serum concentration of bilirubin with increased risk of coronary artery disease. Clin Chem, 1994; 40:18–23.

134. Ettinger W, Harris T, Verdery R, Tracy R, Kouba E. Evidence for inflammation as a cause of hypocholesterolemia in older people. JAGS 1995; 43:264–266.

135. Salonen J, Nyyssonen K, Korpela H, Tuomilehto J, Seppanen R, Salonen R. High stored iron levels are associated with excess risk of myocardial infarction in eastern Finnish men. Circulation 1992; 86:803–811.

136. Ascherio A, Willett W, Rimm E, Giovannucci E, Stampfer M. Dietary iron intake and risk of coronary disease among men. Circulation 1994; 89:969–974.

137. Corit M-C, Guralnick J, Salive M, Ferrucci L, Pahor M, Wallace R, Hennekens C. Serum iron level, coronary artery disease, and all-cause mortality in older men and women. Am J Cardiol 1997; 79:120–127.

6
Role of Mechanical Stress in Plaque Rupture
Mechanical and Biological Interactions

Luis E. P. Rohde and Richard T. Lee
Brigham and Women's Hospital and Harvard Medical School, Boston, Massachusetts

I. INTRODUCTION

Atherosclerotic vascular disease is predominantly a clinically silent process. Approximately half of patients with atherosclerotic disease will first be aware of its consequences through the acute and catastrophic event of thrombosis. Through extensive research in the 1990s, it became apparent that mechanical plaque disruption initiates most thrombosis events, particularly in the coronary tree (1–4). Enormous attention has now focused on specific features that increase vulnerability of plaques to disruption, because determination of these features may allow prediction of plaques that are most likely to cause symptoms and acute events in the future.

Postmortem morphologic studies have described features characteristic of the unstable atheromatous plaque (5–7). Lesions with thin eccentric fibrous caps covering large lipid cores appear to be particularly predisposed to develop intimal tears and become unstable (8). Several investigators, notably Born, Richardson, and Davies, recognized the inherent structural instability of this configuration and proposed fundamental mechanical causes of plaque disruption (9, 10). These theories have led to additional proposed theories of the role of extracellular matrix in plaque stability (7). In the absence of readily available imaging tools to study plaque disruption in vivo, evaluation of these proposed mechanisms has depended on circumstantial evidence. However, the circumstantial evidence has been remarkably consistent, and it appears inevitable that additional clinical research will demonstrate the roles of mechanical forces and matrix biology in vivo.

In addition, the success of cholesterol-lowering therapy in reducing clinical events despite no clear angiographic lesion regression emphasizes that understanding the interplay of plaque architecture and composition, mechanical properties, and matrix biology may lead to new therapies that will change the natural history of the atheroma. This chapter introduces basic principles of vascular mechanics, focusing on topics related to the biomechanical behavior of normal and diseased vascular tissue, to provide the appropriate background for understanding the complex interactions of mechanical forces and matrix biology that lead to plaque rupture.

II. VASCULAR MECHANICS—BASIC PRINCIPLES

An important goal of studying the mechanics of materials is to ensure that a structure will be mechanically sound when confronted with the combined effect of applied forces. By understanding the behavior of different materials under distinct conditions, we can estimate the probability that a structure can withstand the stresses it will face in the future. It is important to realize that with all materials, fracture (or rupture) is a probability distribution determined by the nature of the imposed stresses and the strength of the material. Strength is a property that results from the material's structure, which includes the distribution, orientation, and interconnection of its constituents. First, we will introduce basic concepts and terms of solid mechanics to provide the common-ground understanding and vocabulary for a more detailed discussion of the mechanical and biological interactions that take place during atherosclerotic plaque initiation, progression, and rupture.

A. Stress, Strain, and the Stress–Strain Relationship

Stress is defined as force acting on a surface and is expressed in units of force divided by the area of the surface (Figure 1a, Table 1). Stress can be characterized by the direction (vector) of forces: "normal" or "radial" stresses represent forces applied perpendicular to a surface, whereas "shear" or "tangential" stresses represent forces applied parallel to a surface. Normal stresses may be compressive (when the structure tends to shrink) or tensile (when the structure tends to elongate). It is important to realize that stresses may be applied in any direction, and one type of stress can lead to other types of stresses. When a cylinder is pressurized, for example, the radial stress must be counterbalanced by a circumferential tensile stress in the vessel wall. Under the assumption that

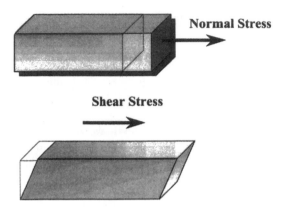

Figure 1 Top panel, Normal vs. shear stress. On a given block of a material stress can be applied perpendicular or normal to one of the faces on the block. A shear or tangential stress is applied parallel to a face. Bottom panel, Strain occurs as a result of stress, but the two terms should not be used interchangeably. In its simplest form, strain in one dimension can be expressed as the percentage of its initial length that a structure increases in length when stress is applied (From Rohde L, Lee R. Mechanical stress and strain and the vulnerable atherosclerotic lesion. In: Fuster V, ed. The Vulnerable Atherosclerotic Plaque: Understanding, Identification, and Modification. Armonk, NY: Futura Publishing Company Inc., 1998.)

Table 1 Definitions of Important Terms in Vascular Mechanics.

Stress	Force acting on a surface, per unit of area. Stress is directional: normal/radial, tangential/shear, or circumferential.
Strain	Deformation resulting from a force, usually expressed as a fraction or a percentage of the change in length.
Stiffness	General term describing resistance to deformation.
Compliance	Change in volume per change in pressure.
Elastic modulus	Fundamental material property that describes the relation between stress and strain.
Linear behavior	Occurs when the stress-strain relations are constant over the range of stresses.
Nonlinear elasticity	Occurs when increments in strain are changed for each increment in stress; common in biological materials.
Isotropy	Property that describes materials in which the direction of stresses does not alter the stress-strain relation.
Anisotropy	Property that describes materials in which the direction of stresses interferes with the stress-strain relation; common in biological materials.
Viscoelasticity	Time-dependence of the stress-strain responses.

the wall of the cylinder is thin relative to the diameter of the vessel, it can be demonstrated that:

$$\sigma = Pr/h$$

where σ is the tensile wall stress, P is the pressure in the vessel, r is the radius of the vessel, and h is the thickness of the vessel. This well-known equation is Laplace's relation, or Lame's equation.

Laplace's relation greatly oversimplifies the forces in the vessel, and much more complex equations are required to understand thick cylinders or cylinders with asymmetric lumens. However, Laplace's relation is a useful way of considering some common clinical problems. For example, Laplace's relation helps to explain why the probability of rupture of aortic aneurysms is closely related to the maximal diameter of the aneurysm (because stress is directly proportional to radius) and why blood pressure control is essential for the management of patients with aortic aneurysms (because stress is also directly proportional to pressure). In heterogeneous structures, such as the atherosclerotic coronary artery, the stresses become quite complex, but the concept of the thin fibrous cap (causing increased stress as thickness "h" decreases) still holds true.

It is common—and useful—to focus on the dominant stress in a given configuration. For example, blood flow in a normal artery creates a shear stress on the surface of the endothelium in the direction of blood flow. Similarly, blood pressure causes circumferential tension in the wall of the vessel. In reality, the stresses on the vessel and vascular cells are much more complex. Normal and shear stresses interact throughout the vessel and even within a given cell. For example, shear stress on the luminal surface of an endothelial cell subjects cytoskeletal elements inside the cell to tensile stress. Thus, even with sophisticated modern engineering techniques, we tend to simplify the mechanics of the artery.

When a surface is subjected to a force (such as the effects of blood pressure on endothelial cells), the resulting deformation is the *strain* (Figure 1b, Table 1). Strain is usually expressed as a fraction or a percentage of the change in length:

Strain $= \Delta$ *length/original length*

Strains can also be tensile (positive strain) or compressive (negative strain). For the same amount of stress acting on two materials with different mechanical properties, the amount of deformation (strains) will differ. A simple demonstration of strain is the stretching of a rubber band by a gentle tug; the amount of elongation of the rubber band divided by its original length is the strain. When we consider three-dimensional structures, a more comprehensive description of strain using matrices is required; these are often called Green strains, or LaGrangian strains, after the mathematicians that described their use.

The stress-strain relationship of a material is a fundamental characterization of its mechanical behavior. Stiff materials (such as thick fibrous caps of an atherosclerotic lesion) will respond to large stresses with minimal deformation. E is the ratio of stress to strain and is called the *elastic modulus* or the *Young's modulus*:

$$E = stress/strain$$

In many circumstances the ratio between stress and strain is constant over the range of stresses imposed on a structure (*linear elastic behavior*). If the vessel wall were made of a uniform, incompressible, linear elastic material, the elastic modulus (E) would describe most of its mechanical behavior. In most biological materials, however, the increments in strain decrease for each increment of stress, so that the material actually becomes stiffer when exposed to higher levels of stress (*nonlinear elasticity*, Table 1). In addition, most biological materials, including the vessel wall, have complex geometrical structures that have different stress-strain relationships in different directions, an important property called *anisotropy* (Table 1). The highly anisotropic nature of the vessel makes its biomechanical characterization much more difficult, and relatively few measurements of the critical variables needed to describe anisotropy have been made in diseased human arteries.

Another important factor that must be considered to understand the stress-strain relation is the time-dependence of the stress-strain responses. When stress is removed from a perfectly elastic material, strain will decrease and the material will immediately assume its unstressed shape. On the other hand, strains in *viscoelastic* materials (such as most of the constituents of the vessel wall) will gradually decrease over time, a phenomenon called creep. Numerous mathematical models can be used to describe this time dependence of the stress-strain relation (11).

III. NORMAL VESSELS

The arterial wall consists of three layers: tunica intima, media, and adventitia. The intima has a one-cell-thick layer of axially oriented endothelial cells over a thin basal membrane that probably bears little of the stress load of the vessel. The adventitia is composed primarily of loose collagen fibers with admixed elastin, fibroblasts, and vasa vasorum that helps to anchor the artery, particularly in the longitudinal direction. It is generally accepted that the structural integrity of the arterial wall results primarily from layers of smooth muscle cells, collagen, and elastin, which are the main components of the tunica media. Elastin is a highly extensible fiber that can be stretched to many times its initial length without rupturing, although it can fracture at relatively low levels of stress (12). Elastin behaves much like a linear elastic material (hence its name), because it deforms with strain proportional to stress and rapidly returns to its initial shape when stresses are removed. Although elastin is an important contributor to the normal pulsatile behavior of the vessel, it is much less important in determining its overall strength, because elastin fibers are easily broken.

Collagen fibers, in contrast, have much higher fracture stresses compared with elastin. Collagen has a tensile modulus several thousand times higher than that of elastin and can tolerate stresses more than 100 times greater than levels that usually would fracture elastin fibers (13, 14). Roach and Burton suggested that elastin and collagen are the main components that govern the passive arterial responses at low and high pressures, respectively (15). At low stresses and strain, collagen fibers are not under tension, and the "rubber-band-like" properties of elastin fibers dominate the mechanical behavior of the artery. At higher stresses and strains, elastin fibers stretch to their limit, and collagen fibers are sequentially recruited so that the vessel becomes stiffer and more resistant to rupture. This type of fiber network leads to highly nonlinear material behavior but is well suited to the task of the artery.

Smooth muscle cells also play an essential role in the active behavior of the vessel. By vasoconstricting or vasodilating, the vessel can adjust its luminal diameter and influence both wall stiffness and blood flow. In addition, smooth muscle cells are the major source of vascular extracellular matrix, including collagen, elastin, and proteoglycans.

A. Behavior of Normal Arteries

1. Residual Stress

For any given solid structure, identification of a reference configuration (the original stress-free configuration to which the material will return after any reversible process) is essential for stress analyses. Residual stress is the stress that exists in a body in the absence of externally applied forces. Several investigators, notably Fung and Vaishnay, studied the influence and importance of residual stress in determining arterial biomechanical behavior along the vascular tree (16–19). They observed that intact unloaded artery rings open up at different angles in response to longitudinal cuts. Several of their experiments demonstrate that these different opening angles (representing distinct levels of residual stress) vary with species and with the location along the vascular tree and that they usually continue to gradually increase after the cuts are made, suggesting a viscoelastic component (20, 21).

2. Passive Behavior and Active Behavior

The behavior of an artery, both in active (dependent on smooth muscle cell activity) and passive states, is nonlinear over finite strains, irrespective of location along the vascular tree. In the absence of smooth muscle tone, most arteries demonstrate stress relaxation under constant extension and creep under constant loads (indicating viscoelastic behavior) (22). Interestingly, some experiments indicate that axial extension tends to make the vessel stiffer in the circumferential direction after cyclic pressurization (23). This pattern of interaction between forces acting in different directions may represent mechanisms by which the vessel protects itself against acute hemodynamic challenges.

The active behavior of normal arteries has been evaluated by pressure-diameter and axial force-length tests on cylindrical segments, because these experiments can mimic in vivo loads (24, 25). Norepinephrine and potassium chloride infusions or baths are most commonly used to evoke these responses. If the passive stress is subtracted from the active stress at each strain state, one can obtain the active stress-strain behavior. It appears that the active response is similar for various arteries, is length-dependent, and peaks at a particular circumferential stretch (L_{max}). This type of behavior is similar to Frank-Starling behavior exhibited by skeletal and cardiac muscles (22).

IV. THE DISEASED VESSEL

A. General Structure

The atheroma is a complex structure of many cells and matrix components with great spatial heterogeneity. Understanding mechanical behavior of such a complex structure is facilitated by breaking down the structure into simpler components. Thus, we can consider typical atherosclerotic lesions as consisting of three predominant components: (a) *plaque cap*, composed mainly of dense collagen fibers; (b) the *necrotic plaque core*, usually consisting of a disorganized mass of lipid material, cholesterol clefts, cellular debris and fibrin; and (c) the underlying vessel wall, including the media and adventitia (similar to those of the healthy vessel). Plaque composition may in fact vary as a function of the percentage of stenosis, age, gender, and clinical presentation. Kragel et al., for example, found that the amount of dense fibrous tissue and calcium increases progressively as the vessel narrows, whereas the percentage of cellular fibrous tissue tends to decrease (26).

The mechanics of the atherosclerotic lesion are not easily considered with simple formulas such as the Laplace equation. However, progress has been made in determining some of the important mechanical properties of the different components of the human atheroma, and these data have allowed further understanding of the atheroma as a whole.

B. The Plaque Cap

Several studies have evaluated mechanical properties of the atherosclerotic vessel by comparing diseased arteries and nondiseased control vessels. Most of these studies used uniaxial tension tests on vessel strips or passive pressure-diameter experiments. These reports were consistent in demonstrating that the atherosclerotic vessel wall is stiffer than the nondiseased wall. Many of these experiments evaluated the entire vessel, rather than comparing separate data on the atherosclerotic plaque or its components. Kinney et al., for example, evaluated the response of diseased and nondiseased vessels after angioplasty and reported the percentage change in the luminal cross-sectional area as a function of pressure. Nondiseased specimens exhibited greater distensibility than diseased vessels, and most of the changes in luminal area (>85%) were due to plaque disruption rather than to tissue compaction or content extrusion. Interestingly, points of sudden change in compliance occurred at lower stresses in calcified lesions compared with noncalcified vessels, probably indicating microscopic tears in the artery near calcium deposits (27).

These studies were useful for understanding the hemodynamics of the arterial system as a whole, because gradual stiffening leads to changes in systemic vascular impedance and pulse wave reflection. However, to understand the atheroma, we need to consider the individual components of the atheroma. Lendon et al. investigated both ulcerated and non-ulcerated plaque caps from human aorta and observed that only non-ulcerated lesions demonstrated significant associations between vessel stiffness, collagen content, and stress (28). Born and Richardson tested the hypothesis that the propensity to rupture depends on the structural and physical properties of the atherosclerotic lesion (9). They subjected human coronary artery plaque caps from diseased vessels and the near nondiseased intima to uniaxial tensile tests. Plaque caps demonstrated less elongation than normal intima for a given level of stress (load) and a distinctive sudden rise in stress values with negligible increases in elongation. Supporting the concept that biological features influence the mechanical behavior of atherosclerotic lesions, Lendon et al. evaluated whether macrophage density reduces plaque cap strength (29). Aortic strips from ulcerated and nonulcerated plaque caps were subjected to mechanical testing and analyzed to evaluate macrophage density. Plaque caps without tearing had significantly fewer macrophages than lesions with fissures. In addition, nonulcerated plaques needed approximately three times higher levels of stress to fracture than intact lesions. Stress-strain data from these samples clearly reveal the nonlinear behavior of plaque caps and the influence of cellular aspects on the mechanical behavior of the lesion.

We and others have reported experiments evaluating the role of the fibrous cap composition and thickness as a critical factor in determining lesion stress and propensity to rupture (30). We performed dynamic and static uniaxial compression tests in aortic atherosclerotic lesions and reported mechanical data as a function of plaque cap type, classified by standard histological studies as primarily cellular, hypocellular, or calcific. Overall, it was demonstrated that stiffness is significantly greater (two to five times) in calcific lesions compared with hypocellular and cellular caps, that the viscoelastic component is prominent in plaque caps with cellular dominance, and that plaque stiffness increases as the loading frequency is increased. Loree et al. evaluated the tensile behavior of aortic plaque caps and also correlated this behavior with the underlying plaque composition (cellular, hypocellular, or calcific). At a physiological applied circumferential tensile stress of 25 kPa, the tangential moduli of cellular, hypocellular, and calcified specimens was 927 ± 468 kPa, 2323 ± 2180 kPa, and 1466 ± 1284 kPa, respectively. Although no statistical significant differences in static tensile stiffness were observed among histologically different plaque groups, the tangential modulus increased progressively with the percent strain, providing direct evidence of the nonlinear tensile behavior of plaque caps (31). Taken together, these studies indicate that the stress-strain behavior of atherosclerotic plaques is, in fact, composition dependent, anisotropic, and nonlinear.

C. The Lipid Core

Description of plaque cap mechanical properties has been a great focus of attention from biomechanical investigations, but other regions from the atherosclerotic lesion may also influence its mechanical behavior. Kaltenbach et al. examined core morphology of atherosclerotic lesions and evaluated the effects of prolonged pressure compression (5 atm for 3–60 seconds) during transluminal coronary angioplasty. Lesions classified as lipoid by histological analysis had a twofold greater reduction in thickness after angioplasty than fibrotic plaques (32). Similarly, Loree et al. hypothesized that the lipid composition of the plaque core could interfere with the mechanical properties of the atheroma. In this study, four types of plaque lipid pools were artificially created, primarily composed of different amounts of cholesterol monohydrate, phospholipids, and triglycerides. The specimens were subject to cyclic shear loading, and the dynamic shear modulus was measured. A significant positive association was observed between the dynamic shear moduli and the concentration of cholesterol monohydrate in each specimen, indicating that mechanical behavior of the lipid core is also composition-dependent (33).

D. Calcified Plaques

Arterial calcification is a common feature of atherosclerosis, occurring in most angiographically significant lesions. Most plaques that rupture, however, are not heavily calcified (34), and focal calcifications probably are not as important as fibrous plaque cap thickness in predisposing to plaque rupture. Calcification of lesions, however, can have a significant impact on the outcome of balloon angioplasty, in which calcium deposits may accentuate the dissection that generally accompanies successful procedures. Vogt et al. recently suggested that the presence of calcification was a favorable prognostic characteristic that could predict which lesions would remain patent after peripheral angioplasty (35). It is important to recognize that balloon angioplasty, in most cases, is successful, in part, because of shear created between layers of the artery as the balloon expands to diameters that the artery does not experience under normal conditions. The mechanisms that control calcium deposition in the vascular system are not well understood, but recent evidence suggests that development of atherosclerotic calcification is under regulatory controls similar to osteogenesis (36). Data from genetically engineered mice also indicate that vascular calcification has an inherited component, with incomplete penetrance (37).

E. Finite Element Analysis

Another approach that some investigators have used to study the mechanical properties of the vulnerable lesion is through *finite element analysis*. Finite element analysis is a widely used engineering technique used to study complex three-dimensional structures. By subdividing a complex structure into much smaller sections and assigning specific mechanical properties for each element, the distribution of stresses within the original structure can be calculated (Figure 2). As described later, such an approach has provided important insight into the nature of the vulnerable lesion, being supported by postmortem findings and as clinical data.

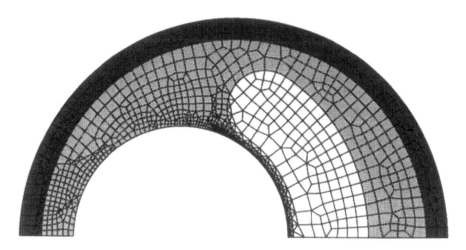

Figure 2   Representative example of a finite element mesh from a vessel wall. The vessel wall is subdivided in much smaller sections, and specific mechanical properties can be assigned for each element, allowing the estimation of the distribution of stresses within the original structure. Different shades of gray represent areas where distinct mechanical properties will be assigned to reach the final stress solution (From Ref. 38.)

Loree et al. used the finite element method to study two-dimensional cross-sections of diseased vessels similar to intravascular ultrasonographic images. In this study, it was hypothesized that subintimal plaque structural features such as thickness of the fibrous cap could be more important factors in the distribution of stress in the plaque than stenosis severity. With a constant luminal area reduction (70%), maximum circumferential stress had a fourfold increase as the thickness of the lipid pool was increased because of a thinner fibrous cap. Conversely, increasing the stenosis severity solely by incrementing the fibrous cap thickness induced a fivefold decrease in maximum circumferential stress (38). Figure 3 illustrates the effect of plaque cap thickness on maximum circumferential stress normalized to luminal pressure. Note that when fibrous cap thickness falls below 200 μm, stress increases to levels that have been shown to be necessary to fracture human atherosclerotic tissue.

Using the finite element method, Richardson et al. published landmark data on the association of vulnerable lesion pathological conditions, mechanical stress, and plaque rupture (39). In this study of human coronary plaque fissures, these investigators suggested that the particularly common configuration of a fissure

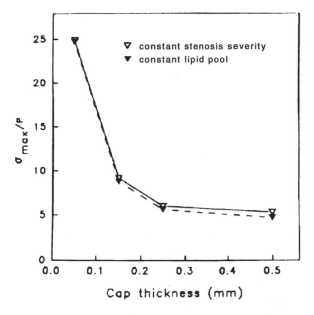

Figure 3 The effect of plaque cap thickness on maximum circumferential stress normalized to luminal pressure. When fibrous cap thickness falls below 0.2 mm, circumferential stress increases exponentially, reaching levels shown to be necessary to fracture human atherosclerotic tissue. (From Ref. 38.)

through the edge of a fibrous cap was due to high circumferential tensile stress in the fibrous cap. Evaluating different plaque geometries that caused lethal coronary thrombosis, they observed increased levels of circumferential stress concentrating at the edges of the fibrous cap near the border of normal intima, mainly in lesions with large lipid pools. This concentration of stress was due to the inability of the soft lipid core to bear the large mechanical stresses that develop during blood pressure elevations or repetitive dynamic stresses caused by the pulsatile blood pressure. Supporting these results, Cheng et al. demonstrated that the magnitude of circumferential stress in plaques of patients who died of acute coronary events was significantly greater than maximum stress in stable control lesions (4091 $\pm$ 1199 vs. 1444 $\pm$ 485 mmHg; $p < 0.001$). In most lesions, the actual plaque ruptures occurred in high-stress locations, defined as regions with stresses greater than 2250 mmHg. Interestingly, it was also observed that the location of plaque rupture was not always the area of greatest stress in an individual lesion (40). This observation suggests that local variations in plaque strength may determine which regions of high stress actually evolve to rupture.

F. Plaque Fatigue

Most studies of mechanical properties of atherosclerotic lesions indicate that isolated oscillations of heart rate or blood pressure may not be sufficient to cause a plaque to fissure. Plaque fracture may be in fact an insidious process that culminates with structural damage induced by the cumulative effects of cyclic stresses. The repetitive deformations caused by the cardiac cycle may play an important role in lesion stability. Supporting this concept, McCord and Ku studied arterial rings subjected to cyclic bending loads and evaluated microscopical sections to look for indications of mechanical failure. Histological analysis revealed that fatigued sections had much more structural changes than control specimens. In addition, during mechanical tests after fatigue loading, plaque fracture was significantly more common in the previously fatigued sections compared with controls (41).

G. Imaging, Mechanical Behavior, and Atherosclerosis

Recently, high-frequency intravascular ultrasonographic imaging has received great attention as a potentially useful and safe method to evaluate atherosclerotic lesions in vivo. Several investigators described the most common morphological features are present in lesions from patients with acute myocardial and stable angina, such as the presence of thrombus, fissures, dissection, degree of stenosis, and eccentricity of the lesion (42, 43).

We used high-frequency intravascular ultrasonographic imaging as a surrogate technique to evaluate the composition of human atherosclerotic tissue. Intravascular ultrasonographic analyses of plaque cap composition (as nonfibrous,

fibrous, or calcified lesions) had good agreement with histological analysis (44). Static compressive stiffness from plaque caps and the time required to reach equilibrium at a constant load were shown to correlate with intravascular ultrasound plaque classifications, suggesting that intravascular imaging could be eventually applied to identify specific lesions predisposed to instability. Structural analysis based on intravascular ultrasonographic imaging performed before in vitro balloon angioplasty was also studied to evaluate whether it could predict unstable regions from atherosclerotic lesions. This approach was able to predict most (82%) of the locations of plaque fracture, an event that usually accompanies angioplasty (Figure 4) (45).

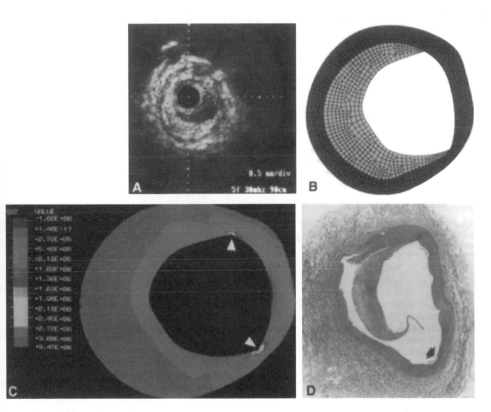

Figure 4   (A) Intravascular ultrasonographic image of atherosclerotic iliac artery. (B) Finite element mesh of ultrasonographic image. The dark elements represent near normal vessel; the lighter elements are fibrous plaque. (C) Finite element solution demonstrating high circumferential stress locations >3 MPa (arrowheads). Values at left in Pascal. (D) Photomicrograph (~x12) of vessel after angioplasty, stained with hematoxylin-eosin. Arrow denotes the site of intimal plaque fracture. (From Ref. 45.)

Current clinical tools are unable to measure the thickness of the atherosclerotic plaque layers in vivo, particularly in the submillimeter range. Because current data indicate that lesion area reduction is not a dominant factor in determining stress in the fibrous cap, our most routinely used method of coronary artery analyses, angiography, is not a good tool for determining plaque stability. This may be one of the reasons that some of the plaques that rupture and cause myocardial infarction are frequently not angiographically severe. Advances in techniques such as optical coherence tomography, magnetic resonance, and intravascular ultrasonography may provide sufficient vessel wall resolution in the future to estimate plaque stability.

H. High-Stress Regions and the Atheroma Matrix

It is important to note that nonbiological materials may undergo fatigue when subjected to deformation, whereas biological materials may compensate under some circumstances to increase tissue strength. It is possible that failure of the fibrous cap cells to adequately compensate for increased mechanical challenges may be a major factor in plaque instability. In fact, it is becoming apparent that these processes (fatigue, fissure, and rupture) depend on the interplay of plaque architecture and composition, mechanical properties, and extracellular matrix biology.

The variable and seemingly unpredictable nature of plaque rupture has focused attention on the atherosclerotic lesion as an active biological structure, particularly within the extracellular matrix. In the absence of inflammation or injury, many connective tissues have little evidence of active extracellular matrix synthesis and degradation; instead, they appear to be dormant or with a very slow rate of remodeling. Nonetheless, when tissues are injured and the repair process begins, both synthetic and degradative pathways greatly accelerate. Complex interactions among biological factors regulate the synthesis and breakdown of extracellular matrix. Several observations demonstrate that increased density of T-lymphocytes and macrophage-derived foam cells accumulate "in the shoulder area" of atheromas (46). These inflammatory cells secrete cytokines and proteolytic enzymes, resulting in both decreased synthesis and an enhanced destruction of extracellular matrix.

Matrix metalloproteinases are an important family of proteolytic enzymes that participate in the initial stages of matrix remodeling and have been the focus of intense research (47, 48). We recently demonstrated that regions of high circumferential stress in the shoulder area of atherosclerotic plaques have a twofold to fivefold increase in matrix metalloproteinase expression, an enzyme that initiates fibrillar collagen degradation (49). Although statistical associations like this do not prove a cause-and-effect relationship, it raises the intriguing possibility that mechanical forces acting in specific regions of the atheroma could actually induce an active biological process rather than promote weakening of the extracellular matrix. Several lines of evidence support this hypothesis. One possible source of matrix metalloproteinases in the fibrous cap shoulders is the vascular smooth muscle cell, although the absolute number of smooth muscle cells in unstable fibrous caps is not high. Mechanical signals are powerful regulators of cellular functions, and it has been known for more than 20 years that mechanical deformation regulates extracellular matrix synthesis by vascular smooth muscle cells in vivo. In 1976, Leung et al. reported that mechanical stretch increased matrix synthesis by vascular smooth muscle cells (50).

Recent studies also demonstrate that mechanical modulation of molecular signs may influence vascular remodeling We recently tested the hypothesis that very small mechanical strains interact with growth factors in the regulation of matrix metalloproteinase-1 (MMP-1) secreted by human vascular smooth muscle cells. Unexpectedly, small biaxial strains did not induce MMP-1 in vascular smooth muscle cells, but strain was a potent inhibitor of platelet-derived growth factor and tumor necrosis factor-α induced synthesis of MMP-1. Although this study did not support a direct positive induction of MMP-1 by small mechanical forces on human smooth muscle cells, it demonstrated an exquisite sensitivity of the cell to mechanical stimuli (51).

An alternative explanation for the increase in MMP-1 at high-stress atheroma regions is that MMP-1 expression in the atherosclerotic lesions is increased directly or through paracrine mechanisms involving the macrophage. In fact, several recent reports indicate that monocytes and macrophages are also mechanically responsive. For example, Martin et al. hypothesized that changes in morphology are a common feature of the macrophage activation and that stretch-activated ion channels may play an important role in these processes. They identified an outwardly rectifying potassium channel that is inactive at rest but activated by adhesion of cells or stretch of the membrane (52). Mastsumoto et al. also studied the morphology of monocyte-like cell lines and rat peritoneal macrophages with a uniaxial stretch device. They found evidence suggesting that cyclic stretch inhibits the differentiation to vacuolized cells and facilitates the differentiation to spindle cells (53). We recently reported that mechanical deformation of monocytes/macrophages through biaxial strains rapidly induce the PU.1 transcription factor, an ets-family transcription factor that is essential in monocyte differentiation. In addition, MMP-1 and MMP-3 expression were also induced by cyclic strain (54).

The cellular mechanisms by which mechanical stimuli are translated into biological processes are not fully understood. Multiple transduction pathways may participate in converting mechanical signals into biochemical products, including stretch-activated ion channels, paracrine growth factors, G proteins, MAP kinases, integrins, tyrosine kinases, and phospholipid metabolism (55–58). No single gene or signaling pathway seems to be responsible for all mechanotransduction; in different experimental conditions, different pathways may predominate. It is likely that these studies have only begun to characterize the molecular response of different cell lines to mechanical stimuli.

V. SUMMARY AND CONCLUSIONS

Although much of our insight into the mechanism of plaque formation, progression, and rupture is based on circumstantial evidence, a plausible pathophysiological pathway has emerged in the last few years. Accumulation of a lipid core beneath a fibrous cap sets the stage for instability by gradually increasing the mechanical stresses in the fibrous cap. If the plaque cap is thin and weak and after the cumulative effects of cyclic challenges, high mechanical stresses may approach fracture levels in the fibrous cap, culminating with structural damage in somewhat predictable regions of the plaque. For reasons not fully understood, inflammation and matrix degradation are particularly increased at these high-stress locations. Recent evidence strongly suggests that mechanical forces and biologically active processes are not separate factors in this process, but rather are intricately associated components that can greatly influence the stability of atherosclerotic lesions.

Several clinical observations are consistent with this model of plaque instability and rupture. Because stenosis severity is not a major determinant of stress in atherosclerotic lesions, it is not surprising that angiography has been a disappointing method of identifying vulnerable lesions. In fact, clinical identification of the unstable plaque has been an elusive task. It is expected that newer imagining techniques, such as intravascular ultrasonography and optical coherence tomography, will have enough resolution to evaluate and identify specific features that increase vulnerability to disruption, such as thin fibrous caps over large lipid cores and high-stress locations with increased inflammatory responses. Angiographic studies also suggest that the huge benefits of lipid-lowering therapy in reducing cardiovascular morbidity and mortality (59) are not associated with major changes in lesion severity. This raises the intriguing possibility that the benefits of lipid-lowering therapy are related to modifications of plaque structure and biology rather than to absolute lesion regression. When Aikawa et al. studied aortic atherosclerosis in rabbits with high- and low-cholesterol diets, they found that rabbits fed low-cholesterol diets had less inflammation and less expression of proteolytic enzymes, whereas the amount of dense collagen increased (60). Furthermore, recent epidemiological studies suggest that the inflammatory process precedes clinical events by many years (61). This potentially provides us with a prolonged window of opportunity to intervene before atherosclerotic lesions culminate in acute events. The combination of early detection of vulnerable lesions and implementation of therapies aimed to improve the integrity of the vulnerable lesion may be the foundations for a new strategy to prevent acute catastrophic vascular events.

REFERENCES

1. Constantinides P. Plaque fissure in human coronary thrombosis. J Atheroscler Res 1966; 6:1–17.
2. Davies MJ, Thomas A. Thrombosis and acute coronary-artery lesions in sudden cardiac ischemic death. N Engl J Med 1984; 310:1137–1140.
3. Farb A, Tang AL, Burke AP, Sessums L, Liang Y, Virmani R. Sudden coronary death: frequency of active coronary lesions, inactive coronary lesions, and myocardial infarction. Circulation 1995; 92:1701–1709.
4. Davies MJ, Bland JM, Hangartener JRW, Angelini A, Thomas AC. Factors influencing the presence or absence of acute coronary artery thrombi in sudden cardiac ischemic death. Eur Heart J 1989; 10:203–208.
5. Lee RT, Schoen FJ. Pathology of unstable coronary plaque. In: Rutherford JD, ed. Unstable Angina. New York: Marcel Dekker, Inc. 1991:1–25.
6. Barger AC, Beeuwkes R, Lainey LL, Silverman KJ. Hypothesis: Vasa vasorum and neo-vascularization of human coronary arteries: A possible role in the pathophysiology of atherosclerosis. N Engl J Med 1991; 88:8154–8158.
7. Lee RT, Libby P. The unstable atheoma. Artherioscler Thromb Vasc Biol 1997; 17: 1859–1867.
8. Farb A, Burke AP, Tang AL, Liang Y Mannan P, Smialek J, Virmani R. Coronary plaque erosion without rupture into a lipid core: a frequent cause of coronary thrombosis in sudden coronary death. Circulation 1996; 93:1354–1363.
9. Born GVR, Richardson PD. Mechanical properties of human atherosclerosis. In: Glagov S, Newman W, Schaffer S, eds. Pathobiology of the Human Atherosclerotic Plaques. New York: Springer-Verlag. 1990:413–424.
10. Davies MJ, Thomas AC. Plaque fissuring—the cause of acute myocardial infarction, sudden ischemic death, and crescendo angina. Br Heart J 1985; 53:363–373.
11. Lee RT, Kamm RD. Vascular mechanics for the cardiologists. J Am Coll Cardiol 1994; 23:1289–1295.
12. Mukherjee DP, Kagan HM Jordan RE, Franzblau C. Effects of hydrophobic elastin ligans on the stress-strain properties of elastin fibers. Connect Tissue Res 1976; 4: 177–179.
13. Kato YP, Christiansen DL, Hahn RA, Shien JJ, Golstein JD, Silver FH. Mechanical properties of collagen fibers: a comparison of reconstituted and rat tail tendon fibers. Biomaterials 1989; 10:38–42.
14. Kato YP, Silver FH. Formation of continuous collagen fibers: evaluation of biocompatibility and mechanical properties. Biomaterials 1990; 11:169–75.
15. Roach MR, Burton AC. The reason for the shape of the distensibility curve of arteries. Can J Biochem Physiol 1957; 35:681–690.
16. Chuong CJ, Fung YC. On residual stress in arteries. ASME J Biomech Engr 1986; 108:189–192.

17. Vaishnav RN, Vossoughi J. Residual stress and strain in aortic segments. J Biomech 1987; 20:235–239.
18. Liu SQ, Fung YC. Zero-stress states of arteries. ASME J Biomech Engr 1988; 110: 82–84.
19. Liu SQ, Fung YC. Change in residual strains in arteries due to hypertrophy caused by aortic constriction. Circ Res 1989; 65:1340–1349.
20. Han HC, Fung YC. Species dependence of the zero-stress state of aorta: pigs versus rat. ASME J Biomech Engr 1991; 113:446–451.
21. Fung YC, Liu SQ. Changes in zero-stress state of rat pulmonary arteries in hypoxic hypertension. J Appl Physiol 1991; 70:2455–2470.
22. Humphrey JD. Mechanics of arterial wall: reviews and directions. Crit Rev Biomed Eng 1995; 23(1–2):1–162.
23. Weizsacker HW, Lambert H, Pascale K. Analysis of the passive mechanical properties of rat carotid arteries. J Biomech 1983; 16:703–715.
24. Dobrin PB. Biaxial anisotropy of dog carotid artery: estimation of circumferential elastic modulus. J Biomech 1986; 19:351–358.
25. Cox RH. Comparison of carotid artery mechanics in rat, rabbit and dog. Am J Physiol 1978; 234:H280–288.
26. Kragel AH, Reddy SG, Wittes JT, Roberts WC. Morphometric analysis of the composition of atherosclerotic plaques in the four major epicardial coronary arteries in acute myocardial infarction and in sudden coronary death. Circulation 1989; 80: 1747–1756.
27. Kinney TB, Chin AK, Rurik GW, Finn JC, Shoor FM, Hayden WG, Fogarty TJ. Transluminal angioplasty: a mechanical, pathological correlation of its physical mechanism. Radiology 1984; 153:85–89.
28. Lendon CL, Briggs AD, Born GVR, Burleigh MC, Davies MJ. Mechanical testing of the connective tissue in the search for determinants of atherosclerotic plaque cap rupture. Biochem Soc Trans 1988; 16(6):1032–1033.
29. Lendon Cl, Davies MJ, Born GVR, Richardson PD. Atherosclerotic plaque caps are locally weakened when macrophages density is increased. Atherosclerosis 1991; 87: 87–90.
30. Lee RT, Grodzinsky AJ, Franf EH, Kamm RD, Schoen FJ. Structure dependent dynamic mechanical behavior of fibrous caps from human atherosclerotic plaque. Circulation 1991; 83:1764–1770.
31. Loree HM, Grodzinsky AJ, Park SY, Gibson LJ, Lee RT. Static circumferential modulus of human atherosclerotic tissue. J Biomechanics 1994; 27:195–204.
32. Kaltenbach M, Beyer J, Waltr S, Klepzig H, Schmidts L. Prolonged application of pressure in transluminal coronary angioplasty. Catheterization Cardiovasc Diagn 1984; 10:213–219.
33. Loree HM, Tobias BJ, Gibson LJ, Kamm RD, Small DM, Lee RT. Mechanical properties of model atherosclerotic lesion lipid pools. Arterioscler Thromb 1994; 14:230–234.
34. Moriuchi M, Saito S, Takaiwa Y, Honye J, Fukui T, Horiuchi K, Takayama T, Yajima J, Shimizu T, Chiku M, Komaki K, Tanigawa N, Ozawa Y, Kanmatsuse K. Assessment of plaque rupture by intravascular ultrasound. Heart Vessels 1997; 12: 178–181.

35. Vogt KC, Just S, Rasmussen JG, Schroeder TV. Prediction of outcome after femoro-popliteal balloon angioplasty by intravascular ultrasound. Eur J Vasc Endovasc Surg 1997;6:563–568.

36. Watson KE, Abrolat ML, Malone LL, Hoeg JM, Doherty T, Detrano R, Demmer LL. Active serum vitamin D levels are inversely correlated with coronary calcification. Circulation 1997; 6:1755–1760.

37. Qiao JH, Xie PZ, Fishbein MC, Kreuzer J, Drake TA, Demer LL, Lusis AJ. Pathology of atheromatous lesions in inbred and genetically engineered mice. Genetic determination of arterial calcification. Arterioscler Thromb 1994; 9:1480–1497.

38. Loree HM, Kamm RD, Stringfellow RG, Lee RT. Effects of fibrous cap thickness on peak circumferential stress in model atherosclerotic vessels. Circ Res 1992; 71:850–858.

39. Richardson PD, Davies MJ, Born GVR. Influence of plaque configuration and stress distribution on fissuring of coronary atherosclerotic plaques. Lancet 1989; 2:941–944.

40. Cheng GC, Loree HM, Kamm RD, Fishbein MC, Lee RT. Distribution of circumferential mechanical stress in ruptured and stable atherosclerotic lesions: A structural analysis with histopathological correlation. Circulation 1993; 87(4):1179–1187.

41. McCord BN, Ku DN. Mechanical rupture of the atherosclerotic plaque fibrous cap. Trans 1993 ASME Bioeng Conf 1993; 24:324–326.

42. Kimura BJ, Bhargava V, DeMaria AN. Value and limitations of intravascular ultrasound imaging in characterizing coronary atherosclerotic plaque. Am Heart J 1995; 130:386–396.

43. Bocksch WG, Schardtl M, Beckmann SH, Dreysse S, Paeprer H. Intravascular ultrasound imaging in patients with acute myocardial infarction: comparison with chronic stable angina pectoris. Coron Artery Dis 1994; 9:727–735.

44. Lee TR, Richardson G, Loree HM, Grodzinsky AJ, Gharib SA, Schoen FJ, Pandian N. Prediction of mechanical properties of human atherosclerotic tissue by high-frequency intravascular ultrasound imaging. Arterioscler Thromb 1992; 12:1–5.

45. Lee RT, Lorree HM, Cheng GC, Lieberman EH, Jaramillo N, Schoen FJ. Computational structural analysis based on intravascular ultrasound imaging before in vitro angioplasty: prediction of plaque fracture location. J Am Coll Cardiol 1993; 21:777–782.

46. Libby P, Lee RT. Role of activated macrophages and T-lymphocytes in rupture of coronary plaques. In: Braumwald E, ed. Heart Disease: A Textbook of Cardiovascular Medicine (Suppl 2). Philadelphia: W.B. Saunders, 1995:1–9.

47. Nikkari ST, O'Brien KD, Ferguson M, Hatsukami T, Welgus HG, Alpers CE, Clowes AW. Interstitial collagenase (MMP-1) expression in human carotid atherosclerosis. Circulation 1995; 92:1393–1398.

48. Galis Z, Sukhova G, Kranzhofer R, Clark S, Libby P. Macrophage foam cells from experimental atheroma constitutively produce matrix-degrading proteinases. Proc Natl Acad Sci USA 1995; 92:402–406.

49. Lee RT, Schoen FJ, Loree HM, Lark MW, Libby P. Circumferential stress and matrix metalloproteinase 1 in human coronary atherosclerosis. Implications for plaque rupture. Arterioscler Thromb Vasc Biol 1996; 16:1070–1073.

50. Leung DY, Glagov S, Mathews MB. Cyclic stretching stimulates synthesis of matrix components by arterial smooth muscle cells in vitro. Science 1976; 191:475–477.

51. Yang J-H, Briggs WH, Libby P, Lee RT. Small mechanical strains selectively suppress matrix metalloproteinase-1 expression by human vascular smooth muscle cells. J Biol Chem 1998; 273:6550–6555.

52. Martin DK, Bootcov MR, Campbell TJ, French PW, Breit SN. Human macrophages contain a stretch-sensitive potassium channel that is activated by adherence and cytokines. J Membrane Biol 1995; 147:305–315.

53. Matsumoto T, Delafontaine P, Schnetzer KJ, Tong BC, Nerem RM. Effect of uniaxial, cyclic stretch on the morphology of monocytes/macrophages in culture. J Biomech Engin 1996; 118:420–422.

54. Yang J-H, Lee RT. Small mechanical deformations induce immediate-early gene expression and augment matrix metalloproteinase expression by human monocyte/macrophages. Circulation 1998; 98:I47.

55. Banes AJ, Tauzaki M, Yamamoto J, Fischer T, Brigman B, Brown T, Miller L. Mechanoreception at the cellular level: the detection, interpretation, and diversity of responses to mechanical signals. Biochem Cell Biol 1995; 73:349–365.

56. Davies PF, Barbee KA, Volin MV, Robotewskyj A, Chen J, Joseph L, Griem ML, Wernick MN, Jacobs E, Polacek DC, DePaola N, Barakat AI. Spatial relationships in early signaling events of flow-mediated endothelial mechanotransduction. Annu Rev Physiol 1997; 59:527–749.

57. Takahashi M, Ishida I, Traub O, Corson MA, Berk BC. Mechanotransduction in endothelial cells: temporal signaling events in response to shear stress. J Vasc Res 1997; 34:212–219.

58. Dopico, AM, Kirber MT, Singer JJ, Walsh JV. Membrane stretch directly activates large conductance Ca^{2+}-activated K^+ channels in mesenteric artery smooth muscle cells. Am J Hypertens 1994; 7:82–89.

59. Scandinavian Simvastatin Survival Study Group. Scandinavian simvastatin survival study (4S). Lancet 1994; 334:1383–1389.

60. Aikawa M, Rabkin E, Okada Y, Voglic SJ, Clinton SK, Brinckerhoff CE, Sukhova GK, Libby P. Lipid lowering by diet reduces matrix metalloproteinase activity and increases collagen content of rabbit atheroma. Circulation 1998; 97:2433–2444.

61. Ridker PM, Cushman M, Stampfer MJ, Tracy RP, Hennekens CH. Inflammation, aspirin, and the risk of cardiovascular disease in apparently healthy men. N Engl J Med 1997; 336:973–979.

7
Determinants of Thrombosis After Plaque Rupture

Juan Jose Badimon, James H. Chesebro, and Valentin Fuster
Zena and Michael A. Wiener Cardiovascular Institute, Mount Sinai School of Medicine, New York, New York

Lina Badimon
CSIC–Hospital Santa Cruz y San Pablo, Universidad Autònoma de Barcelona, Barcelona, Spain

Atherosclerotic disease is the most frequent underlying cause of ischemic heart and cerebrovascular disease, and its thrombotic complications are the major cause of mortality and morbidity in the United States and Western countries. The most up-to-date statistical data suggest that cardiovascular diseases are responsible for one of four deaths in the United States. However, atherosclerotic disease, defined as thickening of the arterial wall caused by the accumulation of intracellular and extracellular lipids, macrophages, T cells, smooth muscle cells, proteoglycans, collagen, calcium, and necrotic debris, is rarely fatal. The mechanisms responsible for the conversion of a stable and clinically silent atherosclerotic lesion to a life-threatening condition is plaque disruption. The important socioeconomic implications of atherosclerotic disease arise from the impact of the acute plaque disruption syndromes (unstable angina, acute myocardial infarction, stroke, and even sudden death). Clinical, experimental, and postmortem evidence has clearly demonstrated the critical role of acute thrombosis after plaque disruption, not only in the pathogenesis of atherosclerotic disease but also in the onset of acute coronary syndromes. Because of these observations, the more relevant therapeutic approaches to reduce the impact of atherosclerosis on our society are those directed against the conditions involved in the instability or disruption of plaques and, those specifically directed toward reducing the thrombotic consequences of plaque disruption.

I. ATHEROSCLEROTIC DISEASE: ORIGIN AND PROGRESSION

Several theories have been postulated to explain the origin and progression of atherosclerotic disease. The two major hypotheses regarding its pathogenesis, the thrombogenic and the lipidic, were formulated in the nineteenth century. The thrombogenic or incrustation theory of von Rokitansky (1), later modified by Duguid and Robertson(2), suggests that fibrin deposition and its subsequent organization by fibroblasts, with secondary lipid enrichment, would lead to intimal thickening. This initial theory has recently been extended to include the observations that platelet deposition on de-endothelialized areas may trigger the migration and proliferation of vascular smooth muscle (3).

The lipidic theory was initially postulated in 1856 by Virchow and later supported by the pioneering work of Anistkchow (4), who induced atherosclerotic-like lesions in rabbits by feeding them a cholesterol-rich diet. This theory suggests that lipid accumulation within the arterial wall is the consequence of an imbalance between the influx and efflux of cholesterol.

At present, these two theories may be integrated into a more complex and unified theory (Figure 1) (5–6). The most likely sequence of events involves early endothelial dysfunction caused mainly by disturbances in the blood flow pattern. The areas of the arterial tree that are generally located in tortuous and outer edges of branching points demonstrate an increased permeability to blood cells and proteins. Endothelial dysfunction may be further potentiated by the coexistence of the so-called cardiovascular risk factors, such as, hypercholesterolemia, tobacco, diabetes, hypertension, sedentary lifestyle, obesity, and other yet to be discovered factors. The activated endothelial cells express a series of molecules (selectins) that induce flowing monocytes to marginate, roll, and attach to the endothelial surface. The expression of selectins is followed by synthesis of adhesive proteins, vascular cell adhesion molecule (VCAM) and intracellular adhesion molecule (ICAM), that result in the adherence and spreading of monocytes. These monocytes, together with plasma lipids, enter the arterial wall and accumulate in the subendothelial space. The entry of monocytes into the arterial wall is enhanced by specific chemotactic agents such as oxidized low-density lipoproten (LDL) and monocyte chemotactic proten-1 (MCP-1). Once in the arterial wall, the monocytes are capable of acting as lipoprotein modifiers and scavengers, transforming themselves into macrophages and foam cells resulting from the internalization of lipid material. In addition, the dysfunctional endothelial cells, monocytes, and aggregated platelets act as a source of chemotactic, inhibitory, and stimulatory growth factor for monocytes and smooth muscle cells. The increased receptor-mediated lipid accumulation and connective tissue synthesis will construct the typical atherosclerotic plaque. The perpetuation these processer

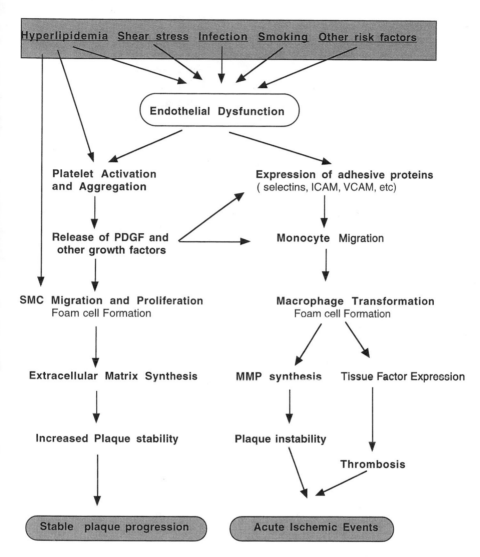

Figure 1   Sequence of processes involved in the genesis and progression of atherosclerotic disease.

will result in the classical slow and relentless progression of the disease. However, a faster process has also been indicated by angiographic and pathological studies. Serial angiographic studies have indicated that mild or moderately stenotic plaques are most frequently the cause of acute ischemic events (7–11). Postmortem analysis of patients who died of acute ischemic events concluded that the culprit atherosclerotic lesions shared some common characteristics (11–16). These "vulnerable" plaques defined as plaques more prone to disruption, are histologically characterized by the presence of an eccentric plaque, containing a soft lipid-rich core that is separated from the arterial lumen by a thin cap of fibrous tissue. The fibrous cap is generally infiltrated by macrophages and T cells. The presence of activated macrophages and T cells around the disrupted areas of the vulnerable plaques led to the hypothesis of an important inflammatory component in plaque disruption.

Other theories have also been postulated to explain the origin of atherosclerosis, such as the monoclonal theory of Benditt (17). This theory is based on the monoclonal origin of the smooth muscle cell population that constitutes the atherosclerotic lesion. In light of the presence of T-lymphocytes in both initial and more advanced atherosclerotic lesions, these observations have been used to postulate an immunologic origin of this disease (18). A viral origin has also been reported based on the possibility of inducing atherosclerotic-like disease in avians by means of Marek's disease virus (19). The role of infection in the pathogenesis of atherosclerosis is currently being revisited (20–22).

Despite a common and generalized hypothesis for the origin and progression of atherosclerotic disease, the heterogeneity of different atherosclerotic plaques is clearly demonstrated not only between different subjects but also within the same individual (11).

The effects of different phenotypic, genotypic, and other risk factors have been correlated with the progression of atherosclerotic plaques, but little is known about a specific relation between risk factors and composition of the atherosclerotic lesion (23–24). These observations are important because several studies have demonstrated that plaque composition, rather that severity of luminal narrowing, is the critical determinant of the risk for disruption and subsequent thrombosis.

The major determinants of plaque disruption could be divided into *intrinsic* and *extrinsic* factors (25). Included among the more important extrinsic factors, are the geographical location of the specific plaque, its exposure to fluid dynamics, the circumferential tensile stress, compressive stress, circumferential bending stress, and longitudinal flexion stress. The intrinsic factors depend on the structure of the atherosclerotic lesions relating specifically to the cell type (smooth muscle cells vs. macrophages) and extracellular composition (lipid vs. fibrotic material) (11–16).

II. PATHOPHYSIOLOGY OF THROMBUS FORMATION

In the initial stages of endothelial injury manifested by functional abnormalities but without major morphological changes, no significant platelet deposition or thrombus formation can be demonstrated. A few scattered platelets may interact with mildly injured or dysfunctional endothelium and contribute, through the release of growth factors, to very mild intimal hyperplasia. In contrast, after endothelial denudation and mild intimal injury, platelets ranging from a monolayer to several layers may deposit on the lesion, with or without subsequent mural thrombus formation. The release of platelet growth factors may contribute significantly to an accelerated intimal hyperplasia as occurs in coronary vein grafts within the first postoperative year. In severe injury, with exposure of components of deeper layers of the vessel, as in spontaneous plaque rupture or after angioplasty, marked platelet aggregation with mural thrombus formation is seen. Vascular injury of this magnitude also stimulates thrombin formation through both the intrinsic (surface-activated) and extrinsic (tissue factor–dependent) coagulation pathways, in which the platelet membrane facilitates interactions between clotting factors. This concept of vascular injury as a trigger of the platelet coagulation response is important in understanding the pathogenesis of various vascular diseases associated with atherosclerosis and coronary artery disease (3, 5–6).

Growing thrombi may locally occlude the arterial lumen or embolize and be washed away by the blood flow to occlude distal vessels. However, thrombi may also be physiologically and spontaneously lysed by mechanisms that block thrombus propagation. Thrombus size, location, and composition are regulated by hemodynamic forces (mechanical effects), thrombogenicity of exposed substrate (local molecular effects), relative concentration of fluid phase and cellular blood components (local cellular effects), and the efficiency of the physiological mechanisms of control of the system, mainly fibrinolysis (6, 7, 25).

III. MODULATION OF ACUTE THROMBOSIS AFTER
PLAQUE DISRUPTION

The presence of intraluminal thrombi in unstable angina and acute myocardial infarction patients has been documented by numerous pathological, angiographic, and angioscopic reports (11–14, 26, 27). In contrast with the high incidence of thrombi in acute myocardial infarction, the incidence in unstable angina varied significantly among different studies, in part related to the interval between the onset of ischemic symptoms and the angiographic study (28–31). Accordingly, when cardiac catheterization was delayed for weeks, the incidence of thrombi was low; on the other hand, if the angiographic procedure was performed early

Table 1 Typical Ranges of Wall Shear Rates and Wall Shear Stresses in Human Blood Vessels

Blood vessels	Wall shear rate[a]	Wall shear stress[b]
Large arteries	300–800	11.4–30.4
Arterioles	500–1,600	19.0–60.8
Veins	20–200	0.76–7.6
Stenotic vessels	800–10,000	30.4–380

[a] Wall shear rates expressed as seconds^{-1} and shear stress as dynes/cm^2.
[b] Assuming a blood viscosity of 0.038 Poise.
Source: Modified from Ref. 32.

after the onset of symptoms, Thrombus was present in approximately two thirds of cases. Presumably, thrombus is nearly occlusive at the time of anginal pain, later becomes subocclusive, and is ultimately lysed.

Platelet-arterial wall interaction and thrombosis are modulated by the interaction of several factors (Table 1). These factors are related to the *local fluid dynamics*, the *exposed substrate*, and the presence of *systemic* "thrombogenic risk factors."

IV. EFFECT OF LOCAL FLUID DYNAMICS ON ACUTE THROMBUS FORMATION

An investigation into the local fluid dynamics is essential for an understanding of events occurring at the blood–vessel wall interface. Blood flow determines the rate of transport of cells to and away from the substrate and imposes fluid forces that affect the removal of material deposited at the surface. These forces may also lead to physical activation of release processes (32, 33).

From the rheological point of view, blood is essentially incompressible and viscous. Because it is incompressible, it is insensitive to the pressure to which it is subjected, responding only to differences among neighboring points (34, 35). Therefore, the mechanical forces produced in blood vessels may result from (a) luminal pressure changes that cause blood flow (which yields *shear stress*), or (b) transmural pressure changes that cause circumferential deformation of the layers of the vessel wall during the cardiac cycle (*tensile stress*). Fluid shear stress is the force per unit area generated by flow of a viscous liquid. Tensile stress produces strain, which is a measure of the percent change in vessel circumference generated by the expansion and contraction of the vascular lumen. Strain is the force that can tear components of the vessel wall.

The term *shear* has the precise physical meaning of a sliding motion between two adjacent planes. Blood flow can be described as an infinite number of laminae sliding across one another, each lamina suffering some frictional interference with the other laminae. Blood flow in a tubular chamber generates a parabolic flow profile. This results in maximal velocity and minimal shear at the center of the blood flow stream and minimal velocity and maximal shear rate at the vessel wall. Shearing forces are generated by the different velocities between the laminae of the blood flow.

The shear rate, according to its definition for one-dimensional flow, is the velocity gradient in the direction perpendicular to the flow. The magnitude of the shear rate at the wall (*wall shear rate*) is particularly important in that it reflects the movement near the wall where most of the mass transport and reaction processes occur. In tubular vessels, wall shear stress of newtonian fluid can be calculated as a function of the volumetric flow rate: $\tau = 4\mu \, Q/\Pi r^3$, where μ is viscosity, Q is the volumetric flow, and r is the radius of the tubular chamber. Shear rate is directly correlated with the blood flow and inversely related to the third power of the radius; thus, a small change in the lumen of an artery will be associated with a significant increase in the local shear rates. Shear stress, which is mathematically the product of the fluid viscosity and the shear rate, is another basic parameter. According to this formula, Table 2 presents the typical ranges of wall shear rates and wall shear stresses (36).

The value of wall shear rate represents the force per unit area applied by the fluid on the vascular wall. Although these two parameters differ only in magnitude by a coefficient of viscosity [shear stress $\tau = -\mu \, (dv_z/dr)$; where μ is viscosity and (dv_z/dr) is shear rate], from a physical point of view, they have different functions in events at the wall. It is the shear stress that directly exerts a force on substances, tending to strip them from the wall, whereas the shear rate contributes to the convective transport of material to the area and the removal of detached (soluble) material from the area.

A. Effect of Flow on Thrombus Formation in a Tubular Perfusion Chamber

Platelet–vessel wall interactions and thrombus formation in vivo take place under flow conditions. Several in vitro systems capable of modeling the different flow conditions present in blood vessels have been developed to investigate the mechanisms by which mechanical forces affect platelet-thrombus formation (37–44). Table 2 presents a summary of different flow systems. The effects of local rheological conditions on platelet-thrombus formation have been similar among all the different perfusion systems described. Therefore, in the following discussion we will mainly focus on data generated by our group using our original perfusion chamber.

Table 2 Different Flow Systems for Studying the Effects of Flow on Blood Cell-Surface Interactions

Type	Shear stress	Substrates
Cone viscosimeter (44)	<1–>200	None, cells, proteins, ECM
Annular chamber (45)	<10–800	Everted rabbit aorta
Parallel plate chamber (46)	<10–>500	None, cells, protein, ECM, biomaterials
Flow viscosimeter (47)	>1000	None
Filter aggregation (48)	?	Glass fiber
Flow column (49)	15–52	Proteins
Filtragometry (50)	?	Siliconized nickel filter
Tubular chamber (51)	<10–>250	Aortic tissue, proteins, cells, ECM, biomaterials
Stenotic chambers		
Tubular chamber (52)	<10–>500	Aortic tissue, proteins, ECM biomaterials
Parallel plate chamber (53)	<10–>500	None, cells, protein, ECM, biomaterials

ECM: extracellular matrix.

To investigate the dynamics of platelet deposition and thrombus formation after vascular damage and to study the influence of various biochemical and physical factors, we developed a tubular perfusion chamber that retains the cylindrical shape of the vascular system and permits ex vivo exposure of such surfaces to blood under controlled flow conditions. The description and rheological characterization of the chamber has been previously described (42). To allow for the evaluation of platelet-thrombus formation on the exposed substrate to flowing blood, autologous platelets are labeled with 111-Indium. To study the contribution of fibrin(ogen) deposition to thrombus formation, experiments are performed with double-labeled blood (platelets and fibrinogen). Results are normalized by exposed surface area as previously described (45).

B. Effects of Rheology on Thrombus Formation on Mildly and Severely Injured Arterial Wall

Exposure of de-endothelialized vessel wall (thus mimicking mild vascular injury) to blood has demonstrated the shear-dependence of platelet deposition. At low shear rates, platelet deposition reached a maximum within 5 to 10 minutes of exposure, after which platelet deposition remained relatively constant. At higher wall shear rates (1690/s), The initial platelet deposition rate is higher than at the lower shear rates. Maximum platelet deposition occurs at 5 to 10 minutes of exposure. However, the thrombi can be dislodged from the substrate by the flowing blood, suggesting that the thrombus was labile. At longer perfusion times, platelet deposition decreases to values not significantly different from those seen at the lower shear rate levels.

Exposure of fibrillar collagen (thus mimicking a deeper injury into the vessel wall) to blood produces platelet deposition of more than two orders of magnitude greater than on subendothelium (46). Even at high shear rates, The platelet thrombus was not dislodged but remained adherent to the surface. These observations emphasize the importance not only of the shear rate but also the influence of the depth of injury on platelet deposition and thrombus formation. Overall, it is likely that when injury to the vessel wall is mild, the thrombogenic stimulus is relatively limited, and the resulting thrombotic occlusion is transient, as occurs in unstable angina. On the other hand, deep vessel injury secondary to plaque rupture or ulceration results in exposure of collagen, tissue factor, and other elements of the vessel matrix, leading to relatively persistent thrombotic occlusion.

Most experimental flow studies have been performed in laminar flow conditions. In atherosclerotic vessels, laminar flow conditions are not maintained because the thickening of the arteral wall will induce flow disturbances. These flow disturbances give to modify cell-cell and cell–vessel wall interactions, as well as the local concentrations of fluid-phase chemical mediators necessary for cell interaction. Using a modification of our perfusion chamber allows study of the effects of varying degrees of stenosis on acute platelet deposition (43). We found that platelet deposition on the damaged artery increased with increasing stenosis. In addition, the axial distribution of platelet deposition clearly indicated that platelet thrombi grew preferentially at the apex of the stenosis, where the highest shear rate develops. Similar observations were obtained in an in vivo model developed to study the effects of arterial damage and shear. In this in vivo study, arterial injury was achieved by carotid angioplasty, and progressive degrees of stenosis were produced at the center of the dilated area by using an external ring. In low shear rate conditions, deep arterial injury will lead to mural thrombosis without further thrombus growth. When deep arterial injury occurs under critical local shear conditions, platelet deposition will be enhanced, and thrombosis may progress to total occlusion (47).

Vessel characteristics also regulate fibrin(ogen) deposition kinetics. Differences in fibrin(ogen) deposition (^{125}I-fibrinogen) kinetics are observed on mildly versus severely damaged vessel wall (45). Fibrin(ogen) deposition to damaged vascular wall was studied at a constant laminar flow typical of unobstructed medium size arteries. Mildly damaged (subendothelial) and severely damaged (below the internal elastic lamina) vascular walls were studied as triggers of thrombosis. Firbin deposition per surface area and longitudinal axial dependence of fibrin deposition and its relationship to platelet deposition were studied by segmental analysis of the substrates exposed in the flow chamber placed in an extracorporeal shunt. Fibrin(ogen) deposition was similar in nonanticoagulated and heparinized blood in acute perfusions and significantly higher on severely damaged vessels than on mildly damaged vessels. Segmental dependence analysis showed a significant decrease in fibrin deposition with distal location on both types of lesions. The ratio of fibrin(ogen) to platelet deposition was similar at all perfusion times on mildly injured arteries whereas on severely injured vessels, a higher ratio was found at short perfusion times. That is, fibrin deposition is higher in the thrombus layers closest to the vessel wall after severe injury. Even under low shear conditions of arterial thrombosis, fibrin deposition and fibrin regulate platelet ratio are highly dependent on the degree of vascular damage (45).

Overall, it is likely that when injury to the vessel wall is mild, the thrombogenic stimulus is relatively limited, and the resulting thrombotic occlusion is transient, as occurs in unstable angina. On the other hand, deep vessel injury secondary to plaque rupture or ulceration results in exposure of substrates that may lead to relatively persistent thrombotic occlusion and myocardial infarction (5, 6).

C. Effects of Shear Rate on Vessel Wall

Despite the presence of the same systemic risk factors all over our body, atherosclerosis is seen as a heterogenous disease. It is possible to predict the areas with a higher probability of atherosclerotic lesions developing. These regions, generally located at the outer edges of vascular curvatures and bifurcations, are rheologically characterized by the presence of lower shear stress and flow disturbances. These observations have suggested that elevated levels of shear stress might have a protective effect against atherogenesis (48–52).

The relationship between local shear stress and atheroschelerotic lesions has triggered study of the biological effects of shear on endothelial function. Endothelial cells are capable of responding to local hemodynamic forces (53, 54). These forces include shear stress and shear strain. Flow-induced signals cause endothelial cells to modulate the synthesis and release of a variety of vasoactive and antithrombotic substances. Flow-induced vasoadaptation is mediated by the release of two vasoactive products, prostacyclin (PGI_2) and endothelium-derived relaxing factor (EDRF) as nitric oxide (NO) from shear-exposed endothelial cells (55–58). These molecules, in addition to their vasoactive properties, are also powerful antiplatelet agents. PGI_2 acts by raising intracellular levels of cyclic AMP in vascular smooth muscle cells and platelets.

NO is also a potent vasodilator and antiplatelet agent. Its effects are mediated by elevating the intracellular levels of cyclic GMP in smooth muscle cells and platelets. The release of EDRF by endothelial cells is activated by both shear stress and cyclic strain (57). The release of NO in response to increased shear rates seems mediated by increased production of cNOS messenger RNA (58).

Other indirect mechanisms leading to inhibition of platelet activation and deposition are increasing the levels of tissue type plasminogen actuator (tPA). It has been described that tPA and plasmin inhibit shear-induced platelet aggregation (59). High levels of shear stress stimulate secretion of tPA without modification of the plasminogen actuafor anhibiton-1 (PAI-I) levels (60).

All these actions are mediated by the shear rate stimulation of the shear-stress responsive element (SSRE) regions on the promoter of shear-responsive genes. The transcriptional factor NF-KBβ, which accumulates in the nuclei of endothelial cells exposed to shear stress, binds to the SSRE and has been implicated in the rheological activation of endothelial cells (61).

The recent report of the induction of the tissue factor gene by shear stress indicates that it is not only the genes containing SSRE in their promoter regions that can be induced by shear stress. Shear-stress induction of tissue factor is mediated through increased Sp1 transcriptional activity with a concomitant hyperphosphorylation of Sp1 (62).

V. EFFECT OF ARTERIAL WALL COMPOSITION ON ACUTE THROMBUS FORMATION

Heterogeneity of plaques exists not only between subjects but also within the same individual. Therefore, given the different composition of atherosclerotic plaques, plaque disruption of different persons will be associated with the exposure of different materials. We have studied the relative thrombogenicity of different types of atherosclerotic lesions. Human atherosclerotic plaques, including normal nonatherosclerotic tunica media, collagen-rich matrix, fatty streaks, and lipid-rich plaques obtained at autopsy and surgically prepared to mimic ruptured plaques, were exposed to flowing blood in a perfusion model. Those plaques characterized by the presence of atheromatous gruel and a lipid-rich core were the most thrombogenic plaques. Lipid-rich plaques were up to six times more thrombogenic than the collagen-rich matrix (63). By contrast, collagen-rich fibrotic plaques are less likely to rupture, and have less thrombogens constituents such that when thrombotic complications do occur, they are generally the result of decreased blood flow caused by the severe stenosis of the vessel lumen (64). Our observations clearly suggest that the vulnerable plaques are not only those more prone to disruption, but on disruption, they expose most thrombogenic substrates (63). The exact mechanism(s) responsible for the thrombogenic properties of the various components of atherosclerotic plaques, and specially of the lipid core, is still uncertain. However, the mechanism responsible for the observed thrombogenicity of lipid-rich plaques seems to be related to increased tissue factor (TF) exptession 229 (65).

One of the more important tasks is to delineate the origin of the TF found in the lipid-rich core of atherosclerotic lesions. The expression of TF by monocytes and macrophage-derived foam cells has been demonstrated in atherosclerotic lesions (66, 67). More importantly, studies carried out with directional atherectomy specimens retrieved from patients with unstable coronary syndromes showed a higher population of macrophage-rich areas than specimens from stable angina patients. Furthermore, a highly significant correlation was obtained between macrophage-rich areas and TF-positive stained areas in atherectomy samples from unstable angina vs. stable angina patients (68–70). Even though these observations strongly suggest that the TF present in the lipid core of human atherosclerotic lesions is largely derived from macrophages in the plaque, we cannot rule out the possible contribution of smooth muscle cells and even endothelial cells.

These observations clearly emphasize the role of the monocyte-macrophage system, not only in the early pathogenesis of atherosclerotic disease, but more importantly in both plaque instability and subsequent thrombosis of the disrupted promoting atherosclerotic lesions. Not surprisingly, inflammatory cells have been described at sites of intimal rupture or erosion of thrombosed coronary atherosclerotic plaques (71). In addition, we and others have reported the production of a variety of proteolytic matrix–degrading enzymes that break down collagen by macrophages in human atherosclerotic lesions (72–74). Of particular interest are enzymes of the matrix metalloproteinase family such as interstitial collagenase (MMP-1), stromelysin (MMP-3), gelatinase-B (MMP-9), and others (75, 76).

A. Effect of Fresh Mural Thrombus on Thrombus Growth

Angiographic studies have documented the importance of residual mural thrombus as a risk factor for rethrombosis after successful thrombolysis (77, 78). Factors that may contribute to rethrombosis include re-exposure of damaged vessel wall (46), liberation of thrombin bound to clot or arterial wall matrix (79), platelet secretory products (80), and thrombolysis-induced platelet activation (81) or stimulation of thrombin generation. Increased thrombin generation may persist beyond the acute event of thrombolytic treatment and lead to late reocclussion despite current antithrombotic treatment (82–83). We studied the effects of fresh mural thrombus growth when exposed to flowing blood; our data indicate that residual mural thrombus on a severely damaged arterial wall is very thrombogenic. Its thrombogenicity seems to be mediated by thrombin, because aspirin has little effect on preventing thrombus growth. Heparin dose-dependently reduced thrombus growth, but even the highest dosage was less effective than specific thrombin inhibition by hirudin (84). More recently, under similar experimental conditions, we tested the hypothesis that thrombin activity is necessary for thrombus growth and thrombus cohesion and, therefore, specific thrombin inhibition (but not current heparin-based antithrombotic therapy) is effective in deaggregating fresh platelet-rich mural thrombus (85). Our data clearly indicate that direct inhibition of thrombin activity by r-hirudin totally abolishes thrombus growth and leads to a reduction of the pre-existing mural thrombus. It appears that both thrombus growth and thrombus maintenance are thrombin-dependent processes. R-hirudin is more effective at lower levels of anticoagulation than the highest dose of heparin tested (85). Thus, specific thrombin inhibition appears to remain a promising treatment, but further studies are required to substantiate these potential benefits in humans.

The critical modulatory role of the exposed substrate on acute thrombus formation after atherosclerotic plaque disruption, whether spontaneous or induced by the coronary procedures, highlights the therapeutic possibilities for selecting the optimal antithrombotic treatment on the basis of the composition of the substrate interacting with flowing blood.

VI. SYSTEMIC THROMBOGENIC RISK FACTORS

Focal thrombosis may lead to a local hypercoagulable or thrombogenic state of the circulation that may favor progression or recurrence of the thrombi. In addition, there is increasing experimental and clinical evidence that a primary hypercoagulable or thrombogenic state of the circulation exists that can favor focal thrombosis.

Systemic factors, including alterations in lipid and hormonal metabolism,

Table 3 Factors Modulating Platelet–Arterial Wall Interaction

Local fluid dynamics
   Shear stress
   Tensile stress
Nature of the exposed substrate
   Degree of injury (mild vs. severe arterial injury)
   Composition of atherosclerotic plaque
   Residual mural thrombus
Systemic thrombogenic factors
   Catecholamines
   Smoking
   Hypercholesterolemia
   Homocysteine
   Lipoprotein (a)
   Defective fibrinolytic state
   Hypercoagulable state (fibrinogen, vWF, factor VII)
   Diabetes

hemostasis, fibrinolysis, and platelet and leukocyte function, are associated with an increased blood reactivity and thrombogenicity (Table 3).

Platelet reactivity may be favored by increased plasma catecholamine levels. Platelet aggregation and the generation of thrombin may be experimentally activated by circulating catecholamine (86–88); this interrelationship could be of importance in humans, because it may be a link between conditions of emotional stress (89) or circadian variation (early morning hours) (90–92) with catecholamine effects (93, 94) and the development of myocardial infarction. Anecdotal evidence associated with situations of high stress, such as the 1971 earthquake in Athens or after missile attacks in Israel during the Gulf War in 1991, have been associated with an increased number of hospital admissions because of plaque rupture events.

Of importance is the increasing evidence of enhanced platelet reactivity in cigarette smokers (95–97), which may or may not be related to catecholamine stimulus (98); indeed, in agreement with the thrombogenic role of cigarette smoking, after discontinuation of smoking it has been observed that there is a sharp decrease in acute vascular thrombotic events (99, 100).

Increasing numbers of clinical and experimental investigations in patients with hypercholesterolemia link this condition with hypercoagulability (101, 102) and enhanced platelet reactivity (103–105). Within this context, young patients with a family history of coronary artery disease seem to have an increased platelet reactivity. Our group and others have reported increased platelet reactivity associated with hypercholesterolemia. More importantly, normalization of plasma cholesterol levels by statin treatment seems to normalize the increased platelet reactivity observed during the hyperlipidemic conditions (106, 107).

Homocysteine is also associated with atherosclerosis and arterial thrombosis. It increases tissue factor activity of the endothelial cells, possibly in synergy with lipoprotein(a); it inhibits the expression of endothelial cell surface thrombomodulin, the thrombin cofactor responsible for the activation of protein C; and it inhibits the binding activity of antithrombin III to the endothelial heparan sulfate. Therefore, homocysterm reduces the anticoagulant properties of the normal endothelium (108–111).

Lipoprotein(a) represents an independent risk factor for coronary artery disease (112–116). Apolipoprotein (a), the major apoprotein found in lipoprotein (a), has close structural homology with plasminogen (117). Evidence suggests that high levels of lipoprotein (a) result in competitive inhibition of the fibrinolytic potential of plasminogen (118), thus displacing the hemostatic balance toward thrombosis and predisposing patients to thrombotic complications. Both lipoprotein (a) and LDL compete with plasminogen for binding to extracellular matrix. However, elevated lipoprotein (a) appears to be an atherogenic rather than a thrombogenic risk factor (119).

These observations support the concept that defective fibrinolytic states could be a thrombogenic risk factor in patients with coronary artery disease (120–122). A correlation between high levels of PAI-1, t-PA and cross-linked fibrin with the progression of atherosclerotic disease has been demonstrated in The Atherosclerosis Risk in Communities Study (123). The European Concerted Action on Thrombosis and Disabilities Study showed that in patients with angina pectoris, plasma levels of fibrinogen, von Willebrand factor, and t-PA are independent predictors of subsequent myocardial infarction or sudden death (124). In patients with types IIa, IIb, and IV hyperlipidaemia, high levels, of PAI-1 correlated with triglyceride levels, apoB, and total cholesterol levels. These correlations were dependent on apoB and may reflect the relation between PAI-1 and hyperlipidaemia. Within this scope, another of the components of the fibrinolytic system, plasminogen-activator inhibitor, is now being studied (125, 126). Although some studies have supported the hypothesis that high levels of this inhibitor are a risk factor for ischemic heart disease and myocardial infarction, other studies have been less convincing, casting doubts on the hypothesis (124, 125).

Of no less importance is the increasing clinical and experimental evidence implicating other hemostatic proteins, specifically fibrinogen and factor VII, as thrombogenic risk factors. Several prospective studies have indicated that high plasma fibrinogen concentrations are independent risk factors for coronary artery disease and myocardial infarction (127). The mechanism by which fibrinogen contributes to atherogenesis is not well understood; several hypotheses have been postulated such as increased fibrin formation, viscosity, platelet aggregation, and stimulation of smooth muscle cell proliferation. On the other hand, it is important to remember that high plasma fibrinogen levels are correlated with age, degree of obesity, hyperlipidemia, diabetes, smoking, and emotional stress, conditions themselves associated with atherosclerotic disease.

Platelet aggregation and coagulation are increased in diabetes mellitus. Platelets from diabetic patients demonstrate enhanced adhesiveness and hyperag-gregability in response to a wide range of agonists (128, 129). Synthesis is thromboxane A_2 is increased in diabetic patients, facilitating platelet aggregation and thrombus formation (130). The primary reason for altered platelet behavior in diabetes in not well understood, but evidence exists that the derangement may start at the megakaryocyte level. Other abnormalities in the coagulation system of diabetic patients that could also be implicated in platelet reactivity include increased fibrinogen and von Willebrand factor levels and decreased antithrombin III activity. In addition, a typical feature of insulin resistance and hyperinsulinemia is increased plasminogen activator inhibitor-I activity, resulting in reduced plasma fibrinolytic activity (131).

In addition, diabetes has also been associated with profoundly altered endothelial function. The best characterized abnormality is impaired endothelium-dependent relaxation, which can be induced by even short exposure to high glucose concentrations. Diabetes may impair endothelium-dependent relaxation by increased generation of advanced glycosylation end-products and increased oxygen free radicals in the arterial wall (132). The loss of endothelium-derived relaxing factor has a profound effect on arterial vasomotion and leads to vasospasm and, by increasing local shear rate, to increased platelet aggregation. Furthermore, diabetes seems to reduce the prostacyclin metabolism of the endothelial cells, possibly resulting in higher levels of platelet activation and endothelial adhesion. In addition, high glucose levels seem to affect endothelium regeneration (128–129).

VII.   ARTERIAL THROMBOSIS: THE CLINICAL MANIFESTATIONS OF ATHEROSCLEROTIC VASCULAR DISEASE

The importance of subsequent acute thrombosis on a disrupted or eroded atherosclerotic plaque was highlighted in 1956 by the Norwegian physiologist Dedichen when he said "man lives with arteriosclerosis, and dies of the complicating thrombosis" (131).

Fissure or rupture of an atherosclerotic plaque in the coronary arteries plays a fundamental role in the development of the acute coronary syndromes. The clinical manifestations of atherosclerotic plaque ruptures depend on several factors, including the degree and suddenness of blood flow obstruction, the duration of decreased myocardial perfusion, and the myocardial oxygen demand at the time of blood flow obstruction. The thrombotic response to the disrupted plaque is also a major determinant. Plaque rupture is accompanied by hemorrhage into the plaque and by various amounts of luminal thrombosis. If the thrombus is small, plaque rupture probably proceeds unnoticed, if, on the other hand, the thrombus is large, compromising blood flow to the myocardium, the individual may experience an acute ischemic syndrome ranging from unstable angina to myocardial infarction to sudden death.

REFERENCES

1. Von Rokitansky C. A Manual of Pathological Anatomy. Vol 4. Berlin: Sydenhman Society, 1852:261.
2. Duguid JB, Robertson WB. Mechanical factors in atherosclerosis. Lancet 1957; 1: 1205–1209.
3. Ross R. Pathogenesis of atherosclerosis: An update. N Engl J Med 1986; 314:488.
4. Anistchow N, Chalatov S. Uber experimentelle cholesterinase und ihre bedeutung fur die enthstehung einiger pathologischer prozesse. Zentralbl Allg Pathol Pathol Anat 1913; 24:1.
5. Badimon JJ Fuster V, Chesebro JH, Badimon L. Coronary atherosclerosis. A multifactorial disease. Circulation 1993; 87:(II) 3–(II) 16.
6. Fuster V, Badimon L, Badimon JJ, Chesebro JH. The pathogenesis of coronary artery disease and the acute coronary syndromes. N Engl J Med 1992; 326:242–250; 310–318.
7. Ambrose J, Tannembaum MA, Alexopoulos D, Hjemdahl-Monsen CE, Levay J, Weiss M, Borrico S, Gorlin R, Fuster V. Angiographic progression of coronary artery disease and the development of myocardial infarction. J Am Coll Cardiol 1988; 12:56–62.
8. Little WC, Constantinescu M, Applegate RJ, Kutcher MA, Burrows MT, Kahl FR, Santamore WP. Can coronary angiography predict the site of a subsequent myocardial infarction in patients with mild-to-moderate coronary artery disease? Circulation 1988; 78:1157–1166.
9. Nobuyoshi M, Tanaka M, Nosaka H, Kimura T, Yokoi H, Hamasaki N, Kim K, Shimo T, Kimura K. Progression of coronary atherosclerosis: is coronary spasm related to progression?. J Am Coll Cardiol 1991; 18:904–910.
10. Giroud D, Li JM, Urban P, Meier B, Rutishauer W. Relation of the site of acute myocardila infarction to the most severe coronary arterial stenosis at prior angiography. Am J Cardiol 1992; 69:729–732.
11. Falk E, Shah PK, Fuster V. Coronary Plaque disruption. Circulation 1995; 92:657–671.
12. Davies MJ, Thomas AC. Plque fissuring: the cause of acute myocardial infarction, sudden ischemic death, and crescendo angina. Br Heart J 1985; 53:363–373.
13. Mann HJM, Davies MJ. Vulnerable plaques. Relation of characteristics to degree of stenosis in human coronary arteries. Circulation 1996; 94:928–931.

14. Falk E. Why do plaques rupture? Circulation 1992; 86(suppl III):30–42.
15. Davies MJ. Stability and instability: two faces of coronary atherosclerosis. The Paul Dudley Whiye Lecture 1995. Circulation 1996; 94:2013–2020.
16. Felton CV, Crook D, Davies MJ, Oliver MF. Relation of plaque lipid composition and morphology to the stability of human aortic plaques. Arterioscl Thromb Vasc Biol 1997; 17:1337–1345.
17. Benditt EP, Benditt JM. Evidence for a monoclonal origin of human atherosclerotic plaques. Proc Natl Acad Sci USA 1973; 70:1753–1758.
18. Hansson GK, Jonason L, Seifert PS, Stemme S. immune mechanisms in atherogenesis. Arteriosclerosis 1989; 9:567–578.
19. Fabricant CG. Herpes induced atherosclerosis. Diabetes 1981; 30:29–31.
20. Capron L. Chlamydia in coronary plaques—hidden culprit or harmless hobo? Nat Med 1996; 2:856–857.
21. Gurfinkel E, Bozovich G. *Chlamydia pneumoniae*: inflammation and instability of the atherosclerotic plaque. Atherosclerosis 1998; 140(suppl):S31–35.
22. Noll G. Pathogenesis of atherosclerosis: a possible relation to infection. Atherosclerosis 1998; 140(suppl 1):S3–9.
23. Kragel A, Roberts WC. Composition of atherosclerotic plaques in the coronary arteries in homozygous familial hypercholesterolemia. Am Heart J 1991; 121:210–214.
24. Gertz SD, Malekzadeh S, Dollar AL, Kragel AH, Roberts WC. Composition of atherosclerotic plaques in coronary arteries in women <40 years of age with fatal coronary artery disease and implications for plaque reversibility. Am J Cardiol 1991; 67:1223–1227.
25. Badimon L, Chesebro JH, Badimon JJ. Thrombus formation on ruptured atherosclerotic plaques and rethrombosis on evolving thrombi. Circulation 1992; 86(suppl III):74–85.
26. Constantinides P. Plaque fissures in human coronary thrombosis. J Atheroscler Res 1966; 6I:1–17.
27. DeWood MA, Stifter WF, Simpson CS, Spores J, Eugster GS, Judge TP, Hinnen ML. Coronary arteriographic findings soon after non-Q wave myocardial infarction. N Engl J Med 1986; 315:417–423.
28. Rentrop P, Blanke H, Karsch KR, Kaiser H, Kostering H, Leitz K. Selective intracoronary thrombolysis in acute myocardial infarction and unstable angina pectoris. Circulation 1981; 63:307–317.
29. Rehr R, Disciascio G, Vetrovec G, Crowley M. Angiographic morphology of coronary artery stenoses in prolonged rest angina: evidence of intracoronary thrombosis. J Am Coll Cardiol 1989; 14:1429–1435.
30. Sherman CT, Litvack F, Grundfest W, Lee M, Hickey A, Chaux A, Kass R, Blanche C, Matloff J, Morgenstern L. Coronary angioscopy in patients with unstable angina. N Engl J Med 1986; 315:913–919.
31. Uchida Y, Tomaru T, Nakamura F, Furuse A, Fujimori Y. Percutaneous coronary angioscopy in patients with ischemic heart disease. Am Heart J 1987; 1114:1216–1222.
32. Leonard EF. Rheology of thrombosis. In: Colman RW, Hirsh J, Marder VJ, Salzman EW, eds. Hemostasis and Thrombosis. 3rd Ed. Philadelphia: JB. Lippincott Co., 1994:1211–1223.

33. Goldsmith HL and Turitto VT. Rheological aspects of thrombosis and haemostasis: Basic principles and applications. Thromb, Haemost 1986; 55:415–435.
34. Alevriadou BR, McIntire L. Rheology. In: Loscalzo J, Schaffer A., eds. Thrombosis and Haemorrhage. Blackwell Science, 1995:369.
35. Joist JH, Zeffren DI, Bauman JE. A programmable, computer-controlled cone-plate viscosimeter for the application of pulsatile shear stress to platelet suspensions. Biorheology 1988; 25:449–456.
36. Weiss H, Baumgartner H, Tschopp, Turitto VT, Cohen D. Correction by factor VII of the impaired adhesion to subendothelium in von Willebrand's disease. Blood 1978; 51:267–275.
37. Sakariassen KS, Aarts P, De Groot PG, Houdijk W, Sixma JJ. A perfusion chamber developed to investigate platelet interaction in flowing blood with human vessel wall cells, their extracellular matrix, and purified components. J Lab Clin Med 1983; 102:522–531.
38. Wurzinger LJ, Opiz R, Blasberg P, Schnid-Schonbein H. Platelet and coagulation parameters following milliseconds exposure to laminar shear stress. Thromb Haemost 1985; 54:381–395.
39. O'Brien JR, Salmon GP. Shear stress activation of platelet GP IIb/IIIa plus von Willebrand factor causes aggregation: Filter blockage and the long bleeding time in von Willebrand's disease. Blood 1987; 70:1354–1360.
40. Polanoiwska-Grabowska R, Gear ARL. High-speed platelet adhesion under conditions of high shear rate. Proc Natl Acad Sci USA 1992; 89:5754–5761.
41. Hornstra G, ten Hoor F. The filtragometer: a new device for measuring platelet aggregation in venous blood of man. Thromb Diath Haemorr 1975; 34:531–544.
42. Badimon L, Turitto V, Rosemark J. Characterization of a tubular flow chamber for studying platelet interaction with biologic and prosthetic materials. J Lab Clin Med 1987; 110:706–718.
43. Badimon L, Badimon JJ. Mechanisms of arterial thrombosis in non-parallel streamlines. Platelet thrombi grow on the apex of stenotic severely injured vessel wall. J Clin Invest 1989; 84:1134–1144.
44. Barstard RM, Kierulf P, Sakariassen K. Collagen-induced thrombus formation at the apex of eccentric stenoses. A time-course study with non-anticoagulated human blood. Thromb Haemost 1996; 75:685–692.
45. Mailhac A, Badimon JJ, Fallon JT, Fernandez-Ortiz A, Meyer B, Fuster V, Meyer B, Badimon L. Effect of an eccentric severe stenosis on fibrin(ogen) deposition on severely damaged vessel wall. Circulation 1994; 23:1562–1569.
46. Badimon L, Badimon JJ, Galvez A, Chesebro JH, Fuster V: Influence of arterial damage and wall shear rate on platelet deposition. Ex vivo study in a swine model. Arteriosclerosis 1986; 6:312–320.
47. Merino A, Cohen M, Badimon JJ, Fuster V, Badimon L. Synergistic action of severe wall injury and shear forces on thrombus formation in arterial stenosis: definition of a thrombotic shear rate threshold. Am Coll Cardiol 1994; 24:1091–1097.
48. Caro CG, Fitzgerald JM, Schroter RC. Atheroma and arterial wall shear. Observation, correlation and proposal of a shear dependent mass transfer mechanisms for atherogenesis. Proc R Soc Lond R Biol Soc 1971; 177:109–159.
49. Glagov S, Zarins C, Giddens DP, Ku K. Hemodynamics and atherosclerosis. In-

sights and perspectives gained from studies of human arteries. Arch Pathol Lab Med 1988; 112:1018–1031.

50. Ku KDN, Giddens DP, Zarins CK, Glagov S. Pulsatile flow and atherosclerosis in the human carotid bifurcation. Positive correlation between plaque location and low oscillating shear stress. Arteriosclerosis 1985; 5:293–302.

51. Asakura T, Karino T. Flow patterns and spatial distribution of atherosclerotic lesions in human coronary arteries Circ Res 1990; 1045–1066.

52. Gnasso A, Irace C, Carallo C. in vivo association between low wall shear stress and plaque in subjects with asymmetrical carotid atherosclerosis. Stroke 1997; 28: 993–998.

53. Malek AM, Izumo S. Control of endothelial cell gene expression by flow. J Biochem 1995; 28:1515–1528.

54. Chien S, Li S, Shyi YJ. Effects of mechanical forces on signal transduction and gene expression in endothelial cells. Hypertension 1998; 31:162–169.

55. Alshihabi SN, Chang YS, Frangos JA, Tarbell JM. Shear stress-induced release of PGE2 and PG12 by vascular smooth muscle cells. Biochem Biophys Res Commum 1996; 224:808–814.

56. Rubanyi G, Romero J, Vanhoutte P. Flow-induced release of endothelium derived derived relaxing factor. Am J Physiol 1986; 250:H1145.

57. Awolesi MA, Sessa WC, Sumpio BE: Cyclic-strain upregulates NO-synthase in cultured bovine aortic endothelial cells. J Clin Invest 1995; 96:1449–1456.

58. Nishida K, Harrison D, Navas J, Fisher A, Dockery S, Uematsu M, Nerem R, Alexander W, Murphy T. Molecular cloning and characterization of the constitutive bovine endothelial cell nitric oxyde synthase. J Clin Invest 1992; 90:2092–2097.

59. Coller B. Platelets and thrombolytic therapy. N Engl J Med 1990; 33:322–328.

60. Diamond SL, Eskin SG, McIntire LV. Fluid flow stimulates tissue plasminogen activator secretion by cultured endothelial cell. Science 1989; 243:1483–1486.

61. Khachigian L, Resnick N, Gimbrone M, Collins T. Nuclear factor-kb interacts functionally with the PDGF B-chain shear stress response element in vascular endothelial cells exposed to fluid flow. J Clin Invest 1995; 96:1169–1175.

62. MC Lin, Almus-Jacons F, Chen HH, Parry GCN, Mackman N, Shyy JY, Chien S. Shear stress induction of tissue factor gene. J Clin Invest 1997; 99:737–744.

63. Fernandez-Ortiz A, Badimon JJ, Falk E, Fuster V, Meyer B, Mailhac A, Weng D, Shah PK, Badimon L. Characterization of the relative thrombogenicity of atherosclerotic plaque components: implications for consequences of plaque rupture. J Am Coll Cardiol 1994; 23:1562–1569.

64. Kragel AH, Gertz SD, Roberts WC. Morphologic comparison of frequency and types of acute lesions in the major epicardial coronary arteries in unstable angina pectoris, sudden coronary death and acute myocardial infarction. J Am Coll Cardiol 1991; 18:801–808.

65. Toschi V, Gallo R, Lettino M, Fallon JT, David S. Gertz, Fernandez-Ortiz A, Chesebro J, Badimon L, Nemerson Y, Fuster V, Badimon JJ. Tissue Factor modulates the thrombogenicity of human atherosclerotic plaques. Circulation 1997; 95:594–599.

66. Wilcox JN, Smith KM, Schwartz SM, Gordon D. Localization of tissue factor in normal vessel wall and in the atherosclerotic plaque. Proc Natl Acad Sci USA 1989; 86:2839–2843.

67. Thiruvikraman SV, Guha A, Rebos R, Nemerson Y, Fallon JT. In situ localization of tissue factor in human atherosclerotic plaques by binding of digoxigenin labeled factors Viia and X. Lab Invest 1996; 75:451–461.
68. Moreno PR, Falk E, Palacios IF, Newell JB, Fuster V, Fallon JT. Macrophage infiltration in acute coronary syndromes. Circulation 1994; 90:775–778.
69. Moreno P, Bernardi V, Lopez-Cuellar J, Murcia A, Palacios I, Gold H, Sharma S, Nemerson Y, Fuster V, Fallon J. Macrophages, smooth muscle cells and tissue factor in unstable angina. Implications for cell-mediated thrombogenicity in acute coronary syndromes. Circulation 1996; 94:3090–3097.
70. Annex BH, Denning SM, Channon KM, Sketch MH, Stacks RS, Morrisey JH, Peters KG. Differential expression of tissue factor protein in directional atherectomy specimens from patients with stable and unstable angina coronary syndromes. Circulation 1995; 91:619–622.
71. Van der Waal A, Becker A, Van der Loos C, Das P. Sit. Site of intimal rupture or erosion of thrombosed coronary atherosclerotic plaques is characterized by an inflammatory process irrespective of dominant plaque morphology. Circulation 1994; 89:36–45.
72. Shah PK. Falk E, Badimon JJ, Fernandez-Ortiz A, Mailhac A, Villareal-Levy G, Fallon JT, Regnstrom J, Fuster V. Human minocyte-derived macrophages induce collagen breakdown in fibrous caps of atherosclerotic plaques: potential role of matrix-degrading metalloproteinases and implications for plaque rupture. Circulation 1995; 92:1565–1569.
73. Galis ZS, Sukhova G, Lark MW, Libby P. Increased expression of matrix metalloproteinases and matrix degrading activity in vulnerable regions of human atherosclerotic plaques. J Clin Invest 1994; 2493–2503.
74. Galis ZS, Sukhova GK, Kranzhofer R, Libby P. macrophage foam cells from experimental atheroma constitutively produce matrix-degrading proteinases. Proc Natl Acad Sci USA 1995; 92:402–406.
75. Newby AC, Southgate KM, Davies MJ. Extracellular matrix degrading metalloproteinases in the pathogenesis of arteriosclerosis. Basic Res Cardiol 1994; 89 (Supp I):59–70.
76. Davies MJ. Reactive oxygen species, metalloproteinases, and plaque stability. Circulation 1998; 97:2382–2383.
77. Brown BG, Gallery CA, Badgers RS, Kennedy JW, Mathey D, Bolson EL, Dodge HT. Incomplete lysis of thrombus in the moderate underlying atherosclerotic lesion during intracoronary infusion of streptokinase for acute myocardial infarction. Circulation 1986; 73:653–661.
78. Gulba DC, Westhoff-Bleck M, Claus G, Piper J,Lichten PR. Residual coronary thrombus; a major risk factor for early reocclussion after thrombolysis in acute myocardial infarction. Circulation 1991; 84 (suppl II):572–561.
79. Weitz JI, Hudoba M, Massel D, Maraganore J, Hirsh J. Clot-bound thrombin is protected from inhibition by heparin-antithrombin III but is susceptible to inactivation by antithrombin III-independent inhibitors. J Clin Invest 1989; 84:1096–1104.
80. Golino P, Ashton JH, Glass-Greenwalt P, McNatt J, Buja M, Willerson JT. Mediation of reoclussion by thromboxane A2 and serotonin after thrombolysis with tissue-type plasminogen activator in a canine preparation of coronary thrombosis. Circulation 1988; 77:678–684.

81. Fitzgerald DJ, Catella F, Roy L, Fitzgerald GA. Marked platelet activation in vivo after intravenous streptokinase in patients with acute myocardial infarction. Circulation 1988; 77:142–150.
82. Merlini P, Ardissino D, Bauer K, Oltrona L, Pezzano A, Botasso B, Rosenberg R, Mannucci P, Persistent thrombin generation during heparin therapy in patients with acute coronary syndromes. Arterioscler Thromb Vasc Biol 1997; 17:1325–1330.
83. Merlini P, Ardissino D. Current status of activation markers in ischemic heart disease: markers of coagulation activation. Thromb Haemost 1977 78:276–279.
84. Meyer B, Badimon JJ, Mailhac A, Fernandez-Ortiz A, Chesebro JH, Fuster V, Badimon L. Inhibition of thrombus growth on fresh mural thrombus. Targeting optimal therapy. Circulation 1994; 90:2432–2438.
85. Meyer B, Badimon JJ, Chesebro JH, Fallon JT, Fuster V, Badimon L. Dissolution of mural thrombus by specific thrombin inhibition with r-hirudin. Comparison with heparin and aspirin. Circulation 1998; 97:681–685.
86. Rowsell HC, Hegardt B, Downie HG, Mustard JF, Murphy EA. Adrenaline and experimental thrombosis. Br J Haematol 1966; 12:66–73.
87. Goto S, Handa S, Takahashi E, Abe S, Handa M, Ikeda Y. Synergistic effect of epinephrine and shearing on platelet activation. Thromb Res 1996; 84:351–359.
88. Spalding A, Vaitkevicius H, Dill S, MacKenzie S, Schmaier A, Lockette W. Mechanism of epinephrine-induced platelet aggregation. Hypertension 1998 31:603–607.
89. Krantz DS, Kop WJ, Santiago HT, Gottdiener JS. Mental stress as a trigger of myocardial ischemia and infarction. Cardiol Clin 1996; 14:271–287.
90. Mueller JE, Stone PH, Turi ZG, et al. The MILIS Study Group. Circadian variation in the frequency of onset of acute myocardial infarction. N Engl J Med 1985; 313:1315–1322.
91. Johnstone MT, Mittleman M, Tofler G, Muller JE. The pathophysiology of the onset of morning cardiovascular events. Am J Hypertens 1996; 9:22S–28S.
92. Willich SN, Linderer T, Wegscheider K, Leizorovicz A, Alamercery I, Schroder R. Increased morning incidence of myocardial infarction in the ISAM study: absence with prior beta-adrenergic blockade. Circulation 1989; 80:853–858.
93. T Tofler GH, Brezinski D, Schafer AI, Czeisler CA, Rutherford JD, Willich SN, Gleason RE, Williams GH, Muller JE. Morning increase in platelet response to ADP and epinephrine: association with the time of increased risk of myocardial infarction and sudden cardiac death. N Engl J Med 1987; 316:1514–1518.
94. Fuster V, Chesebro JH, Frye RL, Elveback L. Platelet survival and development of coronary artery disease in the young adult: effects of cigarette smoking, strong family history and medical therapy. Circulation 1981; 63:546–551.
95. Winniford M, Wheelan K, Kremers M, Ugolini V, van den Berg E, Niggemann E, Jansen D, Hillis L. Smoking-induced coronary vasoconstriction in patients with atherosclerotic coronary artery disease: evidence for adrenergically mediated alterations in coronary artery tone. Circulation 1986; 73:662–667.
96. Blann A, Kirkpatrick U, Devine C, Naser S, McCollum C. The influence of smoking on leucocytes, platelets and the endothelium. Atherosclerosis 1998; 141:133–139.
97. Powell JT. Vascular damage from smoking: disease mechanisms at the arterial wall. Vasc Med 1998; 3:21–28.

98. Buhler FR, Vesanen K, Watters J. Impact of smoking on heart attacks, strokes, blood pressure control, drug dose, and quality of life in the Intern Prospective Primary Prevention Study in Hypertension. Am Heart J 1988; 115:282–288.

99. Paul O. Prevention of cardiovascular disease. II. Arteriosclerosis, hypertension and selected risk factors. Circulation 1989; 80:206–214.

100. Hunt BJ. The relation between abnormal hemostatic function and the progression of coronary disease. Curr Opin Cardiol 1990; 5:758–765.

101. Thompson SG, Kienast J, Pyke SDM, Haverkate F, Van de Loo JCW, for the European Concerted Action on Thrombosis and Disabilities Angina Pectoris Study. Hemostatic factor and the risk of myocardial infarction or sudden death in patients with angina pectoris. N Engl J Med 1995;332(10):635–641.

102. Carvalho ACA, Colman R, Lees R. Platelet function in hyperlipoproteinemia. N Engl J Med 1974; 290:434–438.

103. Badimon JJ, Badimon L, Turitto VT, Fuster V. Platelet deposition at high shear rates is enhanced by high plasma cholesterol levels. In vivo study in the rabbit model. Arteriosclerosis 1991; 11:395–402.

104. Henry PD, Cabello OA, Chen CH. Hypercholesterolemia and endothelial dysfunction. Curr Opin Lipidol 1995; 6(4):190–195.

105. Lacoste L, Lam J, Hung J, Letchacovski G, Solymoss C, Waters D. Hyperlipidemia and coronary artery disease. Correction of the increased thrombogenic potential with cholesterol reduction. Circulation 1995; 92:3172–3177.

106. Rauch U, Osende J, Chesebro JH, Fuster V, Vorchheimer DA, Harris KA, Harris P, Sandler D, Fallon JT, Jayaraman S, Badimon JJ. Statins and cardiovascular diseases: multiple effects of lipid-lowering by statins. Atherosclerosis 2000; 153:181–189.

107. Boers G, Smals A, Trijbels F, Fowler B, Bakeren J, Schoonderwaldt H, Kleijer W, Kloppenborg P. Heterozygosity for homocystinuria in premature peripheral and cerebral occlusive arterial disease. N Engl J Med 1985; 313:709–715.

108. Boers GH Hyperhomocysteinemia as a risk factor for arterial and venous disease. A review of evidence and relevance. Thromb Haemost 1997; 78:520–522.

109. Prasad K. Homocysteine, a risk factor for cardiovascular disease. Int J Angiol 1998; 8:76–86.

110. de Jong S, van den Berg M, Rauwerda J, Stehouwer C. Hyperhomocysteinemia and atherothrombotic disease. Semin Thromb Hemost 1998; 24(4):381–385.

111. Dahlen GH, Guyton JR, Attar M, Farmer JA, Kautz JA, Gotto AM. Association of levels of lipoprotein(a), plasma lipids, and other lipoproteins with coronary artery disease documented by angiography. Circulation 1986; 74:758–765.

112. Seed M, Hoppichler F, Reaveley D, McCarthy S, Thompson GR, Boerwinkle E, Utermann G. Relation of serum lipoprotein(a) and apolipoprotein(a) phenotype to CHD patients with familial hypercholesterolemia. N Engl J Med 1990; 322:1494–1499.

113. Djurovic S, Berg K. Epidemiology of Lp(a) lipoprotein: its role in athero thrombotic disease. Clin Genet 1997; 52:281–292.

114. Hopkins PN, Hunt SC, Schreiner PJ, Eckfeldt JH, Borecki IB, Ellison CR, Williams RR, Siegmund KD. Lipoprotein(a) interactions with lipid and non-lipid risk factors inpatients with early onset coronary artery disease: results from the NHLBI Family Heart Study. Atherosclerosis 1998; 141:333–345.

115. Hajjar KA, Nachmann RL. The role of lipoprotein(a) in atherogenesis and thrombosis. Annu Rev Med 1996; 47:423–442.

116. McLean JW, Tomlinson JE, Kuang WJ, Eaton DL, Chen EY, Fless GM, Scanu AM, Lawn RM. cDNA sequence of human apolipoprotein(a) is homologous to plasminogen. Nature 1987; 330:132–137.

117. Scanu AM. Atherothrombogenicity of lipoprotein(a): the debate. Am J Cardiol 1998; 82(9A):26Q–33Q.

118. Allen S, Khan S, Tam SP, Koschinsky M, Taylor P, Yacoub M. Expression of adhesion molecules by lp(a): a potential novel mechanism for its atherogenicity. FASEB J 1998; 12:1765–1776.

119. Vaughan DE. Plasminogen activator inhibitor-1: a common denominator in cardiovascular disease. J Invest Med 1998; 46(8):370–376.

120. Geppert A, Graf S, Beckmann R, Hornykewycz S, Schuster E, Binder BR, Huber K. Concentration of endogenous tPA antigen in coronary artery disease: relation to thrombotic events, aspirin treatment, hyperlipidemia, and multivessel disease. Arterioscler Thromb Vasc Biol 1998; 18:1634–1642.

121. Olofsson B, Dahlen G, Nilsson T. Evidence for increased levels of plasminogen activator inhibitor and tissue plasminogen activator in plasma of patients with angiographically verified coronary artery disease. Eur Heart J 1989; 10:77–82.

122. Salomaa V, Stinson V, Kark JD, Folsom AR, Davis CE, Wu KK. Association of fibrinolytcparameters with early atherosclerosis. The ARIC Study. Atherosclerotic Risk in Communities Study. Circulation 1995; 91:284–290.

123. Thompsom SG, Kiennast J, Pyke SD, Haverkate F, van de Loo JC. Hemostatic factors and the risk of myoicardila infarction and sudden death in patients with angina pectoris. European Concerted Action on Thrombosis and Disabilities Study Group. N Engl J Med 1995; 332:635–641.

124. Hamsten A, Wilman B, de Faire U, Blomback M. Increased plasma levels of a rapid inhibitor of tissue plasminogen activator in young survivors of myocardial infarction. N Engl J Med 1980; 303:897–902.

125. Oseroff A, Krishnamurti C, Hassett A, Tang D, Alving B. Plasminogen activator and plasminogen activator inhibitor activities in men with coronary artery disease. J Lab Clin Med 1990; 113:88–93.

126. Meade TW. Fibrinogen and cardiovascular disease. J Clin Pathol 1997; 50:13–15.

127. Winocour PD. Platelet abnormalities in diabetes mellitus. Diabetes Metab Rev 1992; 8:53–66.

128. Aronson D, Rayfield EJ, Chesebro JH. Mechanisms determining course and outcome of diabetic patients who have had acute myocardial infarction. Ann Intern Med 1997; 126:296–306.

129. Davi G, Catalano I, Averna M. Thromboxane biosynthesis and platelet function in type II diabetes mellitus. N Engl J Med 1990; 322:1769–1774.

130. McGill JB, Schneider DJ, Arfken CL. Factors responsible for impaired fibrinolysis in obese subjects and NIDDM patients. Diabetes 1994; 43:104–109.

131. Chappey O, Dosquet C, Wautier MP, Wautier JL. Advanced glycosylation end products, oxidant stress and vascular lesions. Eur J Clin Invest 1997; 27:97–108.

132. Dedichen J. Thrombosing atherosclerosis. Result of long-term anticoagulant therapy. BMJ 1956; Nov 3:1038–1039.

8
The Clinical Manifestations of Plaque Rupture

Michael Berlowitz and David L. Brown
Albert Einstein College of Medicine and Montefiore Medical Center, Bronx, New York

I. INTRODUCTION

The acute coronary syndromes of unstable angina, acute myocardial infarction, and sudden ischemic cardiac death share a common pathophysiology: the abrupt development of ischemia caused by the obstruction of a coronary artery by thrombus formed on an acutely disrupted atherosclerotic plaque (1). Together these syndromes affect approximately 2.5 million persons and account for 600,000 or 1 in 5 deaths annually in the United States. This chapter provides an overview of the clinical manifestations of plaque rupture with its main focus on the acute coronary syndromes.

II. PATHOPHYSIOLOGY AND CLINICAL IMPLICATIONS

As early as the 1920s, Benson postulated that coronary thrombosis resulted from disruption of the intima (2). The clinical significance of this finding remained controversial for the next 60 years. In the 1980s, angiographic and angioscopic studies demonstrated the importance of plaque rupture and thrombus formation in the development of myocardial infarction and unstable angina (3, 4). Pathological studies have confirmed atheromatous plaque disruption as responsible for the overlying coronary artery thrombus (5, 6). These studies established the association between plaque disruption, thrombosis, and development of the acute coronary syndrome. Plaque disruption takes two forms, erosion, where the endothelium over a plaque becomes denuded, and rupture, where the fibrous cap is torn through to the underlying lipid core. In the former situation, thrombus forms on the surface of the plaque, whereas in the latter thrombus forms within the plaque itself, later extending into the lumen. It is estimated that 25% of thrombi responsible for sudden cardiac death are due to endothelial erosion, and the remainder are due to plaque disruption.

The unifying concept that unstable angina, myocardial infarction, and sudden death share a common pathophysiology has had a dramatic impact on the identification and management of patients with acute coronary syndromes. Traditional definitions relied on the timing of chest pain, electrocardiographic changes, and the presence of biochemical markers of myocardial necrosis. Relying on these somewhat arbitrary criteria for diagnosis promoted consideration of these syndromes as discrete entities. Rather, the acute coronary syndromes should be thought of in terms of their shared pathophysiology, with each syndrome reflecting different stages of plaque rupture and thrombosis.

The clinical manifestations of plaque rupture form a continuum from silent ischemia to acute infarction and sudden death. The extent of ischemia depends on the distribution of the ischemia-producing artery, the supply of and demand for oxygenated blood, and the severity of stenosis. The clinical presentation depends on the extent and duration of ischemia and the presence of a previous myocardial infarction (7). In general, myocardial infarction is associated with a more complete and flow-limiting occlusion than unstable angina. Unstable angina and sudden death are associated with more transient occlusions that contain less fibrin. The size and composition of these thrombotic occlusions depend on a number of local and systemic factors, including the degree of plaque rupture or erosion, the underlying tissue substrate, metabolic states, activation of the clotting system, and platelets as well as other, as yet less well defined, inflammatory components (8).

The dynamic interplay of thrombosis, endogenous thrombolysis, and endothelial repair determines the amount of luminal obstruction by thrombus (9). After rupture of an atherosclerotic plaque, flowing blood encounters exposed collagen, the lipid core, smooth muscle cells, and macrophages, all of which promote platelet activation (10, 11). Vasoactive substances promote further platelet aggregation (12). As the platelet-rich thrombus increases in size, reductions in blood flow enhance additional thrombus growth. This thrombus may then progress to varying degrees of luminal obstruction or embolize downstream (Fig. 1) (13). Alternatively, the thrombus may organize and become incorporated into the vessel wall, resulting in a residual stenosis. Fig. 2 summarizes the integrated pathogenesis of plaque rupture and subsequent clinical syndromes (14–16).

The clinical manifestations of an arterial occlusion, whether complete or transient, result from an acute imbalance of oxygen supply and demand. Several important factors affect this balance, including vasoconstriction, which tends to

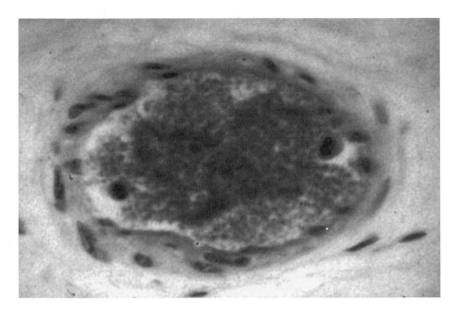

Figure 1 Platelet embolus found distant from a site of coronary plaque rupture in a patient who died of sudden ischemic cardiac death.

reduce oxygen supply and collateral blood flow, which has the opposite effect (17, 18). Likewise, factors that increase oxygen demand, like physical or emotional stress, may precipitate or worsen acute ischemic syndromes. An abrupt reduction in myocardial perfusion caused by plaque rupture and thrombosis may be the cause of unstable angina in two-thirds of patients, whereas one-third of cases may be caused by transient increases in myocardial oxygen demand (8, 19).

The composition of an atherosclerotic plaque and its fibrous cap determine its vulnerability to rupture. The release of proteolytic enzymes by inflammatory cells contributes to plaque disruption by inducing progressive thinning and weakening of the fibrous cap (1). Clinical triggers of plaque rupture and subsequent thrombosis are less clear. The incidence of coronary plaque rupture events peaks in the early morning (20), when enhanced platelet aggregation and higher plasminogen activator inhibitor levels may result in a prothrombotic state (21). The risk of myocardial infarction is increased during emotional and physical stress (22), possibly related to catecholamine excess, the hemodynamic consequences of which may precipitate plaque fissure. However, the identified triggers of plaque rupture are common events, and the incidence of plaque rupture is relatively rare in a given patient. Pre-existing clinical characteristics of patients with

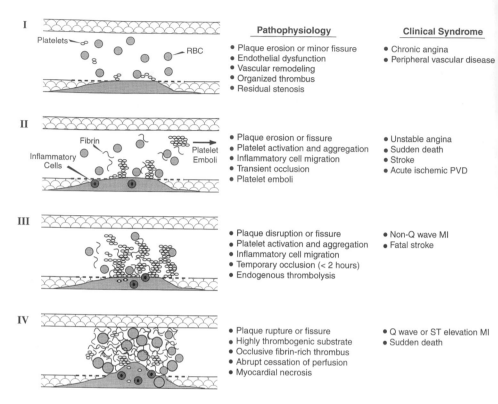

Figure 2 The relationship between degree of plaque disruption, type and extent of thrombus, and the ensuing clinical syndrome.

acute coronary syndromes influence the mode of presentation. Cigarette smoking, advanced age, and renal impairment are associated with myocardial infarction, whereas treatment with aspirin, hypertension, and previous revascularization favor unstable angina (23).

Angiographic studies have permitted correlation of the clinical presentation of an acute coronary syndrome with plaque morphology. These studies have confirmed the paradoxical finding that most plaques that rupture are hemodynamically inconsequential, causing less than 70% diameter stenosis of the artery (24–26). In support of this concept are the angiographic findings in patients after successful thrombolytic treatment of acute myocardial infarction. In these patients the residual luminal narrowing caused by the culprit plaque is often less than 60% (27). New-onset angina at rest and angina after treatment of myocardial infarction are associated with angiographically more complex lesions and evidence of intracoronary thrombus (28). Unstable angina has also been associated

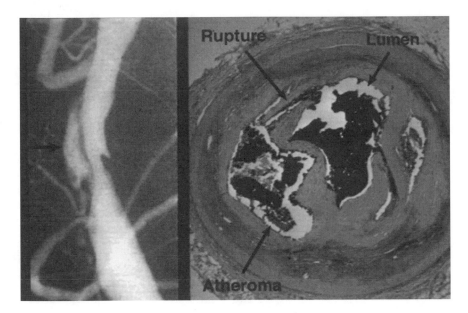

Figure 3 The left panel depicts an angiogram of a coronary artery with a ruptured plaque. The arrow denotes the entry of radiographic contrast media into the plaque through the ruptured fibrous cap. The right panel microscopically depicts a ruptured atherosclerotic plaque with thrombus (dark material) extending from within the atheroma through the rupture in the fibrous cap to occlude the lumen.

with greater amounts of thrombus and atheroma in plaque fragments obtained from directional atherectomy (29).

Angioscopy has corroborated the angiographic findings among patients with acute coronary syndromes (30). In unstable angina, thrombus appears white from platelet clumps. In myocardial infarction, thrombus appears red from an accumulation of red blood cells and fibrin. Complete occlusion by thrombus is present in most patients with acute myocardial infarction and relatively few with unstable angina. These findings may explain differences in response to certain treatments such as thrombolytic or antiplatelet therapy in patients with different acute coronary syndromes (3, 31).

III. CLINICAL APPROACH

Most patients who survive a plaque rupture event have some form of chest pain or its equivalent such as shortness of breath. The character of chest pain varies, and its severity does not predict adverse outcomes or angiographic results (32,

33). The differential diagnosis of chest pain includes peptic ulcer disease and reflux, esophageal spasm, pericarditis, musculoskeletal pain, and anxiety. The physical examination is often not diagnostically helpful. However, the physical examination can detect serious complications of acute myocardial infarction such as ventricular septal rupture, papillary muscle rupture, or the development of cardiogenic shock.

The electrocardiogram (ECG) is an important tool in the identification of acute coronary syndromes. Shifts in the ST segment, although not diagnostic of any particular syndrome, are often the earliest objective evidence of active ischemia. New ST segment depression in three or more leads identifies patients that will progress to myocardial infarction (34). These ECG changes, along with duration of symptoms greater than 4 hours, absence of prior revascularization, and absence of prior beta-blocker therapy identify patients at high risk for acute myocardial infarction. The presence of ST segment elevation predicts the development of Q waves and identifies patients likely to benefit from thrombolytic therapy. A normal ECG does not exclude the diagnosis of unstable angina or infarction.

Cardiac enzymes are often measured on admission and repeated every 4 to 8 hours until symptoms resolve. Elevation of the creatinine phosphokinase (CK) MB isoenzyme denotes myocardial cell necrosis, the extent of which is an important determinant of mortality (35). Myocardial necrosis distinguishes unstable angina from myocardial infarction. Recently, troponin T and I have been introduced as more sensitive and specific markers of myocardial cell injury. Troponin T and I are the tropomyosin-binding proteins located on the contractile apparatus of cardiac myocytes. Elevations in troponin T or I strongly predict adverse short-term and long-term outcomes in patients with acute coronary syndromes, even those without elevations of CK-MB (36, 37). Among patients with normal CK-MB, absence of troponin elevation is associated with low risk (38, 39). Elevation in the inflammatory markers, C-reactive protein and serum amyloid A protein, also predict a poor outcome in patients with unstable angina at the time of hospital admission (40).

Noninvasive imaging has limited value in the initial assessment of patients with unstable coronary syndromes. Two-dimensional echocardiography may detect wall motion abnormalities during ischemia. These abnormalities may occur before pain or electrocardiographic changes (41). An abnormal nuclear perfusion scan during an episode of chest pain is associated with a 71% cardiac event rate compared with a 1.4% rate with a negative scan (42). However, stress testing with or without imaging is usually reserved for risk stratification after patients with acute coronary syndromes are stabilized.

Angiography is capable of rapidly establishing the diagnosis of patients with confusing clinical presentations or nondiagnostic test results. Importantly, angiography also defines the extent of coronary disease. An asymmetrical ulcerated lesion with an overlying, hazy filling defect suggests recent plaque rupture with superimposed thrombus (Fig. 3). These findings are present in more than 70% of patients with persistent, ischemic chest pain despite medical therapy and correlate with a higher frequency of untoward inhospital cardiac events (53).

IV. CLINICAL SYNDROMES

Plaque rupture manifests a broad spectrum of clinical presentations, angiographic findings, and outcomes. The nomenclature and relationship of the different plaque rupture syndromes is presented in Fig. 4. Sequelae of plaque rupture can range from asymptomatic resolution to refractory ischemia, myocardial infarction, or death. These syndromes are not distinct entities but rather exhibit many overlapping features in diagnosis and management.

A. Silent Ischemia

A patient may not have chest pain or other symtpoms during episodes of plaque disruption and thrombosis. In previously healthy patients who die from noncardiac causes, 9% to 22% have asymptomatic disrupted plaques in their coronary arteries (44). In the Framingham Heart Study, 30% of myocardial infarctions

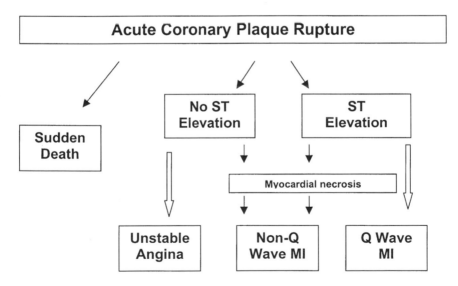

Figure 4 Classification of the acute coronary plaque rupture syndromes. (Adapted from Braunwald EB, et al. Heart Disease: A Textbook of Cardiovascular Medicine. Philadelphia: WB Saunders, 1997.)

identified by ECG and biennial examinations occurred either without symptoms or with mild symptoms that could only be recalled later (45). The 10-year age-adjusted mortality rate in the patients with unrecognized myocardial infarction is 45% compared with 39% in the group in whom myocardial infarction was recognized. The clinical impact of asymptomatic ischemia is particularly significant when it appears after acute myocardial infarction or during or immediately after noncardiac surgery. Patients with silent myocardial ischemia detected by ambulatory ECG monitoring early after acute myocardial infarction possess a twofold increase in the risk of death or nonfatal myocardial infarction over the next year (46). The mortality associated with perioperative infarction can be as high as 30% to 40%. Patients who demonstrate asymptomatic ECG abnormalities perioperatively have a three- to ninefold increase in the risk of cardiac death, myocardial infarction, unstable angina, ventricular tachycardia, or congestive heart failure (47–49).

The mechanism of asymptomatic ischemia is unknown and may be attributed to individual variation in pain threshold, autonomic function, or severity of ischemia. In patients with silent myocardial infarction, postinfarction ischemia, or perioperative ischemia, it is unclear whether the pathogenesis is plaque rupture or myocardial oxygen demand in excess of supply without plaque rupture. Angiographic data in the Asymptomatic Cardiac Ischemia Pilot study suggest that patients with "stable" coronary artery disease and silent ambulatory ischemia have high-risk plaques and more complex and active coronary artery disease (50, 51). Thus, plaque disruption and thrombosis probably account for the increased morbidity and mortality in these groups. In addition, the relationship between silent ischemia and adverse events may reflect a greater plaque burden and thereby a statistically greater likelihood of plaque rupture. In summary, silent ischemia may be a marker for unstable coronary artery disease in patients who appear clinically stable (52).

B. Unstable Angina and Non-Q Wave Myocardial Infarction

Unstable angina accounts for more than 1.2 million hospital admissions in the United States annually (53). These patients present a diagnostic and therapeutic challenge that reflects the heterogeneity of the clinical presentation, severity, and prognosis of unstable angina. Broadly defined, unstable angina is the new onset of chest pain at rest or with exertion or a change in pattern from previously stable chest pain symptoms. It is distinguished from myocardial infarction by the absence of biochemical manifestations of myocardial necrosis.

The prognosis of unstable angina is quite variable. One-year mortality can range from 3% to 22% based on the presence of certain clinical risk factors that include ST segment depression on the ECG, the presence of elevated serum troponin, history of recent infarction, or persistence of rest pain (54–57). The cardiac event rate (death or nonfatal myocardial infarction) can be as low as 3% and as high as 50% in the case of patients with persistent chest pain despite maximal medical therapy (58). To better explain prognosis, Braunwald proposed a classification that divides unstable angina into subgroups on the basis of the presence and timing of chest pain, the history of recent myocardial infarction, and the presence of noncardiac conditions that intensify ischemia (Table 1). Although this classification is useful in the management of patients with unstable angina and in the design of clinical trials, it has only been partially validated prospectively. In the Thrombolysis in Myocardial Ischemia (TIMI) III Registry, there was no difference in the 1-year cardiac event rate between the acute and subacute rest pain subgroups (59). In a prospective validation of the Braunwald classification as a predictor of in-hospital cardiac complications, there was no difference in outcome between patients that had rest pain within or before 48 hours (32). Angiographic studies have failed to demonstrate a relationship between lesion morphology and clinical severity (60).

At the time of presentation, one cannot distinguish unstable angina from non-Q wave myocardial infarction without the results of biochemical markers of cardiac necrosis. Myocardial necrosis in the absence of the development of electrocardiographic Q waves defines non-Q wave myocardial infarction. Although there might be a several-hour delay before the diagnosis of non-Q wave myocardial infarction can be established, it is associated with a worse prognosis than unstable angina (61).

In non-Q wave myocardial infarction, more severe plaque disruption results in more complete thrombotic occlusion (16) of the culprit vessel. The presence of total occlusion at the time of angiography is approximately 20% to 40% in

Table 1 Braunwald Classification of Unstable Angina

Severity
  Class I—new onset of severe or accelerated angina; no pain at rest
  Class II—angina at rest within past month, but not within preceding 48 h
  Class III—angina at rest within 48 h
Clinical setting
  Type A—secondary unstable angina precipitated by extracardiac condition
  Type B—primary unstable angina developed in the absence of extracardiac condition
  Type C—postinfarction unstable angina developed within 2 weeks after myocardial infarction

---

Source: Adapted from Braunwald E. Unstable angina. A classification. Circulation 1989;80:410–414.

non-Q wave myocardial infarction versus 10% to 20% in unstable angina (31). In patients with non-Q wave myocardial infarction and total occlusion of the culprit vessel, collateral blood flow to the infarct zone is often present. Management of non-Q wave myocardial infarction remains similar to the management of unstable angina. A tool for the calculation of prognosis for patients with unstable angina or non-ST segment elevation myocardial infarction is presented in Table 2.

A new category of non-Q wave myocardial infarctions has been created by the successful development of reperfusion therapies for acute ST elevation syndromes. Before the availability of thrombolytic therapy or angioplasty for ST elevation patients, these patients would invariably develop Q waves. However, in a significant fraction of patients who are seen early in the course of their infarction, rapid reperfusion prevents the development of Q waves and leaves the patient with the diagnosis of non-Q wave myocardial infarction. It is unclear

Table 2 Thrombolysis in Myocardial Infarction (TIMI) Risk Score for Unstable Angina and Non-ST Segment Elevation Myocardial Infarction

Feature	Points
Age ≥ 65 y	1
≥ 3 CAD risk factors	1
Known CAD (stenosis ≥ 50%)	1
Aspirin use in the past 7 days	1
Recent (≤24 h) severe angina	1
Elevated cardiac markers	1
ST deviation ≥ 0.5 mm	1

Score	Percent risk of death or MI in next 14 days
0/1	3
2	3
3	5
4	7
5	12
6/7	19

Source: Adapted from Antman EM, Cohen M, Bernink PJ, McCabe CH, Horacek T, Papuchis G, Mautner B, Corbalan R, Radley D, Braunwald E. The TIMI risk score for unstable angina/non-ST elevation MI: A method for prognostication and therapeutic decision making. JAMA 2000;284:835–842.

whether these non-Q wave patients have a better prognosis than patients with either traditionally defined non-Q wave or Q wave infarcts.

C. Q Wave Myocardial Infarction

Q wave myocardial infarction is generally preceded by persistent chest pain accompanied by acute ST elevations or the presence of a new left bundle branch block on the ECG. It represents 50% of all myocardial infarctions and is associated with an in-hospital mortality of 10% to 20% (62). When compared with non-Q wave myocardial infarction, patients with Q wave infarction have larger infarct sizes and increased in-hospital cardiac event rates compared with patients with non-Q wave infarcts. Q wave infarction is associated with a lower risk of reinfarction and improved out-of-hospital survival than non-Q wave myocardial infarction (63). This may be due to a more active and unstable residual plaque in non-Q wave myocardial infarction.

By angiography, patients with Q wave myocardial infarction have fewer collateral vessels supplying the myocardium subtended by the culprit vessel and more complex lesion morphology than patients with non-Q wave infarction (29). The infarct vessel is completely occluded in almost 90% of patients angiographically studied within 4 hours of symptom onset (64). In Q wave infarction, larger plaque fissures result in more persistent fibrin-rich thrombus (65). Total coronary occlusion without collateral blood supply for more than 1 hour results in transmural necrosis of the involved myocardium (8).

In-hospital mortality caused by myocardial infarction is due to either severe left ventricular dysfunction or mechanical complications. These complications include papillary muscle rupture with mitral regurgitation, ventricular septal wall or free wall rupture, and right ventricular infarction. Pump failure caused by extensive myocardial necrosis is the most common cause of in-hospital deaths from myocardial infarction (66). The development of heart failure, advanced age, hypotension, and anterior infarct location are important predictors of poor outcome (67). A tool for prediction of outcome associated with ST elevation myocardial infarction is presented in Table 3.

D. Sudden Cardiac Death

Sudden cardiac death occurs within 6 hours of the onset of chest pain or within 24 hours of a previously normal state of health. Approximately 220,000 persons die of sudden cardiac death annually in the United States. Sudden death is most commonly caused by ischemia-induced fatal ventricular arrhythmias. Patients who experience sudden death tend to have multivessel coronary disease, a culprit lesion without severe stenosis, and the absence of well-developed collateral circu-

Table 3 Thrombolysis in Myocardial Infarction (TIMI) Risk
Score for ST-Elevation Myocardial Infarction

Feature	Points
Age ≤ 75 y	3
Age 65–74 y	2
Diabetes, hypertension, or angina	1
Systolic blood pressure < 100 mmHg	1
Heart rate > 100/min	1
Killip class II–IV	1
Anterior ST elevation or left bundle	1
Time to treatment ≥ 4 h	1

Score	Percent 30-day mortality
0	0.8
1	1.6
2	2.2
3	4.4
4	7.3
5	12
6	16
7	23
8	27
>8	36

Source: Adapted from Morrow DA, Antman EM, Charlesworth A, Cairns R,
Murphy SA, de Lemos JA, Giugliano RP, McCabe CH, Braunwald E. TIMI
risk score for ST-elevation myocardial infarction: a convenient, bedside, clinical score for risk assessment at presentation: an Intravenous nPA for Treatment
of Infarcting Myocardium Early II Trial substudy. Circulation 2000;102:2031–
2037.

lation. Pathological studies have demonstrated considerable variability in the
presence of active coronary lesions and the frequency of plaque rupture (68, 69).
Recently, plaque erosion without rupture has been identified as an important
cause of coronary thrombosis in sudden death (70). In these patients, platelet
microemboli (Fig. 1) and the absence of collateral flow to the jeopardized myocardium contributed to ischemia and fatal arrhythmias (71). Among men with
coronary artery disease who die suddenly, elevated cholesterol is associated
with plaque rupture, whereas cigarette smoking predisposes to plaque erosion
(72).

E.   Peripheral and Cerebrovascular Disease

Atherosclerosis, plaque erosion, and rupture also occur in the carotid arteries, the aorta, and its branches. Occlusive thrombus in these larger caliber arteries is rare, yet plaque rupture is the usual cause of fatal occlusion of the carotid artery (73). More commonly, episodic plaque erosion followed by nonocclusive thrombosis that stimulates plaque progression leads to gradually progressive stenosis and ischemia (74). Thrombus overlying a disrupted plaque may embolize, resulting in ischemic syndromes such as stroke, transient ischemic attacks, or peripheral ischemia manifested by crescendo claudication. After embolization, the residual ulcer crater is capable of repetitively activating platelets and thus can be a recurrent source of microemboli to the brain, kidneys, gastrointestinal tract, and extremities (75). Similar to the acute coronary syndromes, the incidence of stroke has an early morning peak, correlating with the circadian increase in coagulability and vasoconstriction (76).

V.   TREATMENT

The primary goal of treatment for each of the acute coronary syndromes is to restore antegrade flow as rapidly as possible. Achievement of reperfusion will result in control of symptoms and prevention of infarction and death. In addition to specific reperfusion therapies, adjuvant treatments can be categorized into therapics that optimize the balance between oxygen supply and demand, those that inhibit further thrombosis, and those that stabilize plaque.

A.   Pharmacological Reperfusion Therapy

Thrombolytic therapy is first-line therapy in acute myocardial infarction with persistent ST elevation. Since the GUSTO-1 angiographic substudy correlated early restoration of blood flow with a mortality reduction, the goal of thrombolysis has been early and complete reperfusion (77). A pooled analysis of more than 60,000 patients treated in clinical trials of thrombolytic agents has demonstrated an 18% reduction in mortality for patients treated within 12 hours of symptom onset (78). Thromblytic therapy is not indicated in unstable angina or non-Q wave myocardial infarction. In TIMI IIIB, patients with unstable angina or non-Q wave infarction given alteplase had increased rates of death, myocardial infarction, and bleeding (79). Reduction in the degree of stenosis or improvement in coronary flow were modest overall and only apparent in those patients with greater thrombus burdens or more occlusive non-Q wave infarctions (80).

Several mechanisms may explain the differential response to thrombolysis between Q wave myocardial infarction and unstable angina. In myocardial infarction, the thrombus tends to be fibrin-rich, anchored to the plaque, and completely occlusive, thus providing a favorable substrate for thrombolysis. In unstable angina and non-Q wave myocardial infarction the thrombus is more likely to be platelet-rich, adherent only to the plaque surface, less occlusive, and possibly more resistant to thrombolysis. Thrombolytics also promote thrombosis by activating platelets and induce local vasoconstriction (81). Thrombolysis is currently only indicated for the treatment of acute coronary syndromes with ST elevation and is not recommended for unstable angina or non-Q wave myocardial infarction.

B. Mechanical Reperfusion Therapy

Primary percutaneous transluminal coronary angioplasty (PTCA) refers to the use of angioplasty as the primary reperfusion modality for patients with acute myocardial infarction. Despite the limited availability of the facilities and resources to perform primary angioplasty, clinical trial data suggest at least equivalence and perhaps superiority of this form of mechanical treatment compared with thrombolytic treatment. In GUSTO IIb, primary PTCA compared favorably with thrombolytic therapy for acute myocardial infarction, although 6-month outcomes were similar in both groups (82). In PAMI-1, primary angioplasty resulted in a lower occurrence of nonfatal myocardial infarction or death and fewer intracranial hemorrhages than thrombolysis with alteplase (83). Primary stenting, which places a metal scaffold against the plaque wall, further reduces the incidence of recurrent infarction and need for revascularization when compared with balloon angioplasty alone (84). The impact of stenting on mortality in acute myocardial infarction is unclear.

The role of primary PTCA in unstable angina and non-Q wave myocardial infarction is less clear. In the VANQWISH trial, 920 patients with unstable angina or non-Q wave myocardial infarction were randomly assigned to invasive or standard medical therapy with subsequent invasive management if indicated (85). During the first year of follow-up, patients randomly assigned to the invasive arm had higher rates of death and nonfatal myocardial infarction. In this study, however, only 44% of the patients randomly assigned to the invasive arm underwent revascularization compared with 33% in the conservative arm. Median time from presentation to intervention was more than 1 week, and stenting was not approved for clinical use at the time of initial enrollment. TIMI IIIB also demonstrated no benefit with an invasive treatment strategy in patients with unstable angina or non-Q wave infarction (79). Like VANQWISH, TIMI IIIB was conducted in the era before glycoprotein IIb/IIIa inhibitors and stenting. Recently, the FRISC II and TACTICS-TIMI 18 trials have demonstrated superiority of the

Table 4 Comparison of Randomized Trials of Early Invasive Versus Conservative
Approach for Treatment of Patients with Non-ST Elevation Acute Coronary
Syndromes

	TIMI IIIB	VANQWISH	FRISC II	TACTICS-TIMI 18
Stents used?	No	No	Yes	Yes
GP IIb/IIIa Inhibitors used?	No	No	No	Yes
Catheterization timing in invasive arm (hours from admission)	24	48–96	96	24
Exercise stress testing in conservative arm	Nuclear	Nuclear/Echo	ECG	Nuclear/echo
ST segment criteria for positive test (mm)	1	1	3	1
In-hospital catheterization rate in conservative arm (%)	57	24	10	50
Superior approach	Equivalent	Conservative	Invasive	Invasive

early invasive compared with conservative treatment strategies in patients with
unstable angina or non-Q wave myocardial infarction (86, 87). The randomized
trials comparing invasive with conservative therapy in unstable angina and non-
ST elevation myocardial infarction are summarized in Table 4.

Certain subgroups of patients may benefit uniquely from percutaneous
intervention. One such group includes patients with cardiogenic shock. In the
SHOCK trial, patients with cardiogenic shock were randomly assigned to an early
medical stabilization and delayed revascularization versus immediate revascularization strategy (88). There appeared to be a short-term survival advantage for
early intervention in patients younger than 75 years and a 6-month mortality
benefit for all patients in the early revascularization arm. Patients that fail thrombolysis may also benefit from rescue angioplasty. Rescue angioplasty has been
noted to result in superior left ventricular function and improved 30-day survival
compared with conservative treatment (89).

C. Adjuvant Therapy

As negative inotropes and chronotropes, beta-blockers reduce myocardial oxygen
demand and improve survival in patients with acute myocardial infarction and
unstable angina (90–94). Current evidence suggests beta-blockers should be first-

line therapy in acute coronary syndromes. They should be administered cautiously in patients with hypotension, bradycardia, or heart failure.

The vasodilatory nitrates and calcium channel blockers are widely used for the control of symptoms associated with acute coronary syndromes. However, although nitrates reduce myocardial oxygen demand and augment blood flow, there is no convincing data that these agents improve outcome. Likewise, a meta-analysis has demonstrated no reduction in the risk of death or myocardial infarction in unstable angina among patients treated with calcium channel blockers (94). Currently, nitrates and calcium channel blocking agents are recommended for symptomatic relief in the absence of contraindications but are not first-line agents.

Aspirin remains a cornerstone of therapy of the acute coronary syndromes. Irreversible inhibition of the cyclo-oxygenase pathway in platelets, blocking formation of thromboxane A_2 and platelet aggregation, accounts for its benefit. Aspirin reduces the risk of death and myocardial infarction in patients with unstable angina (95, 96) and improves survival when administered for acute myocardial infarction (97). Aspirin is recommended in all patients with unstable coronary syndromes on presentation.

In patients with unstable angina, heparin reduces the incidence of myocardial infarction and refractory angina (98). Likewise heparin administration in addition to thrombolytic agents reduces 30-day mortality from acute myocardial infarction (99). Recently, low molecular weight heparin, offering the advantage of a more predictable anticoagulant effect, has been found to be more effective than unfractionated heparin in reducing the incidence of additional ischemic events in patients with unstable angina or non-Q wave myocardial infarction (100). Unfractionated heparin or low molecular weight heparin is recommended in all patients with unstable coronary syndromes, including myocardial infarction.

Glycoprotein IIb/IIIa receptor blockers inhibit the final step in platelet aggregation. Several recent trials have demonstrated benefit in patients with unstable angina and non-Q wave myocardial infarction. The combination of eptifibatide, unfractionated heparin, and aspirin significantly reduces the incidence of death or myocardial infarction at 30 days compared with the combination of unfractionated heparin and aspirin (101). Likewise, treatment with the combination of tirofiban, aspirin, and unfractionated heparin reduces the incidence of myocardial infarction or death at 7 and 30 days compared with the combination of unfractionated heparin and aspirin alone (102). Neither of these agents has an effect on mortality. Despite inclusion in treatment guidelines, there is no compelling evidence that these agents need to be administered to every patient with an acute coronary syndrome (103).

Optimal medical and interventional strategies for the treatment of acute coronary syndromes require further investigation in the era of more potent antithrombotic agents, glycoprotein IIb/IIIa inhibitors, and stents. Important trials become outdated as newer therapies emerge. Currently, the management of unstable coronary syndromes varies considerably from institution to institution and from community to community and ranges from an aggressive interventional approach to a more conservative medical approach. In either case, the goals remain the same: early reperfusion and plaque stabilization. Plaque stabilization is discussed in other chapters.

REFERENCES

1. Falk E, Shah PK, Fuster V. Coronary plaque disruption. Circulation 1995;92:657–671.
2. Benson RL. Present status of coronary artery disease. Arch Pathol Lab Med 1926:2:876–916.
3. DeWood MA, Spores J, Notske R, Mouser LT, Burroughs R, Golden MS, Lang HT. Prevalence of total coronary occlusion during the early hours of transmural myocardial infarction. N Engl J Med 1980;303:897–902.
4. Ambrose JA, Winters SL, Arora RR, Haft JI, Goldstein J, Rentrop KP, Gorlin R, Fuster V. Angiographic morphology and the pathogenesis of unstable angina pectoris. J Am Coll Cardiol 1985;5:609–618.
5. Falk E. Plaque rupture with severe pre-existing stenosis precipitating coronary thrombosis. Characteristics of coronary atherosclerotic plaques underlying fatal occlusive thrombi. Br Heart J 1983;50:127–134.
6. Davies MF, Thomas AC. Plaque fissuring—the cause of acute myocardial infarction, sudden ischaemic death, and crescendo angina. Br Heart J 1985;53:363–373.
7. White HD. Unstable angina. In: Topol EJ, ed. Textbook of Cardiovascular Medicine. Philadelphia: Lippincott-Raven Publishers, 1998:366.
8. Fuster V, Lewis A. Conner Memorial Lecture. Mechanisms leading to myocardial infarction: insights from studies of vascular biology. Circulation 1994;90:2126–2146.
9. Fuster V, Badimon L, Cohen M, Ambrose JA, Badimon JJ, Chesebro J. Insights into the pathogenesis of acute ischemic syndromes. Circulation 1988;77:1213–1220.
10. Fernandez-Ortiz A, Badimon JJ, Falk E, Fuster V, Meyer B, Mailhac A, Weng D, Shah PK, Badimon L. Characterization of the relative thrombogenicity of atherosclerotic plaque components: implications for consequences of plaque rupture. J Am Coll Cardiol 1994;23:1562–1569.
11. Moreno PR, Bernardi VH, Lopez-Cuellar J, Murcia AM, Palacios IF, Gold HK, Mehran R. Sharma SK, Nemerson Y, Fuster V, Fallot JT. Macrophages, smooth muscle cells, and tissue factor in unstable angina: implications for cell-mediated thrombogenicity in acute coronary syndromes. Circulation 1996;94:3090–3097.
12. Hamm CW, Lorenz RL, Bleifeld W, Kupper W, Wober W, Weber PC. Biochemical evidence of platelet activation in patients with persistent unstable angina. J Am Coll Cardiol 1987;10:998–1004.
13. Davies MJ, Thomas AC, Knapman PA, Hangartner JR. Intramyocardial platelet aggregation in patients with unstable angina suffering sudden ischemic cardiac death. Circulation 1986;73:418–427.

14. Fuster V, Badimon L, Badimon JJ, Chesebro JH. Mechanisms of disease. The pathogenesis of coronary artery disease and the acute coronary syndromes (second of two parts). N Engl J Med 1992;326:310–318.

15. Farb A, Burke AP, Tang AL, Liang Y, Mannan P, Smialek J, Virmani R. Coronary plaque erosion without rupture into a lipid core. A frequent cause of coronary thrombosis in sudden coronary death. Circulation 1996;93:1354–1363.

16. Theroux P, Fuster V. Acute coronary syndromes. Unstable angina and non-Q wave myocardial infarction. Circulation 1998;97:1195–1206.

17. Bogaty P, Hackett D, Davies G, Maseri A. Vasoreactivity of the culprit lesion in unstable angina. Circulation 1994;90:5–11.

18. Fuster V, Frye RL, Kennedy MA, Connolly DC, Mankin HT. The role of collateral circulation in the various coronary syndromes. Circulation 1979;59:1137–1144.

19. Braunwald E, Jones RH, Mark DB, Brown J, Brown L, Cheitlin MD, Concannon CA, Cowan M, Edwards C, Fuster V. Diagnosis and managing stable angina. Circulation 1994;90:613–622.

20. Krantz DS, Kop WJ, Gabbay FH, Rozanski A, Barnard M, Klein J, Pardo Y, Gottdienter JS. Circadian variation of ambulatory myocardial ischemia. Triggering by daily activities and evidence for endogenous circadian component. Circulation 1996; 93:1364–1371.

21. Kono T, Morita H, Nishina T, Fujita M, Hirota Y, Kawamura K, Fujiwara A. Circadian variations of onset of acute myocardial infarction and efficacy of thrombolytic therapy. J Am Coll Cardiol 1996;27:774–778.

22. Leor J, Poole WK, Kloner RA. Sudden cardiac death triggered by an earthquake. N Engl J Med 1996;334:413–419.

23. Kennon S, Suliman A, MacCallum PK, Ranjadayalan K, Wilkinson P, Timmis AD. Clinical characteristics determining the mode of presentation in patients with acute coronary syndromes. J Am Coll Cardiol 1998;32:2018–2022.

24. Ambrose JA, Tannenbaum MA, Alexopoulos D, Hjemdahl-Monsen CE, Leavy J, Weiss M, Borrico S, Gorlin R, Fuster V. Angiographic progression of coronary artery disease and the development of myocardial infarction. J Am Coll Cardiol 1988;12:56–62.

25. Little WC, Constantinescu M, Applegate RJ, Kutcher MA, Burrows MT, Kahl FR, Santamore WP. Can coronary angiography predict the site of a subsequent myocardial infarction in patients with mild to moderate coronary artery disease? Circulation 1988;78:1157–1166.

26. Ambrose JA, Winters SL, Arora RR, Eng A, Riccio A, Gorlin R, Fuster V. Angiographic evolution of coronary morphology in unstable angina. J Am Coll Cardiol 1986;7:472–478.

27. Brown BG, Gallery CA, Badger RS, Kennedy JW, Mathey D, Bolson EL, Dodge HT. Incomplete lysis of thrombus in the moderate underlying atherosclerotic lesion during intracoronary infusion of streptokinase for acute myocardial infarction: quantitative angiographic observations. Circulation 1986;73:653–661.

28. Dangas G, Mehran R, Wallenstein S, Courcoutsakis NA, Kakarala V, Hollywood J, Ambrose JA. Correlation of angiographic morphology and clinical presentation in unstable angina. J Am Coll Cardiol 1997;29:519–525.

29. Dacanay S, Kennedy HL, Uretz E, Parrillo JE, Klein LW. Morphological and quan-

titative angiographic analyses of progression of coronary stenoses. A comparison of Q wave and non-Q wave myocardial infarction. Circulation 1994;90:1739–1746.

30. Mizuno K, Satomura K, Miyamoto A, Arakawa K, Shibuya T, Arai T, Kurita A, Nakamura H, Ambrose JA. Angioscopic evaluation of coronary artery thrombi in acute coronary syndromes. N Engl J Med 1992;26:287–291.

31. DeWood MA, Stifter WF, Simpson CS, Spores J, Eugster GS, Judge TP, Hinnen ML. Coronary arteriographic findings soon after non-Q wave myocardial infarction. N Engl J Med 1986;315:417–423.

32. Calvin JE, Klein LW, Vandenberg BJ, Meyer P, Condon JV, Snell RJ, Ramirez-Morgen LM, Parrillo JE. Risk stratification in unstable angina. Prospective validation of the Braunwald classification. JAMA 1995;273:136–141.

33. Hultgren HN, Peduzzi P, Relation of severity of symptoms to prognosis in stable angina pectoris. Am J Cardiol 1984;54:988–993.

34. Lloyd-Jones DM, Carargo CA, Lapuerta P, Giugliano RP, O'Donnell CJ. Electrocardiographic and clinical predictors of acute myocardial infarction in patients with unstable angina pectoris. Am J Cardiol 1998;81:1182–1186.

35. Geltman EM, Ehsani AA, Campbell MK, Schechtman K, Roberts R, Sobel BE. The influence of location and extent of myocardial infarction on long-term ventricular dysrhythmia and mortality. Circulation 1979;60:805–814.

36. Antman EM, Tanasijevic MJ, Thompson B, Schactman M, McCabe CH, Cannon CP, Fischer GA, Fung AY, Thompson C, Wybenga D, Braunwald E. Cardiac-specific troponin I levels to predict the risk of mortality in patients with acute coronary syndromes. N Engl J Med 1996;335:1342–1349.

37. Ohman EM, Armstrong PW, Christenson RH, Granger CB, Katus HA, Hamm CW, O'Hanesian MA, Wagner GS, Kleiman NS, Harrell FE, Califf RM, Topol EJ, for the GUSTO-IIA Investigators. Cardiac troponin T levels for risk stratification in acute myocardial ischemia. N Engl J Med 1996;335:1333–1341.

38. Lindahl B, Venge P, Wallentin L, for the FRISC Study Group. Relation between troponin T and the risk of subsequent cardiac events in unstable coronary artery disease. Circulation 1996;93:1651–1657.

39. Hamm CW, Goldmann BU, Heeschen C, Kreymann G, Berger J, Meinertz T. Emergency room triage of patients with acute chest pain by means of rapid testing for cardiac troponin T or troponin I. N Engl J Med 1997;337:1648–1653.

40. Liuzzo G, Biasucci LM, Gallimore JR, Grillo RL, Rebuzzi AG, Pepys MB, Maseri A. The prognostic value of C-reactive protein and serum amyloid A protein in severe unstable angina. N Engl J Med 1994;331:417–424.

41. Nixon JV, Brown CN, Smitherman TC. Identification of transient and persistent segmental wall motion abnormalities in patients with unstable angina by two-dimensional echocardiography. Circulation 1982;65:1497–1503.

42. Hilton TC, Thompson RC, Williams HJ, Saylors R, Fulmer H, Stowers SA. Technetium-99m sestamibi myocardial perfusion imaging in the emergency room evaluation of chest pain. J Am Coll Cardiol 1994;23:1016–1022.

43. Freeman MR, Williams AE, Chisholm RJ, Armstrong PW. Intracoronary thrombus and complex morphology in unstable angina. Relation to timing of angiography and in-hospital cardiac events. Circulation 1989;80:17–23.

44. Davies MF, Bland JM, Hangartner JRW, Angelini A, Thomas AC. Factors influ-

encing the presence or absence of acute coronary artery thrombi in sudden ischaemic death. Eur Heart J 1989;10:203–208.

45. Kannel WB, Abbott RD. Incidence and prognosis of unrecognized myocardial infarction. N Engl J Med 1984;311:1144–1147.

46. Gill JB, Gairns JA, Roberts RS, Constantini L, Sealey BJ, Fallen EF, Tomlinson CW, Gent M. Prognostic importance of myocardial ischemia detected by ambulatory monitoring early after acute myocardial infarction. N Engl J Med 1996;334: 65–70.

47. Hollenberg M, Mangano DT. Therapeutic approaches to postoperative ischemia. Am J Cardiol 1994;73:30B–33B.

48. Mangano DT, Browner WS, Hollenberg M, London MJ, Tubau JF, Tateo IM. Association of perioperative myocardial ischemia with cardiac mobility and mortality in men undergoing noncardiac surgery. N Engl J Med 1990; 323:1781–1788.

49. Hollenberg M, Mangano DT, Browner WS, London MJ, Tubau JF, Tateo IM. Predictors of postoperative myocardial ischemia in patients undergoing noncardiac surgery. JAMA 1992;268:205–209.

50. Stone PH, Chairman BR, Forman S, Andrews TC, Bittner V, Bourassa MG, Davies RF, Deanfield JE, Frishman W, Goldberg AD, MacCallum G, Ouyang P, Pepine CJ, Pratt CM, Sharaf B, Steingart R, Knatterud GL, Sopko G, Conti CR, for the ACIP Investigators. Prognostic significance of myocardial ischemia detected by ambulatory electrocardiography, exercise treadmill testing, and electrocardiogram at rest to predict cardiac events by one year (the Asymptomatic Cardiac Ischemia Pilot Study). Am J Cardiol 1997;80:1395–1401.

51. Sharaf BL, Williams DO, Miele NJ, McMahon RP, Stone PH, Bjerregaard P, Davies R, Goldberg AD, Parks M, Pepine CJ, Sopko G, Conti CR, for the ACIP Investigators. A detailed angiographic analysis of patients with ambulatory electrocardiographic ischemia: Results from the Asymptomatic Cardiac Ischemia Pilot (ACIP) study angiographic core laboratory. J Am Coll Cardiol 1997;29:78–84.

52. Pepine CJ. Prognostic implications of silent myocardial ischemia. N Engl J Med 1996;334:113–114.

53. Graves E. National Hospital Discharge Survey. Annual Survey 1996. Series 13 (4). National Center for Health Statistics, 1998.

54. Mulcahy R, Al Awadhi AH, de Buitleor M, Tobin G, Johnson H, Contoy R. Natural history and prognosis of unstable angina. Am Heart J 1985;109:753–758.

55. Lincoff AM, Tcheng JE, Califf RM, Kereiakes DJ, Kelly TA, Timmis GC, Kleiman NS, Booth JE, Balog C, Cabot CF, Anderson KM, Weisman HF, Topol EJ. Sustained suppression of ischemic complications of coronary intervention by platelet GP IIb/IIIa blockade with abdiximab: one-year outcome in the EPILOG trial. Circulation 1999;99:1951–1958.

56. Schechtman KB, Capone RJ, Kleiger RE, Gibson RS, Schwartz DJ, Roberts R, Young PM, Boden WE. Risk stratification of patients with non-Q wave myocardial infarction. The critical role of ST segment depression. The Diltiazem Reinfarction Study Research Group. Circulation 1989;80:1148–1158.

57. Betriu A, Heras M, Cohen M, Fuster V. Unstable angina: Outcome according to clinical presentation. J Am Coll Cardiol 1992;19:1659–1663.

58. Gazes PC, Mobley EM, Faris HM, Duncan RC, Humphries GB. Preinfarctional

(unstable) angina—a prospective study—ten year follow up: Prognostic significance of electrocardiographic changes. Circulation 1973;48:331–337.

59. Canon CP, Thompson B, McCabe CH, Mueller HS, Kirshenbaum JM, Herson S, Nasmith JB, Chaitman BR, Braunwald E. Predictors of non-Q wave acute myocardial infarction in patients with acute ischemic syndromes: an analysis from the Thrombolysis in Myocardial Ischemia (TIMI) III trials. Am J Cardiol 1995;75: 977–981.

60. Ahmed WH, Bittl JA, Braunwald E. Relation between clinical presentation and angiographic findings in unstable angina pectoris, and comparison with that in stable angina. Am J Cardiol 1993;72:544–550.

61. Karlson BW, Herlitz J, Richter A, Sjolin M, Hjalmarson A. Prognosis in patients with ST-T changes but no rise in serum enzyme activity as compared with non-Q wave infarction. Cardiology 1991;79:271–279.

62. Cragg DR, Friedman HZ, Bonema JD, Jaiyesimi IA, Ramos RG, Timmis GC, O'Neill WW, Schreiber TL. Outcome of patients with acute myocardial infarction who are ineligible for thrombolytic therapy. Ann Intern Med 1991;115:173–177.

63. Klein LW, Helfant RH. The Q wave and non Q wave myocardial infarction: differences and similarities. Prog Cardiovasc Dis 1986;29:205–220.

64. DeWood MA, Spores J, Notske R, Mouser LT, Burroughs R, Golden MS, Lang HT. Prevalence of total coronary occlusion during the early hours of transmural myocardial infarction. N Engl J Med 1980;303:897–902.

65. Rentrop KP. Thrombi in acute coronary syndromes. Revisited and revised. Circulation 2000;101:1619–1626.

66. Reeder GS. Identification and treatment of complications of myocardial infarction. Mayo Clin Proc 1995;70:880–884.

67. Lee KL, Woodlief LH, Topol EJ, Weaver WD, Betriu A, Col J, Simoons M, Aylward P. Van de Werf F, Califf RM. Predictors of 30-day mortality in the era of reperfusion for acute myocardial infarction: Results from an international trial of 41,021 patients. Circulation 1995;91:1659–1668.

68. Farb A, Tang AL, Burke AP, Sessums L, Liang Y, Virmani R. Sudden coronary death. Frequency of active coronary lesions, inactive coronary lesions, and myocardial infarction. Circulation 1995;92:1701–1709.

69. Kragel AH, Gertz SD, Roberts WC. Morphologic comparison of frequency and types of acute lesions in the major epicardial coronary arteries in unstable angina pectoris, sudden coronary death and acute myocardial infarction. J Am Coll Cardiol 1991;18:801–818.

70. Farb A, Burke AP, Tang AL, Liang TY, Mannan P, Smialek J, Virmani R. Coronary plaque erosion without rupture into a lipid core: a frequent cause of coronary thrombosis in sudden coronary death. Circulation 1996;93:1354–1363.

71. Fuster V, Stein B, Ambrose JA, Badimon JJ, Chesebro JH. Atherosclerosis plaque rupture and thrombosis: evolving concepts. Circulation 1990;86(suppl III):47–49.

72. Burke AP, Farb A, Malcom GT, Lang YH, Smialek J, Virmani R. Coronary risk factors and plaque morphology in men with coronary artery disease who died suddenly. N Engl J Med 1997;336:1276–1282.

73. Lammie GA, Dandercock PA, Dennis M. Recently occluded intracranial and extra-

cranial carotid arteries. Relevance of the unstable atherosclerotic plaque. Stroke 1999;30:1319–1325.

74. Davies MJ. Arterial thrombosis and acute coronary syndromes. In: Acute Coronary Syndromes. A Continuing Medical Education Monograph. The International Thrombosis Education Initiative and American College of Cardiology 1999;1–6.

75. Wilson JM, Ferguson JJ III. Platelet-endothelial interactions in atherothrombotic disease: therapeutic implications. Clin Cardiol 1999;22:687–698.

76. Johnstone MT, Mittleman M, Tofler G, Muller JE. The pathophysiology of the onset of morning cardiovascular events. Am J Hypertens 1996;9:22S–28S.

77. Simes RJ, Topol EJ, Holmes DR, White HD, Rutsch WR, Vahanian A, Simoons ML, Morris D, Betriu A, Califf RM, Ross AM. Link between the angiographic substudy and mortality outcomes in a large randomized trial of myocardial reperfusion: importance of early and complete infarct artery reperfusion. Circulation 1995; 91:1923–1928.

78. Fibrinolytic therapy trialists' (FTT) collaborative group. Indications for fibrinolytic therapy in suspected acute myocardial infarction: collaborative overview of early mortality and major morbidity results from all randomized trials of more than 1000 patients. Lancet 1994;343:311–322.

79. The TIMI IIIB Investigators. Effects of tissue plasminogen activator and a comparison of early invasive and conservative strategies in unstable angina and non Q wave myocardial infarction. Results of the TIMI IIIB Trial. Circulation 1994;89:1545–1556.

80. The TIMI IIIA Investigators. Early effects of tissue type plasminogen activator added to conventional therapy on the culprit coronary lesion in patients presenting with ischemic cardiac pain at rest. Results of the TIMI IIIA Trial. Circulation 1993; 87:38–52.

81. Waters D, Lam JYT. Is thrombolytic therapy striking out in unstable angina? Circulation 1992;86:1642–1644.

82. The GUSTO IIb Substudy Investigators. A clinical trial comparing primary coronary angioplasty with tissue plasminogen activator for acute myocardial infarction. N Engl J Med 1997;336:1621–1628.

83. Grines CL, Browne KF, Marco J, Rothbaum D, Stone GW, O'Keefe J, Overlie P, Donohue N, Timmis GC, Vlietstra RE, Strzelecki M, Puchrowicz-Ochocki S, O'Neill WW, for the Primary Angioplasty in Myocardial Infarction Study Group. A comparison of immediate angioplasty with thrombolytic therapy for acute myocardial infarction. N Engl J Med 1993;328:673–679.

84. Suryapranata H, Van't Hof AWJ, Hoorntje JCA, de Boer MJ, Zijlstra F. Randomized comparison of coronary stenting with balloon angioplasty in selected patients with acute myocardial infarction. Circulation 1998;97:2502–2505.

85. Boden WE, O'Rourke RA, Crawford MH, Blaustein AS, Deedwania PC, Zoble RG, Wexler LF, Kleiger RE, Pepine CJ, Ferry DR, Chow BK, Lavori PW for the The VANQWISH Trial Investigators. Outcomes in patients with acute non-Q wave myocardial infarction randomly assigned to an invasive as compared with a conservative management strategy. N Engl J Med 1998;338:1785–1792.

86. Fragmin and Fast Revascularisation during InStability in Coronary artery disease

Investigators. Invasive compared with non-invasive treatment in unstable coronary-artery disease: FRISC II prospective randomized multicenter study. Lancet 1999; 354:708–715.

87. Channon CP, Weintraub WS, Demopoulos L, Robertson D, DeLucca P, McCabe CH, Braunwald E. Results of the treat angina with Aggrastat and determine the cost of therapy with an invasive or conservative strategy (TACTICS-TIMI 18) trial. A comparison of invasive vs. conservative strategies in patients with unstable angina and non-ST elevation myocardial infarction. Presented at the Scientific Sessions of the American Heart Association. New Orleans, LA, November 2000.

88. Hochman JS, Sleeper LA, Webb JG, Sanborn TA, White HD, Talley JD, Buller CE, Jacobs AK, Slater JN, Col J, McKinlay SM, LeJemtel TH. Should we emergently revascularize occluded coronary arteries for cardiogenic shock? N Engl J Med 1999;341:624–634.

89. Ross AM, Lundergan CF, Rohrbeck SC, Boyle DH, van den Brand M, Buller CH, Holmes DR, Reiner JS, for the GUSTO-1 Angiographic Investigators. Rescue angioplasty after failed thrombolysis: technical and clinical outcomes in a large thrombolysis trial. J Am Coll Cardiol 1998;31:1511–1517.

90. Basu S, Senior R, Raval U, van der Does R, Bruckner T, Lahiri A. Beneficial effects of intravenous and oral carvedilol treatment in acute myocardial infarction. A placebo controlled, randomized trial. Circulation 1997;96:183–191.

91. Soumerai SB, McLaughlin TJ, Spiegelman D, Hertzmark E, Thibault G, Goldman L. Adverse outcomes of underuse of B-blockers in elderly survivors of acute myocardial infarction. JAMA 1997;277:115–121.

92. Beta-Blocker Heart Attack Trial Research Group. A randomized trial of propranolol in patients with acute myocardial infarction. I. Mortality results. JAMA 1982;247: 1707–1714.

93. ISIS-1 (First International Study of Infarct Survival) Collaborative Group. Randomised trial of intravenous atenolol among 16,027 cases of suspected acute myocardial infarction: ISIS-1. Lancet 1986;2:57–66.

94. Yusuf S, Wittes J, Friedman L. Overview of results of randomized clinical trials in heart disease. II. Unstable angina, heart failure, primary prevention with aspirin, and risk factor modification. JAMA 1988;260:2259–2263.

95. Lewis HD Jr, Davis JW, Archibald DG, Steinke WE, Smitherman TC, Doherty JE, Schnaper HW, LeWinter MM, Linares E, Pouget JM, Sabharwal SC, Chesler E, DeMots H. Protective effects of aspirin against acute myocardial infarction and death in men with unstable angina: results of a Veterans Administration Cooperative Study. N Engl J Med 1983;309:396–403.

96. Cairns JA, Gent M, Singer J, Finnie KJ, Froggart GM, Holder DA, Jablonsky G, Kostuk WJ, Melendez LJ, Myers MG, Sackett DL, Sealey BJ, Tanser PH. Aspirin, sulfinpyrazone, or both in unstable angina: results of a Canadian multicenter trial. N Engl J Med 1985;313:1369–1375.

97. ISIS-2 (Second International Study of Infarct Survival) Collaborative Group. Randomised trial of intravenous streptokinase, oral aspirin, both, or neither among 17,187 cases of suspected acute myocardial infarction: ISIS-2. Lancet 1988;2:349–360.

98. Theroux P, Ouimet H, McCans J, Latour JG, Joly P, Levy G, Pelletier E, Juneau

M, Stasiak J, deGuise P, Pelletier GB, Rinzler D, Waters DD. Aspirin, heparin, or both to treat acute unstable angina. N Engl J Med 1988;319:1105–1111.

99. Granger CB, Hirsch J, Califf RM, Col J, White HD, Betriu A, Woodlief LH, Lee KL, Bovill EG, Simes RJ, Topol EJ. Activated partial thromboplastin time and outcome after thrombolytic therapy of acute myocardial infarction. Circulation 1996;93:870–878.

100. Cohen M, Demers C, Gurfinkel EP, Turpie AGG, Fromell GJ, Goodman S, Langer A, Califf RM, Fox KAA, Premmereur J, Bigonzi F, for the Efficacy and Safety of Subcutaneous Enoxaparin in Non-Q wave Coronary Events Study Group. A comparison of low-molecular-weight heparin with unfractionated heparin for unstable coronary artery disease. N Engl J Med 1997;337:447–452.

101. The PURSUIT Trial Investigators. Inhibition of platelet glycoprotein IIb/IIIa with eptifibatide in patients with acute coronary syndromes. N Engl J Med 1998;339: 436–443.

102. The PRISM-PLUS Investigators. Inhibition of the platelet glycoprotein IIb/IIIa receptor with tirofiban in unstable angina and non-Q wave myocardial infarction. N Engl J Med 1998;388:1488–1497.

103. Zaacks SM, Liebson PR, Calvin JE, Parrillo JE, Klein LW. Unstable angina and non-Q wave myocardial infarction: does the clinical diagnosis have therapeutic implications? J Am Coll Cardiol 1999;33:107–118.

9
Triggers of Coronary Plaque Rupture Syndromes

Jacqueline Müller-Nordhorn and Stefan N. Willich
Charité Hospital, Humboldt University of Berlin, Berlin, Germany

I. INTRODUCTION

Plaque rupture and subsequent thrombosis at the site of the plaque rupture is the most common underlying pathophysiological mechanism of acute coronary syndromes (1). The clinical manifestations of acute coronary syndromes are sudden cardiac death, acute myocardial infarction, and unstable angina. Approximately 90% of cases of nonfatal myocardial infarction and many cases of sudden cardiac death are caused by the rupture of a coronary atherosclerotic plaque (2). Plaque rupture may be precipitated by external stresses or 'triggers' superimposed on vulnerable coronary plaques (3). It is important to differentiate intrinsic long-term changes of coronary plaques, internal triggering mechanisms, and external triggers (Figure 1). Intrinsic long-term changes consist of progressive lipid accumulation in the atheromatous core and degradation of the fibrous cap by proteolytic processes and inflammation (4, 5). An increased vulnerability of the plaque and a proneness to rupture are the consequences. External triggers probably activate internal triggering mechanisms such as biomechanical and hemodynamic stresses and changes in platelet aggregability and blood viscosity; they may thus determine the actual time of coronary plaque rupture (2). External triggers include physical activity, emotional stress, environmental changes, and other factors. A circadian, weekly, and seasonal variation of coronary events has also been observed.

A number of studies have examined the relationship between external triggers and the onset of acute coronary syndromes. For example, the MILIS (Multicenter Investigation of Limitation of Infarct Size) Study (6) showed that

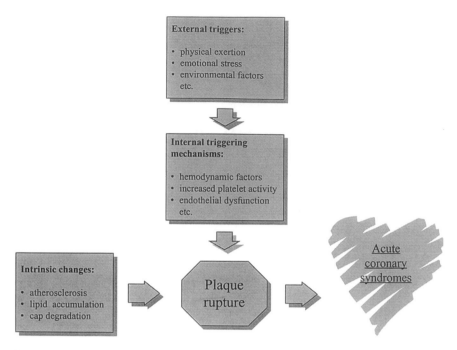

Figure 1   Model of triggering of acute coronary syndromes (see text for details).

50% of 849 patients reported possible triggers preceding the event. The following main triggers were experienced by the patients: emotional stress (19%), moderate physical activity (14%), and heavy physical activity (9%). Sumiyoshi et al. (7) found that among 416 patients admitted to the National Heart Center of Japan, 53% reported that their infarct occurred during moderate to heavy exertion, emotional stress, or excitation. Smith et al. (8) showed that of 186 patients interviewed within 72 hours after admission for myocardial infarction, 40% reported either emotional distress, strenuous exercise, or a sudden change in position, usually in the morning after awakening.

In this chapter, we will review the evidence for the frequency and importance of external triggers of coronary plaque rupture syndromes and their pathophysiological consequences and propose improved preventive strategies.

II.   EXTERNAL TRIGGERS OF PLAQUE RUPTURE

A.   Physical Activity

Physical activity may trigger the rupture of coronary plaques resulting in acute coronary syndromes (7, 9, 10). Several studies of patients with acute coronary events have established that in approximately 5 to 14% of cases, heavy exertion precedes the onset of symptoms (11). In the TRIMM (Triggers and Mechanisms of Myocardial Infarction) Study (9), 1194 patients in Germany were interviewed during their hospital stay for acute myocardial infarction, focusing on the hours before the acute event. Exposure to possible triggers in patients was compared first with matched controls and second, in a case-crossover analysis, with the patient acting as his or her own control (12). In the case-crossover analysis, the frequency of physical exertion in the hours preceding the onset of symptoms was compared with the usual frequency of such exertion over the year before the infarction. Heavy physical exertion at the onset of myocardial infarction was reported by 7.1% of patients compared with 3.9% in the control group. The increase in relative risk associated with physical exertion during and in the 1-hour period after the acute event was approximately twofold [relative risk (RR), 2.1; 95% confidence internal (CI): 1.1, 3.6]. Figure 2 shows the different odds ratios of various physical activity states among patients compared with controls (13). A significant difference ($p < 0.01$) in the relative risk of persons engaging in regular heavy exertion at least four times per week compared with those exercising fewer than four times per week could be detected as well (RR, 1.3 and 6.9, respectively). The risk of myocardial infarction associated with strenuous exercise is therefore particularly increased in individuals with a more sedentary life-

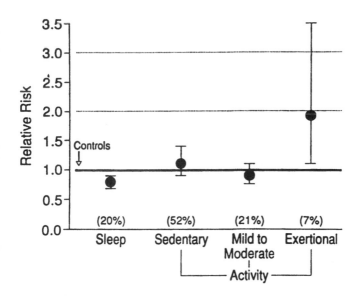

Figure 2 Physical activity at the onset of myocardial infarction. Adjusted odds ratios of physical activity states among patients with myocardial infarction compared with controls. (From Ref. 13.)

style. Similar in design to the TRIMM Study, the Onset Study (10) interviewed 1228 patients in the United States about their activities at the advent of acute myocardial infarction. Heavy physical exertion was reported by 4.4% of the patients; the induction time was usually less than 1 hour, with symptoms beginning during the activity. The estimated relative risk of myocardial infarction in the hour after heavy physical exercise was 5.9 (95% CI: 4.6, 7.7). The relative risk ranged from as high as 104 in patients who exercised less than once per week on average to 2.4 in patients who exercised more than five times per week. Higher levels of habitual physical activity were therefore associated with a lower relative risk during exertional activities. The inherent problem of studies investigating activities preceding acute coronary syndromes is their retrospective nature. Patients may have a tendency to overestimate the amount of physical activity and other possible triggers; recall bias cannot be excluded.

Acute physical exertion as a trigger in the subgroup of sudden cardiac deaths is difficult to assess, because a history of the hours preceding the event can usually not be obtained from the patient (14). Second-hand information by the family and other witnesses is often incomplete and not reliable. Patients who have been successfully resuscitated can be interviewed, but they may not be representative of the whole group of sudden cardiac death patients. In addition, their memory may be obscured by the trauma of the event. Patients with an implantable cardioverter are another potential source of information, but selection bias is difficult to eliminate. Physical fitness is associated with a lower risk of sudden cardiac death, similar to myocardial infarction. In a prospective British cohort study (15), 7735 middle-aged men from 24 British towns with and without pre-existing ischemic heart disease were followed for 8 years. Physical activity was assessed with questionnaires. During this time, 488 major cardiac events occurred, of which 117 (24%) were classified as sudden cardiac deaths. Regular exertion was associated with a decreased risk of sudden cardiac death ($p < 0.05$) in men without pre-existing ischemic heart disease.

Physical activity is thus a double-edged sword for patients with coronary disease. Acute exertion is associated with a marked risk of triggering acute coronary syndromes, particularly if performed by untrained individuals with coronary heart disease. But although the relative risk associated with acute heavy exertion may be high, the absolute risk is relatively small (16). Regular physical activity, on the other hand, has a beneficial effect and reduces mortality from coronary heart disease in the long term (17).

B. Emotional Stress

Acute coronary syndromes may also be triggered by emotional stress. Studies indicate that approximately 4 to 18% of cases of myocardial infarction are immediately preceded by emotional stress (11). In particular, episodes of anger have been reported to trigger acute events. The Onset Study (18) showed a twofold increased relative risk of acute coronary syndromes in the 2 hours after an emotional outburst of anger (Figure 3). Anger was assessed by the Onset anger scale, which is a single item, seven-level, self-reported scale, and by the state anger subscale of the State-Trait Personality Inventory. Thirty-nine of 1623 patients (2.4%) were identified with episodes of anger in the 2 hours before the onset of myocardial infarction. Regular users of aspirin ($p < 0.05$) had a significantly lower relative risk than nonusers (1.9 vs. 2.9%, respectively). The patients of the TRIMM Study were more likely to report emotionally upsetting events as possible triggers of myocardial infarction than the controls ($p < 0.05$). In addition to this subjective reporting, objective unusual life events such as death of a family member or friend, etc., were evaluated. The cumulative frequency of these life events during weeks before myocardial infarction was similar in both groups. The patient group showed a greater tendency to report stress at work than the control group, but this was not statistically significant (9).

Personality structures predisposing to acute coronary events are type A behavior and anxiety (19). The evidence provided by several prospective studies on the relationship between depression and acute coronary syndromes is inconsistent. Components of type A behavior that increase the risk of acute coronary

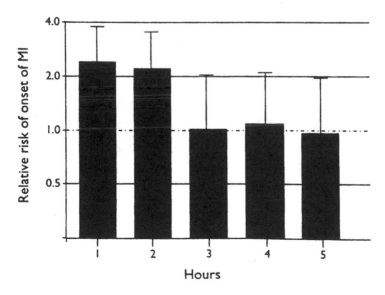

Figure 3 Relative risk of myocardial infarction in the hours after an outburst of anger. The error bars indicate the 95% confidence intervals; the dotted line represents the baseline risk. (From Ref. 18.)

syndromes are hostility, cynicism, and anger (20). A prospective study by Kawachi et al. (21) in 1994 with a cohort of American physicians suggested an
increased risk of sudden cardiac death associated with phobic anxiety.

C.   Other Possible Triggers

Other possible triggers of acute coronary events include sexual activity, war
threats, and earthquakes. They often combine unusual emotional and physical
stress, but other factors may play a role as well.

Sexual activity occasionally serves as a trigger of myocardial infarction,
unstable angina, and sudden cardiac death. The Onset Study, for example, showed
a 2.5-fold increased relative risk of acute coronary syndromes in the 2 hours after
sexual activity (22). But because sexual activity only contributed to about 0.9%
of cases, the authors concluded that the absolute risk was extremely low. Furthermore, the relative risk was not increased in patients with a previous history of
acute coronary syndromes, and regular exercise appeared to prevent triggering.
A number of cardiac deaths have been associated with the new drug sildenafil
(Viagra), which is taken as a treatment for male erectile dysfunction. Because
their risk profile is similar, patients with impotence may also have coronary heart
disease (e.g., they are more likely to be older and to have other underlying diseases such as hypertension and diabetes). Apparently, a combination of nitrates
and other cardiovascular drugs with Viagra can lead to an irreversible drop in
blood pressure, resulting in myocardial infarction and death in men with pre-
existing coronary heart disease (23). Another possible explanation is that men,
who are no longer used to regular sexual activity, suddenly engage again in a
potentially strenuous activity. But further evaluation of the reported deaths is still
needed.

Acute stress such as caused by earthquakes or war threats can result in
acute coronary syndromes as well. Suzuki et al. (24) examined patients with acute
myocardial infarctions after the most severe earthquake ever to occur in Japan
(Hanshin-Awaji district) in January 1995. The number of patients increased by
about 3.5-fold during the first 4 weeks after the earthquake. The mean posttrau-
matic stress disorder reaction index score indicated a severe stress level. The
proportion of women with acute myocardial infarction was significantly higher
than in the preceding years; their mean score on the stress disorder index was
considerably higher than in men. The authors concluded that after an earthquake,
severe emotional stress can trigger acute myocardial infarctions, especially in
women.

Sudden cardiac deaths increased significantly during the Northridge earthquake in California in January 1994 (25). The number of deaths rose from a daily
average of 4.6 (SD $\pm$ 2.1) to 24 on the day of the earthquake (Figure 4). In the
week following the earthquake, there was an unusually low incidence of sudden

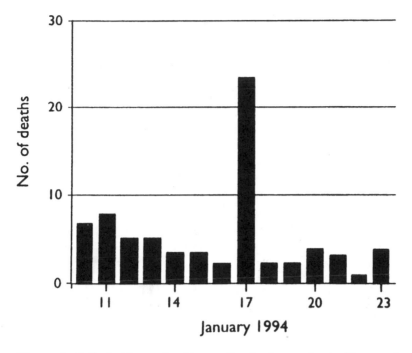

Figure 4 Daily incidence of sudden cardiac deaths associated with an earthquake. A major earthquake occurred in Northridge, California, on January 17, 1994. (From Ref. 25.)

cardiac deaths (2.7 ± 1.2 per day). These findings suggest that stress may precipitate cardiac events in people who were predisposed to such events but would have had them at a later date.

The effect of war on the incidence of acute coronary syndromes has been observed in the Israeli civilian population during the first days of the Gulf War in 1991 (26) (Figure 5). A 58% increment in mortality largely caused by an increase in mortality from cardiovascular diseases could be observed on the day of the first strike on Israeli cities (27). Female mortality showed a more pronounced 77% increase in mortality compared with a 41% increase in mortality for men.

D. Environmental Factors and Smoking

Air pollution as an environmental factor has been consistently associated with increased cardiovascular mortality. For example, in the December 1952 smog disaster in London, a substantial increase in cardiovascular mortality has been

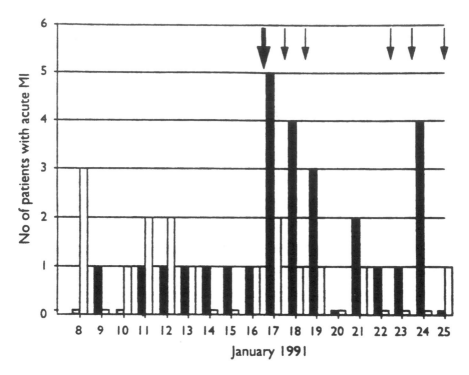

Figure 5   Daily incidence of acute myocardial infarction associated with war threat in a Tel Aviv population from January 8 to 25, 1991, compared with the same period in 1990. Large arrows = beginning of the Gulf war; small arrows = missile attacks on Israel. (From Ref. 26.)

reported (28). Several studies have documented associations between short-term increments of air pollutants such as sulfur dioxide and cardiovascular admissions (29) to the hospital. But because different methods for evaluation have been used, a comparison of the results proved to be difficult. The multinational European Community–funded APHEA (Air Pollution of Health: European Approach) project in 10 different European countries and 12 European cities (30) investigated the relationship between air pollution and mortality from specific causes using a standard statistical method. A time series analysis with the application of Poisson regression to the daily number of deaths from selected causes over several years was performed. Possible confounding factors were taken into account. A positive relationship between increased daily air pollution and the incidence of acute coronary syndromes has been observed by a considerable number of European cities participating in the APHEA trial (31–35), as well as by a number of other trials outside Europe (29, 36–39).

Peters et al. (40) hypothesized that inflammation of the peripheral airways caused by pollution might increase blood coagulability by means of an acute-phase reaction. Plasma viscosity was measured as part of the MONICA Augsburg survey during the winter of 1984–85. Daily mean concentrations of air pollution were recorded by the Bavarian air-quality network in Augsburg. Plasma viscosity was assessed in 324 people during a 13-day period, when high concentrations of sulfur dioxide (mean, 200 $\mu g/m^3$) and total suspended particles (mean 98 $\mu g/m^3$) were reported. In the remaining time period of the survey, plasma viscosity of a further 2932 people was measured. The odds ratio for plasma viscosity above the 95th percentile of the distribution in the 13-day time period was 3.6 (95% CI: 1.6, 8.1) for men and 2.3 (95% CI: 1.0, 5.3) for women.

Some evidence suggests that smoking is not only a long-term risk factor for coronary heart disease but may be a potential trigger for the development of an acute coronary thrombus as well. Burke et al. (41) examined the coronary arteries of 113 patients with sudden cardiac death. Fifty-nine men had an acute coronary thrombus develop, and in the remaining 54 men, narrowing of the coronary arteries by an atherosclerotic plaque without acute thrombosis could be detected. Seventy-five percent of men with an acute thrombus were smokers compared with 41% of those with stable plaques ($p < 0.001$).

III. THE SIGNIFICANCE OF THE CIRCADIAN, WEEKLY, AND SEASONAL VARIATION

A. The Circadian Variation

The presence of a circadian variation in the onset of acute coronary events was originally proposed by Muller et al. (42). On the basis of numerous reports, the circadian pattern with an increased morning risk and a trough during the night is now well established (43–46). A meta-analysis, performed by Cohen et al. (47) in 1997, concluded that approximately 1 of every 11 acute myocardial infarctions and 1 of every 15 sudden cardiac deaths are attributable to the morning excess risk. The TRIMM Study (9) demonstrated a twofold to threefold increased risk of acute coronary syndromes in the 3 hours after awakening ($p < 0.01$) (Figure 6). Two major prospective studies, the ISAM (Intravenous Streptokinase in Acute Myocardial Infarction) Study (48) and the ISIS-2 (Second International Study of Infarct Survival) trial (49), which included 1741 and 12,163 patients, respectively, confirmed the morning peak of coronary events. It was often argued that the morning peak was because patients slept through the onset of symptoms and only reported them after awakening. The MILIS Study (42) used serial creati-

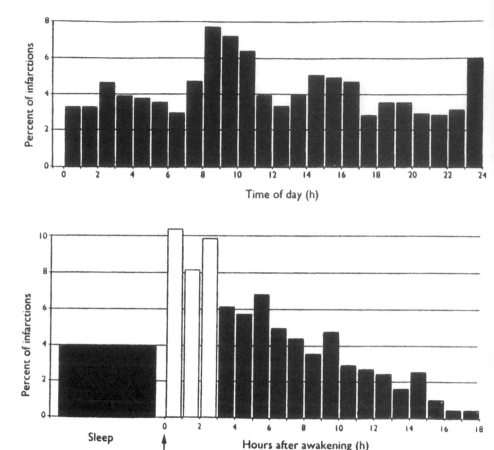

Figure 6 Circadian variation in the onset of myocardial infarction. The upper panel shows the unadjusted circadian pattern of myocardial infarction ($p < 0.01$); the lower panel the circadian pattern adjusted for time of awakening. (From Ref. 9.)

nine kinase levels from 703 patients and extrapolated from the results to define the onset time of the event. Again, a marked morning peak could be shown, and an artefact caused by increased reporting in the morning seems unlikely.

Some studies (50–52) described a second peak of acute coronary events in the afternoon or evening. For example, a Swedish study by Hansen et al. (53), including 10,791 patients, observed a bimodal circadian variation with a peak in the morning (6 AM and 12 AM) and a second peak in the evening (6 PM and

12 PM). A New Zealand Study, the ARCOS Study (54), which was done in collaboration with the WHO MONICA Project ($n = 4983$ patients), demonstrated both an afternoon peak and a secondary morning peak in the subgroup of sudden cardiac death patients. The observed difference in circadian patterns may reflect different lifestyles and/or rest activity patterns. The combination with other triggers of acute coronary syndromes, such as physical activity or emotional stress, appears to increase the morning risk even further. Krantz et al. (55) showed that during the morning, ischemic vs. nonischemic periods were more likely to occur with high levels of activity ($p < 0.001$). High physical activity triggered ischemia to a lesser but still significant extent in the afternoon ($p < 0.05$), but not in the evening ($p < 0.04$).

The circadian variation affects all types of coronary syndromes. Sudden cardiac deaths have an approximately threefold increase in relative risk during the morning (56). The CAST (Cardiac Arrhythmia Suppression Trial) (57) showed that sudden cardiac deaths occurred most frequently within 2 hours after awakening. Ventricular fibrillation and ventricular tachycardia as causes of sudden cardiac death followed the circadian pattern, whereas electromechanical dissociation and asystole were quite evenly distributed throughout the day (50, 58). The circadian variation is also observed in unstable angina and non-Q-wave acute myocardial infarction ($p < 0.001$), as demonstrated by Cannon et al. (43).

Beta-adrenergic blocking agents and aspirin appear to reduce the incidence of myocardial infarction in the morning. The Physicians' Health Study (45), a randomized placebo-controlled trial, compared the incidence of myocardial infarction in 22,071 U.S. men taking either aspirin or placebo. Aspirin was associated with a 59% reduction in the incidence of infarction during the morning hours, compared with a 34% reduction for the remaining hours of the day. A number of studies (42, 48, 53) showed the absence of a circadian variation with β-blocking agents. The importance of these findings is that appropriate pharmacological protection can be directed at the morning hours for patients with coronary heart disease (59). The absence of a circadian pattern in the subgroup of patients with diabetes in the ISIS-2 trial ($n = 12,163$ patients) suggests impairment of the autonomic nervous system (49). The findings of Behar et al. (44), on the other hand, did not confirm the absence of a circadian variation in diabetic patients, only in patients with peripheral vascular disease and those having had a stroke.

The inhibition of fibrinolytic activity in blood peaks in the morning, favoring the development of an arterial thrombus (60). A Japanese study with 244 patients with acute myocardial infarction described a resistance to thrombolytic treatment after a circadian pattern similar to myocardial infarction (52) ($p < 0.05$), with a phase difference of about 2 hours. Similarly, Kurnik (61) claimed that there is a circadian variation in the ability of the tissue-type plasminogen activator to rapidly open coronary arteries, with the highest efficacy between noon and midnight. In the study by Winther et al. (62) with healthy male subjects, assuming the upright position in the morning significantly increased platelet aggregation and produced only a moderate increase in fibrinolytic activity. Compared with exercise, assuming the upright posture increased platelet aggregation to similar levels, but exercise was also associated with a higher protective fibrinolytic activity.

B. The Weekly Variation

The weekly profile shows that the risk of acute coronary syndromes is greater at the beginning of the week than on the other days (46, 63). The New Zealand ARCOS trial (54) found an increased incidence not only on Mondays but also during the weekend for surviving patients, and a Saturday high (18.6%) for sudden cardiac deaths. In a study conducted by the Augsburg MONICA center, 5596 patients were analyzed in a regionally defined population between 1985 and 1990 (64). Patients with myocardial infarction ($n = 2636$) demonstrated a significant weekly variation ($p < 0.01$) with a peak on Monday, whereas patients with sud-

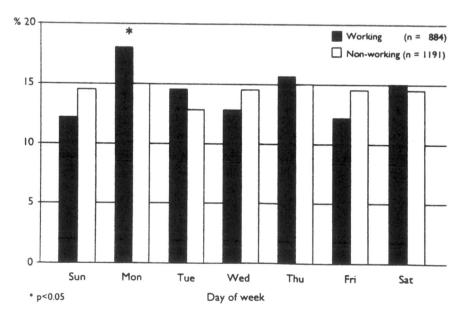

Figure 7 Weekly variation in the onset of myocardial infarction in a working ($n = 884$) and a nonworking ($n = 1191$) population (1985–1990). (From Ref. 64.)

den cardiac death ($n = 2960$) were evenly distributed throughout the week. Information on working status was available for 2074 of the 2636 patients with myocardial infarction. The weekly variation in the incidence could only be seen in the working population, with a 33% increase in relative risk on Mondays ($p < 0.05$) (Figure 7). The weekly pattern was observed in all patients out of the working population, irrespective of age, sex, cardiac risk factors, prior cardiac medication, and infarct characteristics.

C. The Seasonal Variation

Myocardial infarction occurs more frequently in the winter months than in summer months and, generally, on colder days the year around (46, 65, 66). Analyzing a total of 259,891 cases of acute myocardial infarction reported to the second National Registry of Myocardial Infarction (NRMI-2), Spencer et al. (67) confirmed the seasonal variation with increased incidence in winter. Approximately 53% more cases were reported in winter than during the summer months. The same seasonal pattern was seen in men and women, in different age groups and in 9 of 10 geographical areas.

IV. PATHOPHYSIOLOGY

Physical exertion, emotional stress, and the other possible triggers of coronary plaque rupture syndromes may lead to a change in the hemodynamic and biomechanical parameters, as well as to an alteration of the platelet and coagulation systems (68, 69). The activation of the sympathetic nervous system by stress of any kind increases the cardiac output with a higher blood pressure and pulse rate with the secretion of catecholamines. Greater circumferential and flexion stresses on vulnerable plaques are the consequence. Circumferential stress depends, according to Laplace's law (2, 70), on the arterial blood pressure and the vessel radius and is inversely related to the thickness of the vessel wall. Following Laplace's law, mild and moderate lesions are more likely to rupture than the more severe ones; this is confirmed by 60 to 70% of acute coronary syndromes evolving from mildly to moderately obstructive atherosclerotic plaques (4). Flexion stress with axial bending and stretching of the coronary arteries (2) is associated with heart contractions.

 Platelet activity, leading to thrombosis at the site of the ruptured plaque, appears to be increased by acute physical exertion, especially in patients with prior myocardial infarction (71) and in sedentary individuals (72) but not in healthy volunteers. Emotional activity (73) and smoking, similarly, lead to a higher platelet aggregability. Aspirin does not prevent the enhanced platelet activity in smokers (74). Increased catecholamine secretion and shear stress during periods of stress are probably responsible for the activation of the platelet system (75). The benefit of regular dynamic exercise appears to be caused by an improved cardiac output and stroke volume. This leads to a decreased activation of the sympathetic nervous system with lower levels of plasma catecholamines and a lower pulse rate and rate-pressure product at rest and during comparable levels of physical exertion. Regular exercise also has a favorable effect on the lipid profile, causes an inhibition of platelet aggregability (76), and increases the endogenous fibrinolytic response to venous occlusion.

The higher morning incidence of acute coronary events is presumably also caused by an activation of the sympathetic system in the morning (77). Elevation of coagulation factors with a greater tendency to clot during cold weather may, in part, explain the higher mortality from myocardial infarction in winter. A study by Yeh et al. (78) measured coagulating factors including antithrombin III, prothrombin time, activated partial thromboplastin time, fibrinogen, plasminogen, and the factors VII and VIII in 2877 subjects. A statistically significant increment of all parameters, except prothrombin time, could be shown on days with a mean temperature $<20°C$ compared with days with a mean temperature $>20°C$.

V. IMPLICATIONS FOR PREVENTION

External triggers in acute coronary syndromes were identified in previous studies in up to 50% of all patients. Reduction or elimination of triggers could, therefore, play a major role in the prevention of acute events. But whereas certain triggering activities are comparatively easy to avoid, others such as emotional stress or sexual activity belong to human life, and it is neither desirable nor feasible to control them. Pharmacological protection of the population at risk during vulnerable periods will be one of the key issues in the future. Medications, such as β-blockers and aspirin, have already been shown to lower the increased morning risk. Health education about the risks associated, for example, with sudden, strenuous exercise in untrained individuals or with smoking has to be given more emphasis as well. But it has to be taken into account that knowledge about potential triggers might increase anxiety in patients and result in a reduction of activities and in a potential loss of quality of life. It is of note that regular physical activity is not only for long-term protection but also reduces the risk of acute strenuous exercise.

A vulnerable plaque is a "time bomb" with potential catastrophic consequences. To avoid or at least delay plaque rupture by developing appropriate preventive strategies is essential in reducing the incidence and mortality of coronary syndromes. Behavior modification and pharmacological interventions seem equally important.

REFERENCES

1. Fuster V, Badimon J, Chesebro JH, Fallon JT. Plaque rupture, thrombosis, and therapeutic implications. Haemostasis 1996; 26(suppl 4):269–284.
2. Davies MJ, Thomas AC. Plaque fissuring—the cause of myocardial infarction, sudden ischemic death, and crescendo angina. Br Heart J 1985; 53:363–373.
3. Grønholdt ML, Dalager-Pederson S, Falk E. Coronary atherosclerosis: determinants of plaque rupture. Eur Heart J 1998; 19(suppl C):C24–C29.
4. Shah PK. Plaque disruption and coronary thrombosis: new insight into pathogenesis and prevention. Clin Cardiol 1997; 20(suppl 2):II38–44.
5. Bauriedel G, Schmucking I, Hutter R, Luchesi C, Welsch U, Kandolf R, Luderitz B. Increased apoptosis and necrosis in unstable angina. Z Kardiol 1997; 86:902–910.
6. Tofler GH, Stone PH, Maclure M, Edelman E, Davis VG, Robertson T, Antman EM, Muller-JE. Analysis of possible triggers of acute myocardial infarction (The MILIS Study). Am J Cardiol 1990; 66:22–27.
7. Sumiyoshi T, Haze K, Saito M, Fukami K, Goto Y, Hiramori K. Evaluation of clinical factors involved in the onset of myocardial infarction. Jpn Circ J 1986; 50:164–173.
8. Smith M, Little WC. Potential precipitating factors of the onset of myocardial infarction. Am J Med Sci 1992; 303:141–144.
9. Willich SN, Lewis M, Löwel H, Arntz HR, Schubert F, Schröder R. Physical exertion as a trigger of acute myocardial infarction. N Engl J Med 1993; 329:1684–1690.
10. Mittleman MA, Maclure M, Tofler GH, Sherwood JB, Goldberg RJ, Muller JE. Triggering of acute myocardial infarction by heavy physical exertion. N Engl J Med 1993; 329:1677–1683.
11. Mittleman MA. Triggering of myocardial infarction by physical activity, emotional stress and sexual activity. In: Willich SN, Muller JE, eds. Triggering of Acute Coronary Syndromes. Dodrecht, Boston, London: Kluwer Academic Publishers, 1996; 267–283.
12. Maclure M. The case-crossover design: a method for studying transient effects on the risk of acute events. Am J Epidemiol 1991; 133:144–153.
13. Willich SN, Lewis M, Arntz HR, Löwel H, Schubert F, Stern R, Schröder R, und die TRIMM-Studiengruppe. Belastungssituation beim akuten Myokardinfarkt: Die Rolle von körperlicher Anstrengung und ungewöhnlichen Lebensereignissen. Z Kardiol 1994; 83:423–430.
14. Willich SN, Arntz HR. Triggers of sudden cardiac death. In: Willich SN, Muller JE, eds. Triggering of Acute Coronary Syndromes. Dodrecht, Boston, London: Kluwer Academic Publishers, 1996; 267–283.

15. Wannamethee G, Shaper AG, Macfarlane PW, Walker M. Risk factors for sudden cardiac death in middle-aged British men. Circulation 1995; 91:1749–1756.
16. Mittleman MA, Siscovick DS. Physical exertion as a trigger of myocardial infarction and sudden cardiac death. Cardiol Clin 1996; 14:263–270.
17. Pfaffenbarger RS Jr, Hyde RT, Wing AI, Jung DL, Kampert JB. The association of changes in physical-activity level and other lifestyle characteristics with mortality among men. N Engl J Med 1993; 328:538–545.
18. Mittleman MA, Maclure M, Sherwood JB, Mulry RP, Tofler GH, Jacobs SC, Friedman R, Benson H, Muller JE. Triggering of acute myocardial infarction onset by episodes of anger. Circulation 1995; 92:1720–1725.
19. Wassertheil-Smoller. Subacute psychobiological factors. In: Willich SN, Muller JE. Triggering of Acute Coronary Syndromes. Dodrecht, Boston, London: Kluwer Academic Publishers, 1996; 267–283.
20. Williams RB. Psychological factors in coronary artery disease: Epidemiological evidence. Circulation 1987; 76(supply I):I-117–I-23.
21. Kawachi I, Colditz GA, Ascherio A, Rimm EB, Giovannucci E, Stampfer MJ, Willett WC. Prospective study of phobic anxiety and risk of coronary heart disease in men. Circulation 1994; 89:1992–1997.
22. Muller JE, Mittleman A, Maclure M, Sherwood JB, Tofler GH. Triggering myocardial infarction by sexual activity. Low absolute risk and prevention by regular physical exertion. Determinants of Myocardial Infarction Onset Study Investigators. JAMA 1996; 275:1405–1409.
23. Blickpunkt IM. Arzneimittelsicherheit und Viagra—Plädoyer für die einstweilige Marktrücknahme. Arznei-telegramm 1998, 6/53–54.
24. Suzuki S, Sakamoto S, Koide M, Fujita H, Sakuramoto H, Kuroda T, Kintaka T, Matsuo T. Hanshin-Awaji earthquake as a trigger for acute myocardial infarction. Am Heart J 1997; 134(5Pt1):974–977.
25. Leor J, Poole K, Kloner RA. Sudden cardiac deaths triggered by an earthquake. N Engl J Med 1996; 334:413–419.
26. Meisel SR, Kutz I, Dayan KI, Pauzner-H, Chetboun I, Arbel Y, David D. Effect of iraqi missile war on incidence of acute myocardial infarction and sudden death in Israeli civilians. Lancet 1991; 338:660–661.
27. Kark JD, Goldman S, Epstein L. Iraqui missile attacks on Israel. The association of mortality with a life-threatening stressor. JAMA 1995; 273:1208–1210.
28. Schwartz-J. Air pollution and daily mortality: a review and meta-analysis. Environ Res 1994; 64:36–52.
29. Schwartz J. Air pollution and hospital admissions for cardiovascular disease in Tucson. Epidemiology 1997; 8:371–377.
30. Katsouyanni K, Touloumi G, Spix C, Schwartz J, Balducci F, Medina S, Rossi G, Woityniak B, Sunyer J, Bacharova L, Schouten JP, Ponka A, Anderson HR. Short-term effects of ambient sulphur dioxide and particulate matters on mortality in 12 European cities: results from a time series data from the APHEA project. Air Pollution and Health: a European approach. BMJ 1997; 314:1658–1663.
31. Zmirou D, Barumandzadeh T, Balducci F, Ritter P, Laham G, Ghilardi JP. Short term effects of air pollution on mortality in the city of Lyon, France, 1985–1990. J Epidemiol Commun Health 1996; 50(suppl 1):S30–35.

32. Sunyer J, Castellsague J, Saez M, Tobias A, Anto JM. Air pollution and mortality in Barcelona. J Epidemiol Community Health 1996; 50(suppl 1):S76–80.

33. Woityniak B, Piekarski T. Short term effect of air pollution on mortality in Polish urban population—what is different? J Epidemiol Commun Health 1996; 50(suppl 1):36–41.

34. Ballester F, Corella D, Perez-Hoyos S, Hervas A. Air pollution and mortality in Valencia, Spain: a study using the APHEA methodology. J Epidemiol Commun Health 1996; 50:527–533.

35. Ponka A, Savela M, Virtanen M. Mortality and air pollution in Helsinki. Arch Environ Health 1998; 53:281–286.

36. Morgan G, Corbett S, Wlodarczyk J, Lewis P. Air pollution and daily mortality in Sydney, Australia, 1989 through 1993. Am J Public Health 1998; 88:759–764.

37. Schwartz J. Total suspended particulate matter and daily mortality in Cincinnati, Ohio. Environ Health Perspect 1994; 102:186–189.

38. Xu X, Gao J, Dockery DW, Chen Y. Air pollution and daily mortality in residential areas of Beijing, China. Arch Environ Health 1994; 49:216–222.

39. Schwartz J, Morris R. Air pollution and hospital admissions for cardiovascular disease in Detroit, Michigan. Am J Epidemiol 1995; 142:23–35.

40. Peters A, Doring A, Wichmann HE, Koenig W. Increased plasma viscosity during an air pollution episode: a link to mortality? Lancet 1997; 349:1582–1587.

41. Burke AP, Farb A, Malcom GT, Liang YH, Smialek J, Virmani R. Coronary risk factors and plaque morphology in men with coronary disease who died suddenly. N Engl J Med 1997; 336:1312–1314.

42. Muller JE, Stone PH, Turi ZG, Rutherford JD, Czeisler CA, Parker C, Poole WK, Passamani E, Roberts R, Robertson T. Circadian variation in the frequency of onset of acute myocardial infarction. N Engl J Med 1985; 313:1315–1322.

43. Cannon CP, McGabe CH, Stone PH, Schactman M, Thompson B, Theroux P, Gibson RS, Feldman T, Kleiman NS, Tofler GH, Muller JE, Chaitman BR, Braunwald E. Circadian variation in the onset of unstable angina and non-Q-wave acute myocardial infarction (the TIMI III registry and TIMI IIIB). Am J Cardiol 1997; 79:253–258.

44. Behar S, Halabi M, Reicher-Reiss H, Zion M, Kaplinsky E, Mandelzweig L, Goldbourt U. Circadian variation and possible external triggers of onset of myocardial infarction. SPRINT Study Group. Am J Med 1993; 94:395–400.

45. Ridker PM, Manson JE, Buring JE, Muller JE, Hennekens CH. Circadian variation of acute myocardial infarction and the effect of low-dose aspirin in a randomized trial of physicians. Circulation 1990; 82:897–902.

46. Sayer JW, Wilkinson P, Ranjadayalan K, Ray S, Marchant B, Timmis AD. Attenuation or absence of circadian and seasonal rhythms of acute myocardial infarction. Heart 1997; 77:325–329.

47. Cohen MC, Rohtla KM, Lavery CE, Muller JE, Mittleman MA. Meta-analysis of the morning excess of acute myocardial infarction and sudden cardiac death. Am J Cardiol 1997; 79:1512–1516.

48. Willich SN, Linderer T, Wegscheider K, Leizorovicz MD, Alamercery I, Schroder R, and the ISAM Study Group. Increased morning incidence of myocardial infarction in the ISAM Study: absence with prior beta-adrenergic blockade. Circulation 1989; 80:853–858.

49. ISIS-2 (Second International Study of Infarct Survival) Collaborative Group. Morning peak in the incidence of myocardial infarction: experience in the ISIS-2 trial. Eur Heart J 1992; 13:594–598.

50. Hausmann D, Trappe HJ, Bargheer K, Daniel WG, Wenzlaff P, Lichtlen PR. Circadian variation of ventricular tachykardia in patients after myocardial infarction. J Am Coll Cardiol 1992; 19:386A.

51. Tsuda M, Hayashi H, Kanematsu K, Yoshikane M, Saito H. Comparison between diurnal distribution of onset of infarction in patients with acute myocardial infarction and circadian variation of blood pressure in patients with coronary artery disease. Clin Cardiol 1993; 16:543–547.

52. Kono T, Morita H, Nishina T, Fujita M, Hirota Y, Kawamura K, Fujiwara A. Circadian variations of onset of acute myocardial infarction and efficacy of the thrombolytic treatment. J Am Coll Cardiol 1996; 27:774–778.

53. Hansen O, Johansen BW, Gullberg B. Circadian distribution of onset of acute myocardial infarction in subgroups from analysis of 10,791 patients treated in a single center. Am J Cardiol 1992; 69:1003–1008.

54. Van der Palen J, Doggen CJ, Beaglehole R. Variation in the time and day of onset of myocardial infarction and sudden cardiac death. N Z Med J 1995; 108:332–334.

55. Krantz DS, Kop WJ, Gabbay FH, Rozanski A, Barnard M, Klein J, Pardo Y, Gottdiener JS. Circadian variation of ambulatory myocardial ischemia. Triggering by daily activities and evidence for an endogenous circadian component. Circulation 1996; 93:1364–1371.

56. Willich SN, Levy D, Rocco MB, Tofler GM, Stone PH, Muller JE. Circadian variation in the incidence of sudden cardiac death in the Framingham Heart Study Population. Am J Cardiol 1987; 60:801–806.

57. Peters RW, Mitchell LB, Brooks MM, et al. Circadian pattern of arrhythmic death in patients receiving encainide, flecainide or moricizine in the Cardiac Arrythmia Suppression Trial (CAST). J Am Coll Cardiol 1994; 23:283–289.

58. Arntz HR, Willich SN, Oeff M, Bruggemann T, Stern R, Heinzmann A, Matenaer B, Schroder R. Circadian variation of sudden cardiac death reflects age-related variability in ventricular fibrillation. Circulation 1993; 88:2284–2289.

59. Muller JE, Mangel B. Circadian variation and triggers of cardiovascular disease. Cardiology 1994; 85(suppl 2):3–10.

60. Andreotti F, Kluft C, Davies GJ, Huisman LG, de Bart AC, Maseri A. Effect of propranolol (long-acting) on the circadian fluctuation of tissue-plasminogen activator and plasminogen activator inhibitor-1. Am J Cardiol 1991; 68:1295–1299.

61. Kurnik RP. Circadian variation in the efficacy of tissue-type plasminogen activator. Circulation 1995; 91:1341–1346.

62. Winther K, Hillegrass W, Tofler GH, Jimenez A, Brezinski DA, Schafer AI, Loscalzo J, Williams GH, Muller JE. Effects on platelet aggregation and fibrinolytic activity during upright posture and exercise in healthy men. Am J Cardiol 1992; 70:1051–1055.

63. Nicolau GY, Haus E, Popescu M, Sackett-Lundeen L, Petrescu E. Circadian, weekly, and seasonal variations in cardiac mortality, blood pressure, and catecholamine excretion. Chronobiol Int 1991; 8:149–159.

64. Willich SN, Löwel H, Lewis M, Hörmann A, Arntz HR, Keil U. Weekly variation

of acute myocardial infarction. Increased Monday risk in the working population. Circulation 1994; 90:87–93.

65. Marchant B, Ranjadayalan K, Stevenson R, Wilkinson P, Timmis AD. Circadian and seasonal factors in the pathogenesis of acute myocardial infarction: the influence of environmental temperature. Br Heart J 1993; 69:385–387.

66. Enquselassie F, Dobson AJ, Alexander HM, Steele PL. Seasons, temperature and coronary disease. Int J Epidemiol 1993; 22:632–636.

67. Spencer FA, Goldberg RJ, Becker RC, Gore JM. Seasonal distribution of acute myocardial infarction in the second National Registry of Myocardial Infarction. J Am Coll Cardiol 1998; 31:1226–1233.

68. Jern C, Eriksson E, Tengborn L, Risberg B, Wadenvik H, Jern S. Changes of plasma coagulation and fibrinolysis in response to mental stress. Thrombosis Hemostasis 1989; 62:767–771.

69. Benowitz NL, Fitzgerald GA, Wilson M, Zhang Q. Nicotine effects on eicosanoid formation and hemostatic function: comparison of transdermal nicotine and cigarette smoking. J Am Coll Cardiol 1993; 22:1159–1167.

70. Moreno PR, Shah PK, Falk E. Determinants of rupture of atherosclerotic coronary lesions. In: Willich SN, Muller JE, eds. Triggering of acute coronary syndromes: Implications for prevention. Dodrecht, Boston, London: Kluwer Academic Publishers, 1996.

71. Douste-Blazy P, Sie P, Boneau B, Marco J, Eche N, Bernadet P. Exercise-induced platelet activation in myocardial infarction survivors with normal coronary arteriogram. Thromb Haemostas 1984; 52:297–300.

72. Kestin AS, Ellis PA, Barnard MR, Errichetti A, Rosner BA, Michelson AD. Effect of strenous exercise on platelet activation state and reactivity. Circulation 1993; 88: 1502–1511.

73. Levine SP, Towell BL, Saurez AM, Khieriem LK, Harris MM, George JN. Platelet activation and secretion associated with emotional stress. Circulation 1985; 71: 1129–1134.

74. Hung J, Lam JY, Lacoste L, Letchacovski G. Cigarette smoking acutely increases platelet thrombus formation in patients with coronary artery disease taking aspirin. Circulation 1995; 92:2432–2436.

75. Markovitz JH, Matthews KA. Platelets and coronary heart disease: potential psychophysiologic mechanisms. Psychosom Med 1991; 53:643–668.

76. Rauramaa R, Salonen JT, Seppanen K, et al. Inhibition of platelet aggregability by moderate-intensity physical exercise: a randomized clinical trial in overweight men. Circulation 1986; 74:939–944.

77. Feng DL, Tofler GH. Diurnal physiological processes and circadian variation of acute myocardial infarction. J Cardiovasc Risk 1995; 2:494–498.

78. Yeh CJ, Chan P, Pan WH. Values of blood coagulation factors vary with ambient temperature: the Cardiovascular Disease Risk Factor Two-Township Study in Taiwan. Chin J Physiol 1996; 39:111–116.

10
Lessons About Plaque Rupture Learned from Angiography

Kevin M. Rankin, Robert J. Applegate, and William C. Little
*Wake Forest University School of Medicine, Winston-Salem,
North Carolina*

I. INTRODUCTION

Coronary angiography provides detailed, dynamic images of the coronary artery lumen. It has been the "gold standard" for evaluation of patients with coronary artery disease. The compelling images of stenotic lesions provides the explanation for myocardial ischemia experienced by patients with angina and a guide to direct surgical or catheter-based revascularization (1, 2). In addition, the extent and severity of the angiographic stenoses along with left ventricular function are indicators of the patient's prognosis.

Unstable angina and/or myocardial infarction are usually caused by a sudden, partial, or complete thrombotic occlusion of a coronary artery at the site of a fissured atherosclerotic plaque (3). This rupture of an eccentric lipid-rich plaque at the shoulders or hinge point is thought to be the classic pathophysiological phenomenon leading to an acute coronary syndrome. However, it must be kept in mind that this is a syndrome resulting from coronary artery pathology with significant heterogeneity. Although significant strides have been made in understanding the coronary pathophysiology underlying plaque rupture in an acute coronary syndrome, substantial gaps in our understanding still exist. Coronary angiography has provided many insights into our understanding of the pathological process of coronary artery disease. This chapter will review the lessons that have been learned from coronary angiography with respect to plaque rupture and the unstable coronary syndrome.

Features that can be analyzed on coronary angiography are the extent and severity of coronary stenosis and stenosis morphology (1, 2). The presence of a high-grade stenosis (i.e., greater than 80–90% diameter narrowing) is an angiographic risk factor for subsequent occlusion of a coronary artery (4, 5). It is attractive to assume that stenotic sites are at risk for thrombotic occlusion that will produce an unstable coronary event and that coronary arteries, which do not contain obstructive lesions (i.e., < 50%), are nearly free of the risk of occlusion. On the basis of these considerations, it may be assumed that a cardiologist viewing a coronary angiogram has a good understanding of the clinical problem and prognosis enabling appropriate strategies to relieve angina and prevent subsequent myocardial infarctions (6). However, this intuitively appealing concept has been challenged. Studies performed in the late 1980s revealed that the residual stenosis after thrombolysis of superimposed clot was frequently nonobstructive (7, 8). This observation suggests that rupture of a nonobstructive lesion may trigger a thrombotic coronary artery occlusion, resulting in myocardial infarction.

II. SERIAL ANGIOGRAPHIC STUDIES

Serial angiographic studies have reported observations in patients who had undergone coronary angiography both before and after myocardial infarction. Little et

Before MI

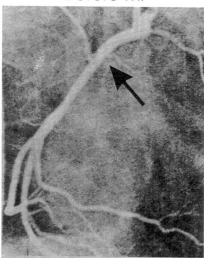

After MI

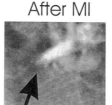

Figure 1   Angiograms before and after an inferior myocardial infarction.

al. (9) and Ambrose et al. (10) demonstrated that a coronary artery does not have to contain an angiographically severe stenosis to suddenly occlude and cause myocardial infarction (Figure 1). In fact, the coronary artery that previously contained the most severe stenosis is usually not the culprit, whereas most myocardial infarctions occur because of occlusion of arteries that previously did not contain significant stenoses.

III. WHICH SEGMENTS OCCLUDE?

This seemingly paradoxical finding that most coronary events (myocardial infarctions) arise from previously nonobstructive lesions, when it is presumed that severely stenosed segments are at high risk of occlusion, can be understood by evaluating both the risk of subsequent occlusion and the frequency of the presence of stenotic and nonstenotic coronary artery segments. Segments of coronary arteries that contain a severe stenosis are severalfold more likely to occlude than segments without a significant stenosis. However, the risk of occlusion of a nonsignificantly stenosed segment is not zero, and these are far more numerous (11). Thus, the bulk of obstructing thrombotic occlusions overlying a ruptured plaque occur in nonstenotic but diseased segments.

A great deal of emphasis has been placed on the risk of occlusion of a stenotic lesion, whereas the risk of occlusion of the nonstenotic segments has been underestimated. This apparent dichotomy underscores the fact that coronary atherosclerosis is a disease of the arterial wall. Coronary angiography can be misleading as to the extent and severity of coronary atherosclerosis, because coronary artery disease is visible angiographically only as focal areas of luminal narrowing. However, pathological examination and studies using intravascular ultrasonography indicate that coronary artery disease is usually a diffuse process with extensive involvement of the arterial wall (12–16).

There is difficulty directly comparing pathological and angiographic analyses of coronary artery disease. The definition of stenosis severity used by the two techniques differs in two ways. First, in pathological studies, the severity of a stenosis is determined by the reduction in vessel cross-sectional area, whereas angiographically the stenosis is quantitated as a reduction in luminal diameter. A 68% reduction in luminal diameter produces a 90% reduction in cross-sectional area. The second difference between the methods occurs in determining the reference area or diameter (Figure 2). The pathologist uses the area contained within the elastic lumen, whereas the angiographer uses the diameter of an adjacent segment with a normal-appearing lumen. This reference segment usually has atherosclerosis within the vessel wall. Because of these considerations, the culprit lesion in myocardial infarction, quantified as a 90% reduction in cross-sectional area in a pathological study, may have been apparent only as a 40% or smaller

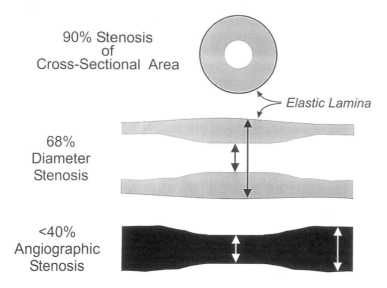

Figure 2 Representations of different methods used to quantify the severity of coronary atherosclerosis. A 90% reduction in cross-sectional area is caused by a 48% reduction in human diameter. Furthermore, diameter stenosis is based on an adjacent reference segment that may itself be diseased.

diameter stenosis on an angiogram (Figure 2). Therefore, the observation that myocardial infarction can occur in the absence of an angiographically apparent stenosis and the autopsy data suggesting severely atherosclerotic vessels are not in conflict. Moreover, because of the limitations of coronary angiography in detecting the extent of atherosclerosis, the occlusion of an area of "angiographically insignificant" narrowing is actually thrombosis at a site of advanced atherosclerosis, albeit without narrowing of the lumen.

As atherosclerosis develops in the arterial wall, the initial response is usually an outward expansion of the artery that accommodates the atheroma while preserving the lumen area (17, 18). Thus, there is usually a substantial amount of atherosclerosis in the coronary artery wall before there is any significant narrowing of the lumen. A single stenosis can be a marker that diffuse atherosclerosis is present in other coronary arteries (Figure 3). In addition, intravascular ultrasonography demonstrates significant atherosclerosis in patients whose coronary angiograms are normal or contain only minimal irregularities (19). Consistent with this concept, even patients with minor irregularities of the coronary artery walls, but without any angiographically apparent stenoses, have a substantially lower survival rate than patients with completely normal coronary arteries (20, 21).

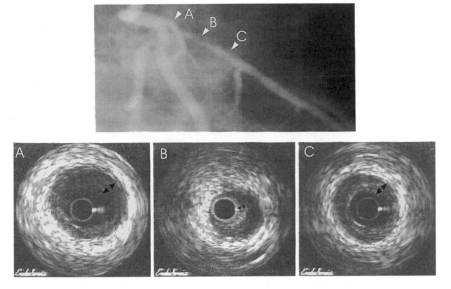

Figure 3   Angiogram of left coronary artery, and intravascular ultrasonographic cross-sectional images in proximal (A) and distal (C) normal-appearing site in the left anterior descending coronary artery and in an area of severe stenosis (B). The arrows indicate the thickness of atherosclerosis in the wall, which is similar in the three sites.

Although coronary atherosclerosis produces its clinical manifestations by narrowing or occluding the lumen, it is difficult to accurately predict potential plaque rupture and occlusion by assessment of angiographic stenosis severity. However, even small changes in severity of lesions by coronary angiography may indicate active disease in the arterial wall, which may be associated with subsequent development of myocardial infarction (22). Coronary angiography also has prognostic implications related to the number of severely stenosed coronary arteries and left ventricular ejection fraction (21).

IV.   ANGIOGRAPHIC CHARACTERISTICS

Because stenosis severity alone does not adequately define the risk of myocardial infarction, subsequent studies have carefully evaluated features of individual stenoses to characterize lesion-specific factors predisposing to thrombotic occlusion. Therefore, angiographic morphology is the second major feature that can be analyzed with respect to identifying vulnerable plaques. Unfortunately, these studies have not all yielded consistent findings.

Frequently the endothelium of the plaque underlying the coronary thrombosis of patients with myocardial infarction or unstable angina has been disrupted, exposing the thrombotic components of the plaque to the bloodstream. The fissured plaque with overlying thrombosis in patients with unstable angina, non-Q-wave myocardial infarction, or after thrombolytic therapy of myocardial infarction may be angiographically apparent as a convex, intraluminal obstruction with overhanging edges, irregularities, or intraluminal defects. Lesions believed to be "culprits" in acute coronary syndromes often exhibit these angiographic characteristics (23, 24).

Some studies suggest that the more complex the morphology of the culprit stenosis responsible for an unstable syndrome, the more likely there will be further progression. Davies et al. (25) found that in patients who had received successful thrombolytic treatment for acute myocardial infarction, need for urgent revascularization because of unstable symptoms in the hospital was significantly greater in patients with an increased degree of angiographic irregularity.

Chen et al. (26) found that in patients who initially were stabilized on medical therapy after a major coronary event, but subsequently required revascularization, more complex lesions (irregular borders, overhanging edges, or thrombus) progressed than did smooth lesions. It is postulated that stenoses with complex morphological characteristics in patients without myocardial infarction or unstable angina may have a greater subsequent risk of myocardial infarction (27), especially in occlusion that produces a Q-wave myocardial infarction (28).

Subgroup analysis of the Coronary Artery Surgery Study (CASS) patients by Ellis et al. (5) found stenosis roughness to be an independent predictor of subsequent myocardial infarction. However, in other studies the culprit lesions may not have been complex on an angiogram performed before the event. Haft and Al-Zarka (29) demonstrated that irregular lesions, likely representing ruptured atherosclerotic plaques, frequently originated from mildly occlusive smooth lesions. Similarly, the angiographic morphology of the culprit lesion after thrombolytic therapy may not predict subsequent reocclusion as demonstrated by Ellis et al. (30) and later by Taeymans et al. (31). These investigators did not find that irregular lesion contours were associated with the risk of subsequent occlusion.

Much still needs to be learned regarding the importance of lesion morphology. Recently, Ledru et al. (32) found in a serial angiographic study that coronary artery narrowings with steeper outflow angles were more likely to occlude and that symmetrical narrowings are more likely to occlude than eccentric lesions. This differs from the previous finding that eccentric stenoses are an angiographic sign of unstable or ruptured plaque. However, this is not incongruous with the findings of Haft and Al-Zarka (29), in which mildly stenotic smooth lesions often progress to complex lesions. In addition, irregularity, and not necessarily eccentricity, has been the marker for progressive lesions (5). Thus, angiographically complex or irregular stenoses may have some increased risk for subsequent occlusion, but these morphologic features are not sufficient to accurately predict which area will subsequently cause a myocardial infarction. Moreover, there are far more smooth areas (with and without angiographic stenoses) that are at risk for causing a subsequent myocardial infarction.

V. LIMITATIONS OF CORONARY ANGIOGRAPHY

There are clear limitations of coronary angiography to predict vulnerable atherosclerotic plaques. First, angiography provides a two-dimensional depiction of the coronary artery lumen with only indirect and limited information about the atherosclerotic process within the arterial wall. No matter how well multiple angiographic characteristics correlate with coronary occlusion, it seems unlikely that coronary angiography will ever be able to precisely define all potentially dangerous vulnerable plaques within the arterial wall (1). It is possible that improved direct imaging at the arterial wall with intravascular ultrasonography or magnetic resonance imaging, or characterizing the plaque by spectroscopy (33) or thermal imaging (34, 35) will be more successful in evaluating the status of disease within the wall of the artery, which ultimately is the predictor of clinical outcomes. Second, all serial angiographic studies have limitations in that patients are highly selected and typically do not include patients who have had angiograms both before and after their myocardial infarction. Thus, most patients with myocardial infarction are not included in these studies. These limitations point out the flaw in attempting to use coronary angiograms to help direct therapy aimed at preventing subsequent coronary events.

VI. CONCLUSION

Coronary angiography can help direct appropriate revascularization. However, because most occlusions occur at sites that did not previously contain a flow-limiting stenosis, interventions such as coronary artery bypass surgery or percutaneous transluminal coronary intervention are not likely to be effective in preventing many subsequent myocardial infarctions. Coronary angiography, however, can provide a clear roadmap to guide appropriate interventions that are effective in eliminating ischemia and improving exertional capacity. Especially in combination with newer imaging modalities, coronary angiography will remain an important tool in the evaluation of patients at risk for, or with, acute coronary syndromes.

REFERENCES

1. Little WC, Applegate RJ. The shadows leave a doubt. The angiographic recognition of vulnerable coronary artery plaques. J Am Coll Cardiol 1999; 33:1362–1364.
2. Little WC, Applegate RJ. Coronary angiography before myocardial infarction: can the culprit site be prospectively recognized? Am Heart J 1998; 136(3):368–370.
3. Fuster V, Lewis A. Conner Memorial Lecture: Mechanisms leading to myocardial infarction: insights from studies of vascular biology. Circulation 1994; 90(4):2126–2146.
4. Moise A, Lesperance J, Theroux P, Taeymans Y, Goulet C, Bourassa MG. Clinical and angiographic predictors of new total coronary occlusion in coronary artery disease: analysis of 313 nonoperated patients. Am J Cardiol 1984; 54(10):1176–1181.
5. Ellis S, Alderman E, Cain K, Fisher L, Sanders W, Bourassa M, the CASS investigators. Prediction of risk of anterior myocardial infarction by lesion severity and measurement method of stenoses in the left anterior descending coronary distribution: a CASS Registry Study. J Am Coll Cardiol 1988; 11(5):908–916.
6. Topol EJ, Nissen SE. Our preoccupation with coronary luminology. The dissociation between clinical and angiographic findings in ischemic heart disease. Circulation 1995; 92(8):2333–2342.
7. Brown BG, Gallery CA, Badger RS, Kennedy JW, Mathey D, Bolson EL, Dodge HT. Incomplete lysis of thrombus in the moderate underlying atherosclerotic lesion during intracoronary infusion of streptokinase for acute myocardial infarction: quantitative angiographic observations. Circulation 1986; 73(4):653–661.
8. Hackett D, Davies G, Maseri A. Pre-existing coronary stenoses in patients with first myocardial infarction are not necessarily severe. Eur Heart J 1988; 9:1317–1323.
9. Little WC, Constantinescu M, Applegate RJ, Kutcher MA, Burrows MT, Kahl FR, Santamore WP. Can coronary angiography predict the site of a subsequent myocardial infarction in patients with mild to moderate coronary artery disease? Circulation 1988; 78(5 Pt 1):1157–1166.
10. Ambrose JA, Tannenbaum MA, Alexopoulos D, Hjemdahl-Monsen CE, Leavy J, Weiss M, Borrico S, Gorlin R, Fuster V. Angiographic progression of coronary artery disease and the development of myocardial infarction. J Am Coll Cardiol 1988; 12(1):56–62.
11. Little WC, Downes TR, Applegate RJ. The underlying coronary lesion in myocardial infarction: implications for coronary angiography. Clin Cardiol 1991; 14(11):868–874.
12. Roberts WC, Jones AA. Quantification of coronary arterial narrowing at necropsy in sudden coronary death. Analysis of 31 patients and comparison with 25 control subjects. Am J Cardiol 1979; 44:39–45.
13. Roberts WC, Jones AA. Quantification of coronary arterial narrowing at necropsy in acute transmural myocardial infarction. Analysis and comparison of findings in 27 patients and 22 controls. Circulation 1980; 61(4):786–790.
14. Vlodaver Z, Frech R, Van Tassel RA, Edwards JE. Correlation of the antemortem coronary arteriogram and the postmortem specimen. Circulation 1973; 47:162–169.
15. Dietz WA, Tobis JM, Isner JM. Failure of angiography to accurately depict the

extent of coronary artery narrowing in three fatal cases of percutaneous transluminal coronary angioplasty. J Am Coll Cardiol 1992; 19(6):1261–1270.

16. Braden GA, Herrington DM, Downes TR, Kutcher MA, Little WC. Qualitative and quantitative contrasts in the mechanisms of lumen enlargement by coronary balloon angioplasty and directional coronary atherectomy. J Am Coll Cardiol 1994; 23(1): 40–48.

17. Glagov S, Weisenberg E, Zarins CK, Stankunavicius R, Kolettis GJ. Compensatory enlargement of human atherosclerotic coronary arteries. N Engl J Med 1987; 316(22):1371–1375.

18. Stiel GM, Stiel LS, Schofer J, Donath K, Mathey DG. Impact of compensatory enlargement of atherosclerotic coronary arteries on angiographic assessment of coronary artery disease. Circulation 1989; 80(6):1603–1609.

19. Porter TR, Sears T, Xie F, Michels A, Mata J, Welsh D, Shurmur S. Intravascular ultrasound study of angiographically mildly diseased coronary arteries. J Am Coll Cardiol 1993; 22(7):1858–1865.

20. Kemp HG, Kronmal RA, Vlietstra RE, Frye RL. Seven year survival of patients with normal or near normal coronary arteriograms: a CASS Registry Study. J Am Coll Cardiol 1986; 7(3):479–483.

21. Mock MB, Ringqvist I, Fisher LD, Davis KB, Chaitman BR, Kouchoukos NT, Kaiser GC, Alderman E, Ryan TJ, Russell RO, Mullin S, Fray D, Killip T, III. Survival of medically treated patients in the coronary artery surgery study (CASS) registry. Circulation 1982; 66(3):562–568.

22. Applegate RJ, Herrington DM, Little WC. Coronary angiography: more than meets the eye. Circulation 1993; 87(4):1399–1401.

23. Nakagawa S, Hanada Y, Koiwaya Y, Tanaka K. Angiographic features in the infarct related artery after intracoronary urokinase followed by prolonged anticoagulation. Circulation 1988; 78(6):1335–1344.

24. Ambrose JA. Coronary arteriographic analysis and angiographic morphology. J Am Coll Cardiol 1989; 13(7):1492–1494.

25. Davies SW, Marchant B, Lyons JP, Timmis AD, Rothman MT, Layton CA, Balcon R. Irregular coronary lesion morphology after thrombolysis predicts early clinical instability. J Am Coll Cardiol 1991; 18(3):669–674.

26. Chen L, Chester MR, Redwood S, Huang J, Leatham E, Kaski JC. Angiographic stenosis progression and coronary events in patients with 'stabilized' unstable angina. Circulation 1995; 91(9):2319–2324.

27. Ambrose JA. Prognostic implications of lesion irregularity on coronary angiography. J Am Coll Cardiol 1991; 18(3):675–676.

28. Dacanay S, Kennedy HL, Uretz E, Parrillo JE, Klein LW. Morphological and quantitative angiographic analyses of progression of coronary stenoses: a comparison of Q-wave and non-Q-wave myocardial infarction. Circulation 1994; 90(4):1739–1746.

29. Haft JI, Al-Zarka AM. The origin and fate of complex coronary lesions. Am Heart J 1991; 121(4 Pt 1):1050–1061.

30. Ellis SG, Topol EJ, George BS, Kereiakes DJ, Debowey D, Sigmon KN, Pickel A, Lee KL, Califf RM. Recurrent ischemia without warning: analysis of risk factors for in-hospital ischemic events following successful thrombolysis with intravenous issue plasminogen activator. Circulation 1989; 80:1159–1165.

31. Taeymans Y, Theroux P, Lesperance J, Waters D. Quantitative angiographic morphology of the coronary artery lesions at risk of thrombotic occlusion. Circulation 1992; 85(1):78–85.

32. Ledru F, Theroux P, Lesperance J, Laurier J, Ducimetiere P, Guermonprez JL, Diebold B, Blanchard D. Geometric features of coronary artery lesions favoring acute occlusion and myocardial infarction: a quantitative angiographic study. J Am Coll Cardiol 1999; 33:1353–1361.

33. Moreno PR, Lodder RA, Muller JE, Muller J. Characterization of composition and vulnerability of atherosclerotic plaques by near-infrared spectroscopy (abstr). Circulation 1998; 98:1473.

34. Casscells W, Hathorn B, David M, Krabach T, Vaughn WK, McAllister HA, Bearman G, Willerson JT. Thermal detection of cellular infiltrates in living atherosclerotic plaques: possible implications for plaque rupture and thrombosis. Lancet 1996; 347(9013):1447–1449.

35. Stefanadis C, Diamantopoulos L, Vlachopoulos C, Tsiamis E, Dernellis J, Toutouzas K, Stefanadi E, Toutouzas P. Thermal heterogeneity within human atherosclerotic coronary arteries detected in vivo. A new method of detection by application of a special thermography catheter. Circulation 1999; 99:1965–1971.

11
Intravascular Ultrasonography to Diagnose Vulnerable Plaque

Allen Jeremias, Peter J. Fitzgerald, and Paul G. Yock
Stanford University School of Medicine, Stanford, California

I. CHARACTERIZING CORONARY ATHEROSCLEROTIC PLAQUE

The greatest challenge of vascular imaging of any type is the early detection of unstable plaques. This year, in the United States alone, approximately 500,000 deaths will result from rupture of plaques that would be classified as nonsignificant by angiographic evaluation (1). Of the different imaging modalities under investigation for their ability to identify ''vulnerable plaque,'' intravascular ultrasonography is the most widely applied clinically. This chapter will focus on the promise and limitations of intravascular ultrasonography in the early visualization of plaques at risk.

II. CORONARY ANGIOGRAPHY—THE "GOLD STANDARD" FOR THE DIAGNOSIS OF CORONARY ATHEROSCLEROSIS?

Coronary angiography is still the standard imaging modality for the detection of coronary plaque and lesion assessment in vivo. However, angiography represents a luminographic method visualizing only the silhouette of the lumen. In complex lesions with distorted or highly eccentric luminal shapes, angiography may fail to demonstrate the true extent of disease severity. Even when orthogonal views are obtained, imaging angles are frequently suboptimal because of superimposed vessels or foreshortening, resulting in the impaired ability to delineate true coronary structure (Figure 1). Furthermore, no information can be obtained regarding plaque burden, degree of remodeling, plaque structure, or composition. Because atherosclerosis is a disease of the vessel wall, angiographic detection of lumen encroachment is only a surrogate for the actual burden of disease and provides very little information about the likely course of disease progression. In one study that compared the angiograms of 25 patients before and after an episode of unstable angina, 18 of the 25 lesions (72%) were previously insignificant (less than 50% luminal narrowing) (2). Similar results have been documented in other studies of acute coronary syndromes (3, 4). Only in those occasional cases where there is clear thrombus or deep ulceration can coronary angiography clearly show signs of plaque rupture (5, 6). An additional limitation of angiography is that the quantification of disease severity is expressed as the ratio of the diseased segment to an angiographically ''normal'' reference segment. In a recent study, Mintz et al. showed that the angiographic ''normal'' reference segment contained signifi-

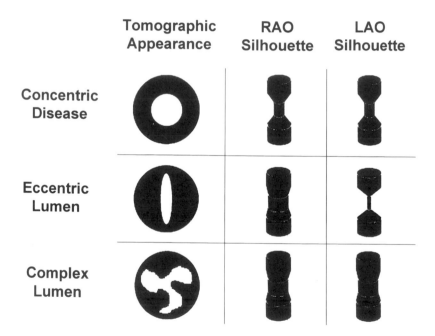

Figure 1   Differences between intravascular ultrasonography and angiography for imaging atherosclerotic lesions. Depending on luminal shape and projection angle, angiography can significantly underestimate lesion severity. RAO = right anterior oblique; LAO = left anterior oblique. (Adapted from Nissen SE, et al. Intravascular ultrasound, angioscopy, Doppler, and pressure measurements. In: Topol EJ, ed. Textbook of Cardiovascular Medicine. Philadelphia: Lippincott Williams & Wilkins, 1997:2121.)

cant plaque formation with more than 50% plaque area in the cross-section as visualized by intravascular ultrasonography (7). Because of vascular remodeling, significant plaque volume can be accommodated without compromising luminal size and causing obstruction (8). Angiography, therefore, cannot help in identifying many "early" lesions that may undergo rupture and contribute to significant morbidity and mortality.

III. INTRAVASCULAR ULTRASONOGRAPHY—IMAGING THE VESSEL WALL

The introduction of catheter-based intravascular ultrasonographic imaging has enabled the direct in vivo visualization of the vessel wall and has revolutionized our understanding of coronary artery disease. Intravascular ultrasonography creates cross-sectional images and allows tomographic assessment of the different layers of the arterial wall and atherosclerotic plaque. Detailed information can be obtained regarding vessel and lumen size and important insights gained about plaque structure and composition.

Early studies that used this technique demonstrated that the architecture of normal and diseased vessels could be characterized for the first time in vivo (9,

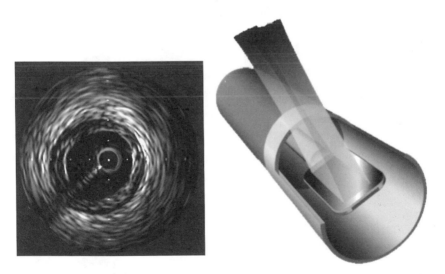

Figure 2 Intravascular ultrasonographic catheter design. In this design, the transducer is mechanically rotated to create cross-sectional images.

10). Reproducibility and comparison to histological findings yielded excellent results for both coronary and peripheral arteries (11–13).

A. Equipment and Imaging

Intravascular ultrasound probes contain a small (<1 mm) ultrasound crystal at the tip of a 140-cm long, flexible catheter that is introduced with a guidewire into the coronary artery during cardiac catheterization. Coronary arteries are imaged perpendicular to the axis of the catheter at the level of the transducer in a cross-sectional fashion (Figure 2). The images show the catheter as a blank in the middle, surrounded by blood and the layers of the vessel wall (Figure 3). The cross-sectional image is created by either rotating a single ultrasound element at a certain speed around the axis of the catheter (mechanical device) or by the consecutive activation of multiple transducers located in a cylindrical array around the catheter tip (solid-state device). In both approaches sound waves are emitted from the ultrasound transducer, and the reflected backscatter signals are

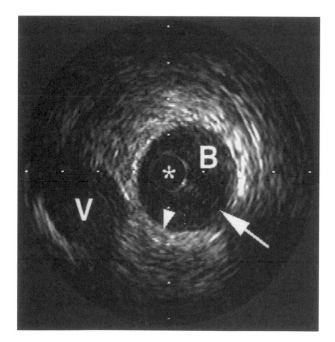

Figure 3 Typical intravascular ultrasonogram cross-sectional image of a normal coronary artery. Asterisk = catheter; arrow = guidewire artifact; arrowhead = vessel wall; B = blood; V = vein.

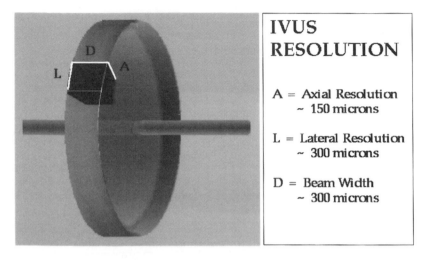

Figure 4   Intravascular ultrasonographic resolution within the focal zone of the ultrasonographic beam.

processed to create ultrasonographic images. The intensity of the scattered signal depends on the acoustic impedance mismatch of structures transversed by the ultrasound beam. Therefore, higher backscatter amplitudes are created at distinct tissue interfaces (blood/intima/media/adventitia), resulting in sharp echo signals in the ultrasonographic image. The resolution of the system varies with transducer size, imaging frequency, and impulse duration. Depending on these parameters, with the best current catheters the lateral resolution (ability to distinguish two separate objects next to each other at similar distance from the transducer) approaches approximately 180 μm, and the axial resolution (ability to distinguish two separate objects next to each other in the line of the beam) is about 150 μm. At each point of imaging, the reflected ultrasound signal is a composition of backscatter from a volume whose dimensions are defined by its lateral and axial resolution and overall beam thickness (Figure 4). Resolution between different catheter systems varies, so it is important to know the characteristics of the particular system in use.

B.   Basic Intravascular Ultrasonographic Image Interpretation

Intravascular ultrasonography allows interrogation of finite elements (between 0.15–0.2 mm) over a depth of approximately 5 mm from the transducer. A typical image of a coronary artery shows a three-layered appearance of the arterial wall

(14) (Figure 5). The outermost layer, the adventitia, is a strong echo-reflector and has a bright appearance in the image because of its high content of collagen and fibrous tissue. The relative brightness of the adventitia can be used as an internal standard to compare the gray level appearance of other tissue (15). With this technique, different plaque types can be discriminated on the basis of their echogenicity in relation to the adventitia. This compensates for differences in image acquisition settings (time gain compensation, compression, etc.) and allows a standardized classification. Postmortem studies on excised vessels have found a close correlation between an increase in echogenicity and the amount of fibrous tissue content.

The middle layer, representing the media, is usually a dark echolucent band. The intima (together with the internal elastic lamina) constitutes the inner layer and is usually echo intense compared with the low echos of the blood speckles in the lumen. In diseased vessels, plaque is included in this layer. Because the minimal intimal thickness necessary for detection with the resolution of current 30-MHz transducers is approximately 180 μm (14), intimal changes below this

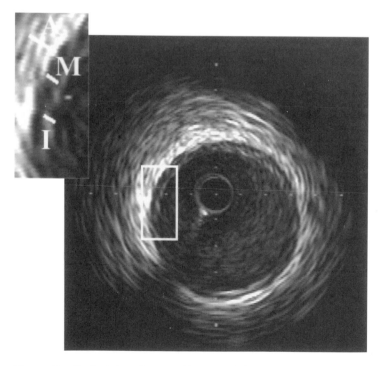

Figure 5 Typical three-layer architecture of the arterial wall. I = intima; M = media; A = adventitia.

Table 1 Intravascular Ultrasonographic Characterization of Different Plaque Types

Plaque type	Intravascular ultrasound characterization	Pitfalls in image interpretation
Calcified	Bright echo similar or brighter than the adventitia with shadowing	Underlying tissue "hidden" by the shadow Degree of calcium-arc varies with distance of transducer to vessel wall
Fibrous	Bright echo similar to adventitia without typical shadowing	Gradual attenuation of signal may occur behind the fibrous plaque Comparison with adventitia depends on the gain-settings
Fibro-fatty	"Soft" echos with less echogenicity than the adventitia Dark, "echolucent" zones may occur	Difficult to distinguish from other plaque types (thrombus) or artifact (echo dropout, shadowing) Highly gain dependent

resolution will not be detected, and the vessel will appear single layered. Fibrous and fibrocalcific plaques are highly echo reflective and are called "hard" plaque. Echos weaker than that of the adventitia represent "soft" plaque, composed of fibro-fatty plaque, thrombus, and/or loose connective tissue (Table 1). This is a reflection of the physical properties of these tissues. A recent study compared the compression stiffness constant (K) for different plaque types (16). K among minimally diseased arterial wall, hypoechogenic "soft" plaque, and fibrous plaque was not significantly different. The authors also pointed out that these tissues were not physically soft compared with adipose tissue. It is, therefore, important to note that "soft" plaque, as judged by intravascular ultrasonography, is not physically soft (i.e., not to the surgeon's touch). It would be technically more correct to refer to soft and hard ultrasonographic patterns.

IV. IMAGING ATHEROSCLEROTIC PLAQUE

A. Calcified Plaque

The deposition of calcium in atherosclerotic plaques is believed to represent a more advanced stage of the disease. It may occur after plaque rupture or thrombus formation and is at that point usually associated with a stable coronary lesion. Calcification is easily identified by intravascular ultrasonography and is characterized by a bright echo signal with complete attenuation of the signal beyond, resulting in shadow formation (Figure 6). Structures located deeper in relation to the calcific region are therefore hidden in the shadow and cannot be imaged. For that reason, intravascular ultrasonography is not a good tool to assess the total volume of calcium in a vessel. The calcium arc angle, which is often used as a surrogate measure of the degree of calcification on intravascular ultrasonography, is highly dependent on the distance from the transducer to the arc (the angle enlarges with proximity to the transducer). Displacement of the catheter by 1 mm toward or away from the calcific region can change a 45-degree arc to 30 or 80 degrees (17). In a histological validation study, intravascular ultrasonography underestimated the calcified cross-sectional area by 16% (18).

The detection of intralesional calcium by intravascular ultrasonography depends on the histological pattern. In a study by Friedrich et al. intravascular ultrasonography correctly detected dense calcific plaques in 89% of cases compared with histological analysis and yielded a sensitivity of 90% with a specificity of 100%. However, microcalcifications (with a calcium fleck size of ≤0.05 mm)

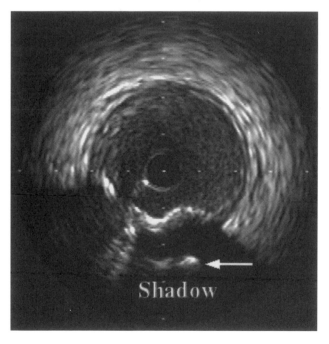

Figure 6 Intravascular ultrasonographic image of superficial calcific plaque. Note the shadowing behind the calcium and the characteristic reverberation (arrow) equidistant from the transducer-plaque length.

were detected in only 17%, and sensitivity dropped to 64% (19). Identifying calcified plaques may be of importance in coronary interventional procedures (20, 21). Arterial calcification can be the reason for noncompliance of the lesion, requiring a different interventional approach (higher balloon pressure, rotational atherectomy) and resulting in increased rates of dissections (22, 23). Comparing intravascular ultrasonography to fluoroscopy for the detection of target lesion calcification revealed a significant difference between the two methods; whereas calcifications were observed in 60 to 80% of the cases by intravascular ultrasonography, only 30 to 40% were identified by fluoroscopy (21, 24).

B. Fibrous Plaque

Dense fibrous tissue can be found in advanced coronary lesions, and these plaque types are usually recognized by an overall echogenicity similar to the adventitia. It can be differentiated from calcific lesions by the absence of shadowing, although a marked attenuation of the signal can occur with an increase in collagen

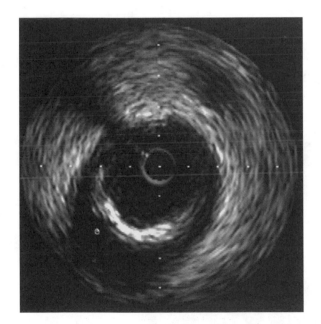

Figure 7   Intravascular ultrasonographic image of a fibrous plaque. Note the signal attenuation by the plaque. Unlike the calcified plaque, complete shadowing is not seen in this example.

and elastic fibers. In general, fibrous plaques are associated with symptoms of stable angina. They can cause severe luminal obstruction but are not prone to rupture. Because fibrous plaques are excellent reflectors, their appearance is bright and fairly homogenous (Figure 7). This stands in contrast to fibro-fatty plaque, which is a worse echo-reflector and diffusely scatters the ultrasound beam. However, brightness of the ultrasonographic image is a relative measure and is highly affected by power, attenuation by tissue components, and time gain compensation. Analysis of plaque brightness for quantifying the relative amount of fibrous versus fatty tissue in any given plaque is influenced by all of these factors. It is, therefore, not surprising that a significant overlap exists in identifying tissue types compared with the histological "gold standard." Nevertheless, in histological studies a good correlation has been found between intravascular ultrasonographic identification of fibrous plaque and histology in vitro (12).

C. Fibro-Fatty Plaque

Fibro-fatty plaques are characterized by a relatively echolucent appearance on intravascular ultrasonography images (Figure 8). Because of the tissue composi-

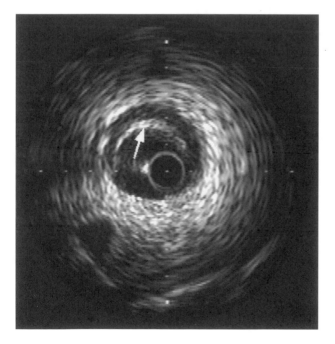

Figure 8   Fibro-fatty plaque with echolucent appearance and fibrous cap (arrow).

tion, attenuation is minimal, and consequently the visualization of the surrounding adventitia and perivascular structures is excellent. It is tempting to identify echolucent regions within the plaque as "lipid lakes" composed of extracellular lipid cores (Figure 9). However, there are many other reasons for the presence of echolucent regions besides lipid accumulation, such as loose collagen and fibromuscular tissue. Sometimes, shadowing from a heavily fibrotic or calcified plaque can be mistaken for lipid. Also a low dynamic range of the imaging system can cause an echo dropout and mimic the presence of a "lipid lake" (25). In addition to these technical considerations from the intravascular ultrasonography standpoint, it is difficult to obtain a firm histological confirmation of lipid. With the standard histological preparation of dehydrating the tissue specimen before embedding in paraffin, lipid is dissolved, leaving an empty cavity as evidence of previous lipid accumulation. This further complicates studies using histological confirmation for intravascular ultrasonographic analysis of fibro-fatty plaque.

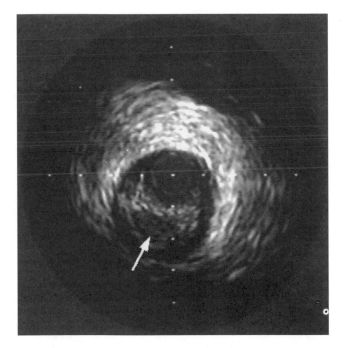

Figure 9 Echolucent region within the plaque (arrow), possibly representing a "lipid lake" composed of extracellular lipid.

V. CHARACTERIZATION OF PLAQUES
BY INTRAVASCULAR ULTRASONOGRAPHY

A. Identification of Different Plaque Components

Multiple studies have focused on the detection of different plaque types on the basis of intravascular ultrasonographic morphology (Table 2). Di Mario et al. used high-frequency intravascular ultrasonography (30 and 40 MHz) to study 112 human vascular specimen and compare them to histological specimen (12). Histologically proven fibrous intimal thickening was echographically detected in 32 of 48 specimen (67%). There was a good correlation between plaque area as seen by intravascular ultrasonography and histological studies ($r = 0.87$, $p < 0.001$). Histologically evident calcium deposits were detected with intravascular ultrasonography in 35 of 36 specimen (97%), and hypoechogenic areas of lipid deposits were detected in 32 of 36 specimen (89%). Intravascular ultrasonography had 88.9% sensitivity and 100% specificity for lipid deposits and 97.2% sensitivity and 98.7% specificity for calcification. In a similar in vitro study, Potkin et al. compared 21 human coronary arteries by intravascular ultrasonography and histological studies (26). Of the 84 fibrous plaque quadrant areas, 81 (96%) were correctly identified by ultrasonography. Of the 19 calcific regions, all were correctly identified, and of the 9 lipid quadrant areas, 7 (78%) were correctly identified by ultrasonography. Thus, ultrasonography accurately predicted histological plaque composition in 96% of quadrants analyzed. Sechtem et al. examined 35 coronary arteries of 18 human autopsy hearts with a 20-MHz device (27). There

Table 2 Intravascular Ultrasonographic Sensitivity and Specificity for Different Atherosclerotic Plaque Types

Study	No. of specimen	Plaque type	Sensitivity (%)	Specificity (%)
DiMario (12)	112	Fibro-fatty	89	97
		Fibrous	67	100
		Calcified	97	98
Potkin (27)	21	Fibro-fatty	78	97
		Fibrous	96	93
		Calcified	100	100
Sechtem (28)	35	Fibro-fatty	26	92
		Fibrous	100	56
		Calcified	86	95
Rasheed (29)	44	"Soft"	95	76
		"Mixed"	67	93
		"Calcific"	86	100

were 114 plaques by histology, which were correctly visualized by ultrasonography as plaques in all instances. Plaque calcification was correctly diagnosed in 54 of 63 (86%) sections, but large calcifications were more reliably identified by ultrasonography than small speckled calcium deposits [43 of 44 (98%) vs. 11 of 19 (58%)]. Fibrous elements were present in all plaques and were identified by intravascular ultrasonography in all instances. Lipid accumulations, however, were detected with a sensitivity of only 26% (16 of 62) and a specificity of 92% (71 of 77). When lipids were diagnosed on the basis of the criterion that more than a quarter of the plaque area showed lower signal intensity than the tissue surrounding the vessel, the sensitivity of ultrasonography improved to 73% (45 of 62), but specificity fell to 30% (23 of 77). The entire histological composition of a section was correctly diagnosed by ultrasonography in only 42% of the 139 sections. The main reason for the poor correlation between histological composition and intravascular ultrasonography was the insufficient detection of fibro-fatty plaques. The usefulness of intravascular ultrasonography in classifying lesions in vivo was assessed in 44 patients undergoing directional coronary atherectomy (28). Atheromateous plaque was classified as soft, mixed, and calcified and evaluated by conventional intravascular ultrasonography and by a computer-assisted analysis of gray-level distribution. Intravascular ultrasonography was found to be 95% sensitive but only 76% specific for the identification of soft plaque. The variability in the detection of different plaque types was examined in a comparison of four different intravascular ultrasonography systems (29). All three mechanically rotating systems in that analysis had fair to good sensitivities for identifying calcification (57–73%) or lipid-filled areas (50–83%). The sensitivity of discriminating fibrous tissue from fatty areas, however, was low (39–52%). The only solid-state device tested (not the current generation system) had a significantly lower sensitivity for identifying all tissue types (4–21%).

B. Detection of Thrombus

Nishimura et al. studied 130 segments of freshly excised peripheral arteries (11). They were able to detect two segments that were involved by a rupture of a soft necrotic plaque and secondary luminal thrombus formation. In both cases the thrombi were visualized on the ultrasound image as an echo density with low echo reflectance. Other studies have investigated the ability of intravascular ultrasonography to detect thrombus formation (30–33). Frimerman et al. designed an in vitro model to test the hypothesis that thrombi of varying composition have different echogenic patterns (32). Platelet-rich thrombi showed low echogenicity similar to saline solution and were therefore virtually undetectable by intravascular ultrasonography. With an increasing amount of red blood cells in the thrombus, there was an increase in echogenic reflections of the image (Figure 10). Whole blood thrombi appeared uniformly "speckled" and were readily identifi-

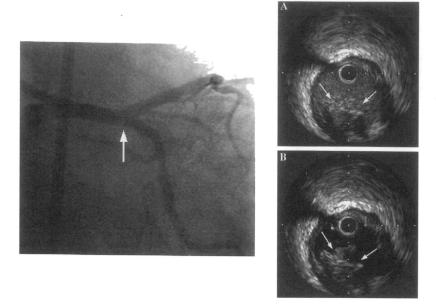

Figure 10 Demonstration of an intraluminal thrombus. Note the subtle appearance by angiography (arrow). (A) Intravascular ultrasonographic image of a large thrombus (arrows), at one side adherent to the vessel wall. (B) Saline injection temporarily clears the lumen of blood cells, allowing a better delineation of the thrombus (arrows).

able by intravascular ultrasonography. Pandian et al. found angioscopy and intravascular ultrasonography to be 100% and 80% sensitive, respectively (31). However, they studied normal vessels with ex vivo prepared thrombi placed in the vessel segments. Siegel et al., studying explanted human vessels, found that the sensitivity of intravascular ultrasonography for detecting thrombi was only 57% with a specificity of 95% because of false-negative interpretation of laminar clots in normal vessels and the inability to distinguish disrupted atheroma from intraluminal thrombus (30).

C. Detection of Plaque at Risk by Intravascular Ultrasonography

In a recently published case report, an intermittent stage of a ruptured plaque with thrombus formation in the emptied cavity was visualized by intravascular ultrasonography (33). The authors suggest that this stage might represent a step toward plaque healing as the thrombus fills the emptied cavity, ultimately leading to the organization of the lesion. Using intravascular ultrasonography in serial studies of plaque rupture has led to a better understanding of the healing process in vivo. Ge et al. demonstrated that a free-floating ruptured intimal flap in the right coronary artery was found adjacent to the arterial wall at follow-up, resulting in an increase in plaque thickness and echodensity (34). Another report described a patient with a plaque rupture and subsequent myocardial stunning, who had a complete healing of the lesion after 2 months with a normal coronary angiogram (35).

Only a relatively small number of studies have correlated intravascular ultrasonography–derived parameters of plaque morphology to clinical variables or clinical outcome in patients with unstable coronary syndromes. In a study of 55 subjects, Nissen et al. investigated plaque composition and structure in patients with stable and unstable angina (36). In patients with unstable syndromes, the maximal thickness of the intimal leading edge was less (0.27 vs. 0.41 mm) and the sonolucent zone greater (0.44 vs. 0.32 mm) than in stable angina. Conversely, dense fibrous tissue was present at 35% of the sites in stable angina but in only 13% of unstable patients. In a similar protocol, Hodgson and colleagues reported that patients with unstable syndromes had more soft lesions (74% vs. 41%), fewer calcified and mixed plaques (25% vs. 59%), and fewer intralesional calcium deposits (16% vs. 45%) compared with stable angina patients (15). Ultrasonography also demonstrated greater sensitivity than angiography for identifying unstable lesions (74% vs. 40%). Another study by the same group also demonstrated predominance of soft atheroma on intravascular ultrasonography images in patients with unstable angina by clinical criteria (37). Kearney et al. identified the presence of a demarcated inner layer in unstable lesions, delimited by a fine circumferential line, as the only significant morphological difference between stable and unstable lesions (38). This pattern was noted in 77% of unstable plaques but in only 7% of stable lesions and was believed by the authors to most likely represent layering of recurrent thrombus.

In an attempt to classify plaque morphology as visualized by intravascular ultrasonography according to the American Heart Association (AHA) guidelines (39, 40), Erbel and colleagues evaluated 49 patients with normal coronary angiograms (41). Normal vessel or early stages of atherosclerosis (AHA class III–V) were found in 63% of the lesions, and advanced atherosclerosis (AHA class VI–VIII) was observed in 23% of the segments. Early signs of atherosclerosis were mainly seen in young people, whereas advanced lesions were found predominantly with an increase in age.

To explain the mechanism of unstable plaque rupture, an intravascular ultrasonography study was performed in 121 patients with unstable angina or acute myocardial infarction (42). Twenty-nine patients were found to have plaque rupture, which was confirmed by injecting contrast material in the ulcerated plaque. All but two rupture sites were identified in the middle of the plaque. The average thickness of the fibrous cap was 0.47 mm, and 83% of the lesions were eccentric. By angiography, only 8 of the 29 patients had signs of an intimal flap, and 5 lesions were misdiagnosed as coronary artery aneurysms.

The major limitation of all studies comparing intravascular ultrasonographic imaging criteria to clinical or angiographic variables is the lack of follow-up. The only prospective follow-up study correlating morphological features of vulnerable atherosclerotic plaque to patient outcome was performed in Japan (43). A total of 105 patients with angiographically insignificant lesions underwent intravascular ultrasonographic imaging; these patients were then prospectively followed for 18 ± 14 months (range, 1–48 months). During this follow-up period, 12 patients developed unstable angina or had an acute myocardial infarction. All lesions related to the acute event were eccentric by intravascular ultrasonography, and 10 of the 12 plaques contained low echogenic areas within the diseased segment as identified on the initial ultrasonographic examination. The percent plaque area of the occluded segments was greater than that of nonoccluded segments, but no statistical significance was achieved. The authors concluded that larger, more eccentric plaque ($>60\%$) with intraplaque low echogenic areas could become vulnerable during the course of disease even though the lumen area is preserved. The sensitivity and specificity of intravascular ultrasonography in predicting clinical events, however, has yet to be determined.

In summary, intravascular ultrasonographic imaging has brought us one step closer to the characterization of atheromateous lesions in vivo and is a promising technique for the detection of plaque at risk for rupture. However, a precise identification of fibro-fatty plaque by intravascular ultrasonography is subject to current limitation by the resolution and dynamic range of the imaging systems. This is the main reason for the heterogeneous data resulting from all the studies investigating the sensitivity of intravascular ultrasonography in the detection of vulnerable plaque.

VI. FUTURE DIRECTIONS

A. High-Frequency Imaging

Recently, transducers working at the 40- to 45-MHz range became available. Figure 11 shows a comparison between intravascular ultrasonographic images at 30 MHz and 40 MHz. Although the detail of the fine structure is greatly improved at 40 MHz, the blood backscatter noise is more prominent and can affect image interpretation. At present, different techniques are under development to filter or subtract the blood signal and allow easier delineation of the blood-intima border. Note also that the penetration of the signal decreases with the increased frequency, and, as a result, perivascular structures are less visible. These limitations have to be addressed before approaching even higher frequency ultrasound trans-

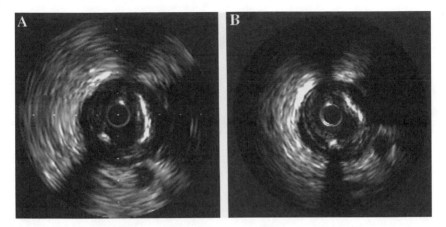

Figure 11 Comparison of intravascular ultrasonographic images at 30 MHz (A) and 40 MHz (B). Note the greater detail of plaque characteristics in the 40-MHz image but also an increase in blood noise and less penetration.

ducers. Nevertheless, there is potential to substantially increase the resolution (at least in the near-field) using higher transducer frequency and ultimately increase sensitivity in the distinction of plaque types.

B. Intravascular Ultrasonographic Tissue Characterization

The main reason for the relatively low sensitivity of intravascular ultrasonography to identify fibro-fatty plaque is the postprocessing of the ultrasonographic signal. The ultrasound image is created by a number of image processing steps, including filtering and amplification of the signal and time gain compensation. During these processes, some information inherent in the signal is lost. By collecting the "raw," unprocessed radiofrequency signal, all postprocessing of the ultrasound signal can be bypassed, and thus the complete information of the original data set is preserved (Figure 12). Theoretically, the characteristics of radiofrequency signals are directly related to the tissue properties. "Ultrasonographic tissue characterization" is a generated term used to describe computer-based approaches to investigate subtle and complex aspects of the interaction between the ultrasound signal and the tissue in question. It is now theoretically possible to analyze these factors, including the effects of a range of frequencies and the distribution of the power spectrum of the signal, in a sufficiently short period of time to accurately identify the composition of a plaque during the course of a clinical intravascular ultrasound examination. A multitude of different statistical approaches have been used in the past to analyze the radiofrequency data, includ-

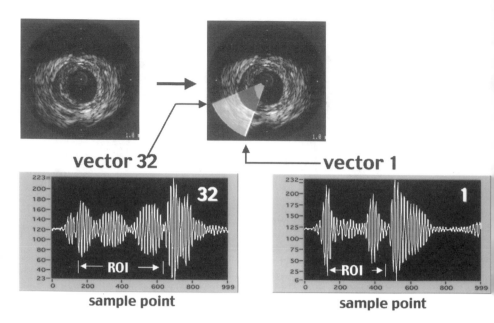

Figure 12 Example of a radiofrequency backscatter analysis of an intravascular ultra-sonographic image. Each vector (line of data) is analyzed separately within a region of interest (ROI).

ing analysis of absolute backscatter power, angular dependency of backscatter, mean/standard deviation ratio of the signal envelope, and attenuation measurements. All statistical analyses are based on three distinct characteristics of the tissue: the average acoustic impedance difference, which determines the magnitude of backscatter from interfaces; the distribution of scatterers, which influences the frequency and angle dependency of the backscatter; and the absorption characteristics of the tissue, which affects the attenuation of the ultrasound signal (44).

Several studies have shown that radiofrequency signal analysis has the potential to discriminate between tissue types in the diseased arterial wall. Picano et al. analyzed backscatter signals derived from human aorta and found that integrated backscatter power from fatty streaks or normal wall was significantly lower than from fibrous or calcified plaque (45). Wickline et al. demonstrated the efficacy of backscatter analysis in the discrimination among normal, fatty, and fibrous tissues in an animal model (46). By use of intravascular ultrasonography, Wilson et al. showed that an abnormally high attenuation slope is seen in areas of plaques that have undergone degeneration (47). This includes lipid pools, cholesterol clefts, necrosis, and microcalcification. Most of these changes were not appreciated by analysis of the gray-scale images. In a recent study, lipid could be differentiated from other types of plaque tissue on the basis of spectral slope analysis in pressure-perfused human coronary arteries (48). Other tissue types (dense fibrotic tissue and calcium) could also be identified with high accuracy. The distinction between fibro-fatty plaque and thrombus by intravascular ultrasonographic tissue characterization has been demonstrated in an in vitro model using the average radiofrequency envelope probability distribution function (49). Distinct changes in the distribution function morphology for plaque compared with thrombus were detected. By means of texture analysis of radiofrequency data, Ramo et al. distinguished thrombi of different ages and cell composition (50). In that study, the more heterogeneous structure of white cell clots was differentiated from that of platelet-rich thrombus by variance analysis, skewness, and kurtosis.

At present, the major limitation of this set of methods is the relatively long acquisition and processing time of the radiofrequency signal. Thus, most of the studies that use intravascular ultrasonographic tissue characterization have been performed in the in vitro setting. Recently, the first results of intravascular ultrasonographic radiofrequency signal analysis in vivo were published (51). The radiofrequency ultrasound signals from each cross section were sampled in real-time at a rate of 500 MHz with 8-bit resolution by use of a personal computer-based digitizer. The unprocessed signal was obtained after preamplification but before time-gain compensation or any other signal manipulation. For each cross section complete 360-degree scans, consisting of 256 vectors (received signal from a single acoustic pulse), were acquired digitally and stored. The technique was applied in a primate model of graft rejection in which aortic segments were transplanted to immunologically mismatched animals. Attenuation was found to be significantly lower in the allografts compared with the host aorta, allowing a discrimination of the different structures. In the future, these methods may be applicable in discriminating plaque types in vivo and in real-time.

In conclusion, intravascular ultrasonography is a useful technique for the detection and localization of coronary atherosclerosis in vivo. However, the precise plaque morphology as seen histologically is difficult to assess by the analysis of the gray-scale images alone. Intravascular ultrasound tissue characterization has the potential to detect plaque vulnerability, but sufficiently powerful analysis systems are just now becoming available for in vivo applications.

REFERENCES

1. Yock PG, Fitzgerald PJ. Intravascular ultrasound: state of the art and future directions. Am J Cardiol 1998; 81:27E–32E.

2. Ambrose JA, Winters SL, Arora RR, Eng A, Riccio A, Gorlin R, Fuster V. Angiographic evolution of coronary artery morphology in unstable angina. J Am Coll Cardiol 1986; 7:472–478.
3. Giroud D, Li JM, Urban P, Meier B, Rutishauer W. Relation of the site of acute myocardial infarction to the most severe coronary arterial stenosis at prior angiography. Am J Cardiol 1992; 69:729–732.
4. Hackett D, Davies G, Maseri A. Pre-existing coronary stenoses in patients with first myocardial infarction are not necessarily severe. Eur Heart J 1988; 9:1317–1323.
5. Ambrose JA, Winters SL, Stern A, Eng A, Teichholz LE, Gorlin R, Fuster V. Angiographic morphology and the pathogenesis of unstable angina pectoris. J Am Coll Cardiol 1985; 5:609–616.
6. MacIsaac AI, Thomas JD, Topol EJ. Toward the quiescent coronary plaque. J Am Coll Cardiol 1993; 22:1228–1241.
7. Mintz GS, Painter JA, Pichard AD, Kent KM, Satler LF, Popma JJ, Chuang YC, Bucher TA, Sokolowicz LE, Leon MB. Atherosclerosis in angiographically "normal" coronary artery reference segments: an intravascular ultrasound study with clinical correlations. J Am Coll Cardiol 1995; 25:1479–1485.
8. Glagov S, Weisenberg E, Zarins CK, Stankunavicius R, Kolettis GJ. Compensatory enlargement of human atherosclerotic coronary arteries. N Engl J Med 1987; 316: 1371–1375.
9. Nissen SE, Gurley JC, DeMaria AN. Assessment of vascular disease by intravascular ultrasound. Cardiology 1990; 77:398–410.
10. Yock PG, Linker DT. Intravascular ultrasound. Looking below the surface of vascular disease. Circulation 1990; 81:1715–1718.
11. Nishimura RA, Edwards WD, Warnes CA, Reeder GS, Holmes DR, Jr., Tajik AJ, Yock PG. Intravascular ultrasound imaging: in vitro validation and pathologic correlation. J Am Coll Cardiol 1990; 16:145–154.
12. Di Mario C, The SH, Madretsma S, van Suylen RJ, Wilson RA, Bom N, Serruys PW, Gussenhoven EJ, Roelandt JR. Detection and characterization of vascular lesions by intravascular ultrasound: an in vitro study correlated with histology. J Am Soc Echocardiogr 1992; 5:135–146.
13. Gussenhoven EJ, Essed CE, Lancee CT, Mastik F, Frietman P, van Egmond FC, Reiber J, Bosch H, van Urk H, Roelandt J, et al. Arterial wall characteristics determined by intravascular ultrasound imaging: an in vitro study. J Am Coll Cardiol 1989; 14:947–952.
14. Fitzgerald PJ, St. Goar FG, Connolly AJ, Pinto FJ, Billingham ME, Popp RL, Yock PG. Intravascular ultrasound imaging of coronary arteries. Is three layers the norm? Circulation 1992; 86:154–158.
15. Hodgson JM, Reddy KG, Suneja R, Nair RN, Lesnefsky EJ, Sheehan HM. Intracoronary ultrasound imaging: correlation of plaque morphology with angiography, clinical syndrome and procedural results in patients undergoing coronary angioplasty. J Am Coll Cardiol 1993; 21:35–44.
16. Hiro T, Leung CY, De Guzman S, Caiozzo VJ, Farvid AR, Karimi H, Helfant RH, Tobis JM. Are soft echoes really soft? Intravascular ultrasound assessment of mechanical properties in human atherosclerotic tissue. Am Heart J 1997; 133:1–7.
17. Kimura BJ, Bhargava V, DeMaria AN. Value and limitations of intravascular ultra-

sound imaging in characterizing coronary atherosclerotic plaque. Am Heart J 1995; 130:386–396.

18. Gutfinger DE, Leung CY, Hiro T, Maheswaran B, Nakamura S, Detrano R, Kang X, Tang W, Tobis JM. In vitro atherosclerotic plaque and calcium quantitation by intravascular ultrasound and electron-beam computed tomography. Am Heart J 1996; 131:899–906.

19. Friedrich GJ, Moes NY, Muhlberger VA, Gabl C, Mikuz G, Hausmann D, Fitzgerald PJ, Yock PG. Detection of intralesional calcium by intracoronary ultrasound depends on the histologic pattern. Am Heart J 1994; 128:435–441.

20. Fitzgerald PJ, Ports TA, Yock PG. Contribution of localized calcium deposits to dissection after angioplasty. An observational study using intravascular ultrasound. Circulation 1992; 86:64–70.

21. Mintz GS, Douek P, Pichard AD, Kent KM, Satler LF, Popma JJ, Leon MB. Target lesion calcification in coronary artery disease: an intravascular ultrasound study. J Am Coll Cardiol 1992; 20:1149–1155.

22. Demer LL. Effect of calcification on in vivo mechanical response of rabbit arteries to balloon dilation. Circulation 1991; 83:2083–2093.

23. Richardson PD, Davies MJ, Born GV. Influence of plaque configuration and stress distribution on fissuring of coronary atherosclerotic plaques. Lancet 1989; 2:941–944.

24. Tuzcu EM, Berkalp B, De Franco AC, Ellis SG, Goormastic M, Whitlow PL, Franco I, Raymond RE, Nissen SE. The dilemma of diagnosing coronary calcification: angiography versus intravascular ultrasound. J Am Coll Cardiol 1996; 27:832–838.

25. Fitzgerald PJ, Brisken AF, Brennan JM, Hargrave VK, MacGregor JS, Yock PG. Errors in intravascular ultrasound image interpretation and measurements due to limited dynamic range (abstr). Circulation 1991; 84:II–438.

26. Potkin BN, Bartorelli AL, Gessert JM, Neville RF, Almagor Y, Roberts WC, Leon MB. Coronary artery imaging with intravascular high-frequency ultrasound. Circulation 1990; 81:1575–1585.

27. Sechtem U, Arnold G, Keweloh T, Casper C, Curtius JM. In vitro diagnosis of coronary plaque morphology with intravascular ultrasound: comparison with histopathologic findings. Z Kardiol 1993; 82:618–627.

28. Rasheed Q, Dhawale PJ, Anderson J, Hodgson JM. Intracoronary ultrasound-defined plaque composition: computer-aided plaque characterization and correlation with histologic samples obtained during directional coronary atherectomy. Am Heart J 1995; 129:631–637.

29. Hiro T, Leung CY, Russo RJ, Moussa I, Karimi H, Farvid AR, Tobis JM. Variability in tissue characterization of atherosclerotic plaque by intravascular ultrasound: a comparison of four intravascular ultrasound systems. Am J Card Imaging 1996; 10: 209–218.

30. Siegel RJ, Ariani M, Fishbein MC, Chae JS, Park JC, Maurer G, Forrester JS. Histopathologic validation of angioscopy and intravascular ultrasound. Circulation 1991; 84:109–117.

31. Pandian NG, Kreis A, Brockway B. Detection of intraarterial thrombus by intravascular high frequency two-dimensional ultrasound imaging in vitro and in vivo studies. Am J Cardiol 1990; 65:1280–1283.

32. Frimerman A, Miller HI, Hallman M, Laniado S, Keren G. Intravascular ultrasound characterization of thrombi of different composition. Am J Cardiol 1994; 73:1053–1057.

33. Jeremias A, Ge J, Erbel R. New insight into plaque healing after plaque rupture with subsequent thrombus formation detected by intravascular ultrasound. Heart 1997; 77:293.

34. Ge J, Haude M, Gorge G, Liu F, Erbel R. Silent healing of spontaneous plaque disruption demonstrated by intracoronary ultrasound. Eur Heart J 1995; 16:1149–1151.

35. Baumgart D, Liu F, Haude M, Gorge G, Ge J, Erbel R. Acute plaque rupture and myocardial stunning in a patient with normal coronary arteriography. Lancet 1995; 346:193–194.

36. Nissen SE, Gurley JC, Booth DC, Berk MR, Yamagishi M, Fischer C, DeMaria AN. Differences in intravascular ultrasound plaque morphology in stable and unstable patients. Circulation 1991; 84:II–436.

37. Rasheed Q, Nair R, Sheehan H, Hodgson JM. Correlation of intracoronary ultrasound plaque characteristics in atherosclerotic coronary artery disease patients with clinical variables. Am J Cardiol 1994; 73:753–758.

38. Kearney P, Erbel R, Rupprecht HJ, Ge J, Koch L, Voigtlander T, Stahr P, Gorge G, Meyer J. Differences in the morphology of unstable and stable coronary lesions and their impact on the mechanisms of angioplasty. An in vivo study with intravascular ultrasound. Eur Heart J 1996; 17:721–730.

39. Stary HC, Chandler AB, Glagov S, Guyton JR, Insull W, Jr., Rosenfeld ME, Schaffer SA, Schwartz CJ, Wagner WD, Wissler RW. A definition of initial, fatty streak, and intermediate lesions of atherosclerosis. A report from the Committee on Vascular Lesions of the Council on Arteriosclerosis, American Heart Association. Arterioscler Thromb 1994; 14:840–856.

40. Stary HC, Chandler AB, Dinsmore RE, Fuster V, Glagov S, Insull W, Jr., Rosenfeld ME, Schwartz CJ, Wagner WD, Wissler RW. A definition of advanced types of atherosclerotic lesions and a histological classification of atherosclerosis. A report from the Committee on Vascular Lesions of the Council on Arteriosclerosis, American Heart Association. Circulation 1995; 92:1355–1374.

41. Erbel R, Ge J, Gorge G, Baumgart D, Haude M, Jeremias A, von Birgelen C, Jollet N, Schwedtmann J. Intravascular ultrasound classification of atherosclerotic lesions according to American Heart Association guidelines. Cor Art Disease 1999; 10:489–499.

42. Ge J, Chirillo F, Schwedtmann J, Gorge G, Haude M, Baumgart D, Shah V, von Birgelen C, Sack S, Boudoulas H, Erbel R. Screening of ruptured plaques in patients with coronary artery disease by intravascular ultrasound. Heart 1999; 81:621–627.

43. Yamagishi M, Terashima M, Awano K, Kijima M, Nakatani S, Daikoku S, Ito K, Yasumura Y, Miyatake K. Morphology of vulnerable coronary plaque: insights from follow-up of patients examined by intravascular ultrasound before an acute coronary syndrome. J Am Coll Cardiol 2000; 35:106–111.

44. Linker DT, Kleven A, Gronningsaether A, Yock PG, Angelsen BA. Tissue characterization with intra-arterial ultrasound: special promise and problems. Int J Card Imaging 1991; 6:255–263.

45. Picano E, Landini L, Distante A, Sarnelli R, Benassi A, L'Abbate A. Different degrees of atherosclerosis detected by backscattered ultrasound: an in vitro study on fixed human aortic walls. JCU J Clin Ultrasound 1983; 11:375–379.
46. Wickline SA, Shepard RK, Daugherty A. Quantitative ultrasonic characterization of lesion composition and remodeling in atherosclerotic rabbit aorta. Arterioscler Thromb 1993; 13:1543–1550.
47. Wilson LS, Neale ML, Talhami HE, Appleberg M. Preliminary results from attenuation-slope mapping of plaque using intravascular ultrasound. Ultrasound Med Biol 1994; 20:529–542.
48. Moore MP, Spencer T, Salter DM, Kearney PP, Shaw TR, Starkey IR, Fitzgerald PJ, Erbel R, Lange A, McDicken NW, Sutherland GR, Fox KA. Characterisation of coronary atherosclerotic morphology by spectral analysis of radiofrequency signal: in vitro intravascular ultrasound study with histological and radiological validation. Heart 1998; 79:459–467.
49. Fitzgerald PJ, Connolly AJ, Watkins RD, Hargrave VK, Yock PG. Distinction between soft plaque and thrombus by intravascular ultrasound tissue characterization. J Am Coll Cardiol 1991; 17:111A. Abstract
50. Ramo MP, Spencer T, Kearney PP, Shaw ST, Starkey IR, McDicken WN, Fox KA. Characterization of red and white thrombus by intravascular ultrasound using radiofrequency and videodensitometric data-based texture analysis. Ultrasound Med Biol 1997; 23:1195–1199.
51. Jeremias A, Kolz ML, Ikonen TS, Gummert JF, Oshima A, Hayase M, Honda Y, Komiyama N, Berry GJ, Morris RE, Yock PG, Fitzgerald PJ. Feasibility of in vivo intravascular ultrasound tissue characterization in the detection of early vascular transplant rejection. Circulation 1999; 100:2127–2130.

12

Detection of Plaque Vulnerability with Intravascular Palpography
Principle and Potentials

Chris L. de Korte and Anton F. W. van der Steen
Thoraxcentre, Rotterdam, The Netherlands

E. Ignacio Céspedes
Jomed Inc., Rancho Cordova, California

I. INTRODUCTION

A great variation exists in the stability of coronary atherosclerotic plaques. When coronary flow is limited by plaque, patients have angina develop, which can be stable for years. However, abrupt disruption of previously stable coronary plaques with superimposed thrombosis is the main cause of acute coronary events, such as unstable angina pectoris, sudden coronary death, and acute myocardial infarction (1–4). Therefore, for event-free survival, the vital question is not why atherosclerosis develops but rather why some plaques remain rupture-resistant and innocuous, whereas other plaques, after years of indolent growth, become rupture-prone and life-threatening (5). There are two major mechanisms of plaque disruption (6, 7): through and through rupture of the fibrous cap of a lipid-rich plaque (8) and superficial denudation and erosion of the endothelial surface (9, 10).

An unstable plaque can be characterized by several morphological features, including a thin fibrous cap and a large necrotic core of lipid and cellular debris (11). The instability of these plaques is mainly caused by the large mechanical stresses that will develop in the thinnest part of the fibrous cap (12, 13). Because the soft lipid core is unable to bear these mechanical forces, all the stress is concentrated in the fibrous cap. Rupture of the cap may be further enhanced by local weakening of the fibrous cap caused by macrophage infiltration. An increased density of macrophages is found in caps of ruptured plaques compared with caps of intact plaques (14). Furthermore, macrophage-rich areas are more prevalent in plaque tissue from patients with acute coronary syndromes than those with stable angina (15). Thus, it is both the geometrical features of the cap and the biology of the underlying lipid core that determine the vulnerability of a plaque.

A major challenge facing medicine is the diagnosis of vulnerable plaques. At present, identification of plaque vulnerability in vivo is impossible. With coronary angiography, advanced lesions, thrombosis, and calcifications may be revealed, but other qualitative features of the plaque cannot be assessed with this imaging technique (8). It is now widely accepted that the propensity of a lesion to rupture is poorly predicted by coronary angiography (11). A major problem is that vulnerability of plaque is not directly related to plaque size (10, 16, 17) but rather the plaque composition (7, 11).

Using intravascular ultrasonography (IVUS), the geometry of lumen, plaque, and vessel wall can be obtained, resulting in an accurate measure of plaque volume that correlates with chronic impairment of coronary flow and the clinical manifestation of angina (18). However, identification of the different plaque components is still limited (19, 20), although some promising techniques are currently being developed (21–27).

Imaging of atherosclerotic plaque with scintigraphy is possible, but the relation with plaque instability is still limited (28–30). Other potential techniques may be magnetic resonance imaging (31) and optical coherence tomography (32). With spectroscopy, certain plaque components may be detectable (33). Also promising are angioscopy (34, 35), electrical impedance imaging (36), and thermal examination (37) of plaque surfaces, because positive correlation between plaque vulnerability and these techniques has been proposed. The main disadvantage of the preceding techniques is that they assume that plaque vulnerability is related to plaque geometry, content, color, or temperature. However, plaque vulnerability may be best described as a mechanical phenomenon. By use of computer simulations, concentrations of circumferential tensile stress are more frequently found in unstable plaque than in stable plaque (12, 38).

In 1991, a new technique was proposed to measure the mechanical properties of tissue by ultrasonography: elastography (39). This technique was initially developed using phantom studies (40) followed by in vivo evaluation (41). The underlying principle is that when tissue is compressed, the rate of compression is related to the local mechanical properties. Measurement of local plaque compression is obtained with ultrasonographic images.

At present, this technique is being developed for intravascular purposes (42–45). For intravascular purposes, a derivative of elastography called palpography may be a suitable tool (46). In this approach, one strain value per angle is determined and plotted as a color-coded contour at the lumen–vessel wall boundary. Because radial strain is obtained, the technique may have the potential to detect regions with elevated stress: increased circumferential stress results in an increased radial compression of the plaque material.

In this chapter, the principle of intravascular palpography is discussed. In addition, the potential of the technique to detect vulnerable lesions is investigated. With phantom studies, the power of the technique to characterize soft and hard materials is demonstrated. Finally, the potential of the technique to characterize different plaque components is discussed.

II. MATERIALS AND METHODS

Vessel phantoms with the structure of atherosclerotic vessels were constructed from solutions of agar and gelatin. These solutions have similar acoustic and mechanical properties as vascular tissues (47). Carborundum (SiC) particles were used for scattering; hyperechoic and hypoechoic regions were constructed by modifying the carborundum concentration. A vessel containing a soft lesion with echogenicity contrast between the wall and plaque and a vessel with no echogenicity contrast between wall and plaque were formed. Atherosclerotic human femoral arteries were obtained postmortem.

The ultrasonography experiments were performed in a water tank (Figure 1) (43). The vessels (phantoms and arteries) were connected to both the insertion sheaths and tied with suture. The intraluminal pressure was adjusted by means of a water column system connected to the proximal sheath. The phantoms were scanned at intraluminal pressures of 50 and 54 mmHg, the artery specimen at pressures at 80 and 100 mmHg. This sheath was also used the insert a Princeps® 30-MHz IVUS catheter (EndoSonics, Rijswijk, The Netherlands). The catheter was connected to a modified IntraSound® motor unit. This unit contains the pulser and receiver of the echographic system and a stepper motor to rotate the single-element transducer. The transducer is rotated in 400 steps per revolution. At each angle, 12 traces of 10.0 µs radiofrequency (rf) data were acquired. These data were stored in an industrial grade Pentium computer, equipped with a 200-MHz sampling frequency acquisition board (43).

After the ultrasonography experiments, the arterial specimens were fixed, processed for histology, and stained with Picrosirius red to identify the collagen. Anti-α-actin was used to counterstain the smooth muscle cells. With these two

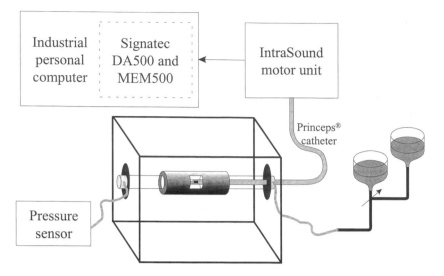

Figure 1 Experimental perfusion setup containing a water tank with two sheaths. The vessels are connected between the two sheaths. The intraluminal pressure is varied by the water column system. The IVUS catheter is inserted into the lumen to acquire the rf data that is stored in the personal computer for off-line processing.

stains, a distinction between fibrous and fatty material was made. Finally, anti-CD68-antibody was used to identify macrophages.

Palpograms were calculated by means of the IVUS frames acquired at the different intravascular pressures. With cross-correlation techniques, the local strain was calculated from the rf traces representing different parts of the vessel wall and plaque (43). The strain values were color-coded from red for low strain to yellow to green for 1% strain and plotted in the IVUS echogram as a color-coded line at the boundary between lumen and vessel wall. The alignment of the ultrasonographic data and histological cross-sections was performed using the IVUS echogram and histology. A region was identified as being rupture prone using four markers for plaque instability: a large lipid core, a low concentration of smooth muscle cells, a thin cap, and an increased number of macrophages (7).

III. RESULTS

Intravascular echograms with palpograms of vessel-mimicking phantoms with the morphology of a vessel wall with a soft eccentric plaque are presented in

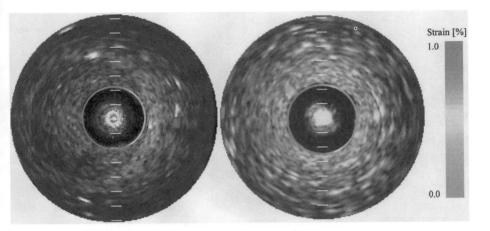

Figure 2 Intravascular echograms with strain palpograms of phantoms with a soft eccentric plaque in a hard vessel. The echogenicity of the plaque in the left phantom is lower than the echogenicity in the vessel wall. The right phantom has no difference in echogenicity between plaque and vessel wall. In both the phantoms, the soft plaque is identified by the palpogram. (See also color insert.)

Figure 2. It is clear from this figure that the soft plaque can be identified from the palpogram, independently of the echogenicity contrast between vessel wall and plaque. This experiment indicates that elastography has the potential to characterize fibrous and fatty plaque components, because fatty plaque components are supposed to be softer than fibrous plaques (48, 49).

An intravascular echogram with palpogram of a human femoral artery is presented in Figure 3. The echogram clearly reveals an eccentric plaque between the 2 and 11 o'clock positions. Although it is clear that the plaque can be divided into two parts, the echogenicity of both the parts is similar. Therefore, no distinction in plaque components in these two parts can be made on the basis of the IVUS echogram alone. The palpogram, however, clearly shows that the plaque can be divided into two parts: a part with high strain values (region II) and a part with low strain values (region III), both compared with the slightly diseased vessel wall (region I). On the basis of the observed strain values, fatty material is expected in region II, whereas fibrous material is expected in region III. The histological sections corroborate these elastographic findings. Region I contains a lipid pool with a very thin fibrous cap. In addition, macrophages are present in this region of the plaque. Region II is mainly composed of fibrous material: a large amount of collagen and smooth muscle cells.

The results from another artery are presented in Figure 4. The echogram reveals a small plaque deposit between the 7 and 11 o'clock positions. The strain

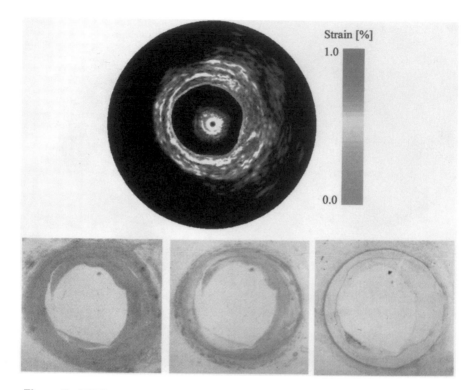

Figure 3 IVUS echogram with strain palpogram and histology of human femoral artery. The echogram shows an eccentric plaque from the 11 to 7 o'clock position. The palpogram reveals that the plaque contains a hard (region II) and a soft part (region III), both compared with the nondiseased vessel wall (region I). The histological findings reveal that the dominant tissue type in region II is fibrous material (collagen and smooth muscle cells). Fatty components are found in region III (no collagen and smooth muscle cells). In addition, macrophages are present in region III. (See also color insert.)

in this plaque has moderate to low values. On the basis of the strain value, fibrous material is expected. The histology confirms fibrous material (a high amount of collagen and smooth muscle cells).

IV. DISCUSSION

Intravascular ultrasonic palpation, an elastographic method for assessing the mechanical properties of the vessel wall and plaque, has been developed. This method is based on local cross-correlation of two IVUS echograms, acquired at

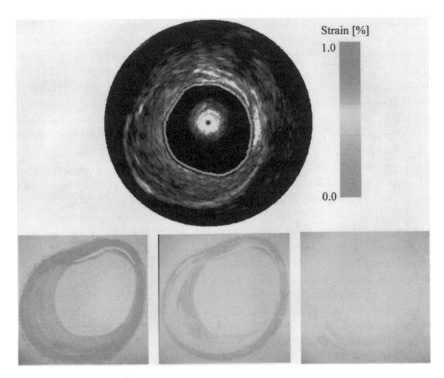

Figure 4 IVUS echogram with strain palpogram and histology of human femoral artery. The eccentric plaque has low strain values, indicating fibrous material. This finding is corroborated by the histological findings. (See also color insert.)

different intraluminal pressures. Because the mechanical information is plotted on the conventional echogram, a direct relation between the geometry and the mechanical information can be made from the resulting image, the palpogram.

The palpogram reveals information that may be inconclusive or unavailable from the IVUS echogram, because mechanical information is unequivocally related to echogenicity. The plaque in the phantom can only be identified in the echogram if a difference in echogenicity is present. In clinical practice, characterization of different plaque components on the basis of the echogenicity still remains limited (19, 50, 51). Figure 3 clearly illustrates that identification of the plaque composition based on the echogram is difficult. The echogenicity in region II is similar to the echogenicity in region III. The palpogram, however, makes it possible to differentiate the two regions: Region II is soft and region III is hard.

The ability to distinguish between hard and soft material may be an important tool to identify plaque vulnerability. Fatty tissue is significantly softer than fibrous tissue as measured with elastography (52). Because the presence of a lipid pool is one of the markers for rupture-prone plaques, palpography reveals prognostically important information. Furthermore, because the radial strain is determined, palpography is able to detect regions with elevated circumferential stress. These regions may be predictive of the location where the plaque will fracture (12, 13, 53). In principle, it is not important to know the thickness of a fibrous cap overlying a fatty pool: the important parameter is the capability of the cap to withstand the forces applied on it. A thin strong cap without inflammation may be more stable than a thicker cap with inflammation. Palpography provides a parameter that is directly related to the stress in the cap. The two arteries presented in this study reveal that at regions with abundant macrophage infiltration present, the strain is increased. The increase in strain may be caused by local weakening of the tissue caused by these macrophages (14, 15).

Because palpography is based on clinically available IVUS catheters, the technique may be easily introduced in the catheterization laboratory. In clinical practice, the intracoronary systolic and diastolic pressures can be used as the mechanical stimuli to strain the tissue. Using time-gated acquisition, different levels of intracoronary pressure are obtained. Motion of the catheter will influence the performance of the technique, but initial experiments in the catheterization laboratory revealed that motion of the catheter near end-diastole is minimal (54).

V. CONCLUSION

Intravascular palpography is a new technique capable of providing local mechanical information of the vessel wall and plaque. With this information, fibrous and fatty plaque components can be characterized. In addition, it has the potential to identify regions with increased circumferential stress. Because plaque composition and regions with increased circumferential stress are markers for plaque vulnerability, intravascular palpography may turn out to be a unique tool to identify the rupture-prone plaque.

REFERENCES

1.   Falk E. Coronary thrombosis: pathogenesis and clinical manifestations. Am J Cardiol 1991; 68:28B–35B.
2.   Fuster V, Badimon L, Badimon JJ, Chesebro JH. The pathogenesis of coronary artery disease and the acute coronary syndromes. N Engl J Med 1992; 326:242–250.
3.   Fuster V. Mechanisms leading to myocardial infarction: Insights from studies of vascular biology. Circulation 1994; 90:2126–2146.

4. Kragel AH, Gertz SD, Roberts WC. Morphologic comparison of frequency and types of acute lesions in the major epicardial coronary arteries in unstable angina pectoris, sudden coronary death and acute myocardial infarction. J Am Coll Cardiol 1991; 18:801–808.

5. Dalager-Pedersen S, Pedersen EM, Ringgaard S, Falk E. Coronary artery disease: plaque vulnerability, disruption, and thrombosis. In: Fuster V, ed. The Vulnerable Atherosclerotic Plaque: Understanding, Identification and Modification. New York: Futura Publishing Company, Inc.; 1999: 1–23.

6. Burke AP, Farb A, Malcolm GT, Liang Y, Smialek J, Virmanu R. Coronary risk factors and plaque morphology in men with coronary disease who died suddenly. N Engl J Med 1997; 336:1276–1282.

7. Davies MJ. Stability and instability: two faces of coronary atherosclerosis. Circulation 1996; 94:2013–2020.

8. Falk E, Shah P, Fuster V. Coronary plaque disruption. Circulation 1995; 92:657–671.

9. Farb A, Burke AP, Tang AL, Liang Y, Mannam P, Smialek J, Virmani R. Coronary plaque erosion without rupture into a lipid core: a frequent cause of coronary thrombosis in sudden coronary death. Circulation 1996; 93:1354–1363.

10. Fishbein MC, Sighel RJ. How big are coronary atherosclerotic plaques that rupture. Circulation 1996; 94:2662–2666.

11. Lee RT, Libby P. The unstable atheroma. Arterioscl Thromb Vasc Res 1997; 17: 1859–1867.

12. Richardson PD, Davies MJ, Born GVR. Influence of plaque configuration and stress distribution on fissuring of coronary atherosclerotic plaques. Lancet 1989; 21:941–944.

13. Loree HM, Kamm RD, Stringfellow RG, Lee RT. Effects of fibrous cap thickness on peak circumferential stress in model atherosclerotic vessels. Circ Res 1992; 71: 850–858.

14. Lendon CL, Davies MJ, Born GVR, Richardson PD. Atherosclerotic plaque caps are locally weakened when macrophage density is increased. Atherosclerosis 1991; 87:87–90.

15. Moreno PR, Falk E, Palacios IF, Newell JB, Fuster V, Fallon JT. Macrophage infiltration in acute coronary syndromes: implications for plaque rupture. Circulation 1994; 90:775–778.

16. Topol EJ, Nissen SE. Our preoccupation with coronary luminology: the dissociation between clinical and angiographic findings in ischemic heart disease. Circulation 1995; 92:2333–2442.

17. Ambrose JA, Tannenbaum MA, Alexopoulos D, Monsen CS, Weiss M, Borriw S, Gorlin R, Fuster V. Angiographic progression of coronary artery disease and the development of myocardial infarction. J Am Coll Cardiol 1988; 12:56–62.

18. Hodgson JMB, Reddy KR, Suneja R, Nair RN, Lesnefsky EJ, Sheehan HM. Intracoronary ultrasound imaging: correlation of plaque morphology with angiograph, clinical syndrome and procedural results in patients undergoing angioplasty. J Am Coll Cardiol 1993; 21:35–44.

19. di Mario C, The SHK, Madrestma S, van Suylen RJ, Wilson RA, Bom N, Serruys PW, Gussenhoven EJ, Roelandt JRTC. Detection and characterization of vascular

lesions by intravascular ultrasound: an in vitro study correlated with histology. J Am Soc Echo 1992; 5:135–146.

20. Potkin BN, Keren G, Mintz GS, Douek PC, Pichard AD, Satler LF, Kent KM, Leon MB. Arterial responses to balloon coronary angioplasty: an intravascular ultrasound study. J Am Coll Cardiol 1992; 20:942–951.

21. Barzilai B, Saffitz JE, Miller JG, Sobel BE. Quantitative ultrasonic characterization of the nature of atherosclerotic plaques in human aorta. Circ Res 1987; 60:459–463.

22. Bridal SL, Fornes P, Bruneval P, Berger G. Correlation of ultrasonic attenuation (30 to 50 MHz) and constituents of atherosclerotic plaque. Ultrasound Med Biol 1997; 23:691–703.

23. Bridal SL, Fornes P, Bruneval P, Berger G. Parametric (integrated backscatter and attenuation) images constructed using backscattered radio frequency signals (25–56 MHz) from human aortae in vitro. Ultrasound Med Biol 1997; 23:215–229.

24. Landini L, Sarnelli R, Picano E, Salvadori M. Evaluation of frequency dependence of backscatter coefficient in normal and atherosclerotic aortic walls. Ultrasound Med Biol 1986; 12:397–401.

25. Spencer T, Ramo MP, Salter DM, Anderson T, Kearney PP, Sutherland GR, Fox KAA, McDicken WN. Assessment of regional vascular distensibility in deceased iliofemoral arteries by intravascular ultrasound. Ultrasound Med Biol 1997; 20:529–542.

26. Wilson LS, Neale ML, Talhami HE, Appleberg M. Preliminary results from attenuation-slope mapping of plaque using intravascular ultrasound. Ultrasound Med Biol 1994; 20:529–542.

27. Pasterkamp G, Schoneveld AH, van der Wal AC, Haudenschild CC, Clarijs RJ, Becker AE, Hillen B, Borst C. Relation of arterial geometry to luminal narrowing and histologic markers for plaque vulnerability: the remodeling paradox. J Am Coll Cardiol 1998; 32:655–662.

28. Vallabhajosula S, Paidi M, Badimon JJ, Le N, Goldsmith SJ, Fuster V, Ginsberg HN. Radiotracers for low density lipoprotein biodistribution studies in vivo: technetium-99m low density lipoprotein versus radioiodinated low density lipoprotein preparations. J Nucl Med 1988; 29:1237–1245.

29. Lees AM, Lees RS, Scoen F, Isaacsohn JS, Fischman AJ, McKusick KA, Strauss HW. Imaging human atherosclerosis with 99mTc-labeled low density lipoproteins. Arteriosclerosis 1988; 8:461–470.

30. Miller DD, Rivera FJ, Garcia OJ, Palmaz JC, Berger HJ, Weisman HF. Imaging of vascular injury with 99m Tc-labeled monoclonal antiplatelet antibody S12: Preliminary experience in human percutaneous transluminal angioplasty. Circulation 1991; 85:1354–1363.

31. Merickel MB, Berr S, Spetz K, Jackson TR, Snell J, Gillies P, Shimshick E, Hainer J, Brookeman JR, Ayers CR. Noninvasive quantitative evaluation of atherosclerosis using MRI and image analysis. Arterioscl Thromb 1993; 13:1180–1186.

32. Brezinski ME, Tearney GJ, Weissman NJ, Boppart SA, Bouma BE, Hee MR, Weyman AE, Swanson EA, Southern JF, Fujimoto JG. Assessing atherosclerotic plaque morphology: comparison of optical coherence tomography and high frequency ultrasound. Heart 1997; 77:397–403.

33. Toussaint JF, Southern JM, Fuster V, Kantor HL. 13 C-NMR spectroscopy of human atherosclerotic lesions: relation between fatty acid saturation, cholesteryl ester content and luminal obstruction. Circulation 1994; 14:1951–1957.

34. Feld S, Ganim M, Carell ES, Kjellgern O, Kirkeeide RL, Vaughn WK, Kelly R, McGhie AI, Kramer N, Loyd D, Anderson HV, Schroth G, Smalling RW. Comparison of angioscopy, intravascular ultrasound imaging and quantitative coronary angiography in predicting clinical outcome after coronary intervention in high risk patients. J Am Coll Cardiol 1996; 28:97–105.

35. Thieme T, Wernecke KD, Meyer R, Brandenstein E, Habedank D, Hintz A, Felix SB, Baumann G, Kleber FX. Angioscopic evaluation of atherosclerotic plaques: validation by histomorphologic analysis and association with stable and unstable coronary syndromes. J Am Coll Cardiol 1996; 28:1–6.

36. Bouma C. Lipid detection in atherosclerotic lesions by intravascular impedance imaging. In: Image Sciences Institute. Utrecht: Utrecht University; 1998.

37. Casscells W, Hathorn B, David M, Krabach T, Vaughn WK, McAllister HA, Bearman G, Willerson JT. Thermal detection of cellular infiltrates in living atherosclerotic plaques: possible implications for plaque rupture and thrombosis. Lancet 1996; 347:1447–1449.

38. Cheng GC, Loree HM, Kamm RD, Fishbein MC, Lee RT. Distribution of circumferential stress in ruptured and stable atherosclerotic lesions. A structural analysis with histopathological correlation. Circulation 1993; 87:1179–1187.

39. Ophir J, Céspedes EI, Ponnekanti H, Yazdi Y, Li X. Elastography: a method for imaging the elasticity in biological tissues. Ultrasonic Imag 1991; 13:111–134.

40. Céspedes EI. Elastography: imaging of biological tissue elasticity. In: Houston, TX: University of Houston; 1993.

41. Céspedes EI, Ophir J, Ponnekanti H, Maklad N. Elastography: elasticity imaging using ultrasound with application to muscle and breast in vivo. Ultrasonic Imag 1993; 17:73–88.

42. de Korte CL, Céspedes EI, van der Steen AFW, Lancée CT. Intravascular elasticity imaging using ultrasound: feasibility studies in phantoms. Ultrasound Med Biol 1997; 23:735–746.

43. de Korte CL, van der Steen AFW, Céspedes EI, Pasterkamp G. Intravascular ultrasound elastography of human arteries: initial experience in vitro. Ultrasound Med Biol 1998; 24:401–408.

44. Ryan LK, Foster FS. Ultrasonic measurement of differential displacement and strain in a vascular model. Ultrasonic Imag 1997; 19:19–38.

45. Shapo BM, Crowe JR, Erkamp R, Emelianov SY, Eberle M, O'Donnell M. Strain imaging of coronary arteries with intraluminal ultrasound: experiments on an inhomogeneous phantom. Ultrasonic Imag 1996; 18:173–191.

46. Céspedes EI, de Korte CL, van der Steen AFW. Intraluminal ultrasonic palpation: assessment of local and cross-sectional tissue stiffness. Ultrasound Med Biol 1999: submitted.

47. de Korte CL, Céspedes EI, van der Steen AFW, Norder B, te Nijenhuis K. Elastic and acoustic properties of vessel mimicking material for elasticity imaging. Ultrasonic Imag 1997; 19:112–126.

48. Lee RT, Gordzinsky AJ, Frank EH, Kamm RD, Schoen FJ. Structure-dependent

dynamic mechanical behavior of fibrous caps from human atherosclerotic plaques. Circulation 1991; 83:1764–1770.

49. Lee RT, Richardson G, Loree HM, Gordzinsky AJ, Gharib SA, Schoen FJ, Pandian N. Prediction of mechanical properties of human atherosclerotic tissue by high-frequency intravascular ultrasound imaging. Arterioscl Thromb 1992; 12:1–5.

50. Potkin BN, Bartorelli AL, Gessert JM, Neville RF, Almagor Y, Roberts WC, Leon MB. Coronary artery imaging with intravascular high-frequency ultrasound. Circulation 1990; 81:1575–1585.

51. Yock PG, Linker DT. Intravascular ultrasound. Looking below the surface of vascular disease. Circulation 1990; 81:1715–1718.

52. de Korte CL, Woutman HA, van der Steen AFW, Pasterkamp G, Bom N. Characterization of plaque components with intravascular ultrasound elastography: a validation study in vitro. Circulation. 2000; 102:617–623.

53. Lee RT, Loree HM, Cheng GC, Lieberman EH, Jaramillo N, Schoen FJ. Computational structural analysis based on intravascular ultrasound imaging before in vitro angioplasty: prediction of plaque fracture locations. J Am Coll Cardiol 1993; 21: 777–782.

54. De Korte CL, Carlier SG, Mastik F, Doyley MM, van der Steen AFW, Serruys PW, Bom N. Morphologic and mechanic information of coronary arteries obtained with intravascular elastography: A feasibility study in vivo. Eur Heart J 2001: in press.

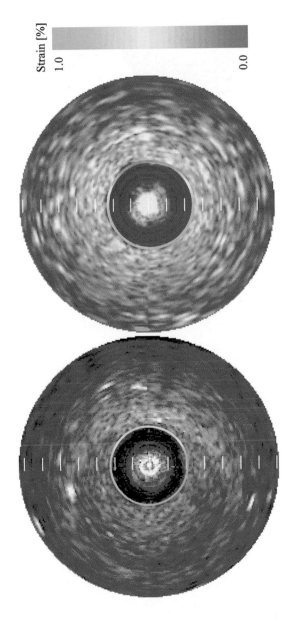

Figure 12.2 Intravascular echograms with strain palpograms of phantoms with a soft eccentric plaque in a hard vessel. The echogenicity of the plaque in the left phantom is lower than the echogenicity in the vessel wall. The right phantom has no difference in echogenicity between plaque and vessel wall. In both the phantoms, the soft plaque is identified by the palpogram.

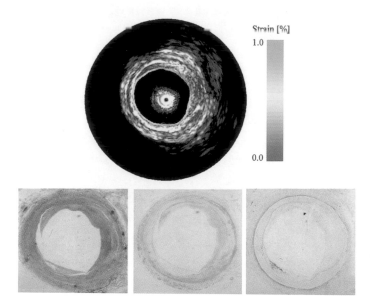

Figure 12.3 IVUS echogram with strain palpogram and histology of human femoral artery. The echogram shows an eccentric plaque from the 11 to 7 o'clock position. The palpogram reveals that the plaque contains a hard (region II) and a soft part (region III), both compared with the nondiseased vessel wall (region I). The histological findings reveal that the dominant tissue type in region II is fibrous material (collagen and smooth muscle cells). Fatty components are found in region III (no collagen and smooth muscle cells). In addition, macrophages are present in region III.

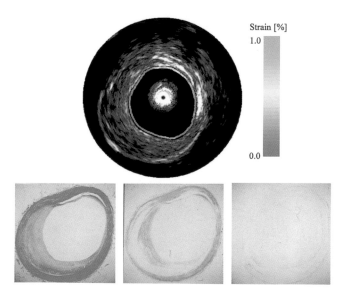

Figure 12.4 IVUS echogram with strain palpogram and histology of human femoral artery. The eccentric plaque has low strain values indicating fibrous material. This finding is corroborated by the histological findings.

13

Prospects of Laser Spectroscopy to Detect Vulnerable Plaque

Sweder W. E. van de Poll
Cleveland Clinic Foundation, Cleveland, Ohio, and Leiden University Medical Center, Leiden, The Netherlands

Jason T. Motz and Michael S. Feld
George R. Harrison Spectroscopy Laboratory, Massachusetts Institute of Technology, Cambridge, Massachusetts

John R. Kramer, Jr.
Cleveland Clinic Foundation, Cleveland, Ohio

I. INTRODUCTION

Atherosclerosis affects most muscular and elastic arteries (1), but its consequences in coronary vessels are particularly severe. Acute obstruction of the coronary artery lumen caused by intraluminal thrombosis overlying a ruptured or fissured atherosclerotic plaque leads to a reduction in coronary blood flow, thereby causing a cardiac event (2). At present, it is believed that the risk of plaque rupture is related to biochemical lesion composition rather than its area or volume (3, 4). Other factors that determine the instability of a plaque include fibrous cap thickness and the presence of compositional junctions (i.e., borders between atheromatous areas and calcifications or nondiseased areas). At present, however, it is not possible to predict whether a plaque will rupture and cause clinical symptoms.

Clinical techniques capable of evaluating atherosclerosis in a safe, valid, and reproducible manner are of critical importance for diagnosis, for the selection and evaluation of the effects of various interventional and pharmaceutical therapies, and for use in epidemiological and clinical research relating to the pathophysiology of atherosclerosis (5). Until now, the standard method of evaluating the extent and location of atherosclerotic lesions has been x-ray angiography (6). This technique can quantify the severity of a stenosis and recognize severe thrombus formation, as well as dense calcification. However, by imaging the contrast medium rather than the artery, it provides little information about the biochemical composition of a lesion. Histopathological examination does provide biochemical information on atherosclerosis, but requires excision of tissue. Angioscopy reveals plaque surface features that are not seen angiographically. In addition, it allows for observation of the arterial color, but because it only views the lesion surface, it does not reveal the internal heterogeneity of the plaque. External ultrasonography, spiral tomography, and magnetic resonance imaging or magnetic resonance angiography can identify fibrous caps and large calcification and provide information about vessel thickness but cannot detect more specific biochemical moieties. Intravascular ultrasonography is the most accurate modality available to assess the biochemistry of the arterial wall. However, identification of small amounts of lipids or calcium is still not possible, and sensitivity in detecting lipid pools is low (7).

Clearly, there is a need for instruments to study the in situ biochemical composition of atherosclerotic lesions. Rapid advances in laser spectroscopy are leading to new methods for the diagnostic imaging of human artery tissue. Optical spectroscopy can provide detailed information about arterial disease. The incident light can interact with tissue constituents in a variety of ways, providing information about the chemical and structural composition of a lesion that is encoded in the spectrum of the re-emitted light. These features can be measured accurately with sensitive equipment, and quality spectra can be collected in less than a second.

In the past two decades it has been shown that such spectra can provide important information about the chemical composition and histology of the arterial wall (8–11). Because spectroscopy does not require tissue removal, it can be exploited as an in vivo tool. It is rapid and safe and thus will be useful for clinicians and researchers in many applications. Recently developed catheters and compact light sources for performing in vivo studies will make it possible to develop laser spectroscopy into a powerful, percutaneous technique for the diagnosis and treatment of atherosclerosis. It may predict lesion progression or plaque rupture, and it may help us in understanding the pathogenesis of atherosclerosis in vivo. In addition, it may be useful in determining the optimum form of medical intervention and as a guidance system for laser angiosurgery catheters. Certainly, laser spectroscopy has the potential of providing diagnostic capabilities that are not available in current medical techniques.

This chapter reviews the basic principles and applications of optical spectroscopy in the study of atherosclerosis and its future directions in cardiovascular medicine, especially its role in the detection of vulnerable plaque. The research has been driven by the use of lasers to study biological tissue, resulting in a field that is referred to as laser spectroscopy. However, some of the techniques that have been developed can be applied using conventional light sources, as well, with the potential of reducing the cost of future commercial instruments. The application of such spectroscopic techniques, based on the insights provided by laser spectroscopy, has the potential to provide a new degree of information for use in the diagnosis and treatment of atherosclerosis.

II. LASER SPECTROSCOPY

Spectroscopy is the study of the interaction of light with matter and is largely based on decomposing light into its spectral components (12). A spectrometer can be used to extract the spectral features. This instrument works on the same principle by which a prism divides sunlight into a rainbow of different colors, or wavelengths, although most spectrometers use diffraction gratings rather than prisms. It measures the intensity of the light at each wavelength and displays this as a spectrum. Depending on the methods of excitation and detection, different types of spectroscopic information can be obtained.

A wide variety of optical spectroscopy techniques can be used to study biological tissue. Those that have proven to be the most useful to date are fluorescence, reflectance, and Raman spectroscopy. In this chapter, we review the basic principles of these tools and their application to the study of atherosclerosis.

A. Fluorescence and Reflectance

1. Basic Principles

Light is made up of photons, which carry energy. As is well known, the energy of a photon is proportional to its frequency or inversely to its wavelength. Optical photons span the ultraviolet (UV), visible, and infrared (IR) spectral range. UV photons have the highest energy, hence the shortest wavelengths, and IR photons have the lowest energy, hence the longest wavelengths. Visible wavelengths range from about 350 nm (violet) to 700 nm (red). UV wavelengths are shorter, and IR wavelengths are longer.

This energy can be transferred to a molecule, raising it to an excited state. Molecules can store energy in discrete states called energy levels. Figure 1 is a simplified diagram showing the relevant molecular states caused by the vibrations and electronic motions of the molecules. Vibrational levels are spaced by energies that correspond to those of IR photons, whereas electronic levels correspond to energies of visible or ultraviolet photons.

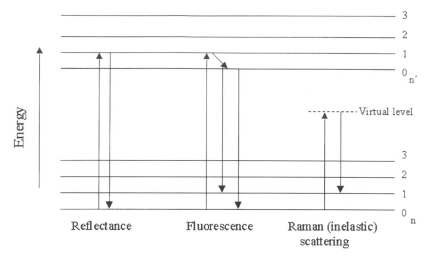

Figure 1 Reflectance, fluorescence, and Raman scattering.

a. Reflectance

Reflectance spectroscopy is based on studying the spectral content of white light
diffusely reflected from biological tissue. (Diffuse reflectance emanates in all
directions and is distinct from the specular reflection of light from smooth surfaces, which occurs at particular angles.) The diffusely reflected light contains
information about the absorbing molecules in the tissue and is responsible for
the color of objects.

Of the many spectroscopic processes that can occur when biological tissue
is exposed to optical radiation, absorption is perhaps the simplest. In this process,
a photon can transfer its energy to a molecule, raising it to an excited state (Figure 1). For energy to be conserved, this transfer requires the photon energy to
be the same as the energy change in the molecule. The photon can then be ''ab-
sorbed.'' If a molecule is subjected to white light, which is composed of light
of all visible wavelengths, and absorption occurs, certain frequency components
of the light will be attenuated. Because these frequencies are specific to the molecule, the absorption spectrum contains information about the absorbing molecules.

Hemoglobin is the predominant absorber in biological tissue in the visible
range. Melanin is another important absorber, particularly in skin. Water, proteins, nucleic acids, and lipids are other important absorbers in the UV and IR
spectral regions.

A second important process is elastic scattering. Elastic scattering, which is pervasive in biological tissue, causes incident photons to be redirected and randomized as they encounter cellular or extracellular tissue structures. ("Elastic" means that the photon energy, and thus the wavelength, is not changed.) An incident light beam thus loses its collimation as it propagates into the tissue and becomes diffused. Some of this light makes its way back to the tissue surface and emerges as "diffuse reflectance," which can be conveniently detected. Thus, when white light is incident on tissue, the diffusely reflected light will be attenuated at certain wavelengths. As with white light absorption, its spectrum contains information about the absorbing molecules in the tissue, which, in turn, relates to chemical composition (13). In addition, the distribution of the scattered light emerging from the tissue can provide information about the structure of the tissue scatterers (14, 15).

b. Fluorescence

Most of the excited state energy resulting from absorption is converted into heat. However, in many molecules a portion of the stored energy can be re-emitted as light (Figure 1). This emission is known as "fluorescence," and molecules that undergo this process are termed "fluorophores."

Substances only fluoresce when excitation light is present; fluorescence ceases in the absence of excitation. For example, a faint blue glow is sometimes visible from a glass of tonic exposed to sunlight. The quinine present in tonic is excited by ultraviolet light from the sun. On return to its ground state, the quinine emits blue light at wavelengths near 450 nm. When the glass of tonic is moved out of the sunlight, the fluorescence disappears.

Tissue fluorescence is never emitted at a single wavelength but rather over a wavelength band. Different fluorophores exhibit emission bands at wavelengths characteristic of their energy level structure, and some fluoresce more than others. As an example, the fluorescence spectrum of elastin, an important arterial fluorophore, excited using 325-nm excitation light is shown in Figure 2 (16). Other important arterial fluorophores are collagen (actually the cross-linking compound pyridinoline) and tryptophan. NAD(P)H may also make minor contributions. In atherosclerotic lesions a unique fluorescence associated with ceroid contributes to the fluorescence of the arterial wall (Table 1) (17, 18).

If several fluorophores are present in a tissue sample, the characteristic fluorescence bands of the constituent molecules will be present. Thus, by analyzing the fluorescence spectrum of a tissue sample, information about the chemical makeup can be extracted. Knowledge of the tissue absorption, which can be obtained from the diffuse reflectance, is also important in evaluating this information, because constituents of tissue such as hemoglobin can strongly absorb the

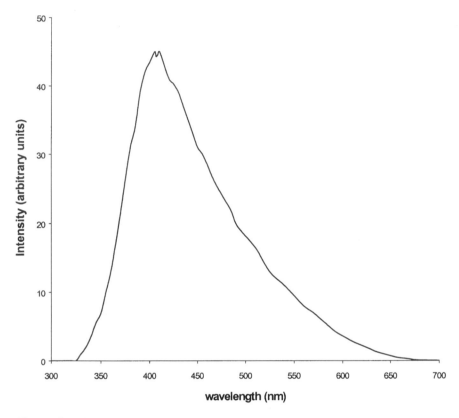

Figure 2 Fluorescence spectrum of elastin, excited using 325-nm laser light.

fluorescence at particular wavelengths and substantially distort the fluorescence spectrum.

Because absorption is frequency dependent, the fluorescence of a given fluorophore depends strongly on the wavelength of the exciting light. For example, the quinine in tonic fluoresces optimally when excited by UV light (at ~400 nm) but only weakly when illuminated by visible light. Moreover, by using different excitation wavelengths, quite different fluorescence spectra can be obtained. Thus, to completely characterize the fluorescence of a molecule, spectra must be collected at a number of excitation wavelengths. Multiple excitation spectra are also required to fully evaluate the fluorescence diagnostic potential of a given type of tissue. An excitation-emission matrix (EEM), a three-dimensional plot displaying the fluorescence intensity (vertical axis) as a function of the excitation and emission wavelengths (horizontal axes), is a convenient

Table 1 Fluorescence Maxima for the Major
Fluorescent Tissue Components in Coronary Arteries
Determined from In Vitro Collected EEMs

Component	Excitation emission maxima (nm)	Fluorophore
Tryptophan	(290,330)	Tryptophan
Collagen (I)	(350,420)	Pyridinoline
(III)	(340,390)	Pyridinoline
(III)	(450,510)	
Elastin	(460,520)	
	(360,410)	Pyridinoline
	(425,490)	
Ceroid	(340,440)	
	(460,520)	
NAD(P)H	(350,465)	

way of exhibiting such information (Figure 3). Such EEMs provide a full characterization of the fluorescent properties of a tissue sample.

2. Instrumentation

Cathctcr-bascd systcms havc bccn developed for accurately and rapidly acquiring
reflectance and fluorescence spectra in biological tissue. These systems contain
four main elements, (a) a light source, (b) an optical fiber spectral probe or catheter, (c) a spectrometer, and (d) a detector. The light source can be either a laser
or narrow-band conventional source for fluorescence and a white light lamp for
reflectance. The detector is typically an intensified photodiode array with 500 to
1000 elements. The catheter contains long, flexible, optical fibers that deliver the
excitation light to the tissue and return the re-emitted light (either fluorescence
or reflectance) to the spectrometer. In our catheters, the distal tip contains several
collection fibers, circularly arranged around a single delivery fiber and terminated
by a short transparent "optical shield," which expands and overlaps excitation
and collection spots and has certain other advantages (19, 20). The outside diameter of these catheters is typically about 1 mm (3–5F). Light from the excitation
source is focused into the proximal end of the catheter, the distal tip of which
is brought into contact with the tissue site to be sampled. The re-emitted light
from the tissue is collected and returned to the spectrometer where it is spectrally
dispersed and then detected. The resulting spectrum is usually then transmitted
to a computer, where it can be stored and analyzed. For fluorescence detection,
a long wavelength-pass filter with a sharp cutoff is used to prevent the excitation
light from flooding the detector.

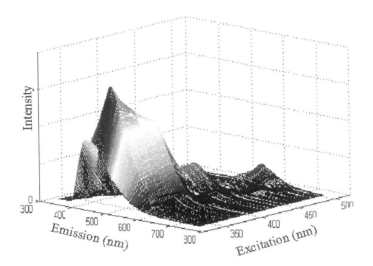

Figure 3 Excitation emission matrix surface plot of a sample of normal aorta. This
EEM was collected with the compact clinical Fast-EEM system in less than 1 second.

In the past, collecting tissue fluorescence at multiple excitation wavelengths
was a tedious process, requiring collection times of the order of an hour, and
thus limited to in vitro samples, which can exhibit substantial artifacts. Recently,
Zangaro et al. have developed a compact clinical instrument, called the Fast-
EEM, for obtaining EEMs. The system uses a sequence of dyes placed in cuvettes
on a rotating wheel (21). As the wheel rotates, the dyes are successively pumped
by a pulsed nitrogen laser ($\lambda = 337$ nm), producing 11 excitation wavelengths
in less than 1 second (Figure 4). The resulting spectra can then be displayed as
an EEM. At the same time, a white light reflectance spectrum is generated by
means of a (xenon) lamp.

Such compact portable systems can collect reflectance spectra, single wavelength fluorescence spectra, and fluorescence EEMs of biological tissue in vivo in
about one-half of a second. When carefully examined, these spectra can provide a
wealth of specific information on the character of human tissue.

3. Advances in Fluorescence Spectroscopy and the Detection of Atherosclerosis

Because the emission of fluorescence from a substance reflects the local environment and the concentrations of the fluorescent species present and is therefore
sensitive to changes in these moieties, one would expect fluorescence to be a
sensitive marker of disease in tissue.

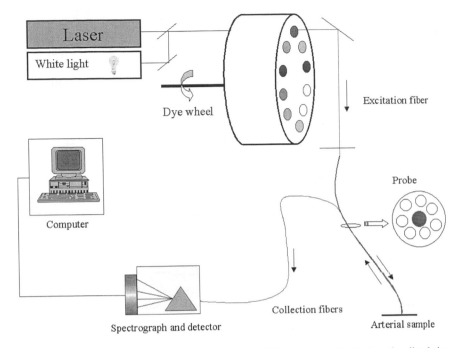

Figure 4 Schematic diagram of the clinical Fast-EEM system, illustrating the distal tip of the optical-fiber spectral probe in the inset.

The possibility of exploiting fluorescence spectroscopy for diagnosing pathological conditions in human tissue has been discussed by many authors. Its ability to identify diseased tissue in vitro and in vivo has been studied in oncology, dentistry, and gasteroenterology (17, 22–25). In addition, promising results have been achieved using fluorescence in human arterial wall to differentiate between normal and atherosclerotic tissue.

Several groups have studied fluorescence from human arterial tissue to identify and investigate differences between healthy and atherosclerotic tissue. In addition to its value as a diagnostic tool, one goal of these studies has been to develop a fluorescence-based guidance system for laser angiosurgery catheters. These studies have sought to determine whether fluorescence spectroscopy can be used to develop a diagnostic algorithm for atherosclerotic plaque detection. This detection may prevent transmural perforations, while also limiting vessel wall injury, thereby reducing the advent of restenosis (26, 27).

Using 480-nm excitation light, Kittrel et al. (8) and Sartori et al. (28) were the first to show that native fluorescence at visible wavelengths could be used to differentiate normal aorta from fibrous atherosclerotic plaque and calcified plaque in vitro. Later studies (16, 27, 29) showed that fluorescence spectroscopy could differentiate normal aorta from white fibrous plaque and yellow fatty atherosclerotic plaques when excited with UV light at 337 or 325 nm. Clarke et al. empirically correlated the fluorescence signal at 325-nm excitation wavelength with the intimal thickness and the relative proportions of fibrous, fatty, and calcified tissue within coronary atherosclerotic lesions (30). Laifer et al. (16) developed a classification algorithm based on elastin and collagen spectral decomposition. Each aortic spectrum was normalized to unit area and then mathematically resolved into a linear combination of pure elastin and collagen spectra, thereby assuming that elastin and collagen are the only fluorescent properties at this excitation wavelength. With 325-nm laser excitation, using the total fluorescence intensity (defined as the sum of arterial fluorescence emission at 380 and 440 nm) as a parameter, Deckelbaum et al. (31) demonstrated 97% correct classification of nonatherosclerotic tissue in vitro. Using 337-nm excitation, this group had previously shown that spectral line shape differences could be used to distinguish between atherosclerotic and normal tissue (29). However, at these excitation wavelengths, calcified plaques could not be detected, because in situ calcium phosphate and calcium hydroxyapatite deposits did not exhibit fluorescence. Moreover, these experiments showed that it was more difficult to distinguish between normal and atherosclerotic tissue in coronary arteries than in aorta. Although this approach often leads to a reasonably accurate diagnosis in vitro, it produces little biophysical information regarding tissue composition. To develop a meaningful diagnostic algorithm, it is important to understand the physical and biochemical basis for the observed emission lineshapes and to use this knowledge to extract specific, quantitative biochemical and morphological tissue information from the fluorescence spectra.

The structural proteins collagen and elastin are thought to be the major histochemical components of the fluorescence spectrum of arterial tissue at 325 nm excitation (16). Baraga et al. developed diagnostic algorithms, which indicate the presence of noncalcified and calcified atherosclerosis in human aorta, based on fluorescence emission spectra at 308-nm excitation. They showed that this differentiation is due to differences in the contributions of collagen, elastin, and tryptophan (32).

Based on an in vitro EEM study, Richards-Kortum et al. concluded that normal, noncalcified atherosclerotic and calcified atherosclerotic coronary artery lesions could best be differentiated using excitation at 476 nm (33). An algorithm was developed on the basis of the relative histochemical contributions of structural proteins and ceroid, a fluorescent protein complex associated with insoluble lipid oxidation products, which correlates with the formation of irreversible atherosclerotic lesions. Its exact identity is unknown (34). Normal coronary arteries fluoresced in the green, and this was attributed to the structural proteins elastin and collagen. In noncalcified plaques, an increase in intensity of the collagen band was observed, and this was attributed to its denser packing in the intima. When an atheromatous core was present, intense yellow fluorescence was observed, and this was attributed to ceroid deposits. In calcified plaques, the intense yellow and green fluorescence is mainly due to ceroid and an increased amount of collagenous fibrous tissue. This in vitro diagnostic algorithm for detecting coronary atherosclerosis, developed with optical fiber catheters for light delivery and collection, had a sensitivity of 95% and a specificity of 97% for detecting atherosclerosis, with a positive predictive value of 97% (17).

Initial clinical studies have shown that atherosclerotic tissue can be differentiated in vivo using 325-nm excitation light. Successful percutaneous detection of atherosclerotic plaque has also been reported (26). Despite this initial success, calcified tissue remains difficult to detect at 325-nm excitation, and therefore its clinical use is limited.

Clinical studies using 476-nm excitation light, based on the algorithm successfully developed in vitro (33), have not been successful in differentiating atherosclerosis. It is believed that this is due to issues related to probe geometry (35). Successful application of fluorescence spectroscopy requires that the spectral catheter be in good contact with the arterial wall, without the presence of intervening blood. Hemoglobin does not fluoresce, but its frequency-dependent reabsorption can severely distort the observed fluorescence spectrum. This suggests developing clinical catheters with improved contact and/or the use of an approach that combines information obtained from diffuse reflectance (which monitors absorption) and fluorescence.

Interestingly, little work has been reported to date on the use of diffuse reflectance as a tool for diagnosing atherosclerosis, although its use to identify cancer and dysplasia in various organs has been studied (36, 37).

Fluorescence is a potentially powerful tool for detecting atherosclerosis. However, its in vivo capability depends on developing improved catheters and broader diagnostic algorithms. We are developing side-looking catheters and using a compact EEM-fluorescence system to improve in vivo detection of atherosclerosis (21). At present, this system is being tested at the Cleveland Clinic Foundation to determine whether in vivo EEM fluorescence data and diffuse reflectance will enable us to detect and completely characterize the absorption and fluorescence properties of atherosclerosis.

B. Raman Scattering

1. Basic Principles

In addition to reflectance and fluorescence, the Raman effect is an important spectroscopic tool for tissue analysis. Compared with diffuse reflectance, which is brought about by *elastic* scattering, the Raman effect is an *inelastic* scattering process (Figure 1). Many molecules, when subjected to optical radiation, can be set into vibrational motion. The energy for this comes from the incident photon, whose energy is thereby reduced. Photon energy is proportional to frequency, and thus to conserve energy, the frequency reduction of the photon must exactly equal to the frequency of the excited molecular vibration. Because any given molecule has a unique set of vibrations (i.e., a unique set vibrational energy levels, Figure 1), its Raman spectrum acts as a fingerprint. In other words, the molecular structure of the tissue sample under study is encoded in the Raman-scattered light. By analyzing the spectrum of this inelastically scattered light, it is possible to determine the molecules present in the tissue. Thus, considering that plaque stability is believed to be related to chemical composition, Raman scattering is one of the most promising evaluation techniques.

Unlike tissue fluorescence, wherein the spectra of various molecules are broad, relatively featureless, and difficult to distinguish from one another, Raman spectra are composed of distinct, narrow bands with high information content. Figure 5 shows the Raman spectrum of elastin, which can be contrasted with the

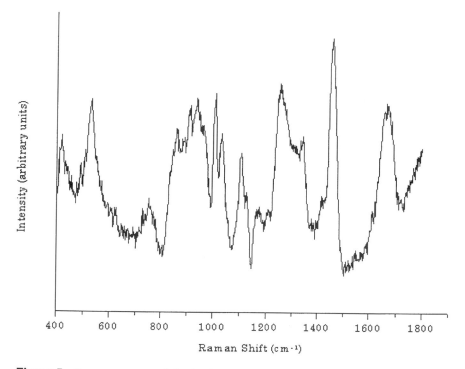

Figure 5 Raman spectrum of elastin, demonstrating the sharp vibrational band structure. The Raman shifts are measured in units of reciprocal wavelength, called wavenumbers (the number of waves per cm) and are a measure of energy.

broad elastin fluorescence spectrum of Figure 2. The sharp Raman features are sensitive to the chemical environment under investigation. However, it is possible to identify individual components by studying them in whole tissue in vitro or microscopically by confocal techniques.

Unlike excitation of fluorescence, which requires an exact match between the incident photon energy and the molecular energy change, Raman scattering can be excited by light of any frequency higher than the vibrational frequency itself. However, Raman scattering is much weaker than fluorescence, typically by a factor of a million. The weakness of such signals is a particularly severe problem in biological tissue, which fluoresces strongly, giving rise to a large background (38). Nevertheless, relatively recent technological advances, described later, have made Raman spectroscopy a clinically viable tool.

Seminal research has been conducted on the use of Raman spectroscopy to study biological tissue in vitro (39–41). This work has led to the almost exclusive use of near infrared (NIR) laser excitation (750–1064 nm wavelength range) for tissue diagnosis, in which background fluorescence is absent or minimal (41, 42). [Deep UV excitation (43) is another method by which background fluorescence can also be avoided, although such wavelengths are mutagenic and therefore not suitable for clinical use.] Additional advantages of these longer wavelengths include the relatively deep penetration of light into tissue (≥ 1 mm), thus yielding a larger sampling volume, and negligible photolytic decomposition of the tissue (38, 41).

2. Instrumentation

The most desirable situation for Raman spectroscopy of biological tissue would be to use excitation wavelengths beyond 1000 nm, where tissue fluorescence is not excited. In fact, the first useful work in this field used Nd:YAG laser excitation at 1064 nm, with Raman scattered light collected out to about 1200 nm using Fourier-transform (FT) Raman spectroscopy. FT instruments spectrally analyze light by means of interferometric techniques, as opposed to the dispersive techniques on which prism and grating spectrometers are based (44). The two well-known advantages of FT instruments are large light collection ability and the so-called multiplex advantage, by which light at all wavelengths can be collected simultaneously, thus significantly reducing data collection time. Thus, FT instruments are well suited for collecting weak signals in the NIR spectral range. Unfortunately, detectors in this wavelength range have large dark current and poor quantum efficiency, and FT-Raman studies on artery tissue required data collection times of the order of 30 minutes, acceptable for proof of principle studies, but clearly unacceptable for clinical use.

As first pointed out by Hirschfield and Chase (44) charge coupled device (CCD) array detectors used with dispersive spectrometers equivalently offer the same two advantages as FT instruments, and CCD offers superior detection capability. Unfortunately, the useful spectral response of these detectors extends to only about 1000 nm, thus necessitating the use of excitation wavelengths below 850 nm. Experiments in arterial tissue (41) showed that the amount of tissue background fluorescence generated by excitation wavelengths in the range 750 to 850 nm was tolerable and could be removed from the raw data by one of several techniques. The shot noise from this fluorescence was the main determinant of the signal-to-noise (S/N) ratio, and spectra with acceptable S/N could be obtained in a few seconds or less (42). CCD detection using excitation wavelengths in this range strikes a balance between reduced fluorescence and acceptable data collection capabilities, while minimizing the effects of radiation damage to the tissue. And so, in the past few years, research in Raman tissue spectroscopy has shifted to the use of the latter systems.

An instrument for NIR Raman spectroscopy contains the same four basic elements as for fluorescence or reflectance: (a) an excitation laser, (b) an optical fiber probe or catheter, (c) a grating spectrometer, and (d) a detector. Excitation can be provided by a tunable Ti:sapphire laser or, in the case of clinical applications where size is a limiting factor, a diode laser. The spectrometer collects and disperses light scattered from the tissue, as described earlier. A "Raman edge" filter with a very sharp cutoff wavelength is placed between the sample and the spectrograph to prevent the intense elastically scattered laser light from flooding the detector. The dispersed light is then collected by a CCD detector and subsequently fed to a computer for storage and analysis. To conduct in vivo studies an optical fiber probe is required. The laser light is coupled to the proximal end of the probe, which is incorporated into a catheter so that studies can be carried out in parallel with traditional angiography. The major limitation to conducting in vivo Raman spectroscopic studies at present is the availability of suitable probes. As the laser light is guided down the optical fibers, the fused silica material of the probe produces a strong unwanted Raman background signal of its own. Over the several meter length required for catheterization, this signal becomes intense, distorting the tissue spectra and adding shot noise to the background. Clinically useful probes that overcome this problem are under development in our laboratory and elsewhere.

3. Advances in Raman Spectroscopy and the Detection of Atherosclerosis

The intensity of the Raman spectrum for a given moiety is linearly proportional to its concentration (39). Thus, with careful calibration of the data collection process, it is possible to obtain precise information regarding what is currently believed to be the most accurate predictor of the instability of atherosclerotic plaques: the chemical constituents and their concentrations present in the diseased vessel (45–47).

To date, in vivo research into using Raman spectroscopy to diagnose atherosclerosis has been limited (48). However, the successful results of extensive in vitro research, along with the success of other spectroscopic techniques (e.g., fluorescence) in vivo, provide high likelihood that the extension to clinical studies will be successful.

As discussed earlier, initial in vitro studies used Fourier-transform Raman spectroscopy with 1064 nm Nd:YAG laser light for excitation. Baraga et al. examined human aorta with this technique and identified the chemical contributions from the various peaks in the spectra (10). For example, the major component of the internal elastic lamina, elastin, was identified by a unique peak at 1335 cm^{-1}. Similarly, calcifications were readily identifiable through two intense Raman bands (960 cm^{-1} and 1072 cm^{-1}), which are caused by a stretching the phosphate bond in calcium hydroxyapatite. They have also indicated that imaging by Raman spectroscopy should be possible.

Using the full Raman spectra and techniques of quantitative histochemistry, Manoharan et al. then went on to measure the concentrations of proteins (collagen and elastin) and lipids (cholesterol and cholesterol esters) in human aorta (39). Comparing these two techniques and relying on the linearity of the process, they were able to establish the relative strengths of the various Raman scattering moieties, and thus to demonstrate that Raman spectroscopy can obtain clinically relevant information. The comparison of concentration values obtained using Raman spectroscopy with those obtained using standard techniques resulted in 94 to 98% agreement between the methods.

Following the foundations laid in aortic tissue, recent studies have extended Raman histochemical analysis to coronary arteries and peripheral vessels. Brennan et al. examined minces of coronary arteries for their chemical makeup (49). The use of CCD detection allowed them to collect spectra comparable in quality with those obtained by FT-Raman in less than 1 minute, rather than longer than 1 hour. Minces were used in this initial study to ensure that the volume examined was homogeneous, thus facilitating comparison with traditional, chemically based analysis techniques. From these data, a model for atherosclerosis based on seven spectral components was developed. The usefulness of this technique was demonstrated by applying the model to intact coronary arteries. The accuracy of the fits to the intact artery data was only limited by the noise of the system (Figure 6).

Römer et al. then went on to apply this same model to a large set of Raman spectra collected from fresh, intact coronary arteries exhibiting a wide variety of disease states (11). Using the extracted concentration of total cholesterol lipids (cholesterol plus cholesterol esters) and the percentage of calcification, they were able to accurately classify the tissue into three disease categories: normal/intimal fibroplasia, noncalcified plaques, and calcified plaques. In a prospective study, using an algorithm derived with logistic regression, they were able to correctly

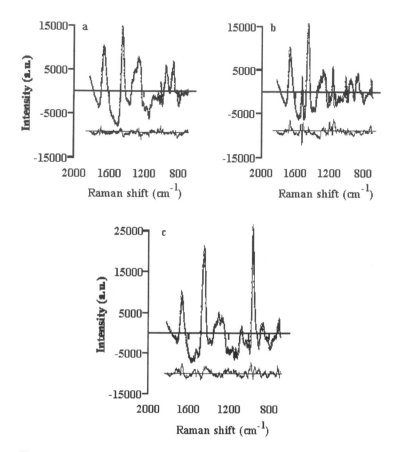

Figure 6 A comparison between the model of Brennan et al. (line) and spectra (dots) of coronary artery that exhibited intimal fibroplasia (a), noncalcified atheromatous plaque (b), and calcified plaque (c). The differences between a spectrum and its model fit are displayed below each comparison (same scale).

classify 64 of 68 samples (94%). Extension of the algorithm into a more elaborate diagnostic scheme was not possible because of the limited number of samples available.

As suggested by Baraga et al., it should be possible to use Raman spectroscopy to create images of various tissues (10). Using APOE*3 Leiden transgenic mice, which have been shown to develop atherosclerosis in a manner similar to that in humans, Römer et al. have conducted such a study (50, 51). Examining the first 7 to 8 mm of aorta from mice fed two different diets, they were able to create image maps of atherosclerotic lesions. They verified that calcium salt deposition in mice occurs exclusively within the area of cholesterol accumulation and that plaque development consistently occurs within the first 5 mm of the aortic arch.

A recent in vitro study by Salenius et al. is also worthy of note (52). This study applied the Raman modeling scheme of Brennan, developed for studying coronary arteries, to peripheral vessels (carotid and femoral arteries). Atherosclerosis in those vessels was successfully diagnosed according to the same three categories described previously. This demonstrates the robustness of this technique and is further indicative that the model already developed will be readily extendible to in vivo studies.

III. FUTURE DIRECTIONS

A. Extension of Current Techniques to In Vivo Work

As discussed in this chapter, methods using Raman and fluorescence spectroscopy have been developed for studying atherosclerosis, and their success has been demonstrated in a variety of in vitro studies. Substantial advances in instrumentation, methods of spectral analysis, and diagnostic algorithms have all been made. In this section, we consider the extension of these techniques to in vivo applications. To achieve this, some outstanding issues must be addressed.

The availability of small, flexible optical fiber probes that collect spectra without adding appreciable noise or background is essential if spectroscopic techniques are to become clinically useful. Flexible, small-diameter catheters are important to access small arteries, such as the coronary arteries, without injuring the endothelium. In vitro fluorescence studies have demonstrated that contact pressure and angle of the probe with the tissue can influence the quality of the spectra, thereby altering the prediction of the diagnostic algorithm. The optimal probe-tissue orientation (in fluorescence spectroscopy) is perpendicular (35). It can therefore be concluded that side-looking catheters will perform better in the confined environment of a blood vessel. We are developing such probes for operating room and percutaneous procedures with improved light collection capabilities based on imaging and nonimaging optics. Moreover, the influence of blood interference on spectral quality is still unknown; most in vitro algorithms have been developed on tissue immersed in saline. It may therefore be useful to develop probes that flush saline between probe and tissue, although designs to ensure good contact may also serve to displace intervening fluid.

B. Fluorescence and Reflectance

Until now, fluorescence diagnosis of atherosclerosis has been based on single wavelength excitation. As discussed in section II.A, a multiexcitation fluorescence system for clinical use has recently been developed (the Fast-EEM). This instrument collects fluorescence spectra at 11 different excitation wavelengths in less than 1 second, from which an excitation-emission matrix can be constructed that fully characterizes the fluorescent properties of the arterial site being sampled. At the same time, a white light reflectance spectrum is obtained, which provides important information about the presence of hemoglobin and other absorbers, and thus the interplay of absorption and fluorescence. The information obtained may lead to a deeper understanding of the spectral properties of in vivo artery tissue and better algorithms for classifying arterial disease more precisely. This system is currently being used for in vitro studies of aorta and coronary artery tissue. Preliminary results show substantial differences in the EEMs from samples at various stages of disease. In the near future, in vivo research during open heart surgery and aortic aneurysmectomy will be performed to further explore its potential.

Fluorescence microscopy of arterial tissue is another important area for future investigation. The bulk fluorescence from a macroscopic tissue sample originates in its constituent microstructures: collagen and elastin fibers, foam cells, macrophages, endothelium, fibroblasts, smooth muscle cells, etc. It would be interesting to determine which of these structures fluoresce, and their EEM spectra would be particularly valuable. Such information might make it possible to develop an algorithm that provides microscopic information from in vivo spectra.

C. Raman

A major limitation to conducting in vivo Raman spectroscopic studies is the availability of suitable optical fiber probes. Fiberoptic probes are necessary to reach arterial sites in vivo. Fiber fluorescence, however, has the potential for obscuring faint Raman signals. Special filters designed to reduce fiber fluorescence and improve the detection of Raman signals are needed. Such devices are currently under development in our laboratory. Initial studies will be performed on abdominal aorta, where the tissue can be removed after the spectra are obtained, and the Raman diagnostic predictions then compared with traditional histological studies.

Morphological modeling of coronary artery is another area of Raman spectroscopy that is under investigation. The quantitative studies performed to date extract the chemical makeup of the tissue from the spectra. It may also be possible to extract the relative abundance of individual arterial morphological structures (foam cells, smooth muscle cells, collagen fibers, etc.). The advantage of this approach is that the results would provide the same type of information that is used by pathologists to classify the degree of atherosclerosis in arterial tissue. Indeed, recent unpublished results from our laboratory indicate that such a model will be successful. Our study uses confocal Raman microscopy to characterize the Raman spectra of the morphological structures in coronary artery tissue and to model the bulk spectra as a linear combination of these. We have found that the Raman spectra of morphological structures of a given type (e.g., foam cells) are quite homogeneous, both within a single tissue sample and among samples from different patients. In addition, in most cases the Raman spectra of different morphological structures exhibit clearly distinguishable features. This type of analysis could allow for true optical "nonbiopsy," providing in vivo diagnosis by means of information currently used to assess the severity of atherosclerosis but presently possible only through in vitro techniques requiring the removal of tissue.

D. Combining Techniques

The spectra of Raman scattering, fluorescence, and reflectance reveal different chemical and morphological information about the composition of the arterial wall. Fluorescence is easily detectable, but the features are relatively broad, and fluorophores are often difficult to distinguish. Raman spectra are much weaker, but their narrow, high-resolution bands directly provide molecular information. Fluorescence easily detects ceroid, which is a good marker of necrotic core in atherosclerotic plaques, whereas Raman spectroscopy cannot. However, in contrast to fluorescence, Raman spectroscopy is able to detect calcium deposits, even small ones. Thus, combining these techniques, perhaps in a single instrument, would combine the advantages of each spectroscopic technique and provide complementary information. A study will soon be started to evaluate the possibilities of combining the different spectroscopy techniques.

It is also worthwhile to consider combining these spectroscopic techniques with contemporary medical diagnostics, such as IVUS, angioscopy, or x-ray angiography, and magnetic resonance imaging. This could lead to improved physicochemical imaging techniques. Some research to evaluate these possibilities has already been performed. Warren et al. used a combined ultrasonic and spectroscopic system to show that chemical cross-sections of aorta could be obtained that resembled the histological cross-section. The chemical image successfully identified regions of ceroid, increased collagen deposition, and normal aorta tissue (53). A system of this type would make possible studies to determine the likelihood of restenosis after percutaneous transluminal coronary angioplasty, based on the chemical composition of the atherosclerotic lesion. In addition, Römer et al. imaged the histochemistry of the arterial wall of human coronary artery in vitro, using both Raman spectroscopy and IVUS, thereby demonstrating the additional value of using Raman histochemical information in combination with ultrasonography for the purpose of diagnosing and studying atherosclerosis.

IV. CONCLUSIONS

In vitro spectroscopy studies done on human atherosclerosis suggest that unstable plaques might be detected in the future by their chemical heterogeneity, which helps identify plaques with relatively thin fibrous caps, marked inflammation, and adjacent lipid pools. Spectroscopy can add important information about the structure of vulnerable plaques. This technique may help in understanding the role of progression and regression of atherosclerotic plaque (e.g., calcification, lipid deposition, macrophage, and smooth muscle cell proliferation). It is clear that spectroscopy has the capability to be developed into a powerful technique to study and treat atherosclerosis. Its role in the detection of vulnerable plaques is an important aspect of present spectroscopic research. We are now embarking on the necessary clinical tests needed to establish the value of laser spectroscopy in clinical cardiovascular medicine.

REFERENCES

1. Cotran RS, Kumar V, Robbins SL. Pathologic basis of disease. Philadelphia: W.B. Saunders Company, 1989.
2. Davies MJ. Acute coronary thrombosis—the role of plaque disruption and its initiation and prevention. Eur Heart J 1995; 16:3–7.
3. Felton CV, Crook D, Davies MJ, Oliver MF. Relation of plaque lipid composition and morphology to the stability of human aortic plaques. Arteriosler Thromb Vasc Biol 1997; 17:1337–1345.
4. Libby P, Schoenbeck U, Mach F, Selwyn AP, Ganz P. Current concepts in cardiovascular pathology: the role of LDL cholesterol in plaque rupture and stabilization. A J Med 1998; 104:14S–18S.
5. Dzau V. Pathobiology of atherosclerosis and plaque complications. Am Heart J 1994; 128:1300–1304.
6. Vallabhasjoula S, Fuster V. Atherosclerosis: imaging techniques and the evolving role of nuclear medicine. J Nucl Med 1997; 28:1788–1796.
7. Benseker PJ, Chrchwell AL, Lee C, Abouelnasr DM. Resolution limitations in intravascular ultrasound imaging. J Am Soc Echocardiogr 1993; 6:158–165.
8. Kittrell C, Willet RL, de los Santos Pacheo C, et al. Diagnosis of fibrous arterial atherosclerosis using fluorescence. Applied Optics 1985; 24:2280–2281.
9. Brennan JF, Tercyak AM, Wang Y, et al. In situ histochemical analysis of human coronary artery by Raman spectroscopy compared with biochemical assay. Proc BIOS/SPIE 1995; 2388:105–109.
10. Baraga JJ, Feld MS, Rava RP. In situ optical histochemistry of human artery using near infrared Fourier transform Raman spectroscopy. Proc Natl Acad Sci USA 1992; 89:3473–3477.
11. Römer TJ, Brennan JF, 3rd, Fitzmaurice M, et al. Histopathology of human coronary

atherosclerosis by quantifying its chemical composition with Raman spectroscopy. Circulation 1998; 97:878–85.

12. Dasari RR, Feld MS. Spectroscopy. In: Collier's Encyclopedia. Vol. 21. New York: Colliers, 1993:414–424.

13. Campbell I, Dwek R. Biological Spectroscopy. Menlo Park, CA: Benjamin/Cummings, 1984.

14. Ferdman A, Yannis IV. Scattering of light from histologic sections: a new method for the analysis of connective tissue. J Invest Dermatol 1993; 100:710–716.

15. Perelman LT, Backman V, Wallace M, et al. Observation of periodic fine structure in reflectance from biological tissue: a new technique for measuring nuclear size distribution. Phys Rev Lett 1998; 80:627–630.

16. Laifer LI, O'Brien KM, Stetz ML, Gindi GR, Garrand TJ, Deckelbaum LI. Biochemical basis for the difference between normal and atherosclerotic arterial fluorescence. Circulation 1989; 80:1893–1901.

17. Richards-Kortum R. Fluorescence spectroscopy as a technique for diagnosis of pathologic conditions in human arterial wall, urinary bladder and gastrointestinal tissues. Ph.D. dissertation. Massachusetts Institute of Technology, Cambridge, MA, 1990.

18. Baraga JJ. Ultraviolet laser induced fluorescence spectroscopy of normal and atherosclerotic human arterial wall. Master's thesis. Massachusetts Institute of Technology, Cambridge, 1989.

19. Kramer JR, Brennan JF, Römer TJ, Wang Y, Dasari RR, Feld MS. Spectral diagnosis of human coronary artery: a clinical system for real time analysis. BIOS/SPIE Biomed Soc 1995; 2385:376–382.

20. Brennan JF, Zonios GI, Wang TD, et al. Portable laser spectrofluorimeter system for in vivo human tissue fluorescence studies. Appl Spectrosc 1993; 47:2082–2085.

21. Zangaro RA, Silveira L, Manoharan R, et al. Rapid multiexcitation fluorescence spectroscopy system for in vivo tissue diagnosis. Applied Optics 1996; 35:5211–5219.

22. Alfano RR, Lam W, Zarabbi H, et al. Human teeth with and without caries studied by laser scattering, fluorescence, and absorption spectroscopy. IEEE J Quantum Electron 1984; 20:1512–1516.

23. Andersson-Engels S, Johansson J, Stenram U, Svanberg K, Svanberg S. Malignant tumor and atherosclerotic plaque diagnosis using laser-induced fluorescence. IEEE J Quantum Electron 1990; 26:2207–2217.

24. Römer TJ, Fitzmaurice M, Cothren RM, et al. Laser-induced fluorescence microscopy of normal colon and dysplasia in colonic adenomas: implications for spectroscopic diagnosis. Am J Gastroenterol 1995; 90:81–87.

25. Richards-Kortum R, Sevick-Muraca E. Quantitative optical spectroscopy for tissue diagnosis. [review]. Ann Rev Phys Chem 1996; 47:555–606.

26. Bartorelli AL, Leon MB, Almagor Y, et al. In vivo human atherosclerotic plaque recognition by laser-excited fluorescence spectroscopy. J Am Coll Cardiol 1991; 17:160B–168B.

27. Leon MB, Lu DY, Prevosti LG, et al. Human arterial surface fluorescence: atherosclerotic plaque identification and effects of laser atheroma ablation. J Am Coll Cardiol 1988; 12:94–102.

28. Sartori M, Sauerbrey R, Kubodera S, Tittel F, Roberts R, Henry PD. Autofluorescence maps of atherosclerotic human arteries—a new technique in medical imaging. IEEE J Quantum Electron 1987; QE-23:1794–1797.

29. Deckelbaum LI, Lam JK, Cabin HS, Clubb KS, Long MB. Discrimination of normal and atherosclerotic aorta by laser-induced florescence. Lasers Surg Med 1987; 7: 330–335.

30. Clarke RH, Isner JM, Gauthier T, et al. Spectroscopic characterization of cardiovascular tissue. Lasers Surg Med 1988; 8:45–59.

31. Deckelbaum LI, Desai SP, Kim C, Scott JJ. Evaluation of a fluorescence feedback system for guidance of laser angioplasty. Lasers Surg Med 1995; 16:226–234.

32. Baraga JJ, Rava RP, Fitzmaurice M, et al. Characterization of the fluorescent morphological structures in human arterial wall using ultraviolet-excited microspectrofluorimetry. Atherosclerosis 1991; 88:1–14.

33. Richards-Kortum R, Rava RP, Fitzmaurice M, Kramer JR, Feld MS. 476 nm Excited laser-induced fluorescence spectroscopy of human coronary arteries: applications in cardiology. Am Heart J 1991; 122:1141–1150.

34. Verbunt R, Fitzmaurice MA, Kramer JR, et al. Characterization of ultraviolet laser-induced autofluorescence of ceroid deposits and other structures in atherosclerotic plaques as a potential diagnostic for laser angiosurgery. Am Heart J 1992; 123:208–216.

35. Römer TJ. Raman spectroscopy and the arterial wall. Ph.D. dissertation. Leiden University Medical Center, Leiden, The Netherlands, 1999.

36. Mourant JR, Bigio IJ, Boyer J, Conn RL, Johnson T, Shimada T. Spectroscopic diagnosis of bladder cancer with elastic light scattering. Lasers Surg Med 1995; 17: 350–357.

37. Bigio IJ, Mourant JR. Ultraviolet and visible spectroscopies for tissue diagnostics: fluorescence spectroscopy and elastic-scattering spectroscopy. Physics Med Biol 1997; 42:803–814.

38. Manoharan R, Wang Y, Feld MS. Review: Histochemical analysis of biological tissues using Raman spectroscopy. Spectrochemica Acta Part A 1996; 52:215–249.

39. Manoharan R, Baraga JJ, Feld MS, Rava RP. Quantitative histochemical analysis of human artery using Raman spectroscopy. J Photochem Photobiol B: Biol 1992; 16:211–233.

40. Manoharan R, Baraga JJ, Rava RP, Dasari RR, Fitzmaurice M, Feld MS. Biochemical analysis and mapping of atherosclerotic human artery using FT-IR microspectroscopy. Atherosclerosis 1993; 103:181–193.

41. Baraga JJ, Feld MS, Rava RP. Rapid near-infrared Raman spectroscopy of human tissue with a spectrograph and CCD detector. Appl Spectrosc 1992; 46:187–190.

42. Brennan JF, Wang Y, Dasari R, Feld MS. Near-infrared Raman spectrometer systems for human tissue studies. Appl Spectrosc 1997; 51:201–207.

43. Manoharan R, Wang Y, Dasari RR, Singer SS, Rava RP, Feld MS. Ultraviolet resonance Raman spectroscopy for detection of colon cancer. Lasers Life Sci 1994; 6: 1–11.

44. Hirschfeld T, Chase B. FT Raman spectroscopy: development and justification. Appl Spectrosc 1986; 40:133–137.

45. Wexler L, Brundage B, Crouse J, et al. Coronary artery calcification: pathophysiol-

ogy, epidemiology, imaging methods, and clinical implications: a statement for health professionals from the American Heart Association. Circulation 1996; 94: 1175–1192.

46. Mann JM, Davies MJ. Vulnerable plaque: relation of characteristics to degree of stenosis in human coronary arteries. Circulation 1996; 94:928–931.

47. Demer LL. Lipid hypothesis of cardiovascular calcification. Circulation 1997; 95: 297–298.

48. Puppels GJ, van Aken T, Wolthuis R, et al. In vivo tissue characterization by Raman spectroscopy. Proc BIOS/SPIE 1998; 3257:78–83.

49. Brennan JF, 3rd, Römer TJ, Lees RS, Tercyak AM, Kramer JR, Jr., Feld MS. Determination of human coronary artery composition by Raman spectroscopy. Circulation 1997; 96:99–105.

50. Groot PHE, van Vlijmen BJM, Benson GM, et al. Quantitative assessment of aortic atherosclerosis in APOE*3 Leiden Transgenic Mice and its relationship to serum cholesterol exposure. Arterioscler Thromb Vasc Biol 1996; 16:926–933.

51. Römer TJ, Brennan JF, Puppels GJ, et al. Raman spectroscopy provides chemical mappings of atherosclerotic plaques in APOE*3 Leiden transgenic mice. JACC 1998; 31:500–501A.

52. Salenius JP, Brennan JF, 3rd, Miller A, et al. Biochemical composition of human peripheral arteries examined with near-infrared Raman spectroscopy. J Vasc Surg 1998; 27:710–719.

53. Warren S, Pope K, Yazdi Y, et al. Combined ultrasound and fluorescence spectroscopy for physico-chemical imaging of atherosclerosis. IEEE Trans Biomed Eng 1995; 42:121–132.

14

Optical Coherence Tomography to Assess Plaque Vulnerability

Neil J. Weissman
Washington Hospital Center, Washington, D.C.

James G. Fujimoto
Massachusetts Institute of Technology, Cambridge, Massachusetts

Mark E. Brezinski
Brigham and Women's Hospital, Boston, Massachusetts

I. INTRODUCTION

Effective in vivo identification of a vulnerable plaque requires an intravascular imaging modality that is portable, uses a catheter of less than 1 mm in diameter, ideally has a resolution <50 μm, and can differentiate a lipid-rich core. Furthermore, the imaging equipment and disposable parts (i.e., catheters) have to be fairly inexpensive if this technology is to be used widely. Optical coherence tomography (OCT) has all of these components (1, 2). OCT has already demonstrated the ability to image in vivo intravascular structures with a resolution of less than 20 μm with a 2.9F catheter (3). OCT's exceptional resolution can identify the fine structural details in the artery, including a thin fibrous cap, fissures, and lipid cores (2). This chapter will review the applications of OCT technology to the assessment of cardiovascular microstructure. Although OCT has the potential to accurately, reliably, and inexpensively identify vulnerable plaques in humans, technical challenges to initiating clinical trials will also be discussed.

II. OCT TECHNOLOGY

Image production from OCT is somewhat analogous to image production from high-frequency ultrasonography. An ultrasonographic image (whether from transthoracic echocardiography or intravascular ultrasonogram) is the result of ultrasound reflecting off cardiovascular structures and returning to the transducer. Because sound travels at a known speed, the time it takes for the ultrasonographic signal to return can be translated into the distance from the transducer. A white "spot" is placed on the screen at that location to represent the cardiovascular structure the sound bounced off of, and this process is repeated in multiple directions, several times each second to produce a two-dimensional moving image. Moreover, because sound will reflect better off of denser material, the "whiteness" or "brightness" of the "spot" is crudely related to the cardiovascular structure's density. Current clinical intravascular ultrasonography (IVUS) systems have been limited in producing images with resolution better than 100 μm, which can reliably identify small lipid pools and the fibrous caps. This is due to the wavelength used and a poor correlation between reflected ultrasonographic amplitude and tissue components.

OCT also forms an image by "bouncing a signal" off cardiovascular structures, but instead of using sound, OCT uses light. Because of the properties of light, very high-resolution imaging can be achieved. With OCT, low-coherence infrared light is directed at the sample, and the amplitude of backreflected light is measured. As with ultrasonography, different tissue components will reflect different amounts of light that is then translated into a corresponding image. The time for light to be reflected back from the sample, or delay time, is also used to measure distances. However, light travels much faster than sound, and the small difference in delay time cannot be measured electronically as they can with ultrasonography. Therefore, a technique known as interferometry, which allows differentiation of minuscule differences in delay, must be used to calculate the distance from the infrared source.

The principles behind low-coherence interferometry are illustrated in Fig. 1. With interferometry, light emitted by the source is split evenly between two fibers, one directed at the sample and one toward a mirror on a reference arm. Light reflects off of the sample and the mirror simultaneously (if they are the same distance away) and is reflected back to the source and beam splitter. If reflected light from the sample and mirror arrives at the beam splitter simultaneously (identical delay time), interference will occur. OCT measures the intensity of interference. To obtain interference data from different depths within the tissue, the light path down the reference arm to the mirror must be varied. This was achieved in the original OCT systems by moving the reference mirror. The result is a plot of backreflection intensity as a function of depth. Once data are obtained in a single axial plane, the beam is scanned across the sample to produce

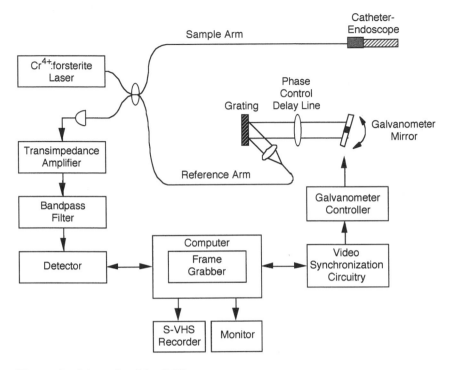

Figure 1 Schematic of the OCT system.

two- and three-dimensional data sets. The backreflection intensity is then converted into an image, where the log amplitude of the backreflection can be displayed with different shades of gray or color coded.

A. Early OCT Imaging

OCT was originally developed to image the transparent tissue of the eye at unprecedented resolution. Multiple studies have demonstrated the potential clinical usefulness of OCT in the diagnosis and management of retinal edema, macular holes, and glaucoma (4–6). Recently, OCT has been applied to the difficult problem of imaging in nontransparent tissue, which has included the cardiovascular system (2, 7, 8). One of the advances was to find an optical window, which is a wavelength of incident light where scattering and absorption is low, allowing increased penetration. Over the last few years, OCT has been used to identify pathologic conditions in other nontransparent organ systems, including the gastrointestinal tract, nervous system, reproductive tract, skin, and urinary tract (9–13).

B. Cardiovascular OCT Imaging

1. Early In Vitro Data

Initial in vitro OCT imaging of cardiovascular tissue was conducted with human aorta obtained postmortem (2). In these studies, OCT images accurately displayed atherosclerotic plaque morphology compared with the corresponding histopathology. The resolution was 16 ± 1 µm, 10X higher than high-frequency ultrasonography. In Fig. 2, an OCT image of a heavily calcified atherosclerotic plaque is seen with the corresponding histopathology (2). Fig. 3 demonstrates a collection of lipid (right with arrow) within the wall of a heavily calcified aorta. Also seen is a thin layer of intima overlying the plaque. In Fig. 4a, an atherosclerotic plaque with a thin intimal cap less than 50 µm in diameter is seen (arrow) over a collection of lipid (2). An imaging technology capable of identifying fine microstructural detail, such as thin intimal walls, will likely be a powerful tool for patient

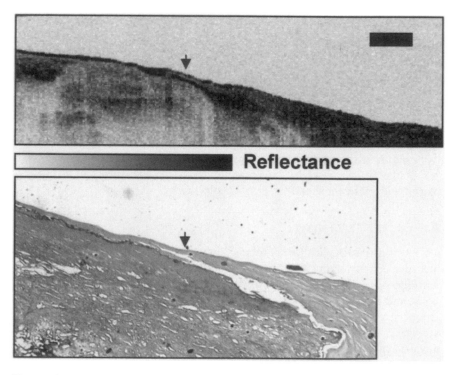

Figure 2   OCT image of atherosclerotic plaque and corresponding histology. (From Ref. 2.)

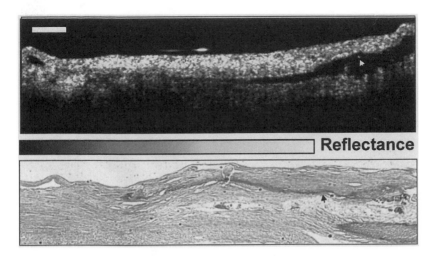

Figure 3 Heavily calcified aorta. (From Ref. 2.)

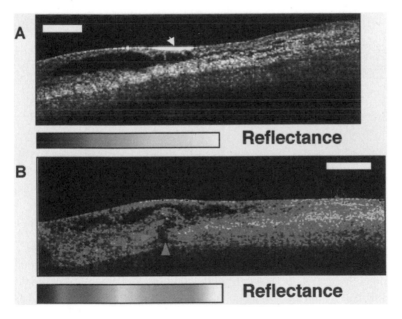

Figure 4 Plaque with fine internal microstructure. (From Ref. 2.)

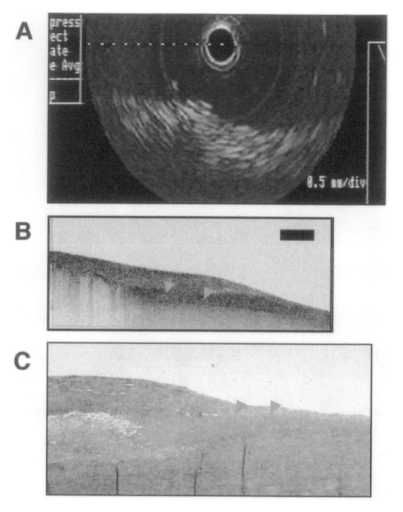

Figure 5 In vitro IVUS and OCT comparison with corresponding histology. (From Ref. 2.)

risk stratification. In Fig. 4b, fissuring (arrows) is occurring at the intimal-medial border, another indication of instability. In addition to demonstrating high-resolution microstructural identification of plaque morphology, OCT also has demonstrated an ability to image through heavily calcified tissue and through the width of a normal coronary artery (2, 8).

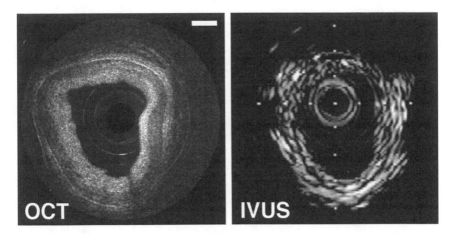

Figure 6 In vitro coronary artery. (From Ref. 14.)

2. Comparison with High-Frequency Ultrasonography

Because IVUS is the only clinically available in vivo intravascular imaging modality with high resolution, it is reasonable to compare OCT with IVUS. OCT and IVUS have undergone direct comparisons qualitatively and quantitatively with histology as the "gold standard" (7). When OCT and IVUS were compared

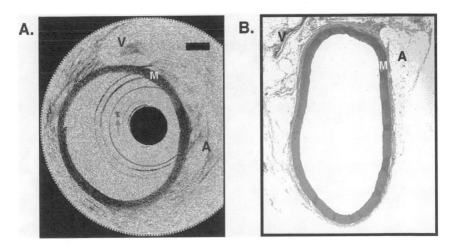

Figure 7 OCT image of aorta with corresponding histology. (From Ref. 3.)

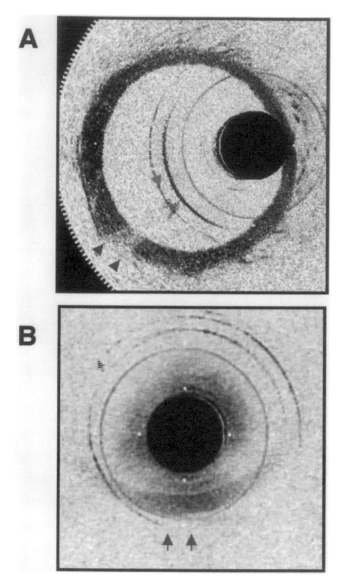

Figure 8   Attenuation by blood. (From Ref. 3.)

qualitatively, OCT consistently demonstrated superior delineation of structural detail. In Fig. 5, an aortic plaque was imaged in vitro with OCT and IVUS. In the IVUS image (A), the presence of the plaque is suggested, but no other structural detail is apparent. In the OCT image (B), in addition to the plaque, a distinct layer (arrows) is seen within the intima that appeared normal by ultrasonography. This layer is confirmed by histopathological finding (C) to represent smooth muscle proliferation. OCT was able to identify focal areas of lipid within a plaque that were not detected by IVUS. Quantitative measurements from OCT were also superior to IVUS. The axial resolution of both OCT and IVUS (30 MHz) was measured directly from the point spread function. The axial resolution of OCT was 16 ± 1 μm compared with 110 ± 7 μm for IVUS. Furthermore, the wall thickness of overlying intima as assessed with OCT strongly correlated with histological findings. Similar comparisons between IVUS and OCT have been confirmed with the 2.9F OCT catheter (14). In Fig. 6, the OCT image of an in vitro coronary artery is on the left; the IVUS image is on the right. The intimal hyperplasia is clearly seen with OCT but not with IVUS.

3. In Vivo OCT Imaging

In vivo OCT imaging has been performed with the aorta of New Zealand White rabbits (3). The OCT imaging catheter was introduced into the aorta through a 7F guiding catheter. Saline flushes were required during imaging at 2 to 3 ml/sec because of light scattering from red blood cells. In Fig. 7, an OCT image of the aorta with corresponding histopathological findings is seen. The media and inferior vena cava are sharply defined. In Fig. 8, the aorta is imaged in the presence (A) and absence (B) of saline flushes. Penetration is limited by blood.

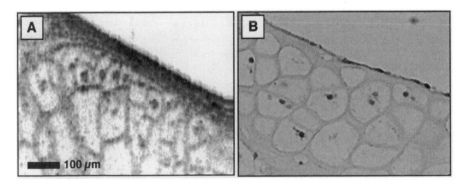

Figure 9   In vivo subcellular imaging of Xenopus laevis with corresponding histology. (From Ref. 15.)

4. Cellular Level Imaging

In vitro studies have been performed that demonstrate OCT imaging at resolutions of 4 μm, approaching the cellular level (15). In Fig. 9, imaging was performed using a living *Xenopus* organism, in which true subcellular imaging is seen. Not only are individual cells identified, but their individual nuclei can be distinguished. Although a catheter-based system is currently not available at this resolution, by use of a more complex catheter design, this level of resolution is possible within coronary arteries (15).

III. TECHNOLOGY

The principles behind OCT have been previously described (1, 2). OCT can be envisioned as analogous to ultrasonography, measuring the intensity of reflected infrared light rather than sound waves. The intensity of backreflection is plotted as a function of depth. Unlike ultrasonography, the echo delay time cannot be measured electronically because of the high speed associated with the propagation of light. Therefore, a technique known as low-coherence interferometry is used. This technique is based on a Michelson interferometer and performs high-resolution measurement of the echo delay time of reflected light by correlating it with light that travels a know reference distance. If the source illuminating the interferometer generates light with a broad bandwidth, the autocorrelation function representing the interference is then proportional to:

$$I(\Delta l) \alpha r_s r_r \; Re[F\{S(\omega)\}] \; cos(\omega_0 \tau_p)$$

where $I(\Delta l)$ is the intensity at the detector, $r_s r_r$ is the product of the reflections off the sample and mirror, $Re[F\{S(\omega)\}]$ is the real component of the Fourier transform of the power spectrum of the source, ω_0 is the center frequency of the source, and τ_p is the phase delay (16). The width of the spectrum and the width of the autocorrelation function (coherence length) are inversely related by means of the Fourier transform. Therefore, the resolution increases (shorter coherence length) with increasing source bandwidth. If the source has a Gaussian spectrum with a full-width half-maximum bandwidth (FWHM), $\Delta\lambda$, and a center λ_0, then the coherence length (Δl) or axial resolution is

$$\Delta l = (2 \ln(2)/\pi)(\lambda^2/\Delta\lambda).$$

through the use of sufficiently broad source bandwidths, resolutions with OCT have been achieved in the range of 4 to 16 μm, up to 25X higher than any technology available in clinical medicine.

The lateral or transverse resolution achieved with an OCT imaging system is determined by the focused spot size in analogy with conventional microscopy. The transverse resolution is

$$\delta x = (4\lambda/\pi)(f/d).$$

where d is the spot size on the objective lens and f is its focal length. High transverse resolution can be obtained by use of a large numerical aperture and focusing the beam to a small spot size. In addition, the transverse resolution is also related to the depth of focus or the confocal parameter b which is $2z_R$, is twice the Raleigh range (17).

$$2z_R = \pi\Delta x^2/2\lambda$$

To obtain data as a function of depth, the optical pathlength in the reference arm needs to be varied. The acquisition rate is generally determined by how rapidly the pathlength can be changed in the reference arm. The maximum frame rate for OCT is currently at 4 to 8 frames per second. All frame rates described in this text will assume an image size of 256 by 512 pixels. In initial OCT systems, the pathlength in the reference arm was changed by means of the use of a moving mirror or galvanometer. However, this embodiment required approximately 40 seconds to perform an image of nontransparent tissue. This system is still in use for systems imaging the transparent tissue of the eye. With second-generation systems, the pathlength in the reference arm was varied by fiber stretching with a piezoelectric crystal (18, 19). Limitations of this embodiment included polarization mode dispersion, hysteresis, crystal breakdown, and voltage requirements unacceptably high for routine clinical use. A recent embodiment showing considerable promise induces a variable optical group delay in the reference arm through the introduction of a linear wavelength-dependent phase ramp (20). Light from the reference arm is Fourier transformed with a grating. The dispersed light is directed onto a mirror. By tilting the mirror, a linear wavelength-dependent phase ramp is introduced. A linear phase ramp in the frequency domain results in an optical group delay in the time domain. An inverse Fourier transform occurs when the light is redirected on the grating. By varying the angle of the mirror, the optical group delay can be varied. In addition to high data acquisition rates (4–8 frames/sec), this system has two addition advantages over previous embodiments. The optical group delay can be varied separately from the phase delay, and the group velocity dispersion can be varied without the introduction of a separate prism (20).

Imaging deep within nontransparent tissue is possible because of the high sensitivity and dynamic range of OCT. The system functions analogously to heterodyne optical detection and achieves nearly quantum-limited performance. OCT has been designed near the shot noise limit by choosing a Doppler frequency (induced by the motion of the mirror or fiber stretching) to avoid low frequency $1/f$ noise and a proper transimpedance amplifier resistance/reference arm voltage to overcome thermal noise. For shot noise detection, the theoretical maximum signal-to-noise ratio that can be achieved with OCT under the assumption of linearity of electronics and high dynamic range of the digitization electronics can be expressed:

$$SNR = 10 \log(\eta P_s/2h\nu NEB)$$

where $\eta P_s/2h\nu$ is the number of electrons per unit time generated by the detector because of returning light and *1/NEB* bandpass filter bandwidth (16).

An additional advantage of OCT, besides high data acquisition rates and high resolution, is the clinical viability of the catheters and endoscopes. The current OCT catheter/endoscopes are 1 mm in diameter (20). A significant advantage of this catheter is that unlike an ultrasonographic catheter, it contains no transducer, making it relatively inexpensive. It consists primarily of relatively simple components, a single mode optical fiber, grins lens, light-directing prism, and speedometer cable. Because the diameter of early prototypes depends primarily on the size of the available speedometer cables, it is likely that commercial devices will be substantially smaller.

IV. DISCUSSION

The greatest limitation in the identification of high-risk plaques is resolution. Through stress analysis studies, it has been determined that plaques with intimal caps of less than 50 µm in diameter have the greatest propensity to rupture (21). This suggests that the 110-µm resolution of 30-MHz IVUS is not sufficient for the identification of high-risk plaques. The axial resolution of OCT, which is between 4 and 16 µm, suggests that it has the magnification necessary for the identification of high-risk plaques.

An imaging modality is not clinically useful unless it can be applied in the patient care setting. OCT's fiberoptic-based design is easily integrated into catheters or endoscopes. A 2.9F OCT imaging catheter has been developed which, unlike ultrasonography, contains no transducer within the catheter body, making it relatively inexpensive (20). OCT is compact and portable, an important consideration within the tight confines of the catheterization laboratory. Finally, OCT can be performed at or near real time. Current systems exist at 4 to 8 frames per second, but video rates are possible with future modifications.

Despite enthusiasm, OCT has not yet been used in clinical trials in humans. One challenge that had to be overcome was scattering of light caused by blood. Simultaneous saline flushing during imaging appears to be a simple and effective solution that has worked well in animals but needs to be tested in patients (3). The current generation of catheter-based OCT appears to have adequate penetration for normal vasculature but remains to be assessed in heavily diseased atherosclerotic arteries.

Future technological development will focus on increasing data acquisition rates and integrating the system with low-cost light sources. Recent studies achieved acquisition rates of 4 frames/sec, but this remains too slow and produces some motion artifacts. For accurate representations of luminal and plaque contour, acquisition rates will need to approach video rates (30 frames/sec). Last, the light source currently used is a mode-locked solid-state laser. This source would be too expensive and complex for routine clinical use. However, compact, inexpensive sources, such as doped fiber lasers or semiconductor diode sources, are currently under development and will likely be available within the next few years.

V. CONCLUSION

OCT identifies plaque microstructure at unprecedented resolution within the aorta and coronary arteries by use of a catheter-based technology that is easily applied clinically. OCT has also been directly compared with IVUS and has demonstrated superior qualitative and quantitative performance. High-speed, catheter-based systems have been developed and applied in vivo with success. In summary, OCT represents a promising new technology; combining high resolution, real-time intravascular imaging for the identification of vulnerable coronary lesions.

ACKNOWLEDGMENTS

This research is supported in part by the National Institutes of Health, contracts NIH-RO1-AR44812-01(MEB), NIH-RO1-HL63953(MEB), NIH-9-RO1-CA75289-01(JGF), NIH-9-RO1-EY11289-10(JGF), and NIH-1-R29-HL55686-01A1 (MEB), the Medical Free Electron Laser Program, Office of Naval Research Contract N00014-94-1-0717 (JGF), and the Whitaker Foundation Contract 96-0205 (MEB). The work on OCT in nontransparent tissue represents the effort of a large number of students, postdoctoral fellows, and collaborators. These include Dr. Michael Hee, Dr. Joseph Izatt, Dr. Gary Tearney, Dr. Stephen Boppart, Dr. Brett Bouma, Dr. James Southern, Dr. Debra Stamper, Dr. Parth Pitwari, and Dr. Jeurgen Herrmann, Costas Pitris. The authors also appreciate the technical support of Ms. Christine Jesser and the secretarial support of Ms. Cindy Kopf.

REFERENCES

1. Huang D, Swanson EA, Lin CP, Schuman JS, Stinson WG, Chang W, Hee MR, Flotte T, Gregory T, Puliafito CA, and Fujimoto JG. Optical coherence tomography. Science 1991; 254:1178–1181.
2. Brezinski ME, Tearney GJ, Bouma BE, Izatt JA, Hee MR, Swanson EA, Southern JF, and Fujimoto JG. Optical coherence tomography for optical biopsy: properties and demonstration of vascular pathology. Circulation 1996; 93:1206–1213.
3. Fujimoto JG, Boppart SA, Tearney GJ, Bouma BE, Pitris C, Brezinski ME. High resolution in vivo intraarterial imaging with optical coherence tomography. Heart. In press.
4. Swanson EA, Izatt JA, Hee MR, Huang D, Fujimoto JG, Lin CP, Schuman JS, and Puliafinto CA. In vivo retinal imaging by optical coherence tomography. Opt Lett 1993; 18:1864–1866.
5. Hee MR, Izatt JA, Swanson EA, Huang D, Lin CP, Schuman JS, Puliafito, and Fujimoto JG. Optical coherence tomography of the human retina. Arch Ophthalmol 1995; 113:325–332.
6. Puliatifo CA, Hee MR, Schumann JS, and Fujimoto JG. Optical Coherence Tomography of Ocular Diseases. New Jersey: Slack Incorporated, 1995.
7. Brezinski ME, Tearney GJ, Weissman NJ, Boppart SA, Bouma BE, Hee MR, Weyman AE, Swanson EA, Southern JF, and Fujimoto JG. Assessing atherosclerotic plaque morphology: comparison of optical coherence tomography and high frequency intravascular ultrasound. Heart 1997; 77:397–403.
8. Brezinski ME, Tearney GJ, Bouma BE, Boppart SA, Hee MR, Swanson EA, Southern JF, and Fujimoto JG. Imaging of coronary artery microstructure (in vitro) with optical coherence tomography. Am J Cardiol 1996; 77:92–93.
9. Fujimoto JG, Brezinski ME, Tearney GJ, Boppart SA, Hee MR, and Swanson EA. Optical biopsy and imaging using optical coherence tomography. Nature Med 1995; 1:970–972.
10. Schmitt JM, Yadlowsky MJ, and Bonner RF. Subsurface imaging of living skin with optical coherence microscopy. Dermatology 1995; 191:93–98.
11. Tearney GJ, Brezinski ME, Southern JF, Bouma BE, Boppart SA, and Fujimoto JG. Optical biopsy in human urologic tissue using optical coherence tomography. J Urol 1997; 157:1915–1919.
12. Tearney GJ, Brezinski ME, Southern JF, Bouma BE, Boppart SA, and Fujimoto JG. Optical biopsy in human gastrointestinal tissue using optical coherence tomography. Am J Gastroenterol 1997; 92:1800–1804.
13. Brezinski ME, Tearney GJ, Boppart SA, Swanson EA, Southern JF, and Fujimoto JG. Optical biopsy with optical coherence tomography, feasibility for surgical diagnostics. J Surg Res 1997; 71:32–38.
14. Tearney GJ, Brezinski ME, Boppart SA, Bouma BE, Weissman NJ, Southern JF, Swanson EA, and Fujimoto JG. Images in cardiovascular medicine. Catheter-based optical imaging of a human coronary artery. Circulation 1996; 94:3013.
15. Boppart SA, Bouma BE, Pitris C, Southern JF, Brezinski ME, and Fujimoto JG. In

vivo subcellular optical coherence tomography imaging in *Xenopus laevis*: Implications for the early diagnosis of neoplasms. Nature Med 1998; 4:861–865.

16. Wiener N. Acta Math 1930; 55:117–122.
17. Wilson T, Confocal Microscopy. California: Academic Press, 1990.
18. Sergeev A, Gelikonov V, Gelikonov A. High-spatial-resolution optical-coherence tomography of human skin and mucous membranes. Conference on Lasers and Electro Optics '95, Anaheim, Ca. May 21–26, 1995.
19. Tearney GJ, Bouma BE, Boppart SA, Golubovic B, Swanson EA, and Fujimoto JG. Rapid acquisition of in vivo biological images by use of optical coherence tomography. Opt Lett 1996; 21:1408–1410.
20. Tearney GJ, Brezinski ME, Bouma BE, Boppart SA, Pitris C, Southern JF, and Fujimoto JG. In vivo endoscopic optical biopsy with optical coherence tomography. Science 1997; 276:2037–2039.
21. Loree HM, Kamm RD, Stringfellow RG, and Lee RT. Effects of fibrous cap thickness on peak circumferential stress in model atherosclerotic vessels. Circ Res 1992; 71:850–858.

15
Magnetic Resonance Imaging of Vulnerable Plaque

Ergin Atalar
Johns Hopkins University, Baltimore, Maryland

I. INTRODUCTION

Conventional x-ray angiography and magnetic resonance (MR) angiography* techniques adequately display the lumen of a vessel. Atherosclerosis, however, is a disease of the vessel wall. Thus, the management of atherosclerosis may be significantly improved if the vessel wall could be imaged directly. For example, recent reports from the literature suggest that the plaques that are vulnerable to rupture are not necessarily large enough to cause a stenosis that is visible with luminography techniques (1, 2). Unfortunately, most imaging techniques are unable to accurately identify the vessel wall and characterize the plaque. Perhaps the most important role for MR imaging in the diagnosis of atherosclerosis is the imaging and characterization of atherosclerotic plaques. Although the components of plaques can be visualized using T1- and T2-weighted MR imaging techniques, with advanced MR imaging techniques, a diffusion map of the plaque can be generated and vessel wall distensibility can be displayed. Research on the development of methods for the imaging and characterization of atherosclerotic plaques is quite extensive. Work in this field began with the introduction of the first MR scanners more than 15 years ago (3). Recently, the development of advanced MR scanners with high-speed gradient systems, high-volume data

---

* Magnetic resonance angiography (MRA) is an excellent tool for imaging luminal narrowing noninvasively at high resolution. With recent advances in three-dimensional contrast-enhanced magnetic resonance (MR) imaging techniques, the quality of MRA images has become equal to or better than standard invasive angiography techniques.

acquisition units, and novel pulse sequences made the imaging of plaques feasible.

In addition to being a noninvasive technique for plaque characterization, advanced MR imaging techniques also have a potential place in the catheterization laboratory. MR scanners with the capability of real-time imaging, as well as MR-compatible catheters and guidewires, are being developed. Small imaging catheter probes that have the capability of increasing imaging resolution beyond what can be achieved with noninvasive techniques have a potential use in the management of atherosclerosis.

II. CHARACTERIZATION OF ATHEROSCLEROTIC PLAQUES USING MRI

In this section, we will discuss methods of characterizing atherosclerotic plaques using different magnetic resonance imaging techniques.* First, we will show that it is possible to characterize atherosclerotic plaques with conventional pulse sequences.

A. T1- and T2-Weighted Imaging Techniques

One of the most commonly used contrast mechanisms in MRI is the acquisition of T1- and T2-weighted MR images.[†] It is, therefore, necessary to understand the appearance of plaques when these types of imaging protocols are used.

Toussaint et al. showed that by combining information obtained from T1- and T2-weighted imaging techniques, it is possible to identify the atheromatous core, collagen cap, calcifications, media, adventitia, and perivascular fat (5). In this study, the authors used three different field strengths, 1.5 Tesla (T), 4.7 Tesla(T), and 9.4T. With all field strengths, identification of the components of the plaques was possible. The measured T1 and T2 values are given in Table 1 for a 9.4T system. Note that pericardial and atheromatous core lipid peaks have significantly different T2 values, which enable easy discrimination in MR images. Although T2 and T1 values of the collagenous cap and the media are similar, other components can be discriminated from each other using T1- and T2-

---

* It is assumed that the reader is familiar with basic MRI terminology. For a complete overview of MRI and the methods used in MRI, readers are referred to other textbooks such as Ref. 4.

[†] By use of conventional spin-echo pulse sequences, T1- and T2-weighted images of plaques can be obtained. In a T1-weighted imaging sequence, the repetition interval (TR) is selected to be short (on the order of 500 ms). In these images, tissues that have long T1 values appear dark, and short T1-valued tissues appear bright. In a T2-weighted imaging technique, data acquisition is delayed (by amount of echo-time or TE, usually more than 40 msec) while maintaining a long repetition interval (>1.5 sec). The tissues that have short T2 values appear dark, whereas long T2 values appear bright.

Table 1 Relaxation Constants at 9.4T of Atherosclerotic
Components. The Accuracy of the Values is Better than 10%.

Component	T1, ms	T2, ms
Atheromatous core (water peak)	1114	20.2
Atheromatous core (lipid peak)	616 ± 240	22.4
Collagenous cap	1834	30.1
Media	1892	29.5
Adventitia	1485	24.7
Periadventitial fat (water peak)	1296	19.3
Periadventitial fat (lipid peak)	636	55.0

Source: Ref. 5.

weighted images. Most commercial MR scanners have a field strength of less than 2.0T. As the field strength decreases, T1 values decrease and T2 values increase. Although the authors did not give T1 values for other field strengths, a T2 comparison was provided, as seen in Table 2. Raynoud et al. (6) showed that the lipid core can be discriminated from the collagenous cap using T2-weighted sequences. They also showed that T2-weighted MRI is rather insensitive to the stage of lipid infiltration. In an independent study, we measured the T2 values for the thickened intima, the media, the adventitia, the collagenous cap, and the necrotic core at 1.5T as 49.5 ms, 101.7 ms, 53.1 ms, 47.6 ms, and 81.5 ms, respectively (7). Our findings are in agreement with Yuan et al. (8) but contradict those of Martin et al. (6) and Toussaint et al. (5). As discussed in Berr et al. (9), the appearance of intraplaque lipids in MR images depends on their physical state, which can vary with factors such as age of the plaque and time of storage. Temperature and the phase of the lipids in the plaque have a significant effect on MRI signal (10). In addition, the composition of the fibrous cap, particularly the amount of collagen, influences the characteristics of the images. Differences in pulse sequences, field strength, and other imaging parameters may also explain differences in image contrast (7).

Table 2 Field Dependence of T2 (in ms)

Component	9.4T	4.7T	1.5T
Atheromatous core	22.2	50.1	54.7
Collagenous cap	30.1	63.3	79.3
Media	29.5	65.4	80.7

Source: Ref. 5.

A recent study (11) verified that at 1.5T, T2-weighted images are quite effective in discrimination of the different components of plaques. In this study, the authors measured the T2 of fibrous caps (T2 = 63 ± 14 ms), restenoses (51 ± 9 ms), lipid cores (36 ± 6 ms, $p < 0.0001$), the media (61 ± 7 ms), and the adventitia (45 ± 6 ms, $p < 0.001$). Furthermore, they showed that the a priori MRI classification can identify collagenous regions in 94% of the cases when T2 > 55 ms. When T2 < 40 ms, lipid cores or fatty streaks are present in 86% of lesions without a fibrous component. For a 40 < T2 < 55 ms, 81% of the regions of interest (ROIs) correspond to collagenous caps or mixed regions; only 8% of these are pure lipid cores. T1s do not provide adequate discrimination. This body of work confirms that MRI classification based on a T2 threshold of 40 ms can correctly identify coronary lesions in vitro and discriminate restenoses from native fatty lesions (11).

It is important to note that the in vitro T2 measurements match with the in vivo measurements (12). This was shown in a study of six patients who required surgical carotid endarterectomy. The plaques were imaged both in vivo and in vitro after surgery. The T2 measurements of the various components of the plaques matched closely.

When arterial specimens were placed inside a container (which was filled with saline to prevent dehydration), they could be imaged at very high resolution (8). In these experiments, scan time optimization was not critical, because the object was not moving. When high field magnets are used, resolution less than 50 μm can be obtained (13). When clinically feasible field strength is desired, it is necessary to use specialized RF (6) and gradient coils (11) to increase the signal-to-noise and image resolution. One such image is shown in Fig. 1. The in-plane image resolution was 78 μm, which was acquired using a 1.5T main magnetic field.

B. Measurement of Water Diffusion Constant of Atherosclerotic Plaques

MRI is a versatile technique. In addition to T1- and T2-weighted imaging, using very strong gradient pulses, diffusion characteristics of the object of interest can be imaged. Using water diffusion characteristics of brain cells, for example, early detection of stroke is possible. The application of this technique for plaque characterization and understanding the nature of the plaques shows very promising results. First, Altbach et al. applied this technique to characterization of plaques (14). Later, Toussaint et al. (15) studied the water diffusion characteristics of the various components of atherosclerotic plaques (see Table 3). Currently, MRI is the only method for generating diffusion maps. These maps may help in understanding the nature of the disease.

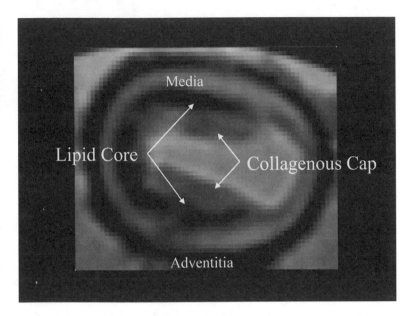

Figure 1 An ultra-high-resolution MR image of coronary artery vessel (11). Image resolution is 78 μm. (Courtesy of Dr. Jean-Francois Toussaint.)

Table 3 Diffusion Coefficients for Various Plaque Components. The Diffusion Coefficient Is Given in Units of $10^{-5}cm^2/s$.

Atheromatous core	0.26
Collagenous cap	1.45
Normal media	1.54
Normal adventitia	1.00
Fresh thrombus	0.72
1-week-old thrombus	0.36
Organized thrombus	1.33
Water	2.33

Source: Ref. 15.

Although diffusion imaging seems to be a very promising technique for basic atherosclerosis research, its use in a clinical setting faces major challenges. The diffusion-weighted pulse sequences are very sensitive to motion. The pulse sequences assume that the object of interest is absolutely still. On the other hand, the quasiperiodic arterial pressure variation causes significant wall motion. In addition, most vessels (including the coronary arteries and thoracic aorta) move about 1 to 2 cm with respiratory motion. Although many methods have been proposed to solve this problem, at the time of publication of this book, the solutions are not robust enough to make this technique a clinically viable technique.

C. Magnetization Transfer and Atherosclerotic Plaques

Magnetization transfer (MT) is another MR image contrast generation technique, which was first developed by Wolff et al. (16). In this method, a long, high-power, off-resonance RF pulse is applied just before imaging. This RF pulse saturates the spins that are bound to the macromolecules (they have a very short T1 value, and using standard MR imaging methods, it is not possible to generate the images). These spins, however, transfer their magnetization to the free spins and cause a reduction of their signal. Therefore, the MR images obtained with a magnetization transfer preparation pulse generate images that are related to the macromolecule distribution of the object of interest.

This method is used in many applications to obtain additional information about tissue characterization (17). The application of this technique to the characterization of plaques, however, is rather new. In a recent article, Pachot-Clouard et al. (18) showed that the MT effect is more pronounced in the collagenous cap and the media than in the lipid core and the adventitia. At this point, there have been no publications on the effects of MT on plaques, in vivo.

There are two drawbacks of this method. First, the length of the RF pulse is rather long and decreases available imaging time significantly in in vivo applications where time is critical. In addition, the high RF power may cause excessive heating of the structure of interest. This limits the applied RF power and amount of MT that can be obtained. Although these are recognized problems with the MT contrast technique, the technique is still used in many applications because of the high contrast of the resultant images.

D. Mechanical Properties of Atherosclerotic Plaques

The motion of the structure of interest in most MR imaging techniques causes image artifacts. In some imaging techniques, however, the sensitivity of MRI to motion (blood flow and motion of the arterial wall) is used to characterize the motion itself. For example, absolute blood flow rate can be measured using MRI. By enhancing the signal generated by the flowing blood, the degree of stenosis can be measured. In addition to these indirect measures of atherosclerotic plaques, mechanical properties of the vessel wall also can be measured with MRI.

Vessel wall distensibility correlates with the stage of atherosclerosis. There are two methods of measurement of aortic wall distensibility. First, the cross-sectional area of the wall is measured under systolic and diastolic pressures. If the change in pressure is known, the local wall distensibility can be calculated (19).

The second method is based on the measurement of the speed of the pressure waveform. It is known that the pressure wave speed, or pulsewave velocity, is inversely proportional to the distensibility of the wall. If one can measure the onset of a velocity waveform at several locations and measure the delay as a function of position, the pulsewave velocity and therefore vessel wall distensibility can be calculated (19). Urchuk et al. (20) measured the pulsewave velocity by acquiring phase-contrast CINE images of two axial slices. Hardy et al. (21) developed a one-dimensional MRI technique to measure pulsewave velocity, which has the capacity to acquire all the necessary information in a single breath-hold. Using this technique, local distensibility changes at the large vessels can be detected (22). This technique may play an important role in the early detection of plaques that are susceptible to rupture.

Another method for measuring distensibility is by a tissue tagging technique that was first developed by Zerhouni et al. (23). The tag lines divide the vessel wall into multiple segments, and the distensibility of individual segments is measured. This method is still under development (24, 25).

E. Multispectral Data Presentation

As discussed previously, the variety of available MR pulse sequences enables the acquisition of multiple images, emphasizing different soft-tissue contrasts obtained at the same slice location, resulting in a multispectral data set. Although it has been recognized that several MR contrasts are necessary for reliable discrimination of different plaque components, a quantitative analysis technique would be helpful to integrate the information obtained from these multiple contrasts. Rutt et al. (26) proposed a multispectral analysis technique that combines the information from each of the MR images with various contrasts and generates color histology-like images of the plaques.

Fig. 2 illustrates the results of multispectral analysis of MR images of atherosclerotic plaques. An endarterectomy specimen was imaged at 1.5T at five different spin-echo weightings. These images formed a five-band MR data set, which was used as input for a multispectral analysis. In the figure, (a) shows a histological section stained with combined Masson's trichrome with elastin (CME) stain near an MR image slice location. (b) represents a "multispectral stain" derived from the five-band MR image. The "multispectral stain" was constructed by performing a principle-component transformation on the five-band

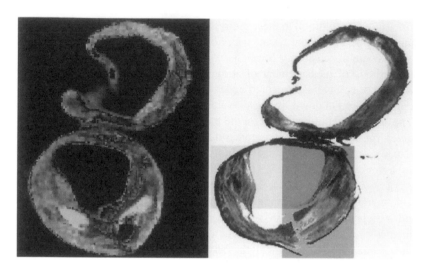

Figure 2   Multispectral MRI (left) versus histology with CME stain. (Courtesy of Brian Rutt, Ross Mitchell, and Sharon Clark, London, Canada.)

MR data set, then extracting the first three principle component images. These principle-component images account for more than 90% of the information in the original 5-band image. The multispectral image was constructed by combining the first three principal components to form a color image for display.

Although direct relationships between the histological stains and the MR multispectral images cannot yet be drawn from this preliminary work, it is apparent that the tissue classes selected by multispectral analysis correspond closely to those seen on the histological stain.

F. Plaque Morphology and MRI

As discussed in the previous section, MRI is a powerful technique for discriminating different components of plaques. In addition, it enables extremely accurate determination of plaque size and plaque morphology. Yuan et al. (27) compared in vivo with ex vivo MRI measurements of plaque size on 14 patients scheduled to have carotid endarterectomy and showed very strong correlation. In addition, these authors showed that plaque position can be determined quite accurately with MRI.*

---

* In MRI, images are formed with respect to the scanner coordinate system. Direct measurements of the position of any structure are possible. In ultrasonography, it is difficult to determine plaque position because of the lack of a frame of reference.

III. MRI AS A NONINVASIVE DIAGNOSTIC TOOL

MRI is a noninvasive imaging technique that uses no ionized radiation. With the advent of new MR imaging pulse sequences and hardware, in vivo imaging of atherosclerotic plaques is now possible. Early MR images of plaques showed the feasibility of imaging plaques (3), but these early images suffered from low SNR and image artifacts.

Dedicated surface coils are especially useful for imaging plaques close to the surface of the body. Hayes et al. designed a phase-array neck coil for high-resolution atherosclerotic carotid plaque imaging (28). Yuan et al. reported an ECG-gated fast-spin-echo (FSE)-based pulse sequence for imaging of plaques in carotid arteries using the phased-array neck coil (29). These investigators showed that the information obtained from high-resolution images of atherosclerotic plaques correlates highly with histological findings. Faro et al. (30) and our group used standard small surface coils for imaging carotid arteries. It is important to note that using standard coils rather than dedicated phased-array coils causes a decrease in SNR, results in difficulties in coil placement, and limits the coverage. For the imaging of vessels deep inside the body, such as the aorta or the coronary artery vessels, the phased-array torso or cardiac coils are most effective (31). Even if the best coil is used, the resolution will be limited by the SNR (32).

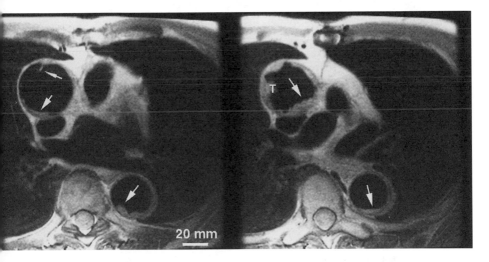

Figure 3   An MR image of thoracic aorta of a patient with severe atherosclerosis. The imaging protocol is ECG-gated, blood suppressed using double inversion recovery, 256 × 256, 2 signal averages, 3-mm slice thickness, 32-cm FOV. (Courtesy of Dr. Zahi Fayad.)

A significant improvement in image quality has been achieved with the development of ECG-gated blood-suppressed fast–spin echo (FSE) pulse sequences. Most of the vessels of interest move significantly with respiratory motion. Arterial pressure variation during a cardiac cycle also causes significant motion of the vessel wall. Flow artifacts are always a problem if no precautions are taken. A simple but effective way to eliminate artifacts caused by respiratory motion is by breath holding. ECG gating is a simple and effective way to eliminate the image blurring caused by wall motion with arterial pressure variation. Blood signal suppression techniques are particularly useful for eliminating flow artifacts and increasing the image contrast between the lumen and the vessel wall. These methods limit the available imaging time; thus, an efficient pulse sequence is necessary. Standard FSE sequences are very susceptible to motion. When, however, the spacing between echoes is decreased, a significant reduction in motion artifacts is observed. An image acquired with this technique is shown in Fig. 3 (33).

IV. INVASIVE MRI FOR HIGH-RESOLUTION IMAGING

The maximum resolution of an MR image is determined by SNR, which is a factor of image quality (34). If one maintains all the MR imaging parameters fixed and decreases all three dimensions of an imaging voxel by a factor of 5 to get an ultra-high-resolution image, the SNR decreases by a factor of 125. It is, therefore, necessary to compensate for this image quality reduction with the other parameters that affect SNR. To regain this 125 factor of SNR reduction, the total scan time must be increased by a factor of 15,625. This is obviously impractical. If the original scan time is, for example, 10 minutes, to get the same quality ultra-high-resolution image, the object would have to be scanned for 100 days. A second approach to increase the image SNR (or quality) is to use improved receiver coil designs. The receiver coils must be small to minimize the noise received from the body, and they must be placed close to the ROI. If, however, the ROI is deep inside the body, a large coil is necessary to increase the sensitivity at the cost of increased noise. Because of this unfortunate problem, the maximum SNR attainable with coils placed on the surface of the object is limited (32). The only way to exceed this limit is to place the antenna inside the object.

A. Intravascular MRI

The first attempt to place MR probes inside the blood vessels is not a recent occurrence (35). Many different coil designs have been tested (36–41). Imaging of atherosclerotic plaques using these devices showed that the the media and adventitia of the normal wall can be discriminated, and various components of plaques can be characterized (7).

The coils that are under investigation are as follows (see Fig. 4):

1. Opposed solenoid design: This design is in the form of two very small opposed solenoidal coils that are placed in a series with a gap between them, which provides an imaging plane with a relatively uniform sensitivity. The tuning and matching circuit is placed next to the coil to improve the performance. This design has been developed by two independent groups (37, 38) and subsequently was investigated by others (42).

2. Rectangular coil: This design has an approximately 2-cm long rectangular shape. This design was tested by Kandarpa et al. (36) for intravascular use. They also placed a circuit next to the coil, which enables remote tuning.

3. Expandable coil design: There are a few versions of this type of design. The first expandable intravascular MRI probe was designed by Martin et al. (43) to enable imaging of the arteries from the probes inserted into the veins. The tuning and matching circuit was placed next to the imaging probe for a coarse tuning. The fine-tuning circuit is placed outside the body. Later this design was incorporated into a balloon angioplasty catheter by Quick et al. (39, 44). These investigators also made an expandable coil design constructed from a Nitinol cable. In these later versions of the probes, the local tuning elements were removed from the circuit to overcome implementation difficulties at the cost of reduced performance.

4. Flexible catheter coil design (40): This design is based on two parallel wires that are short-circuited at one end. Because the tuning of this design does not change according to the condition of the probe inside

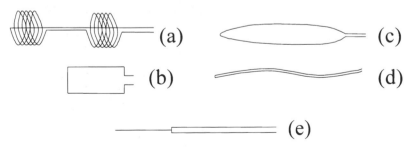

Figure 4   Five experimental intravascular MRI probes. (a) Opposed solenoids; (b) rectangular; (c) expandable; (d) flexible; and (e) loopless intravascular antenna designs.

the body, a fixed tuning/matching circuit is incorporated in this design. The difficulty in placement of the components into a small area without impeding the flexibility of the design is overcome with microcircuit manufacturing techniques. In this design, about 10 cm at the tip of the probe is useful for imaging.

5. Loopless antenna design (41): This design has a very simple structure. It is a coaxial cable with an extended inner conductor. Because there is no electrical loop in this design, it is called the loopless antenna. This design does not require placement of tuning/matching circuit elements next to the antenna. Remote tuning can be done without a significant loss in performance.

These designs and many future designs are in the experimental phase. The experiments are limited to imaging of animals (39) and isolated human vessels (7, 45). Some sample images are shown in Fig. 5.

B. Transesophageal MRI

A less invasive method of imaging plaques involves placing the MR imaging probe next to the target vessel rather than inside it. The aorta and some parts of

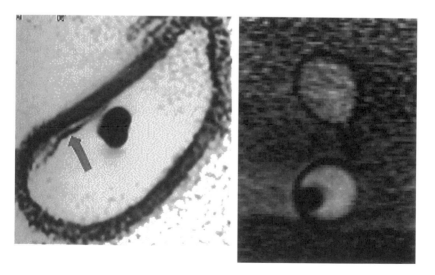

Figure 5 Sample images acquired using intravascular MRI probes. Cross-sectional images of (a) an isolated human aorta, (b) a rabbit aorta, in vivo. All the images were acquired using T2-weighted spin-echo sequences. A fast spin-echo sequence was used in the imaging of coronary artery.

the coronary vessels can be imaged at high resolution with a probe placed inside the esophagus. A similar technique is being used in ultrasonography and is called "transesophageal echo" or TEE. These probes are usually large (more than 1 cm in diameter) in size and require continuous manipulation of their position. They are inserted from the mouth and require patient sedation. They have several drawbacks, including low soft tissue contrast, inability to image regions close to the probe, and the necessity to have an experienced physician in attendance to understand the position and orientation of the probe. Although these are the drawbacks, it is widely used in medicine because it is the only clinically approved reliable way of visualizing aortic plaques.

Transesophageal MRI (TEMRI) is free of some of the drawbacks of TEE but it, too, has some disadvantages. The TEMRI probe is a loopless antenna placed inside a standard nasogastric (NG) tube. Because the TEMRI probes can be made very small, they can easily pass through the patient's nose into the esophagus without the need for sedation. In addition, once the probe is placed, its position does not need to be manipulated during the examination. Sample images acquired from patients with athcrosclerotic plaques can be seen in Fig. 6. Because no physician interaction is required, this method can be performed by technicians in a standard MRI device. Because the cost of the probes is very low, they can be disposed of, which translates to increased patient safety. The main disadvantage of the method compared with TEE is that TEMRI is not a real-time imaging technique. Current imaging protocols enable imaging in a single breath-hold time period.

V. MANAGEMENT OF ATHEROSCLEROSIS USING MRI

Although MRI is known as a purely diagnostic tool, recent advances, including real-time imaging capabilities, small bore sizes, and MRI-compatible interventional devices, make MRI a tool that can be used to guide interventional procedures. Current clinical applications for interventional MRI are limited to nonvascular applications because of the complexity of vascular applications.

MRI, however, is an excellent imaging modality that could replace conventional x-ray in the catheterization laboratory. Researchers have shown that catheters and guidewires can be made visible by simply embedding probes inside these designs (46). Although most scanners are not equipped to handle high-frame-rate data acquisition, the possibility of acquiring images at greater than 10 to 15 frames/sec has been demonstrated (47). In addition to real-time imaging, methods for tracking the position of intravascular devices have been developed (48) and tested on animals (49).

Another aspect of MRI as a noninvasive imaging tool is its functional imaging capabilities for various organs, although in the literature, the term "func-

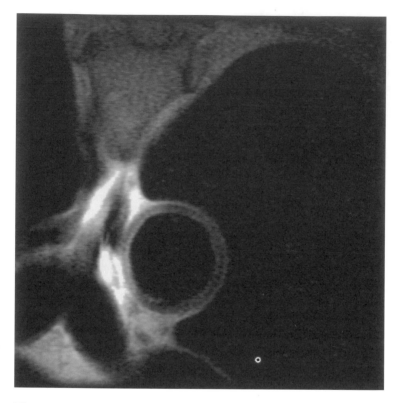

Figure 6 A transesophageal MR image acquired from a patient with atherosclerotic plaques. The cross-sectional image of the arch of the aorta can be seen. The intima of this patient's aorta has been thickened, and a complex plaque at the 6 o'clock position can clearly be seen.

tional MRI'' is associated with brain activation protocols (50). With MRI, a complete functional examination of heart is possible through blood perfusion imaging (51), mechanical function imaging (23), and metabolic imaging (52). Similarly, functional imaging of almost all other organs is possible with MRI. MR angioscopy is another capability of MRI that allows noninvasive imaging of blood flow.

Figure 7 Intravascular MRI-guided balloon angioplasty. (a) Using a cable tie, an artificial stenosis was created in a rabbit aorta (54). (b) An imaging guidewire was placed inside an angioplasty catheter. (c) The inflation of the balloon and removal of the stenosis was monitored using the MR imaging (55).

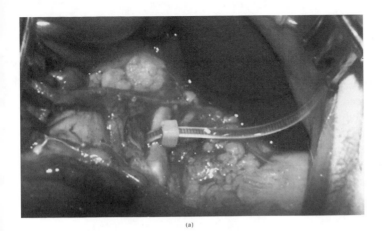

(a)

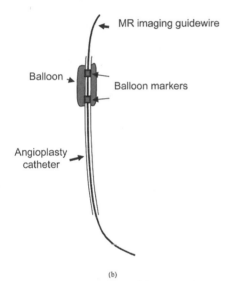

(b)

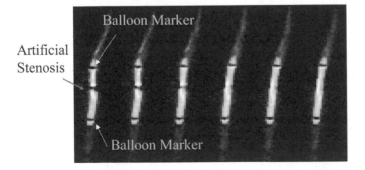

(c)

When these techniques are combined with interventional MRI techniques, a very powerful tool is created. Accordingly, methods for complete management of ischemic diseases with MRI techniques are under investigation. In the feasibility study by Yang (53), an artificial aortic stenosis in a rabbit aorta was first detected with MR angiography, and a renal perfusion deficit was detected with a contrast-enhanced MR perfusion study. Immediately after this diagnosis, the MR-guided balloon angioplasty was performed (see Fig. 7) and recovery of the blood flow in the aorta demonstrated with a subsequent MR angiography. The recovery of renal perfusion was shown with a second contrast-enhanced MR perfusion study. All these procedures were done within a 1-hour period that shows that complete management of the ischemic disease with an MR scanner is feasible.

VI. DISCUSSIONS AND CONCLUSION

The use of MRI for the characterization of atherosclerotic plaques has been investigated for more than 15 years, and more research is required before it becomes an acceptable modality. The progress of MRI in this field has been hampered by the complexity of MR imaging techniques, but MRI still holds great promise for the accurate diagnosis and characterization of atherosclerosis. The primary difficulties with MRI are motion and flow artifacts. With the development of new imaging techniques, however, these difficulties are less of a problem. The low-image resolution and low-image SNR are being resolved by specialized surface coils or probes placed inside the body. In conclusion, MRI shows great potential as a diagnostic tool for the imaging and characterization of atherosclerosis in the near future.

REFERENCES

1. Amarenco P, Cohen A, Tzourio C, Bertrand B, Hommel M, Besson G, Chauvel C, Touboul PJ, Bousser MG. Atherosclerotic disease of the aortic arch and the risk of ischemic stroke. N Engl J Med 1994; 331(22):1474–1479.
2. Cohen A, Tzourio C, Bertrand B, Chauvel C, Bousser MG, Amarenco P. Aortic plaque morphology and vascular events: a follow-up study in patients with ischemic stroke. FAPS Investigators. French Study of Aortic Plaques in Stroke. Circulation 1997; 96(11):3838–3841.
3. Herfkens RJ, Higgins CB, Hricak H, Lipton MJ, Crooks LE, Sheldon PE, Kaufman L. Nuclear magnetic resonance imaging of atherosclerotic disease. Radiology 1983; 148(1):161–166.
4. Higgins CB, Hricak H, Helms CA. Magnetic Resonance Imaging of Body. 2nd ed. New York: Raven Press, 1992.

5. Toussaint JF, Southern JF, Fuster V, Kantor HL. T2-weighted contrast for NMR characterization of human atherosclerosis. Arterioscler Thromb Vasc Biol 1995; 15(10):1533–1542.
6. Martin AJ, Gotlieb AI, Henkelman RM. High-resolution MR imaging of human arteries. J Magn Reson Imaging 1995; 5(1):93–100.
7. Correia LCL, Atalar E, Kelemen MD, Ocali O, Hutchins GM, Flag JL, Gerstenblith G, Zerhouni EA, Lima JAC. Intravascular magnetic resonance imaging of aortic atherosclerotic plaque composition. Arterioscl Thromb Vasc Biol 1997; 17(12): 3626–3632.
8. Yuan C, Tsuruda JS, Beach KN, Hayes CE, Ferguson MS, Alpers CE, Foo TK, Strandness DE. Techniques for high-resolution MR imaging of atherosclerotic plaque. J Magn Reson Imaging 1994; 4(1):43–49.
9. Berr SS, Brookeman JR. On MR imaging of atheromatous lipids in human arteries. J Magn Reson Imaging 1995; 5(3):373–374.
10. Yuan C, Petty C, KD OB, Hatsukami TS, Eary JF, Brown BG. In vitro and in situ magnetic resonance imaging signal features of atherosclerotic plaque-associated lipids. Arterioscl Thromb Vasc Biol 1997; 17(8):1496–1503.
11. Gouya H, Toussaint J-F, Fornès P, Glutron D, Paillard M, Berger G, Bitto J. Coronary wall studied by high-resolution MRI at 1.5T: in vitro T2 contrast characterizes plaques and restenoses. 48th Scientific Sessions of the American College of Cardiology, New Orleans, 1999.
12. Toussaint JF, LaMuraglia GM, Southern JF, Fuster V, Kantor HL. Magnetic resonance images lipid, fibrous, calcified, hemorrhagic, and thrombotic components of human atherosclerosis in vivo. Circulation 1996; 94(5):932–938.
13. Asdente M, Pavesi L, Oreste PL, Colombo A, Kuhn W, Tremoli E. Evaluation of atherosclerotic lesions using NMR microimaging. Atherosclerosis 1990; 80(3):243–253.
14. Altbach MI, Mattingly MA, Brown MF, Gmitro AF. Magnetic resonance imaging of lipid deposits in human atheroma via a stimulated-echo diffusion-weighted technique. Magn Reson Med 1991; 20(2):319–326.
15. Toussaint JF, Southern JF, Fuster V, Kantor HL. Water diffusion properties of human atherosclerosis and thrombosis measured by pulsed field gradient nuclear magnetic resonance. Arterioscl Thromb Vasc Biol 1997; 17(3):542–546.
16. Wolff SD, Balaban RS. Magnetization transfer contrast (MTC) and tissue water proton relaxation in vivo. Magn Reson Med 1989; 10(1):135–144.
17. Wolff SD, Balaban RS. Magnetization transfer imaging: practical aspects and clinical applications. Radiology 1994; 192(3):593–599.
18. Pachot-Clouard M, Vaufrey F, Darrasse L, Toussaint J-F. Magnetization transfer characteristics in atherosclerotic plaque components assessed by adapted binomial preparation pulses. MAGMA 1998; 7(1):9–15.
19. Milnor WR. Hemodynamics. Baltimore: Williams & Wilkins, 1982.
20. Urchuk SN, Plewes DB. A velocity correlation method for measuring vascular compliance using MR imaging. J Magn Reson Imaging 1995; 5(6):628–634.
21. Hardy CJ, Bolster BD, McVeigh ER, Adams WJ, Zerhouni EA. A one-dimensional velocity technique for NMR measurement of aortic distensibility. Magn Reson Med 1994; 31(5):513–520.

22. Bolster BD, Jr., Atalar E, Hardy CJ, McVeigh ER. Accuracy of arterial pulse-wave velocity measurement using MR. J Magn Reson Imaging 1998; 8(4):878–888.

23. Zerhouni EA, Parish DM, Rogers WL, Yang A, Shapiro EP. Human heart: tagging with MR imaging—a method for noninvasive assessment of myocardial motion. Radiology 1988; 169(1):59–63.

24. Shunk KA, Lima JAC, Heldman AW, Atalar E. Transesophageal magnetic resonance imaging. Magn Reson Med 1999; 41(4):722–726.

25. Chu KC, Rutt BK. Polyvinyl alcohol cryogel: an ideal phantom material for MR studies of arterial flow and elasticity. Magn Reson Med 1997; 37(2):314–319.

26. Rutt B, Mitchell JR, Clarke S. Multispectral display of atherosclerotic plaques. in Angio Club. 1998. ???1998.

27. Yuan C, Beach KW, Smith LH, Hatsukami TS. Measurement of atherosclerotic carotid plaque size in vivo using high resolution magnetic resonance imaging. Circulation 1998; 98:2666–2671.

28. Hayes CE, Mathis CM, Yuan C. Surface coil phased arrays for high-resolution imaging of the carotid arteries. J Magn Reson Imaging 1996; 6(1):109–112.

29. Yuan C, Murakami JW, Hayes CE, Tsuruda JS, Hatsukami TS, Wildy KS, Ferguson MS, Strandness DE, Jr. Phased-array magnetic resonance imaging of the carotid artery bifurcation: preliminary results in healthy volunteers and a patient with atherosclerotic disease. J Magn Reson Imaging 1995; 5(5):561–565.

30. Faro, Vinitski, Ortega, Mohamed, Chen, Flanders, Gonzales, Zimmerman. Carotid magnetic resonance angiography: improved image quality with dual 3-inch surface coils. Neuroradiology 1998; 38:403–408.

31. Bottomley PA, Lugo Olivieri CH, Giaquinto R. What is the optimum phased array coil design for cardiac and torso magnetic. Magn Reson Med 1997; 37(4):591–599.

32. Ocali O, Atalar E. Ultimate intrinsic signal-to-noise ratio in MRI. Magn Reson Med 1997; 39(3):462–473.

33. Fayad ZA, Nahar T, Badimon JJ, Goldman M, Weinberger J, Fallon JT, Aguinaldo G, Shinnar M, Chesebro JH, Fuster V. In-vivo characterization of plaques in the thoracic aorta. AHA 71st Scientific Meeting, Dallas, 1998.

34. McVeigh ER, Atalar E. Balancing contrast resolution, and signal-to-noise ratio in magnetic resonance imaging. In Bronskill MJ, Sprawis P, eds. The Physics of MRI. Woodbury, NY: American Association of Physics in Medicine, 1992:235–267.

35. Kantor HL, Briggs RW, Balaban RS. In vivo ^{31}P nuclear magnetic resonance measurements in canine heart using a catheter-coil. Circ Res 1984; 55(2):261–266.

36. Kandarpa K, Jakab P, Patz S, Schoen FJ, Jolesz FA. Prototype miniature endoluminal MR imaging catheter. J Vasc Interv Radiol 1993; 4(3):419–427.

37. Martin AJ, Plewes DB, Henkelman RM. MR imaging of blood vessels with an intravascular coil. J Magn Reson Imaging 1992; 2(4):421–429.

38. Hurst GC, Hua J, Duerk JL, Cohen AM. Intravascular (catheter) NMR receiver probe: preliminary design analysis and application to canine iliofemoral imaging. Magn Reson Med 1992; 24(2):343–357.

39. Zimmermann GG, Quick HH, Hilfiker PR, Schulthess GK, Debatin JF. High-resolution MR imaging in an atherosclerotic rabbit model. Radiology 1997; 205(P):513.

40. Atalar E, Bottomley PA, Ocali O, Correia LCL, Kelemen MD, Lima JAC, Zerhouni

EA. High resolution intravascular MRI and MRS by using a catheter receiver coil. Magn Reson Med 1996; 36(4):596–605.

41. Ocali O, Atalar E. Intravascular magnetic resonance imaging using a loopless catheter antenna. Magn Reson Med 1997; 37(1):112–118.

42. Rogers WL, Prichard JW, Hu YL, Olson PR, Benckart DH, Kramer CM, Reichek N. Intravascular MRI of atherosclerotic plaque: correlation with histology. In ISMRM Sixth Scientific Meeting and Exhibition, Sydney, 1998.

43. Martin AJ, McLoughlin RF, Chu KC, Barberi EA, Rutt BK. An expandable intravenous RF coil for arterial wall imaging. J Magn Reson Imaging 1998; 8(1):226–234.

44. Quick HH, Zimmermann-Paul GG, Hofmann E, vonShulthess GK, Debatin JF. In vitro assessment of a perfused intravascular MR-imaging balloon. In ISMRM Sixth Scientific Meeting and Exhibition, Syndey, Australia, 1998.

45. Zimmermann GG, Erhart P, Schneider J, vonSchulthess GK, Debatin JF. Intravascular MR imaging of atherosclerotic plaque: ex vivo analysis of human femoral arteries with histologic correlation. Radiology 1997; 204(3):769–774.

46. Atalar E, Kraitchman DL, Lesho J, Carkhuff B, Ocali O, Solaiyappan M, Guttman MA. Catheter-tracking FOV MR fluoroscopy. In ISMRM 6th Annual Meeting, Sidney, Australia, 1998.

47. Kerr AB, Pauly JM, Hu BS, Li KC, Hardy CJ, Meyer CH, Macovski A, Nishimura DG. Real-time interactive MRI on a conventional scanner. Magn Reson Med 1997; 38(3):355–367.

48. Dumoulin CL, Souza SP, Darrow RD. Real-time position monitoring of invasive devices using magnetic resonance. Magn Reson Med 1993; 29(3):411–415.

49. Wildermuth S, Debatin JF, Leung DA, Dumoulin CL, Darrow RD, Uhlschmid G, Hofmann E, Thyregod J, Schulthness GKv. MR imaging guided intravascular procedures: initial demonstration in a pig model. Radiology 1997; 202:578–583.

50. Rosen BR, Buckner RL, Dale AM. Event-related functional MRI: past, present, and future. Proc Natl Acad Sci USA 1998; 95(3):773–780.

51. Lima JA, Judd RM, Bazille A, Schulman SP, Atalar E, Zerhouni EA. Regional heterogeneity of human myocardial infarcts demonstrated by contrast-enhanced MRI. Potential mechanisms. Circulation 1995; 92(5):1117–1125.

52. Bottomley PA, Atalar E, Weiss RG. Human cardiac high-energy phosphate metabolite concentrations by 1D-resolved NMR spectroscopy. Magn Reson Med 1996; 35(5):664–670.

53. Yang X, Atalar E. On-line management of ischemic disease using intravascular MR-guided intervention combined with MR perfusion imaging and MR angiography. In ISMRM Seventh Annual Scientific Meeting and Exhibition, Pennsylvania, 1999.

54. Yang X, Kraitchman DL, Bolster BD, Atalar E. Creation of a rabbit model with aortic stenosis for in vivo studies of intravascular MR-guided interventions. In International Society of Magnetic Resonance in Medicine, Sydney, 1998.

55. Yang X, Bolster BD, Kraitchman DL, Atalar E. Intravascular magnetic resonance monitored balloon angioplasty: A feasibility study on rabbit models. J Vasc Intervent Radiol 1998; 9:953–959.

16
In Vivo Thermography of Coronary Arteries

Christodoulos Stefanadis, Leonidas Diamantopoulos, Eleftherios Tsiamis, Konstantinos Toutouzas, and Pavlos Toutouzas
Athens University, Athens, Greece

We have reached the new millennium, and the cause of the most widespread disease of western civilization, coronary artery disease, remains unknown. Starting in childhood, coronary artery disease progresses subclinically until it is exposed by the development of angina pectoris or an acute coronary event. In a few cases, the diagnosis is made by chance during a regular checkup.

I. THE ATHEROSCLEROTIC PROCESS

For many years it was believed that atherosclerosis was a degenerative process caused by aging of the arteries. However, today several pathological factors underlying this disease are well understood. It is now known that smoking, hypercholesterolemia, diabetes, and hypertension are closely related to the atherosclerotic process. However, these factors may not completely explain the development of the disease. Thus, investigators have proposed three theories for the origin of atherosclerosis: The *response-to-injury hypothesis*, the *monoclonal hypothesis*, and the *theory of inflammation* (1–3).

The response-to-injury hypothesis suggests that endothelial damage is the crucial event leading to the formation of atheroma. Each of the primary risk factors for coronary artery disease leads through different events to endothelial injury and dysfunction.

The chain of events leading from endothelial dysfunction to plaque development is intricate. It seems that endothelial injury results in monocyte/macrophage adherence to the endothelium and migration to sunendothelium. Subsequently, macrophages become activated and produce several growth factors that promote the growth of smooth muscle cells. Moreover, macrophages remove oxidized low-density lipoproteins (LDL), which transforming themselves into foam cells. These macrophages accumulate large amounts of lipids, contributing to the formation of the early lesion. In response to the injury, however, platelets also adhere to the damaged endothelium. Platelets aggregate and release platelet-derived growth factor (PDGF) and other growth factors that trigger smooth muscle proliferation and migration, leading to intimal hyperplasia. Smooth muscle cells secrete collagen, elastin, and proteoglycans, promoting the formation of fibrous plaque.

Rupture of the atherosclerotic plaque leads to acute coronary syndromes. Hemodynamic shear forces may trigger plaque rupture. However, it is not clearly defined which plaques are vulnerable to shear forces resulting in thrombus formation and which plaques are stable. Several studies have shown that arteries without severe stenoses are at the greatest risk of rupture, presumably because severe occlusion limits coronary perfusion and the hemodynamic stress required to precipitate rupture (4–8).

The monoclonal hypothesis suggests that the atherosclerotic lesion derives from a single smooth muscle cell that proliferates and acts as a source of all the cells in the lesion (9–10). Accordingly, the plaque is developed just like a tumor. Indeed, some atherosclerotic plaques that appear as isolated nodules surrounded by areas of normal tissue might be monoclonal. However, the pathophysiological process involved in this theory needs to be further clarified.

Recently, several studies have developed evidence for the presence of infectious agents in the atherosclerotic plaque, supporting the theory of inflammation (1, 11–13). *Chlamydia pneumoniae, Helicobacter pylori*, herpes simplex virus, and cytomegalovirus have been associated with coronary artery disease. Despite solid evidence that these agents exist in atherosclerotic lesions, evidence that the presence of organisms is related to disease pathogenesis is circumstantial. If the organisms are involved, their role should fit within the context of events in atherogenesis. Although the underlying mechanism remains unknown, several studies have yielded favorable results on the potential use of antibiotics against infectious agents. These studies have suggested that cardiovascular events were decreased significantly in patients receiving antibiotics. Although a causative role of infection in the process of atherosclerosis has not yet been firmly established, there is growing evidence that infectious agents play a role. The high frequency of infection observed in human atherosclerotic tissue and the results from intervention with antibiotics are consistent with the theory of inflammation (14, 15).

A. Thermal Energy Production

Despite, the different hypotheses regarding the underlying mechanisms of the atherosclerotic process, all investigators seem to agree that the presence of macrophages in the atheromatic plaque is prominent. The infiltration of macrophages into the plaque and the uptake of oxidized LDL generates thermal energy. This was proven in vitro by Casscells et al., who demonstrated that carotid plaques have temperature heterogeneity (16). Our group has investigated whether thermal heterogeneity exists in atherosclerotic coronary arteries in vivo and, if so, whether there is a role for temperature measurement in determining prognosis. Theoretically, the bloodstream should equilibrate any temperature differences within the vascular wall. However, thermal energy, like any other energy, leaks from high to lower levels, and this energy stream degrades from a maximal temperature at the generation point to a minimal temperature, which is the temperature of blood. Complete thermal homogeneity is not possible as long as thermal generation exists. Therefore, thermal heterogeneity should exist in the atherosclerotic arteries as a result of inflammation and macrophage infiltration. The problem is to detect the minimal temperature differences in vivo, because an accurate and feasible method for recording these minimal temperature differences is required. Thus, the temperature sensor should be very accurate, capable of tracing changes less than 0.1°C, and trivial in size to be mounted on a coronary catheter. NTC thermistors (Betatherm, MA) fulfill the above criteria. For this reason we designed an arterial thermography system that consists of a special catheter and a computer-based remote device (17).

B. Temperature Recording

1. The Thermography Catheter

The thermography catheter body is made from polyurethane. The diameter of the catheter is 3F, and its overall length is 120 cm. The distal 10 cm of the catheter has a second lumen for a guidewire, resembling rapid-exchange angioplasty catheters. At the distal tip of the catheter, a NTC thermistor chip (Betatherm, MA, model 100K6MCD368) is attached. The technical characteristics of the thermistor are shown in Table 1. At the opposite side from the thermistor, the tip of the catheter is shaped to form a hydrofoil (HF). Taking advantage of the blood flow, this smooth hydrofoil provides enough hydraulic force to drive the catheter's tip toward the vessel wall, ensuring a contact between the thermistor and the intima (Fig. 1). The proximal tip of the catheter is equipped with a gold-plated connector for low-loss signal passage and easy connection with the rest of the system.

Table 1 Technical Characteristics of the Thermography Catheter

Temperature accuracy	0.05°C
Time constant	300 ms
Spatial resolution	0.5 mm
Correlation of resistance versus temperature	Absolutely linear (over the range of 33°C–43°C)

2. The Computer-Based Device

The temperature-dependent changes of impedance of the thermistor are converted to voltage changes by means of a Wheatstone bridge of resistors. This analog voltage signal is converted into digital form with a 12-bit analog-to-digital converter. Furthermore, digital data are continuously monitored by a computer. Temperature is recorded as individual values in degrees Celsius, with a sampling rate of 3 samples/sec, and is projected in real time on a screen as a continuous succession of connected points (i.e., a temperature line) (Fig. 2). The catheter was tested in vitro and in vivo in experimental studies.

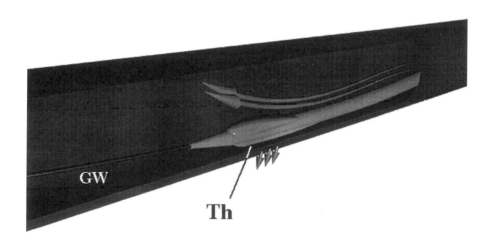

Figure 1 At the opposite side of the thermistor, the tip of the catheter is shaped to form a hydrofoil (HF). Taking advantage of the blood flow (curved arrows), this smooth hydrofoil provides enough hydraulic force to drive the catheter's tip toward the vessel wall (linear arrows), ensuring a contact between the thermistor and the intima.

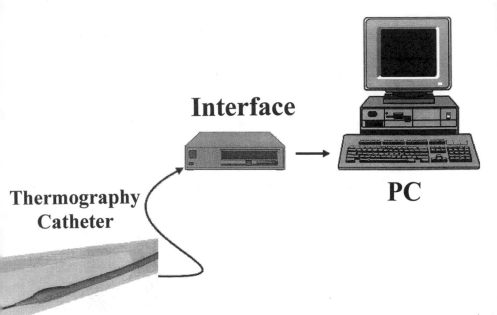

Figure 2 Instrumentation required for the thermography procedure. The analog voltage signal from the thermistor is converted into digital form with a 12-bit analog-to-digital converter (interface). Furthermore, digital data are continuously monitored by computer.

C. In Vitro Testing

To ensure the contact of the thermistor at the distal part of the catheter with the vessel wall, a glass coronary model was used. Heparinized donor whole blood was circulating in the coronary glass model. A Doppler-tip guidewire (FloWire Cardiometrics Inc.) and a catheter-tip micromanometer (Millar Instruments) were used to measure flow and pressure. The pressure and flow were maintained at levels found in human coronary arteries. In all cases, the bloodstream forced the thermistor safely against the wall.

D. In Vivo Testing

The in vivo test was performed in the coronary arteries of pigs. The thermography catheter was inserted through a 7F hockey-stick guiding catheter and positioned in the coronary arteries under fluoroscopic control. Luminal surface temperature was measured at 10 different locations in each vessel. After temperature measurements were performed, the coronary segments were evaluated by light and scanning electron microscopy to observe any possible deleterious effects of the thermistor on the vascular wall. The application of the thermistor to porcine coronary arteries did not induce injury of the vascular wall, including the endothelium.

E. In Vivo Thermography of Coronary Arteries

In humans, the catheter is introduced similarly to a standard angioplasty catheter. The catheter is delivered to the target lesion through a 7F guiding catheter over a conventional guidewire. The catheter remains in place for a few seconds while temperature is being sampled and then is withdrawn. The duration of the procedure is the same as a diagnostic coronary angiogram. The net thermography time is less than 3 minutes.

During the procedure, the blood temperature is measured as the thermistor just emerges from the tip of the guiding catheter so that it is not in contact with the vessel wall. This provides an accurate temperature of the blood. Thereafter, the catheter is advanced to the diseased area, where the plaque temperature is recorded. By retraction of the catheter to a nondiseased area, the background temperature of the arterial wall is obtained. As the catheter is withdrawn in a standard velocity from a distal point to the proximal segment of the vessel, a "thermal map" of the area of interest is recorded.

F. Thermal Heterogeneity of Coronary Arteries: The First Clinical Experience

Temperature measurements were performed in patients with normal coronary arteries, with acute ischemic syndromes, and with stable angina. Forty-five patients catheterized for investigation of valvular heart disease or chest pain with normal coronary arteries served as the control group. In 15 patients with stable angina, temperature measurements were performed during elective coronary angioplasty. Another 15 patients with unstable angina had temperature measurements performed in conjunction with emergency angioplasty. Also, 15 patients with an acute myocardial infarction undergoing primary balloon angioplasty also had thermal measurements.

Temperature was measured at five locations in a nondiseased coronary segment close to the target lesion. The dominant (most frequent) temperature of these measurements was designated as the background temperature. In addition, measurements at five different lesion sites were performed, scanning the lesion both longitudinally and circumferentially. One measurement was made in the proximal part of the lesion, one at the distal, and one at the center. The other two measurements were made in areas between the center and the ends of the plaque. In patients with stable and unstable angina, in whom the thermography catheter could not cross the lesion, measurements spanning the entire lesion were obtained ~5 minutes after successful balloon angioplasty. In patients with acute myocardial infarction, measurements were obtained within 5 minutes of angioplasty.

In control subjects, the absence of atherosclerosis was verified by intravasculary ultrasonography. After blood temperature measurement, five wall temperature measurements in a region ~1-cm long were obtained. This region was designated the control region and its dominant temperature, the background temperature. Subsequently, five temperature measurements were obtained in another region of the same length (randomly selected distally or proximally to the first lesion), which was designated the region of interest (ROI). For control subjects, the absolute values of the differences between ROI and background temperature were taken for analysis. Simultaneous with vessel wall measurements, mouth temperature was measured with a separate thermistor with identical specifications as the thermistor of the thermography catheter.

II. RESULTS

The surface wall temperature was measured in 90 ROIs, 1 in each patient. Two left main coronary arteries, 37 left anterior descending arteries, 18 left circumflex arteries, and 33 right coronary arteries were studied. In the first 10 patients of our series in whom contact of the thermistor on the artery was tested, frame-by-frame analysis in two biplane views during washout of the contrast medium revealed that the radioopaque thermistor was in contact with the edge of the vessel. The temperature of healthy vessel wall was $0.36 \pm 0.11°C$ higher than the oral temperature. Mean coronary artery stenosis was $83 \pm 8\%$ for the stable angina patients and $81 \pm 7\%$ for the unstable angina patients ($p - NS$). The five measurements obtained for determination of background temperature were consistent within each subject of the total study population, varying by only $0.05°C$. The temperature of blood and healthy vessel wall did not differ significantly. Coronary wall temperatures in the ROI of each control subject were constant, varying by only $0.05°C$. In the stable angina or unstable angina patients, there was no difference between maximum and background temperatures before and after angioplasty ($0.470 \pm 0.418°C$ vs. $0.458 \pm 0.415°C$, respectively; $p = NS$). Most atherosclerotic plaques showed higher surface temperatures compared with normal vessel wall. The difference between maximum plaque and background temperatures did not correlate with coronary artery stenosis ($r = -0.10$ and -0.09, respectively; $p = NS$). Greater values in the differences between maximum plaque and background temperatures were observed in unstable angina (maximum, 1.55°C) and acute myocardial infarction (maximum, 2.60°C) patients. Differences between ROI and background temperatures and between maximum ROI and background temperatures were different among the four groups, increasing progressively from stable angina to acute myocardial infarction patients ($p <$ 0.001 for both parameters; for pairwise comparisons). Mean temperature differences between ROI and background temperatures in each group were 0.004 ± 0.009°C in the control subjects, 0.106 ± 0.110°C in stable angina patients, 0.683 ± 0.347°C in unstable angina patients, and 1.472 ± 0.691°C in acute myocardial infarction patients. The mean temperature differences between maximum ROI and background temperatures were 0.010 ± 0.020°C in normal subjects, 0.153 ± 0.134°C in stable angina patients, 0.787 ± 0.360°C in unstable angina patients, and 1.593 ± 0.704°C in acute myocardial infarction patients. There was no statistical difference in the difference from background temperature in terms of its distribution in the five sites of measurement in the coronary artery disease patients. Heterogeneity within the ROI was shown in 20, 40, and 67% of the patients with stable angina, unstable angina, and acute myocardial infarction patients, respectively, whereas no heterogeneity was present in the control subjects. Heterogeneity within the plaque between stable angina, unstable angina, and acute myocardial infarction patients was different ($p < 0.05$), and pairwise comparisons revealed significant differences in heterogeneity between acute myocardial infarction and stable angina patients ($p < 0.05$). Multiple regression analysis revealed that C-reactive protein was the only factor significantly associated with the differences between maximum ROI temperature and background temperature values ($F = 70.2$, multiple $r^2 = 0.55$, B = 0.28, $p < 0.001$). Aspirin intake did not correlate with the difference between maximum ROI and background temperature values in the acute myocardial infarction group ($r = -0.37$, $p = $ NS).

To date we have applied our catheter technique to more than 140 patients without any complication. This population consisted of normal subjects, unstable angina, stable angina, and acute myocardial infarction patients that underwent emergency balloon angioplasty.

A. Color-Coded Thermal Mapping of Coronary Arteries

Using appropriate software developed in our laboratories, we managed to use individual temperature values, recorded at catheter retraction, to reconstruct a thermal "map" of the region of interest. Based on a 256-color palette, each color represents a unique temperature. Cyan-near colors correspond to lower temperatures, whereas red-near ones to higher. Because the thermography catheter is capable of sampling approximately 3 samples/sec, we used a slow-speed automated retraction device. We performed 16 repetitive scans at different angles, 0 to 360 degrees, to secure adequate temperature resolution. The whole procedure is automated and did not take more than 10 minutes.

III. FUTURE PERSPECTIVES

In vitro and in vivo studies have clearly shown that there is temperature heterogeneity in atherosclerotic coronary arteries. Because this heterogeneity is greater in unstable angina and acute myocardial infarction, temperature measurement may be used as a predictive tool for evaluating plaque stability. Thermography could prove useful in identifying the culprit plaque, especially when plaque is extensive, resulting in multiple lesions. The thermistor-based thermography catheter is the first tool in this area, and it has rather limited spatial resolution, but it is the author's belief that in the next years new thermography methods will arise, probably based on infra-red or magnetic reonance technology, capable of making the vision come true: obtaining a thermal snapshot photograph of the heterogenous atherosclerotic plaque.

REFERENCES

1. Ross R. Atherosclerosis—an inflammatory disease. N Engl J Med 1999; 340:115–126.
2. Falk E, Fuster V. Angina pectoris and disease progression. Circulation 1995; 92:2033–2035.
3. Dintefass L. Rheology of Blood in Diagnostic and Preventive Medicine. London, UK: Butterworths, 1976:66–74.
4. Buja LM, Willerson IT. Role of inflammation in coronary plaque disruption. Circulation 1994; 89:503–505.
5. Davies MJ, Thomas AC. Plaque fissuring: the cause of acute myocardial infarction, sudden ischemic death, and crescendo angina. Br Heart J 1985; 53:363–373.
6. Ambrose JA, Tannenbaum MA, Alcxopoulos D, Hjemdahl-Monsen CE, Leavy J, Weiss M, Borrico S, Gnrlin R, Fuster V. Angiographic progression of coronary artery disease in the development of myocardial infarction. J Arn Coli Cardiol 1988; 12:56–62.
7. Alderman EL, Corley SD, Fisher LD, Chaitman BR, Faxon DP, Foster ED, Killip T, Sosa JA, Bourassa MG. Five-year angiographic follow-up of factors associated with progression of coronary artery disease in the Coronary Artery Surgery Study (CASS). J Am Coll Cardiol 1993; 22:1141–1154.
8. De Feyter PJ, Ozaki Y, Baptista J, Escaned J, Di Mario G, de Jacgne PP, Serruys PW, Roelandt JR. Ischemia-related lesion characteristics in patients with stable or unstable angina: a study with intracoronary angioscopy and ultrasound. Circulation 1995; 92:1408–1413.

9. Sakata N, Imanaga Y, Meng J, Tachikawa Y, Takebayashi S, Nagai R, Horiuchi S, Itabe H, Takano T. Immunohistochemical localization of different epitopes of advanced glycation end products in human atherosclerotic lesions. Atherosclerosis 1998 Nov; 141(1):61–75.
10. Khaw BA, Narula J. Antibody imaging in the evaluation of cardiovascular diseases. Nucl Cardiol 1994 Sep-Oct; 1:457–476.
11. Buja LM. Does atherosclerosis have an infectious etiology'? Circulation 1996; 94: 872–873.
12. Maseri A, Crea F. The elusive cause of instability in unstable angina. Am J Cardiol 1991; 68:16B–21B.
13. Liuzzo G, Biasucci IM, Gallimore R, Grill RL, Rebuzzi AG, Pepys MB, Maseri A. The prognostic value of C-reactive protein and serum amyloid A protein in severe unstable angina. N Engl J Med 1994; 331:417–424.
14. Gurfinkel E, Bozovich G, Daroca A, Beck E, Mautner B. Randomised trial of roxithromycin in non-Q-wave coronary syndromes: ROXIS Pilot Study. ROXIS Study Group. Lancet 1997 Aug 9; 350(9075):404–407.
15. Marchioli R, di Pasquale A, Marfisi RM, Tognoni G. Chronic infections and coronary heart disease. The GISSI-Prevenzione Investigators. Lancet 1997; 350:1028–1029.
16. Casscells W, Hathorn B, David M, Krabach T, Vaughn WK, McAllister HA, Bearman G, Willerson T. Thermal detection of cellular infiltrates in living atherosclerotic plaques: possible implications for plaque rupture and thrombosis. Lancet 1996; 347: 1447–1449.
17. Stefanadis C, Diamantopoulos L, Vlachopoulos C, Tsiamis E, Dernellis J, Toutouzas K, Stefanadi E, Toutouzas P. Thermal heterogeneity within human atherosclerotic coronary arteries detected in vivo. A new method of detection by application of a special thermography catheter. Circulation 1999; 99(15):1965–1971.

17
Animal Models of Coronary Artery Disease

Victoria L. M. Herrera, Aram V. Chobanian, and Nelson Ruiz-Opazo
Whitaker Cardiovascular Institute, Boston University School of Medicine, Boston, Massachusetts

I. RATIONALE FOR ANIMAL MODELS—INROADS INTO A UNIFYING FRAMEWORK

Acute coronary syndromes span a spectrum of clinical diagnoses—unstable angina, acute myocardial infarction, and sudden coronary death—caused predominantly by physical disruption or loss of integrity of the atherosclerotic plaque and superimposed thrombosis (1–3). Investigation of mechanisms underlying acute coronary syndromes has shifted toward plaque composition, vulnerability, and thrombogenicity rather than plaque size and stenosis severity (4–6), thus defining the vulnerable atherosclerotic plaque as the biological substrate of acute coronary syndromes (2). The ongoing debate as to terminology, lesion hallmarks, and sequence of events depicts the complexity of the issues, the challenges to investigation, and the need for, and current lack of, a unifying pathogenic framework. The lack of said framework impedes the identification of correlative risk factors, detection parameters, and mechanism-based intervention pathways.

Although inroads have been made into discrete events, the identification of a unifying framework of pathogenic determinants leading to the complication-prone plaque has been limited by the dependence on retrospective association analysis of pathological specimens and clinical events and by the lack of reproducible, accessible animal models that recapitulate acute coronary syndromes (3, 7–8). We recently have developed a transgenic hyperlipidemic–genetic hypertension rat model of coronary artery disease, which exhibits plaque disruption and decreased survival (9) unlike parallel transgenic mouse models (8). This chapter compares this new model with past and recent animal models of coronary artery disease with respect to their similarities with the human disease and to their potential usefulness for studies on the pathogenesis, consequences, and treatment of acute coronary syndromes.

II. BENCHMARKS FOR MODELS OF ACUTE CORONARY SYNDROMES—INTEGRATED CONTEXT SPECIFICITY

A priori, ideal benchmarks of valid animal models of human disease should simulate the context of clinical events and underlying histopathological features. With respect to acute coronary syndromes, benchmarks of the valid animal models should comprise the following:

1. Plaque development, progression, and disruption in the coronary arterial system associated with a pro-atherogenic lipid profile
2. End-stage parallel endpoints of acute coronary syndromes, including cardiac dysfunction, sudden death, and myocardial infarction with resultant decreased survival
3. Pathological hallmarks of plaque disruption such as luminal or intraplaque thrombosis with fissure and/or rupture and/or erosion and/or hemorrhage
4. Identical genetic backgrounds to minimize genetic confounders

Alternative experimental models are available to model surrogate paradigms of acute coronary syndromes, such as: (a) vessel injury to induce plaque rupture and thrombosis in ApoE knockout mouse model (10), (b) viper venom injection to induce acute thrombosis and vessel occlusion in hypercholesterolemic rabbits (11), and (c) mental stress and hypoxia to induce myocardial ischemia in ApoE/LDLr double knockout mice with occlusive coronary lipid-rich lesions (12). However, these have not been useful for studying the determinants of vulnerability to coronary plaque rupture and thrombosis. The limitations of these induced models for molecular analysis of coronary atherosclerotic rupture-prone plaques become increasingly evident in the context of expression profiling studies. Genomic insights from comparative global transcription profiling have demonstrated that integrated biological context-specificity is necessary for accurate modeling of molecular players and determinants of specific developmental or pathogenic events (13). In the event that models recapitulate certain aspects of acute coronary syndromes but not the complete spectrum, validated surrogate endpoints of disease need to be defined to provide an operational experimental frame of reference for the model.

III. CORONARY ARTERY SYSTEM-SPECIFIC MODEL OF ATHEROSCLEROTIC LESION DEVELOPMENT AND PROGRESSION—A REQUIREMENT NOT A NUANCE

A key a priori requirement of valid animal models of acute coronary syndromes is that the lesion phenotype under investigation be in the coronary artery system. As is the case in development, cellular context specificity, hence vessel-specific analysis, is necessary and pertinent to the study of pathological condition. Although earlier paradigmatic analysis may have warranted the study of aortic lesion development as representative of overall atherosclerotic lesion development, it is becoming increasingly evident that vessel-specific vascular biology and biomechanics contribute critical determinants to lesion progression and complication phenotypes. Hence, pathogenic paradigms derived from models that are predominantly aortic root or aortic atherosclerotic disease can be insightful but are not definitive for coronary artery disease determinants.

The experimental standard of vessel-specific modeling is supported by cumulative concordant experimental observations. First, vessel-specific anatomical location and architecture influence biomechanical forces that have been implicated in lesion initiation through shear stress–induced intimal thickening and endothelial activation, lesion destabilization through projected plaque erosion by means of shear stress–induced endothelial apoptosis (14), and/or plaque rupture by extrinsic stress forces on plaque fibrous cap (4). Second, the recent development in genomic analysis of transcription profiles emphasizes the a priori experimental benchmark that reproducible biological context is critical for accurate determination of "transcriptional fingerprints" of pathogenic mechanisms, thus eliminating biological variation as confounders to pathogenic pathway determination (13). Applied to the study of atherosclerotic lesion development, the integrative biology of coronary artery disease needs to be dissected for the elucidation of mechanisms and, ultimately, mechanism-based detection and intervention strategies for the vulnerable plaque. Third, and more importantly, the notion of differential genetic predisposition to lesion development has been experimentally modeled as early as the 1970s in pigeons and nonhuman primates and more recently in rabbits and mice (Table 1).

Comparative analysis of cholesterol levels and lesion predilection site gives insight into their hierarchical relationship. In experimental models listed in Table 1, although hypercholesterolemia is required for atherosclerosis lesion formation, factors other than hypercholesterolemia, such as putative vessel-specific genetic factors, determine lesion predilection sites, because equivalent hypercholesterolemia does not lead to equivalent lesion formation in the aorta and coronary arteries within species. Three main lesion phenotypes are apparent across the different animal models of atherosclerosis (Table 1): (a) predominantly in the aortic, (b)

Table 1 Analysis of Hypercholesterolemia, Lesion Predilection Site

Model	TC (mg/dl)	Coronary lesions	Aortic lesions
Simian			
Macaca arctoides— stumptail (17)	*700	+++	+++
Macaca irus (or *fasicularis*)— cynomolgus (28)	*472	+++ [early]	+ [later]
Saimiri sciureus—squirrel (17)	*450	+++	+++
Macaca mulatta—Rhesus (15)	*450	+++	+
Cercopithecus aethips—African green (17)	*450	+++	+++
Porcine			
Familial hypercholesterolemic swine (35)	245	+++	+
2.8% cholesterol, 1.4% cholate, 0.1% PTU, 2× irradiation miniature swine (41)	*1283	++++	++
Canine			
Cholesterol-thiouracil (29)	1549	++	+++
Avian			
White Carneau pigeons (18)	*1773	+	+++
Show Racer (18)	*1643	+++	+/−
Japanese quail (42)	*1263	+	++
Rabbit			
Hypertensive WHHL rabbit (43)	925	+++ (ostia)	++++
WHHL rabbit (44)	718	++ (prox) + (small)	+++
Cholesterol (0.5%)—fed rabbit (44)	*1400	+ (prox) +++ (small)	++
Inbred mouse			
SM/J (19)	*336	+	+
NZB/BINJ (19)	*306	++	+/−
C57BL/6J (19)	*251	+	++
MRL/lpr (19)	*248	++	+/−
DBA/2J (19)	*193	+	+
Knockout mouse			
ApoE/LDLr (12)	*1017	++	++++
ApoE (45)	400–500	+	+++
Hypertensive ApoE/eNOS (26)	nc	++	++++
Inbred transgenic rat			
Hypertensive Tg53 rat (34)	386	++++	+/−

+ to ++++, relative increasing lesions severity; (+/−), infrequent finding; TC, mean total cholesterol level in mg/dl; *, value obtained on atherogenic cholesterol diet; nc, no change from Apo E knockout mice; ostia, lesion in coronary ostia; prox, lesion in proximal coronary arteries; PTU, propylthiouracil; small, small intramural coronary arteries; 2× irradiation, 2 doses precordial irradiation.

predominantly in the coronary arteries, or (c) equivalent lesion development in both the aorta and coronary arteries.

These studies suggest that differences in atherogenic mechanisms exist between aortic and coronary lesion development in nonhuman primates (15–17), pigeons (18), and mice (19). Differential lesion development mechanisms are also observed in Watanabe rabbits, wherein further increases in cholesterol level increase lesion area in the aorta but not in the coronary artery system (20), and ratio of macrophage to smooth muscle cells is greater in the aorta compared with coronary lesions (21). These studies were not designed, however, to identify putative genetic determinants. A recent study in transgenic mouse atherosclerosis models provides new support for this notion. In apoE-deficient mice back-crossed onto two different inbred strains, C57BL6 and FVB/NJ, the genetic determinants of lesion size were distinct from the determinants of hyperlipidemia, because larger aortic root lesions but less hypercholesterolemia were observed in C57BL6 Apo-deficient mice, in contrast to FVB/NJ ApoE-deficient mice, which exhibited higher cholesterol levels but less aortic root lesion area (22). This model system facilitates genetic analysis.

The pathogenic concept of genetic determinants of coronary vs aortic lesion predilection site is further supported by studies showing that within the aorta, lesion predilection is further stratified to aortic root vs the rest of the aorta in mice (23) or thoracic aorta vs abdominal aorta in dogs (24) and in nonhuman primates (17). In humans, Glagov et al (25) have noted that aortic, coronary, and renal artery atherosclerosis occurred independently.

The fact that genetic predisposition to lesion site predilection is observed in multiple models and in different species reiterates its role as a significant determinant that must be factored into the investigation of mechanisms in human acute coronary syndromes. It also becomes imperative that lesion site predilection should be factored into the analysis of proatherogenic risk factors, because its omission could result in inadvertent false-negative deductions.

IV. COMPARATIVE REVIEW OF ANIMAL MODELS OF CORONARY ATHEROSCLEROSIS AT END STAGE–INSIGHTS INTO PLAQUE RUPTURE AND THROMBOSIS

A review of animal models of coronary atherosclerosis studied until end stage or death reveals that although most animal models of coronary artery disease develop xanthomatous lesions or fatty streaks, atheroma, and fibroatheroma, most do not exhibit rupture and thrombosis (Table 2).

Because these models are studied under regulated experimental conditions, it could be argued that the reproducible lesion phenotype within a model defines

Table 2 Comparative Analysis of Animal Models of Coronary Artery Disease at End-Stage Analysis

Model	End-stage cardiac event	Occlusion	Features of end-stage lesions								
			Neovascularization	Calcification	IEL-defect	Medial thinning	HGE	Erosion ulceration	Rupture fissure	In situ plaque thrombosis
ApoE/LDLr knockout mouse (12)	decreased survival	+	NR	+	NR	NR	(−)	(−)	(−)	(−)
White Carneau (WC) pigeon (18)	2/131 MI	+	NR	+ ao root	NR	NR	NR	+ ao root	NR	(−)
Show Racer [SR] pigeon (18)	9/197 MI	+	NR	+ ao root	NR	NR	NR	+ ao root	NR	(−)
Congenic (WC × SR) pigeon (18)	6/12 MI	+	NR	+ ao root	NR	NR	NR	+ ao root	NR	(−)
Japanese quail (42)	1/15 MI	+	NR	+	+	+	NR	(−)	(−)	(−)
WHHL rabbit (46)	4 MI	+	NR	+	NR	NR	NR	NR	NR	(−)
Cynomolgous monkey (28)	2 early death 1/2 MI	+	+	(−)	+	+	+	(−)	(−)	(−)
African green monkey (17)	1 of 4	+	+	+	+	+	+	NR	NR	(−)
Rhesus monkey (15)	14/160 MI 1/14 early death	+	+	+	+	+	NR	NR	NR	(−), on plaque +, distal to plaque
Cholesterol-thiouracil dog (29)	3/45 MI 1/3 early death	+	NR*	NR*	+	+	NR*	NR*	NR*	+ "Some org. thrombi"
FHC pigs (35)	1/5 early death	+	+	+	NR	NR	+	NR	+	+ "Not a prom. feature"
Cholesterol-thiouracil-Xrad miniature pigs (41)	16/18 MI	+	NR	+	+	+	+	NR	NR	+ Large aa in 2/18 "occl in small aa"
Transgenic hyperlipidemic-hypertensive Tg53 rat (34)	7/7 MI decreased survival	+	+	(−)	+	+	+	+	+	+ Intraplaque in RCA

NOTE: This table is limited to coronary artery disease models followed to end stage.

+, reported/detected as present; (−) reported as not detected; NR, not reported; NR*, not specifically reported but "all stages of lesion" described; ao, aortic; HGE, hemorrhage; IEL, internal elastic lamina; large aa, larger coronary arteries; occl in small aa, occasional thrombus detected in small coronary arteries; RCA, right coronary artery.

a paradigm of lesion pathogenesis. A review of model-delineated lesion paradigms at end stage (experimentally followed until death) supports the hypothesis that end-stage destabilization most likely involves multiple distinct pathways leading to various permutations of endpoints: luminal and/or intraplaque disruption and/or hemorrhage and/or thrombosis. This parallels end-stage lesion phenotype complexity in human coronary artery disease as well (3). It is intriguing that most animal models of atherosclerosis recapitulate lesion initiation and progression, but only a few recapitulate end-stage plaque erosion/rupture and thrombosis, and of these few models, only some of the aspects of human coronary unstable plaques are present (Table 2).

As shown in Table 2, several lesion phenotypes are apparent. One lesion phenotype is depicted in transgenic mouse models. To date, coronary lesion rupture/erosion and thrombosis have not been detected in prototype combinatorial transgenic null mutant mouse models (8), despite cholesterol levels reaching 1000 mg/dL as observed in ApoE/LDLr double knockout mice (12). Even with the addition of known exacerbating risk factors such as hypertension or stress, coronary artery plaque rupture and thrombosis were not detected in ApoE-deficient and ApoE/LDLr deficient mouse models, although critical coronary stenoses were detected (12, 26). It is intriguing to note that plaque rupture and hemorrhage have been detected in ApoE innominate artery plaques, but thrombosis was not detected (27).

A more "advanced" (fibrous cap and lipid/gruel core) but still nonthrombosis-prone lesion phenotype is observed in cynomolgous and African green monkeys (Tables 1 and 2). In cynomolgous monkeys, although foam cell rupture and necrosis were detected, the authors did not detect coronary lesion rupture, ulceration, hemorrhage, or thrombosis, even in the one monkey that died early from a myocardial infarction (28). In African green monkeys, intraplaque hemorrhage and hemosiderin deposits, medial thinning, calcification, vascularization, plaque necrosis, and internal elastic lamina defects were detected, but no lesional thrombus was apparent in the 14 of 160 monkeys shown to have myocardial infarction on electrocardiogram (17). One monkey that died from myocardial infarction exhibited lumen occlusion of the left anterior descending artery and a thrombus distal to this occlusion, but no in situ plaque thrombi (15). These data suggest that in cynomolgus and African green monkey models of coronary atherosclerosis, underlying predispositions to plaque hemorrhage, medial thinning, and significant stenosis are present, but factors leading to plaque rupture and thrombosis are not. In a cholesterol–thiouracil canine model, organized thrombi were detected; however, plaque rupture and hemorrhage were not reported (29).

It is significant to note that the lesion phenotypes in different animal models simulate most of the lesion types deduced from human coronary artery pathological conditions, with different models representing specific lesion types. This classification spans eight main pathological types: type I, initial lesion; type II, fatty streak either progression-prone or progression-resistant; type III, preatheroma; type IV, atheroma; type V, fibroatheroma; type VI, complicated lesion with fissure or erosion (VIa), hemorrhage (VIb), or thrombotic deposit (VIc); type VII, calcific lesion; and type VIII, fibrotic lesion (30). The different lesion phenotypes per model, and the reproducibility of said lesion phenotypes within a model, recapitulate the observation in human coronary artery disease that "lesions may cease to progress at any one of the lesion stages" (30).

In all transgenic mouse models to date, although coronary artery stenosis is observed with increasing xanthomatous development in coronary arteries, rupture and thrombosis have not been reported (8). In innominate artery plaques of ApoE knockout mice, rupture is associated with hemorrhage but not thrombosis (27). The fact that mice do develop thrombotic lesions when plaques are mechanically disrupted (10) helps eliminate the experimental consideration that atherosclerosis mouse models do not develop plaque rupture and thrombosis as a result of a deficiency in thrombotic capacity. It could thus be argued that the natural history of coronary artery disease in mouse models in the C57BL6 strain does not progress to lesion rupture and thrombosis. This distinguishes xanthomatous lesion progression from advanced plaque progression and complication as distinct pathways in lesion pathogenesis. The notion is supported by an extensive study by Falk (31). His recent study of 210 ApoE mice >1 year of age subjected to various experimental manipulations to induce plaque rupture by extrinsic or intrinsic factors resulted in only one rupture with thrombosis of 441 vulnerable-type mature lesions (lipid-rich, thin fibrous cap, heavily macrophage infiltrated) at risk. Recent observations would suggest that plaque disequilibrium toward matrix degradation might be the turnkey toward plaque rupture. In humans, matrix-degrading proteins have been detected in "vulnerable" plaque regions and in unstable plaques but not in stable plaques (32, 33). Recent data from the Tg53 rat model (Table 3) support these observations (34).

The FHC swine model demonstrates plaque rupture in advanced fibroatheromatous plaques in the proximal coronary arteries with a significant inflammatory response to disruption of the plaque surface; however, thrombosis was not detected (35). This is quite puzzling, because thrombotic capacity in swine models has been well demonstrated in injury models (36) and the coronary thrombogenic copper coil model (37). Along with most nonthrombosis animal models of coronary artery disease (Table 2), this model suggests that plaque thrombogenicity necessitates a "threshold mechanism" or turnkey and that it is most likely not a property of all atherosclerotic plaques. This notion would be concordant with the putative role of in situ plaque tissue factor expression in plaque thrombogenesis, deduced from its detection in ruptured human coronary plaques. The hypothesis that plaque tissue factor may be the putative turnkey to acute thrombotic events in acute coronary syndromes is intriguing, because its absence/presence may distinguish asymptomatic from symptomatic (unstable) plaque rupture respectively (38,39). Stary's further classification of type VI lesions indicates that plaque erosion/rupture

Table 3 Morphological Spectrum of Lesions in ACS

Humans		Tg53 rat (34)
Rupture–prone plaques [+/− thrombosis] (47)		
a. Lipid-rich plaque with thin cap; abundant macrophages; few smcs	a.	+
b. Thick fibrous stable plaque with macrophages at shoulder	b.	(−)
* In Tg53 lesions, shoulder thrombosis detected in "vulnerable" but not in stable plaque		
c. Fibrous stable plaque with small focus of macrophages close to surface = erosion prone plaque	c.	(−)
** In Tg53, lesion erosion with neutrophil adhesion and entry in "vulnerable" but not in stable plaque		
Coronary thrombosis plaque substrate (3)		
a. Plaque rupture: thin fibrous caps infiltrated with macrophages	a.	+
b. Plaque erosion		
b-1. Luminal surface is irregular, eroded and lacked endothelial cells	b-1.	+
b-2. Extension into upper layers of the plaque-forming foci of intraplaque thrombi	b-2.	+
c. Calcified nodule	c.	(−)
Type VI. Complicated lesions with thrombotic deposits (30)		
a. Fibroatheroma + fissures	a.	(−)
b. Fibroatheroma + rupture	b.	+
c. Fibroatheroma + erosion	c.	+
		NOTE: associated with foam cell–rich lesions rather than "gruel"-type lesions
Other features:		
d. Breaks of neovessels within lesion: hge + thrombosis	d.	+
e. Dissecting hemorrhage and thrombosis	e.	(−)
Associated cellular and molecular determinants of plaque vulnerability to disruption [rupture/erosion/tear/fissure]		
a. Matrix-degrading proteins (MMP1, MMP3, MMP9) (2, 48)		+ MMP3 in lesion core, macrophage-foam cells and smcs
b. Tissue factor (49)		+ lesion core; macrophage foam cells
c. Apoptosis (50)		+ in macrophage-foam cells
d. Neutrophils (4)		+ site of endothelial erosion and rupture; adhesion only on complicated plaque at end stage
e. T-cell CD40 signaling (51)		+ in areas of intraplaque hemorrhage and thrombosis
f. Abundant macrophage-foam cells (2, 4)		+
g. Paucity of smcs (2)		+
h. Neovascularization (52, 53)		+ in areas of intraplaque hemorrhage and thrombosis

+, detected; (−), not detected; hge, hemorrhage; MMP1, 3, 9: matrix metalloproteinase proteins; smcs, smooth muscle cells.

(VIa) and plaque hemorrhage (VIb) can be detected without plaque thrombosis (VIc), thus concordant with a "turnkey hypothesis." On the other hand, organized thrombi, but not rupture and hemorrhage, were observed in the cholesterol-thiouracil–fed canine coronary atherosclerosis model (29). Conclusions regarding lesion phenotype paradigms are confounded by the use of thiouracil in this canine model, however (29).

The concordance of observations of staged lesion development, progression, and complication in animal models, as well as in human coronary lesions, provides reinforcement for the investigation of pathogenic paradigms of coronary atherosclerosis in animal models. In essence, distinct lesion phenotypes in animal models represent different compartmentalized stages of coronary artery lesion development and progression. With the recent development of the transgenic Tg53 hyperlipidemic–hypertensive rat model (9, 34), a model exhibiting plaque rupture, erosion, hemorrhage, and thrombosis is attained. Further study of this model superimposed on observations of unstable human coronary plaques could begin to provide insight into mechanisms of plaque rupture/erosion and thrombosis.

V. NEW INSIGHTS FROM THE Tg53 RAT MODEL— DYNAMIC END-STAGE LESION COMPLEXITY

Many, but not all, of the features of human lesions associated with acute coronary syndromes are detected in the lesion phenotype of Tg53 rats at end stage. Correlative analysis of pathological cellular and molecular features of plaques associated with acute coronary syndromes in humans and Tg53 rats are presented in Table 3.

This comparison reveals that Tg53 rats exhibit the lesion complication complex of rupture/erosion and thrombosis (34). Tg53 rats exhibit marked hypercholesterolemia, low HDLc, marked hypertriglyceridemia, and polygenic salt-sensitive hypertension, making it the only model with this combination of atherogenic risk factors. Of note, Tg53 rats exhibit lower LDL levels than control nontransgenic Dahl S rats, suggesting the significance of low HDL and hypertriglyceridemia. The significant role of hypertension in this model was demonstrated by the increase in lifespan with blood pressure reduction in 6-month-old Tg53 rats placed on a low-salt diet (0.008% NaCl) while the lipid profile remained unchanged (34).

The tracking of lesions at 6 months and at end stage in this model provides insight into lesion development at different sites. Because stable lesion phenotypes were observed distally and complication-prone plaque phenotypes were detected only in the more proximal coronary artery branches, it becomes apparent that distinct lesion development pathways may exist that lead to stable and complication-prone lesions at the same time. The distinction of stable vs unstable plaque development programs as distinct pathways of lesion development is supported by the differential molecular profile of stable and unstable plaques in the Tg53 rats (34). Immunohistochemical analysis detected differential expression of matrix-degrading proteins and tissue factors that distinguished complication-prone vulnerable plaques proximally from distal stable plaques (34), recapitulating observations in human coronary artery plaques of differential expression of matrix-degrading proteins (32) and tissue factors in stable vs unstable plaques (38, 39).

In addition to the development of a stable fibroatheroma plaque phenotype in the more distal coronary arteries and "vulnerable" plaque phenotype in the proximal coronary arteries, the Tg53 rat model demonstrates another distinct lesion phenotype—lesions with "stable" smooth muscle cell–rich thick fibrous caps but with deep intraplaque hemorrhage, thrombosis, and disruption of the internal elastic lamina in the proximal coronary artery system (34), similar to observations in human lesions (40). Areas of intraplaque hemorrhage and thrombosis were rich in macrophage foam cells exhibiting immunostaining for T-cell activating CD40 ligand, vascular endothelial growth factor, tissue factor, matrix-degrading protein MMP3, and apoptosis caspase-3-enzyme, thus recapitulating many features associated with unstable human coronary plaques (34) but with a very thick fibrous cap. The disrupted internal elastic lamina distinguishes this lesion phenotype (thick fibrous cap, deep intraplaque hemorrhage, and thrombosis) from the other lesion phenotype observed characterized by a thin fibrous cap, foam cell-rich, rupture/erosion-hemorrhage-thrombosis but with intact internal elastic lamina. These observations suggest that another lesion development pathway is detected rather than an interim pathway toward development of complication-prone plaque. Whether this pathway also leads to plaque instability is currently under investigation.

Having controlled genetic background and environmental factors in the Tg53 rat model, it becomes apparent that at end stage, lesion complexity and heterogeneity are apparent, with coronary lesions exhibiting different stages of progression or vulnerability (34). This would imply that a single marker for acute coronary syndromes is highly unlikely and that correlation of multiple molecular and cellular markers will be required to achieve diagnostic accuracy (34).

VI. AN INVESTIGATIVE PERSPECTIVE FOR ACUTE CORONARY SYNDROMES—DYNAMIC MULTIFACTORIAL COMPLEXITY

In summary, although pathogenic paradigms may be inferred segmentally in postmortem analyses of human coronary artery disease and in surrogate cell culture models or animal models of aortic root and aortic atherosclerosis, elucidation of a unifying framework of acute coronary syndrome pathogenesis requires the investigation of validated coronary artery disease models. Such models provide biological contextual accuracy required for the elucidation of the integrative biology of acute coronary syndromes—dissecting genetic determinants of lesion phenotype and global circuits of molecular pathways specific to lesion initiation, progression, destabilization, and disruption, as well as elucidating, while controlling and/or testing for critical environmental risk factors. Biological contextual accuracy facilitates the development of clinically relevant and mechanism-based detection, intervention, and prevention strategies.

The various reproducible lesion phenotypes detected in different animal models of coronary atherosclerosis support the hypothesis that distinct pathogenic pathways most likely underly lesion types. Over the five decades of animal modeling of coronary atherosclerosis, the observed scarcity of animal models of coronary plaque rupture and thrombosis is intriguing. The discovery of such a model could provide important insight into understanding the acute coronary syndrome. Intriguingly, the one model exhibiting coronary plaque disruption, thrombosis, and myocardial infarction to date, the Tg53 rat model (34), depicts heterogeneous lesion complication and destabilization stages, not unlike the heterogeneity of lesions observed in humans at the time of sudden death related to plague rupture (3). Thus, the available data implicate a dynamic multifactorial complex of pathogenic events leading to the acute coronary syndromes.

ACKNOWLEDGMENTS

We thank Sarah E. Traverse for outstanding help. This work is supported by NIH grant HL62857.

REFERENCES

1. Zhou J, Chew M, Ravn HB, Falk E. Plaque pathology and coronary thrombosis in the pathogenesis of acute coronary syndromes. Scan J Clin Lab Invest 1999; 230: 3–11.
2. Libby P, Geng YJ, Sukhova GK, Simon DI, Lee RT. Molecular determinants of atherosclerotic plaque vulnerability. Ann NY Acad Sci 1997; 811:134–142.
3. Virmani R, Kolodgie FD, Burke AP, Farb A, Schwartz SM. Lessons from sudden coronary death: a comprehensive morphological classification scheme for atherosclerotic lesions. Arterioscler Thromb Vasc Biol 2000; 20:1262–1275.
4. Delager-Pedersen S, Pederson EM, Ringgaard S, Falk E. Coronary artery disease: plaque vulnerability, disruption and thrombosis. In: Fuster V, ed. The Vulnerable Atherosclerotic Plaque. New York: Futura, 1999:1–23.

5. Fuster V. Acute coronary syndromes: the degree and morphology of coronary stenoses. J Am Coll Cardiol 1999; 34:1854–1856.

6. Libby P. Changing concepts of atherogenesis. J Intern Med 2000; 247:349–358.

7. Getz GS. Mouse model of unstable atherosclerotic plaque? Arterioscler Thromb Vasc Biol 2000; 20:2503–2505.

8. Lusis AJ. Atherosclerosis. Nature 2000; 407:233–241.

9. Herrera VLM, Makrides SC, Xie HX, Adari H, Krauss RM, Ryan US, Ruiz-Opazo N. Spontaneous combined hyperlipidemia, coronary heart disease and decreased survival in Dahl salt-sensitive hypertensive rats transgenic for human cholesteryl ester transfer protein. Nat Med 1999; 5:1383–1389.

10. Reddick RL, Zjang SH, Maeda N. Aortic atherosclerotic plaque injury in apolipoprotein E deficient mice. Atherosclerosis 1998; 140:297–305.

11. Abela GS, Picon PD, Friedl SE, Bebara OC, Miyamoto A, Federman J, Tofler GH, Muller JE. Triggering of plaque disruption and arterial thrombosis in an atherosclerotic rabbit model. Circulation 1995; 91:776–784.

12. Caligiuri G, Levy B, Pernow J, Thoren P, Hansson GK. Myocardial infarction mediated by endothelin receptor signaling in hypercholesterolemic mice. Proc Natl Acad Sci USA 1999; 96:6920–6924.

13. Lockhart DJ, Winzeler EA. Genomics, gene expression and DNA arrays. Nature 2000; 405:827–836.

14. Tricot O, Mallat Z, Heymes C, Belmin J, Leseche G, Tedgui A. Relation between endothelial apoptosis and blood flow direction in human atherosclerotic plaques. Circulation 2000; 101:2450–2453.

15. Manning PJ, Clarkson TB. Development, distribution and lipid content of diet-induced atheroslcerotic lesions of Rhesus monkeys. Experimental Mol Pathol 1972; 17:38–54.

16. Hollander W, Madoff I, Paddock J, Kirkpatrick B. Aggravation of atherosclerois by hypertension in a subhuman primate model with coarctation of the aorta. Hypertension 1976; 38(suppl II):II-63–II-72.

17. Bullock BC, Lehner NDM, Clarkson TB, Feldner MA, Wagner WD, Lofland IIB. Comparative primate atherosclerosis. Part I. Tissue cholesterol concentration and pathologic anatomy. Exp Mol Pathol 1975; 22:151–175.

18. Wagner WE, Clarkson TB, Feldner MA, Prichard RW. The development of pigeon strains with selected atherosclerosis characteristics. Exp Mol Pathol 1973; 19:304–319.

19. Qiao JH, Xie PZ, Fishbein MC, Kreuzer J, Drake TA, Demer LL, Lusis AJ. Pathology of atheromatous lesions in inbred and genetically engineered mice. Arterioscler Thromb Vasc Biol 1994; 20:1480–1497.

20. Shiomi M, Ito T, Shiraishi M, Watanabe Y. Inheritability of atherosclerosis and the role of lipoproteins as risk factors related to coronary atherosclerosis are different from those related to aortic atherosclerosis. Atherosclerosis 1992; 96:43–52.

21. Shiomi M, Ito T, Tsukada T, Yata T, Ueda M. Cell compositions of coronary and aortic atherosclerotic lesions in WHHL rabbits differ. An immunohistochemical study. Arterioscler Thromb 1994; 14:931–937.

22. Dansky HM, Charlton SA, Sikes JL, Heath SC, Simantov R, Levin LF, Shu P, Moore KJ, Breslow JL, Smith JD. Genetic background determines the extent of atheroscle-

rosis in ApoE-deficient mice. Arterioscler Thromb Vasc Biol 1999; 19:1960–1968.

23. Witting PK, Pettersson K, Letters J, Stocker R. Site-specific antiatherogenic effect of probucol in apolipoprotein E-deficient mice. Arterioscler Thromb Vasc Biol 2000; 20:E26–E33.

24. Haimovici H, Maier N. Role of arterial tissue susceptibility in experimental canine atherosclerosis. J Atheroscler Res 1966; 62–74.

25. Glagov S, Rowley DA, Kohut RI. Atherosclerosis of human aorta and its coronary and renal arteries. Arch Pathol 1961; 72:82–95.

26. Knowles JW, Reddick RL, Jennette JC, Shesely EG, Smithies O, Maeda N. Enhanced atherosclerosis and kidney dysfunction in eNOS$-/-$ ApoE$-/-$ mice are ameliorated by enalapril treatment. J Clin Invest 2000; 105:451–458.

27. Rosenfeld ME, Polinsky P, Virmani R, Kauser K, Rubanyi G, Schwartz SM. Advanced atherosclerotic lesions in the innominate artery of the ApoE knockout mouse. Areterioscler Thromb Vasc Biol 2000; 20:2587–2592.

28. Kramsch DM, Hollander W. Occlusive atherosclerotic disease of the coronary arteries in monkey (Macaca irus) induced by diet. Exp Mol Pathol 1968; 9:1–22.

29. Haimovici H, Maier N. Experimental coronary atherosclerosis in the dog. Bull Soc Int Chir 1962; 6:634–641.

30. Stary HC. The Evolution of Human Atherosclerotic Lesions. West Point: Merck, 1993.

31. Falk E. Plaque remodelling and plaque instability AHA Scientific Conference on Assessing and Modifying the Vulnerable Atherosclerotic Plaque. New York, NY, Sept 16–17, 2000.

32. Galis Z, Sukhova G, Lark M, Libby P. Increased expression of matrix metalloproteinases and matrix degrading activity in vulnerable regions of human atherosclerotic plaques. J Clin Invest 1994; 94:2493–2503.

33. Brown DL, Hibbs MS, Kearney M, Loushin C, Isner JM. Identification of 92-kD gelatinase in human coronary atherosclerotic lesions. Association of active enzyme synthesis with unstable angina. Circulation 1995; 91:2125–2131.

34. Herrera VLM, Didishvili T, Lopez LV, Zander K, Traverse S, Gantz D, Herscovitz H, Ruiz-Opazo N. Hypertension exacerbates coronary plaque progression in transgenic hyperlipidemic Dahl salt-sensitive hypertensive rats. Submitted, 2001.

35. Prescott MF, McBride CH, Hasler-Rapacz J, Von Linden J, Rapacz J. Development of complex atherosclerotic lesions in pigs with inherited hyper-LDL cholesterolemia bearing mutant alleles for ApoB. Am J Pathol 1991; 139:139–147.

36. Zaman AG, Osende JI, Chesebro JH, Fuster V, Padurean A, Gallo R, Worthley SG, Helft G, Rodriguez OX, Fallon JT, Badimon JJ. In vivo dynamic real-time monitoring and quantification of platelet-thrombus formation: use of a local isotope detector. Arterioscler Thromb Vasc Biol 2000; 20:860–865.

37. Uruida Y, Wang QD, Hatori N, Nordlander R, Sjoquist PO, Mattsson C, Ryden L. Coronary thrombosis/thrombolysis in pigs: effects of heparin, ASA, and the thrombin inhibito inogatran. J Pharmacol Toxicol Methods 1998; 39:81–89.

38. Moreno PR, Bernardi VH, Lopez-Cuellar J, Murcia AM, Palacios IF, Gold HK, Mehran R, Sharma SK, Nemerson Y, Fuster V, Fallon JT. Macrophages, smooth

muscle cells, and tissue factor in unstable angina: implications for cell-mediated thrombogenicity in acute coronary syndromes. Circulation 1996; 94:3090–3097.

39. Ardissino D, Merlini PA, Arlens R, Coppola R, Bramucci E, Lucreziotti S, Repetto A, Fetiveau R, Mannucci PM. Tissue factor in human coronary atherosclerotic plaques. Clin Chim Acta 2000; 291:235–240.
40. Gravanis MB. Histopathology of arteriosclerosis. In: Wilson WF, ed. Atlas of Atherosclerosis: Risk Factors and Treatment. Philadelphia: Current Medicine, 2000: 1–19.
41. Lee KT, Jarmolych J, Kim DN, Grant C, Krasney JA, Thomas WA, Bruno AM. Production of advanced coronary atherosclerosis, myocardial infarction and "sudden death" in swine. Exp Mol Pathol 1971; 15:170–190.
42. Ojerio AD, Pucak GJ, Clarkson TB, Bullock BC. Diet-induced atheroslcerosis and myocardial infarction in Japanese quail. Lab Animal Sci 1972; 22:33–39.
43. Nickerson CJ, Haudenschild CC, Chobanian AV. Effects of hypertension and hyperlipidemia on the myocardium and coronary vasculature of the WHHL rabbit. Exp Mol Pathol 1992; 56:173–185.
44. Nakamura M, Abe S, Kinukawa N. Causal relationship between occlusive lesions of the coronary artery and myocardial fibrosis in arteriosclerotic rabbits—differences between cholesterol-fed and heritable hyperlipidemic rabbits. Atherosclerosis 1996; 124:37–47.
45. Breslow JL. Transgenic mouse models of lipoprotein metabolism and atherosclerosis. Proc Natl Acad Sci USA 1993; 90:8314–8318.
46. Hansen BF, Mortensen A, Hansen JF, Ibsen P, Frandsen H, Nordestgaard BG. Atherosclerosis in Watanabe heritable hyperlipidaemic rabbits. APMIS 1994; 102:177–190.
47. van der Wal, AC. Inflammatory cells. AHA Scientific Conference on Assessing and Modifying the Vulnerable Atherosclerotic Plaque. New York, NY, Sept 16–17, 2000.
48. Henney AM, Wakeley PR, Davies MJ, Foster K, Rosalind H, Murphy G, Humphries S. Localization of stromelysin gene expression in atherosclerotic plaques by in situ hybridization. Proc Natl Acad Sci USA 1991; 88:8154–8158.
49. Toschi V, Gallo R, Lettino M, Fallon JT, Gertz SD, Fernandez-Ortiz A, Chesebro JH, Badimon L, Nemerson Y, Fuster V, Badimon JJ. Tissue factor modulates the thrombogenicity of human atherosclerotic plaques. Circulation 1997; 95:594–599.
50. Kockx MM, Herman AG. Apoptosis in atherogenesis: implications for plaque destabilization. Eur Heart J 1998; (supplG):G23–G28.
51. Schonbeck U, Mach F, Sukhova GK, Murphy C, Bonnefoy JY, Fabunmi RP, Libby P. Regulation of matrix metalloproteinase expression in human vascular smooth muscle cells by T lymphocytes: a role for CD40 signaling in plaque rupture. Circ Res 1997; 81:448–454.
52. Depre C, Havaux X, Wijns W. Neovascularization in human coronary atherosclerotic lesions. Cathet Cardiovasc Diagn 1996; 39:215–220.
53. deBoer OJ, van der Wal AC, Teeling P, Becker AE. Leukocyte recruitment in rupture prone regions of lipid-rich plaque: a prominent role for neovascularization? Cardiovasc Res 1999; 41:443–449.

18

Clinical Trial Considerations in the Development of Inhibitors of Cardiovascular Plaque Rupture

David L. Brown
Albert Einstein College of Medicine and Montefiore Medical Center, Bronx, New York

Great strides have been made in the last decade in dissecting the molecular and cellular mechanisms leading to rupture of atherosclerotic plaque. As inhibitors of the cellular and molecular events leading to plaque rupture are developed, it is in the interest of public health to make them available to patients as expeditiously as possible. This chapter reviews the principles of clinical trial design and the steps required to demonstrate the safety and efficacy of new compounds intended to prevent plaque rupture.

I. BASIC PRINCIPLES

Prevention of plaque rupture is an important goal because of the large number of patients afflicted with the clinical manifestations of plaque rupture each year. However, in any group of patients with risk factors for the development of coronary artery disease, or even established coronary artery disease, the risk of a plaque rupture event over any reasonable finite period of time is quite low. Thus, for treatment effects to be detected, any errors in their assessment need to be much smaller than what in all likelihood will be a moderate but worthwhile therapeutic effect (1). Systematic errors or bias in the assessment of treatment can be a result of factors other than the treatment being investigated. They are common in observational studies and can cause either overestimation or underestimation of treatment effects. Random errors may be avoided by studying a large enough sample size or by performing meta-analysis in which data from the undersized studies are combined. Mechanisms to avoid systematic errors include proper randomization, analysis by intention-to-treat principles, and avoidance of subgroup analyses as discussed later (1).

II. RANDOMIZATION

Random allocation of treatment is critical to ensure unbiased assignment of each type of patient to the different treatment strategies under investigation. Randomization must be conducted in irreversible ignorance on the part of the investigators and patients regarding treatment allocation (1). Thus, randomization based on the days of the week or the patient's social security number should be avoided. Nonrandom assignment of treatment introduces the potential for bias that can be at least as large as any moderate effect of treatment on mortality and morbidity.

III. INTENTION-TO-TREAT ANALYSIS

Even in a randomized trial, bias can be introduced by exclusion of certain patients after randomization (1). Thus, the primary statistical analysis of any clinical trial should analyze the outcomes of patients originally assigned to receive the treatment in the treatment group even if they did not actually receive it. Subsequent analyses of on-treatment outcomes, outcomes as a function of compliance, and toxicity may be conducted but should not be included in the primary end point.

IV. AVOIDANCE OF SUBGROUP ANALYSES

Apparent differences between the treatment effects in different study subgroups can often be caused by chance and can either mimic or obscure moderate treatment effects. In the Second International Study of Infarct Survival (ISIS-2), the benefit of aspirin in the prevention of death from myocardial infarction was unequivocally demonstrated in the overall trial (2). However, a post hoc subgroup analysis demonstrated that among patients born under the astrological signs of Libra and Gemini, aspirin was of no benefit (1). Despite these findings, no physician would treat patients differently on the basis of their astrological sign. Nevertheless, clinical recommendations are frequently made on the basis of similarly performed data-derived subgroup analyses. The lack of a statistically significant effect is not always evidence of lack of a clinical effect but rather may be due to a low event rate, resulting in the lack of statistical power to detect a difference.

Thus, the best estimate of risk in a subgroup would be provided by meta-analyses of the treatment in the subgroup of interest (1, 3). Frequently, subgroups seem to have a greater treatment effect than the overall trial population. Again, because of small numbers in the subgroup compared with the overall trial (on which the sample size calculation was based), false-positive results are a likely explanation. In general, it is unlikely that the results in a particular subgroup are qualitatively different from those in the main trial result, although they may be quantitatively different. In fact, a statistically valid method for estimating risk reduction by a treatment in a subgroup is to apply the risk reduction derived from the overall trial and apply this to the absolute risk in the subgroup of interest (3). However, data from subgroup analyses should only be used to generate hypotheses for subsequent trials rather than for making treatment recommendations specific to the subgroup of interest.

V. CLINICAL TRIAL PHASES

The United States Food and Drug Administration (FDA) has specified in its regulations the terminology used to distinguish the phases of research used to bring a new drug to market (4). The initial step in the development of a new compound for human use is to establish safety. A Phase I trial focuses on the safety of a compound and generally involves healthy volunteers being administered single or multiple doses of the new compound. The tolerable dose range is considered in Phase I studies. In the case of new medications for treatment of malignancy, Phase I trials may involve severely ill cancer patients. Pharmacokinetic, pharmacodynamic, and side effect data are collected in Phase I. A Phase I trial usually involves 20 to 80 persons, although the number is highly variable.

The Phase II study is the first controlled study of a novel compound in patients. In a Phase II study, the effectiveness of a drug for a specific therapeutic use is investigated. These trials are usually closely monitored and generally involve only a few hundred patients. The enrollment criteria are narrowly defined and, because of the small number of patients, the end points of the trial may be surrogates for the actual end point of interest. In development of treatments for cardiovascular disease, Phase II trials are usually placebo controlled.

The data from Phase II clinical trials are used to determine whether the extensive resources necessary to mount a Phase III trial are justified (5). Specifically, the results of Phase II trials should at least suggest efficacy and safety, as well as give an idea of the most appropriate dose of a drug to study in Phase III.

A second important goal of a Phase II study is to ascertain the safety profile of a new treatment. Adverse events consist of minor and unexpected complications of treatment such as skin rash that might be deemed acceptable in the face of a drug that reduces death or myocardial infarction. The next type of adverse effect is the predictable consequence of a therapy such as bleeding in the case of a thrombolytic agent. Phase II trials might be large enough to detect an increase in these events if they occur frequently but are unlikely to be able to detect as much as a twofold increase in adverse events. The third category of events includes rare but serious events such as liver failure in the case of troglitazone. Because these types of events are uncommon, they are unlikely to be detected in Phase II trials.

The final goal of a Phase II trial is the selection of a dose to be tested in a larger and more definitive Phase III trial. Thus, Phase II trials frequently use several doses of the drug under investigation. The hope is that the results of the Phase II study will allow the selection of an efficacious dose without safety concerns.

Phase III studies gather information regarding safety and efficacy so that the risk/benefit ratio derived from treatment with the drug can be ascertained. Ultimately, these trials form the basis of FDA approval for marketing and provide the information required for labeling such as indications for and side effects of treatment. Phase III trials examine the use of the drug in a broader patient population than Phase II trials. Some differences between Phase II and III trials are illustrated in Table 1.

In an effort to cut the time and costs associated with drug development, Phase I and II trials may be combined into a single trial. In such a combined Phase I/II trial, assessment of toxicity, dose finding, and some measure of efficacy, usually of a surrogate end point, are the goals. Similarly, Phase II and III trials have been combined into a single large Phase II/III trial. In this design, the study begins with several doses of the drug being evaluated, but at some point in the study a single dose is selected for completion of the trial while enrollment in other arms is terminated.

Table 1 Comparison of Phase II and III Studies

	Phase II studies	Phase III studies
Population	Narrow	Broad
Exclusion criteria	Many	Fewer
End points	Surrogate	Mortality of composite
Size	Dozens to hundreds	Hundreds to thousands
Safety	Common events captured	Uncommon events captured
Duration	Weeks to months	Months to years
Dose-response analysis	Yes	Occasionally
Placebo	Yes	Yes; occasionally with active control

VI. SELECTION OF END POINTS

In any clinical trial, the selection of the most appropriate outcome measure is critical. The initial choice usually hinges around selecting surrogate markers of biological activity or true measures of clinical efficacy (6). A surrogate end point is a measurable quantity, salutary changes in which are expected to be mirrored by changes in clinical outcomes. For example, in a trial of an agent that lowers cholesterol, changes in cholesterol values might be selected as a surrogate end point or reduction in stroke, myocardial infarction, or death might be the clinically relevant primary end points. Obviously, fewer patients are required to demonstrate statistically significant reductions in cholesterol than are required to demonstrate reductions in the harder clinical end points. The risk of using surrogate end points was exemplified in the Cardiac Arrhythmia Suppression Trial (CAST) (7) in which reduction in ventricular ectopy was a surrogate end point used to evaluate antiarrhythmic agents. These agents did suppress arrhythmias but resulted in an increased mortality in the patients who received them. Thus, the validity of surrogates must always be questioned when used as an end point. Prentice has suggested two conditions a surrogate must meet to be considered a valid end point. First, a test of the null hypothesis of no relationship to the treatment group must also be a valid test of the null hypothesis on the basis of the true end point. Second, a surrogate must fully capture a treatment's net effect on the clinical end point when the net effect is the aggregate effect that accounts for all mechanisms of action (6).

True measures of clinical efficacy include death as a solitary end point or the combination of death and a composite of other nonfatal end points. The rationale for the use of composite end points includes statistical consideration, pathophysiology, and the need to evaluate possible clinical benefits of treatment other than reduction in mortality. The statistical rational is related to sample size. The more end points evaluated, the smaller the sample size or the shorter the duration of the trial needs to be. Pathophysiologically, a reduction in certain nonfatal events such as myocardial infarction or stroke may ultimately translate into reduction in mortality. However, the mortality reduction may not be appreciated during the conduct of the original trial. Finally, use of a composite end point allows a broader view of the net clinical benefit of a treatment. Such benefits of interest may include significant improvements in quality of life or reduction in health care costs. However, from the patient's perspective, reduction in mortality is the most important goal of treatment and perhaps should not be weighed equally with prevention of a hospital admission. Most studies do not differentially weight the individual components of composite end points. Regardless, two conditions should be met to use composite end points. First, occurrence of the nonfatal components must have an adverse effect on mortality. Second, therapies that improve the nonfatal end points must also improve mortality (8).

Although death from any cause is easy to define, cardiovascular death, coronary death, and other nonfatal components of composite end points are clinical events and diagnoses, the definitions of which may vary from country to country, institution to institution, or even investigator to investigator. Such variations in definition, if allowed, could introduce bias into the trial. Thus, these end points must be rigorously defined before the trial begins. For example, death from coronary heart disease has been defined as sudden deaths, deaths associated with myocardial infarction, death caused by congestive heart failure, and death caused by complication of an invasive procedure. However, even the components of the definition require defining to ensure informity of event reporting. Ideally, an events commmmittee should be convened to adjudicate both fatal and nonfatal end points.

VII. SAMPLE SIZE CONSIDERATIONS

The sample size required to demonstrate a treatment effect depends on the estimated rate of the end point in the untreated or placebo-treated population, the estimated impact of the treatment on reducing this rate and the power, or statistical precision that one desires to conclude a treatment benefit unrelated to chance. The mortality in cholesterol-lowering trials enrolling patients without prior plaque rupture event (primary prevention) is very low, on the order of 1% annually. Mortality in secondary prevention trials consisting of patients who have had a prior plaque rupture event remains relatively low, ranging from 3% to 10% annually. Adequate power to detect very optimistic treatment effects such as a 50% reduction in clinical events rates requires several hundred to several thousand patients in each arm, depending on the event rate (Table 2). Detection of more realistic benefits on the order of a 20% to 30% reduction in events requires thousands of patients. Because agents that effect plaque stabilization would be expected to reduce myocardial infarction and admission for unstable angina, as well as death, the inclusion of these nonfatal clinical end points would increase the event rate and reduce the sample size.

For example, in the primary prevention Air Force/Texas Coronary Atherosclerosis Prevention Study (AFCAPS/TEXCAPS) of lovastatin, a composite end point of first acute coronary event consisting of fatal or nonfatal myocardial infarction, unstable angina, or sudden death was used (9). This was the first primary prevention study that included unstable angina in a composite end point. After 5.2 years of follow-up, only 5.5% of patients in the placebo group had a first acute coronary event. In contrast, the Veterans Affairs Cooperative Studies Program High-Density Lipoprotein Cholesterol Intervention Trial (VA-HIT) enrolled men with a history of prior myocardial infarction, angina with documented ischemia, coronary revascularization, or angiographic evidence of a stenosis of

Table 2 Sample Sizes Required to Demonstrate Event Reductions of Various Magnitudes

Event rate-placebo (%)	% reduction in treatment arm (%)	Sample size in each arm (power, 0.90)	Sample size in each arm (power, 0.80)
5	50	1291	984
	40	2115	1605
	30	3931	2970
10	50	621	474
	40	1014	771
	30	1881	1422
15	50	398	304
	40	648	493
	30	1197	906
20	50	286	219
	40	464	354
	30	855	647

greater than 50% and randomized them to gemfibrozil or placebo (10). In this secondary prevention study, the primary end point was nonfatal myocardial infarction or death from coronary heart disease. Over a mean follow-up of 5.1 years, 21.7% of placebo-treated patients had a primary end point. If stroke was added to the composite, the event rate increased to 26% or approximately 5% annually. Of note, 35.8% of placebo-treated patients required hospitalization for unstable angina. Thus, as many as 62% of placebo-treated patients may have had nonfatal myocardial infarction, death from coronary heart disease, stroke, or unstable angina over the 5.1-year period. It is likely that the actual event rate is lower, because individual patients probably had more than one end point. Another secondary prevention study compared various warfarin doses with aspirin among patients who had had a myocardial infarction (11). A composite outcome consisting of nonfatal myocardial infarction, nonfatal ischemic stroke, and cardiovascular death was experienced at an annualized event rate of 8.6% in aspirin-treated patients. When all-cause mortality, silent infarction, unstable angina requiring hospitalization, transient ischemic attack, and systemic embolization were added to the original composite end points, the annualized event rate increased to 24%. Thus, it seems that on the basis of the data from a number of studies (the annual rate of a composite end point consisting of death, nonfatal myocardial infarction, ischemic stroke, and unstable angina—all consequences of cardiovascular plaque rupture—would be 7–15% in placebo-treated patients in a secondary prevention trial (10–14) (Table 3). Assuming an annual plaque rupture event rate of 10%,

Table 3 Annualized Rate of Plaque Rupture–Related End Points in Primary and
Secondary Prevention Trials

Trial	Type of trial	N	Total death (%)	CV death (%)	CHD death (%)	Non-fatal MI (%)	Stroke/ TIA (%)	Unstable angina (%)	Total[a] (%)
AFCAPS[9]	1^0	3301	—	0.15	0.1	—	—	0.5	0.65
WOSCOPS[15]	1^0	3293	0.84	0.47	0.35	1.3	0.32	—	2.5
4S[12]	2^0	2223	2.1	1.7	—	4.2	0.80	—	7.1
CARE[13]	2^0	2078	1.9	—	1.1	1.7	0.76	3.5	7.9
CARS[11]	2^0	3393	2.5	2.1	—	5.6	0.52	—	8.6
LIPID[14]	2^0	4502	2.3	1.6	1.4	1.2	0.74	4.0	8.2
VA-HIT[10]	2^0	1267	3.4	—	1.8	2.8	2.0	7.0	15.2

Abbreviations: AFCAPS = Air Force Texas Coronary Atherosclerosis Prevention Study; WOSCOPS
= West of Scotland Prevention Study; 4S = Scandinavian Simvastatin Survival Study; CARE =
Cholesterol and Recurrent Events Trial Investigators; CARS = Coumadin Aspirin Reinfarction
Study; LIPID = the Long-Term Intervention with Pravastatin in Ischaemic Disease Trial; VA-HIT
= Veterans Affairs Cooperative Studies Program High-Density Lipoprotein Cholesterol Intervention
Trial; CV = cardiovascular; CHD = coronary heart disease; MI = myocardial infarction; TIA =
transient ischemic attack.
[a] If multiple definitions of mortality end points are presented, the one with the greatest incidence
was used to calculate the total.

a 2-year study designed to detect a 30% reduction in events with a power of 0.90
would require 855 patients in both the treatment and placebo groups. It must be
borne in mind that many patients eligible for secondary prevention studies will
already be on a statin and thus will have 25% to 33% lower event rates because
of plaque stabilization achieved by cholesterol lowering. Thus, the sample size
will have to be increased accordingly. For a primary prevention trial, where the
annual rate of plaque rupture events is approximately 1%, a 5-year study with
a power of 0.90 to detect a 30% reduction in end points would require 3931
patients.

VIII.   TRIAL DURATION

In a chronic condition such as coronary artery disease, events continue to accure
in the population at risk over time. Thus the duration of a trial is, again, a function
of the frequency of end points and the initial sample size. Trial duration might
also be influenced by the proposed mechanism of action of a plaque-stabilizing
agent. If continuous exposure of the patient to the drug is required to effect plaque

stabilization (such as statin), then the drug should be administered for the duration of the trial. If the mechanism of benefit of a therapeutic agent (such as an antibiotic) is achieved after a brief exposure or there may be toxicity associated with long-term treatment, then the drug may be administered for a shorter duration than the trial. Follow-up of patients treated with active drug after they are taken off the drug may give insight into the mechanism and duration of benefit, if any.

IX. CONCLUSIONS

Following established principles of clinical trial design, the efficacy of new inhibitors of plaque rupture can be accurately determined. End points should reflect the clinical syndromes caused by plaque rupture including sudden death, fatal and nonfatal myocardial infarction, unstable angina and ischemic stroke. Because of the increased freqency of these events in populations with established coronary artery disease, secondary prevention studies will be able to be completed more expeditiously than primary prevention studies.

REFERENCES

1. Collins R, McMahon S. Reliable assessment of the effect of treatment on mortality and major morbidity. Lancet 2001;357:373–380.
2. ISIS-2 (Second International Study of Infarct Survival) Collaborative Group. Randomised trial of intravenous streptokinase, oral aspirin, both or neither among 17 187 cases of suspected acute myocardial infarction: ISIS-2. Lancet 1988;1:397–402.
3. Sleight P. Debate: subgroup analyses in clinical trials–fun to look at, but don't believe them. Curr. Control Trials Cardiovasc Med 2000;1:25–27.
4. Temple R. Current definitions of phases of investigation and the role of the FDA in the conduct of clinical trials. Am Heart J 2000;139.S133–S15.
5. Yusuf S. Challenges in the conduct and interpretation of Phase II (pilot) randomized trials. Am Heart J 2000;129:S136–S142.
6. Fleming TR. Surrogate end points in cardiovascular disease trials. Am Heart J 2000; 139:S193–S196.
7. Echt DS, Liebson PR, Mitchell LB, Peters RW, Obias-Manno D, Barker AH, Arendsberg D, Baker A, Friedman L, Greene HL, Huther ML, Richardson DW. Mortality and morbidity in patients receiving encainide, flecainide, or placebo. The Cardiac Arrhythmia Suppression Trial. N Engl J Med 1991;324:781–788.
8. Cannon CP. Clinical perspectives on the use of composite endpoints. Controlled Clin Trials 1997;18:517–529.
9. Downs JR, Clearfield M, Weis S, Whitney E, Shapiro DR, Beere PA, Langendorfer A, Stein EA, Kruyer W, Gotto Jr. AM. Primary prevention of acute coronary events with lovastatin in men and women with average cholesterol levels. JAMA 1998; 279:1615–1622.

10. Rubins HB, Robins SJ, Collins D, Fye CL, Anderson JW, Elam MB, Faas FH, Linares E, Schaefer EJ, Schectman G, Wilt TJ, Wittes J. Gemfibrozil for the secondary prevention of coronary heart disease in men with low levels of high-density lipoprotein cholesterol. N Engl J Med 1999;341:410–418.

11. Coumadin Aspirin Reinfarction (CARS) Investigators. Randomised double-blind trial of fixed low-dose warfarin with aspirin after myocardial infarction.

12. Scandinavian Simvastatin Survival Study Group. Randomised trial of cholesterol lowering in 444 patients with coronary heart disease: the Scandinavian Simvastatin Survival Study (4S). Lancet 1994;344:1383–1389.

13. Sacks FM, Pfeffer MA, Moye LA, Rouleau JL, Rutherford JD, Cole TG, Brown L, Warnica JW, Arnold JMO, Wun C-C, Davis BR, Braunwald E for the Cholesterol and Recurrent Events Trial Investigators. The effect of pravastatin on coronary events after myocardial infarction in patients with average cholesterol levels. N Engl J Med 1996;335:1001–1009.

14. The Long-Term Intervention with Pravastatin in Ischaemic Heart Disease (LIPID) Study Group. Prevention of cardiovascular events and death with pravastatin in patients with coronary heart disease and a broad range of initial cholesterol levels. N Engl J Med 1996;339:1349–1357.

15. Shepherd J, Cobbe SM, Ford I, Isles CG, Lorimer AR, MacFarlane PW, McKillop JH, Packard CJ. Prevention of coronary heart disease in men with hypercholesterolemia. West of Scotland Coronary Prevention Study Group. N Engl J Med 1995;333:1301–1317.

19
The Relationship Between Cholesterol, Plaque Rupture, and Plaque Stabilization

Babak A. Vakili and David L. Brown
Albert Einstein College of Medicine and Montefiore Medical Center, Bronx, New York

I. INTRODUCTION

The relationship between cholesterol and mortality from cardiovascular disease (CVD) is well established. However, it is not as well appreciated that the increased mortality associated with elevations in the serum cholesterol level is related to an increase in plaque rupture–related events: unstable angina, fatal and nonfatal myocardial infarction (MI), and sudden ischemic cardiac death. Lowering of serum cholesterol levels, whether through diet or medications, reduces mortality from CVD through an ill-defined process known as plaque stabilization. In this chapter we review the epidemiological data linking hyperlipidemia to cardiovascular events, the evidence supporting the efficacy of lipid lowering in reducing plaque rupture–related events in patients with and without established coronary artery disease (CAD) and finally, the proposed mechanisms by which lipid lowering may stabilize the vulnerable plaque.

II. HISTORICAL PERSPECTIVE AND EPIDEMIOLOGICAL STUDIES

Cholesterol in human blood was first demonstrated by Lecanu in 1838, and Vogel in 1843 confirmed its presence in atherosclerotic plaque (1). By the end of the

19th century, a large body of evidence had accumulated linking hyperlipidemic states with CVD. In 1889, Lenzen and Knauss described an 11-year-old girl with xanthomata who at autopsy was found to have xanthomatous involvement of the mitral valve, aorta, and the coronary arteries (2). In 1938, Thannhauser and Magendantz further solidified the association between hypercholesterolemia and xanthomatous vascular disease, and Müller described these patients as having an increased prevalence of premature atherosclerosis and MI (3, 4). These observations, among others, provided the foundation on which future animal and human studies evaluating the relationship between hypercholesterolemia and CVD were based.

Since 1949, the Framingham Heart Study (FHS) has provided continuous epidemiological data on a large cohort of men and women free of CAD at baseline and has contributed substantially to our knowledge of CAD. In 1971, the Framingham investigators reported a significant correlation between total serum cholesterol and the development of CAD in 2282 men and 2845 women followed over a 14-year period (5). The relative risk of reinfarction, coronary mortality, and total mortality were 3.8-, 2.6- and 1.9-fold higher in individuals with serum cholesterol levels >275 mg/dl compared with those with levels <200 mg/dl (6). Similarly, low levels of serum cholesterol were associated with low rates of CAD in this cohort. Although there was a consistent graded relationship between cholesterol and risk of CAD, for the individual patient this risk was not as clear. Figure 1 demonstrates total cholesterol distribution curves for men who developed CAD or those remaining CAD-free in the first 16 years of the FHS (7). Although a shift toward higher cholesterol levels is evident in patients with CAD, there remains a substantial overlap between the two groups. Thus, for the individual patient, cholesterol level alone is not an accurate prognostic marker for the development of CAD (1, 8).

In 1978, the relation between baseline fasting cholesterol levels and subsequent cardiovascular morbidity and mortality was reported in 2789 men with a history of MI enrolled in the placebo arm of the Coronary Drug Project (CDP) (9). Serum cholesterol level was significantly related to all cardiovascular morbid and mortal end points. These data for the first time indicated the possibility of improving prognosis in patients after MI through cholesterol reduction and the importance of preventing the first coronary event.

In the Multiple Risk Factor Intervention Trial (MRFIT), 361,662 men aged 35 to 57 were screened during a 2-year period beginning in 1973. In 1986, the 6-year follow-up of MRFIT was reported, and the age-adjusted CAD death rate was directly proportional to total serum cholesterol levels (Fig. 2) (10). Total mortality was also increased at serum cholesterol levels >200 mg/dl. Between a cholesterol level of 200 mg/dl and 240 mg/dl, there was a linear relationship with death from CAD, which became exponential at cholesterol levels >240 mg/dl (10). There was a fourfold increase in the risk of CAD death among patients

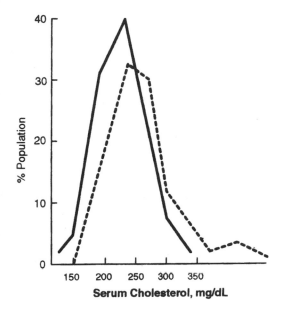

Figure 1   Total cholesterol distribution curves for men having coronary artery disease develop or remaining free of coronary artery disease in the first 16 years of the Framingham study. Dashed line = suffered heart attack; solid line = did not suffer heart attack. (Reprinted with permission from Can J Cardiol).

in the top 10% of serum cholesterol compared with those in the bottom 10% (10). In patients recovering from MI, a high serum cholesterol level was associated with an increase in reinfarction, death from CAD, and all-cause mortality (11).

In addition to the aforementioned studies, numerous other epidemiological studies have confirmed a strong relationship between high serum cholesterol levels and CAD and have further expanded these findings to other segments of the population, including various ethnic groups (1, 12), women (13–16), the elderly (17–20), the young (21), African-Americans, and patients with diabetes mellitus (22, 23).

III. PRIMARY PREVENTION TRIALS

Primary prevention refers to an intervention on patients at risk for the development of CAD but who have not yet had overt manifestations of disease develop. These trials are presented in Table 1 and described in the following. The World

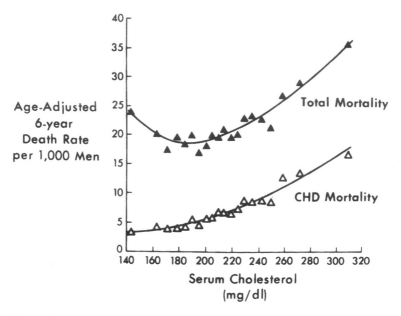

Figure 2 Age-adjusted 6-year coronary heart disease (CHD) and total mortality per 1000 men screened for MRFIT according to serum cholesterol. (Reprinted with permission from Lancet).

Health Organization (WHO) cooperative trial was started in 1965 to test the hypothesis that lowering cholesterol can reduce the incidence of CAD in middle-aged men without previous heart disease (24). In this double-blind study, 15,745 men aged 35 to 59 with elevated cholesterol were randomly assigned to clofibrate or placebo and followed for 5.3 years. There was a 9% reduction in total cholesterol levels in the treatment group and a 25% reduction in nonfatal MI. Of concern, there were 47% more deaths in the clofibrate group. The investigators concluded, "Clofibrate . . . cannot be recommended as a lipid lowering drug for community-wide primary prevention of ischemic heart disease." During the 7.9 years of follow-up after the trial had ended, a 5% increase in mortality was observed in the control group compared with the treatment group (25). Thus, the excess mortality in the clofibrate-treated group did not persist after the end of treatment and was due to a wide variety of causes other than CAD, including cancer of the gastrointestinal tract (25). The increase in noncoronary mortality in the WHO study set back progress in this field for many years by raising concerns about low cholesterol levels increasing mortality and possibly clofibrate-induced drug toxicity as a cause for the increase in mortality observed during the trial period (26).

Table 1 Results of Major Primary Prevention Trials of Cholesterol Modification

Study (year, reference)	N	Gender	Intervention	Duration (yr)	End point in treatment group
WHO (1978; 24)	15,745	Men	Clofibrate	5.3	25% reduction in nonfatal MI 47% higher mortality in treatment group
Oslo Study (1981; 27)	1,232	Men	Diet + smoking cessation	5	47% fewer fatal, nonfatal MI and sudden death
CPPT (1984; 28)	3,806	Men	Cholestyramine	7	19% fewer nonfatal MI 24% reduction in death from CVD
Helsinki Heart Study (1988; 31)	4,081	Men	Gemfibrizol	5	34% fewer deaths from nonfatal MI, fatal MI and coronary death
WOSCOPS (1995; 32)	6,595	Men	Pravastatin	4.9	22% lower all cause mortality 31% reduction in nonfatal MI 28% fewer coronary deaths 33% lower major coronary events
AFCAPS/TexCAPS (1998; 34)	6.605	Men and women	Lovastatin	5.2	37% lower incidence of fatal and nonfatal MI, UA or sudden cardiac death 40% fewer MI 32% fewer UA

MI, myocardial infarction; CVD, cardiovascular disease; UA, unstable angina; WHO, World Health Organization Cooperative Trial of the Prevention of Ischemic Heart Disease; CPPT, Lipid Research Clinics Coronary Primary Prevention Trial; WOSCOPS, The West of Scotland Coronary Prevention Study; AFCAPS/TexCAPS, The Air Force/Texas Coronary Atherosclerosis Prevention Study.

In the Oslo Study 16,202 men, aged 40 to 49 years, were screened for coronary risk factors. Of these, 1232 healthy, normotensive men at high risk of CAD were selected for a 5-year randomized trial to show whether lowering of serum lipids (with diet alone) and cessation of smoking could reduce the incidence of CAD. In the intervention group, total serum cholesterol was lowered by 13%, resulting in a 47% lower incidence of fatal and nonfatal MI and sudden death compared with the control group (27).

In the Lipid Research Clinics Coronary Primary Prevention Trial (CPPT), 3806 middle-aged men were randomly assigned to dietary modification with either placebo or cholestyramine and followed for 7 years (28). The combination of diet and cholestyramine reduced total and low-density lipoprotein (LDL) cholesterol levels by 11.8% and 18.9%, respectively, compared with reductions of 5.0% and 8.6% in the placebo arm. The cholestyramine group had 19% fewer nonfatal MIs and a 24% reduction in deaths from CVD than the placebo group. Patients who took the full dose of the medication reduced their serum cholesterol levels by 25% and lowered their coronary event rate by 50% compared with placebo. The results from the CPPT and Framingham studies together suggest that a 1% reduction in total serum cholesterol translates into an approximate 2% to 3% reduction in CAD risk (29, 30).

The Helsinki Heart Study randomly assigned 4081 men, aged 40 to 55, to treatment with gemfibrozil or placebo (31). Treatment with gemfibrozil resulted in 10% reduction in total cholesterol, 11% reduction in LDL cholesterol and an 11% rise in high-density lipoprotein (HDL) levels. There were 34% fewer coronary events (death from cardiac disease, nonfatal MI, and fatal MI) in the treatment group compared with the placebo group over the 5-year study (31). The results of the Helsinki Heart Study first demonstrated the additional benefit in risk reduction through raising HDL cholesterol levels.

The West of Scotland Coronary Prevention Study (WOSCOPS) randomly assigned 6595 men without a history of CAD to pravastatin or placebo (32). Treatment with pravastatin was associated with 22% reduction in all cause mortality, 31% reduction in the risk of nonfatal MI, and 28% reduction in CAD death after an average follow-up of 4.9 years (32). The number of patients needed to be treated per year to prevent a single fatal or nonfatal coronary event in this study was 217 (33).

The first primary prevention trial to include both men and women was the Air Force/Texas Coronary Atherosclerosis Prevention Study (AFCAPS/TexCAPS), which randomly assigned 6605 men and women without history of CAD to lovastatin or placebo with the goal of achieving an LDL cholesterol level of less than 110 mg/dl (34). After 5.2 years of follow-up, LDL cholesterol was reduced 25%, whereas HDL levels rose 6% in the treatment group compared with the placebo group. This trial was also the first to use a composite end point consisting entirely of coronary plaque rupture events, referred to as major acute coronary events. The incidence of a first major acute coronary event (fatal and nonfatal MI, unstable angina, and sudden cardiac death) was reduced 37% in the lovastatin group compared with the placebo group (34). There were 40% fewer MIs, and the incidence of unstable angina was reduced by 32% in the treatment group. The unique contribution of this trial was to demonstrate the benefit of treatment in a low- to moderate-risk population with average cholesterol and LDL levels and a below-average HDL concentration. The number of patients needed to treat to prevent a single fatal or nonfatal coronary event in this study was 256 (33).

In summary, the primary prevention trials have demonstrated that first coronary plaque rupture events can be reduced by lowering cholesterol levels in patients with elevated cholesterol. Because the event rate in these patients is low, large numbers of patients require treatment to prevent a plaque rupture event.

IV. SECONDARY PREVENTION TRIALS

In secondary prevention trials (Table 2), treatment is initiated in higher risk patients who have already had a plaque rupture event, usually a MI. For example, the Coronary Drug Project (CDP) was a randomized, placebo-controlled, double-blind study of 8341 men with prior MI conducted between 1969 and 1975 (35). After 6 years of follow-up, treatment with clofibrate and niacin lowered total cholesterol by 6% and 10%, respectively. Men in the treatment group had 29% fewer heart attacks than those in the placebo arm (35). Death from CVD and nonfatal MI was reduced by 9% with clofibrate and 15% with niacin (35, 36). At 15 years of follow-up, all-cause mortality in the niacin group was 11% lower than in the placebo group (37).

In the Stockholm Ischemic Heart Disease Study, 555 patients with history of MI were randomly assigned to lipid lowering with a combination of clofibrate and niacin and compared with placebo (38). At the end of the 5-year study period, serum cholesterol and triglyceride levels in the treatment group were lowered by 13% and 19%, respectively. Total mortality was reduced by 26% in the treatment group, and CAD mortality was reduced by 36% (38). In the subset of patients who had a lowering of the serum triglyceride levels by 30% or more, CAD mortality was reduced by 60% (38).

In the Program on the Surgical Control of the Hyperlipidemias (POSCH), 838 men and women with a history of MI were randomly assigned to treatment with partial ileal bypass surgery plus dietary counseling or to dietary counseling alone (39). At 5 years, total cholesterol levels were reduced by 23%, and LDL cholesterol was reduced by 38% in the surgical group compared with the control group. There were 27% fewer CAD-related deaths and 35% fewer total cardiac events in the surgical group.

Table 2 Results of Major Secondary Prevention Trials of Cholesterol Modification

Study (year, reference)	N	Gender	Intervention	Duration (yr)	End point in treatment group
CDP (1975; 35)	8,341	Men	Niacin; clofibrate	6	15% lower coronary death (niacin arm) 9% lower coronary death (clofibrate arm)
Stockholm Study (1988; 38)	555	Men and women	Clofibrate and nicotinic acid	5	36% lower coronary deaths 26% lower all-cause mortality
POSCH (1990; 39)	838	Men and women	Partial ileal bypass	5	27% lower coronary deaths 35% lower total cardiac events
4S (1994; 40, 42)	4,444	Men and women	Simvastatin	5.4	30% lower all-cause mortality 42% lower coronary death 37% lower nonfatal MI 30% lower stroke rate 34% lower major coronary events
CARE (1996; 43)	4,159	Men and women	Pravastatin	5	19% lower coronary death 25% lower fatal/nonfatal MI 24% lower major coronary events 26% lower need for CABG surgery 31% lower stroke rate
LIPID (1998; 44)	9,014	Men and women	Pravastatin	6.1	22% lower all-cause mortality 24% lower coronary deaths 23% lower major coronary events 19% lower rate of stroke

MACE, major adverse coronary events; CABG, coronary artery bypass graft; CDP, Coronary Drug Project; Stockholm Study, The Stockholm Ischemic Heart Disease Study; POSCH, The Program on the Surgical Control of the Hyperlipidemias; 4S, The Scandinavian Simvastatin Survival Study; CARE, The Cholesterol and Recurrent Events Trial; LIPID, The Long-Term Intervention with Pravastatin in Ischemic Disease Study.

In the Scandinavian Simvastatin Survival Study (4S), 4444 men and women with a history of angina pectoris or MI were randomly assigned to treatment with simvastatin or placebo. In the treatment group, total and LDL cholesterol levels were reduced by 25% and 35%, respectively, and there was an 8% rise in HDL cholesterol levels (40). Treatment with simvastatin reduced all-cause mortality by 30% at 5.4 years, coronary death by 42%, and nonfatal MI by 37% (40). Stroke rate in the treatment group was reduced by 30%. From this study, it was estimated that each 1% reduction in LDL cholesterol reduces major coronary event risk by 1.7% (41). Reflecting the higher risk population in secondary prevention trials, the number of patients needed to treat per year to prevent a single fatal or nonfatal coronary event in this study was 63 (33).

Two-year follow-up of the 4S study, bringing the median total follow-up to 7.4 years, revealed that all-cause mortality continued to remain significantly lower in the simvastatin group (11.5%) compared with the placebo group (15.9%) (42). In addition, the numbers of noncardiovascular and other deaths, including cancer, were similar in both groups (42).

The Cholesterol and Recurrent Events (CARE) trial was a randomized, double-blind, placebo-controlled trial of pravastatin in 4159 men and women with a history of MI, total cholesterol levels <240 mg/dl, and LDL levels between 115 and 174 mg/dl (43). After 5 years, there was a 19% reduction in coronary death rate, 25% lower incidence of nonfatal and fatal MI, 24% reduction in the combined cardiac events, and a 26% reduction in the need for coronary bypass surgery. Stroke rate in the treatment group was reduced by 31%. The number needed to treat per year to prevent a single fatal or nonfatal coronary event in this study was 167 (33).

The Long-term Intervention with Pravastatin in Ischemic Disease (LIPID) study, the largest double-blind, randomized, placebo-controlled secondary prevention trial to date, compared treatment with pravastatin with placebo in 9014 men and women with history of MI or unstable angina. After 6.1 years of follow-up, all-cause and coronary mortality rates were reduced by 22% and 24%, respectively, in the treatment group (44). Stroke rate was decreased 19% in the treatment group.

V. META-ANALYSIS OF PRIMARY AND SECONDARY PREVENTION TRIALS

A meta-analysis of 22 primary and secondary prevention trials, involving 40,000 patients with a 4-year follow-up period, found an average reduction in serum cholesterol level of 10% in the treatment group (45). This resulted in a 20% reduction in mortality from cardiac disease and a 17% reduction in the incidence of MI (45). In another meta-analysis by Law et al. (46), a 10% reduction in cholesterol was shown to lower the risk of ischemic heart disease by 50% at age 40 and by 20% at age 70 (46). A third meta-analysis of five primary and secondary prevention trials, which included 30,817 patients with a mean duration of treatment of 5.4 years, was recently reported (47). Treatment with statins reduced total cholesterol by 20%, LDL cholesterol by 28%, triglycerides by 13%, and resulted in a 5% increase in HDL cholesterol levels. Major coronary events were reduced by 31%, and all-cause mortality was reduced by 21%. The risk reduction in major coronary events was similar for women and men (29% vs. 31%, respectively) and for patients older than or younger than 65 years of age (32% vs. 31%, respectively) (47).

VI. ANGIOGRAPHIC TRIALS

In response to the belief that lipid lowering was reducing coronary plaque rupture events by inducing regression of established atherosclerotic lesions, a number of trials were initiated using angiographic end points to assess the mechanism of benefit seen in the primary and secondary prevention studies (Table 3) (48–58). Treatment strategies in angiographic studies have ranged from cholesterol-binding resins to niacin to statins. Careful quantitative angiographic analysis was used to assess regression (reduction in percent or absolute diameter stenosis) or progression (increase in percent or absolute diameter stenosis) of individual atherosclerotic lesions. The lesion-based analysis allowed these trials to be completed with relatively few patients. Several representative trials are summarized in the following.

The National Heart, Lung and Blood Institute Type II (NHLBII) Coronary Intervention Study was a 5-year, double-blind, randomized study in 116 men with significantly elevated LDL cholesterol levels (48). This study was undertaken to compare the effects of diet versus diet plus cholestyramine on the progression of CAD. Atherosclerotic lesions progressed in 49% of the placebo-treated patients compared with 32% of the cholestyramine-treated patients. Approximately 7% of patients in both groups had either probable or definite lesion regression (48).

In the St. Thomas Atherosclerosis Regression Study (STARS), 90 men with angina or previous MI were randomly assigned to receive usual care, dietary intervention, or diet plus cholestyramine with angiography at baseline and 39 months (49). Progression of coronary narrowing occurred in 12% of the diet and cholestyramine group and 15% in the diet group as opposed to 46% of patients receiving usual care. Regression in coronary obstruction by plaque was demonstrated in 4% of patients in the usual care group, 33% in the diet and cholestyramine group, and 38% in the diet group. The mean absolute diameter of the diseased coronary segments studied decreased by 0.2 mm in controls, increased by

Table 3 Results of Major Angiographic Trials Involving Cholesterol Modification

Study (year, reference)	N	Duration (yr)	Control	Treatment	Clinical end point
NHLBII (1984; 48)	116	5	49% Progression 7.1% Regression	32% Progression 6.8% Regression	33% lower CV events
STARS (1992; 49)	90	3.3	46% Progression 11% Regression	Diet: 15% Progression 38% Regression Diet and cholestyramine: 12% Progression 33% Regression	Reduced CV events
FATS (1990; 50)	146	2.5	46% Progression 11% Regression	Lovastatin and colestipol: 21% Progression 32% Regression Niacin and colestipol: 25% Progression 39% Regression	Lovastatin and colestipol: 63% lower death, MI and TVR. Niacin and colestipol: 79% lower death, MI, and TVR.
REGRESS (1995; 51)	885	2	Diameter stenosis increased 0.1 mm	Diameter stenosis increased 0.06 mm	9% absolute lower CV events
CIS (1997; 53)	254	2.3	56% Progression 13% Regression	35% Progression 18% Regression	No significant difference in clinical end points
LCAS (1997; 54)	429	2.5	39% Progression 3% Regression	29% Progression 15% Regression	No significant difference in clinical end points

CV, cardiovascular; MI, myocardial infarction; TVR, target vessel revascularization; NHLBII, The National Heart, Lung and Blood Institute Type II Coronary Intervention Study; STARS, St. Thomas Atherosclerosis Regression Study; FATS, Familial Atherosclerosis Treatment Study; REGRESS, The Regression Growth Evaluation Statin Study; CIS, The Multicenter Coronary Intervention Study; LCAS, Lipoprotein and Coronary Atherosclerosis Study.

0.003 mm and 0.103 mm in the treatment groups. Both interventions significantly reduced the frequency of total cardiovascular events.

In the Familial Atherosclerosis Treatment Study (FATS) trial (50), 120 patients with apolipoprotein-B levels $\geq$ 125 mg/dl completed the 2.5-year double-blind study, which included quantitative angiography at baseline and after treatment. All patients were given dietary counseling and were randomly assigned to one of three treatments: lovastatin and colestipol, niacin and colestipol, or conventional therapy with placebo. In the conventional-therapy group, 46% of the patients had lesion progression, and 11% had lesion regression. Lesion progression was observed in 21% of patients who received lovastatin and colestipol and 25% of those who received niacin and colestipol. Lesion regression was noted in 32% of the lovastatin and colestipol group and in 39% of the niacin and colestipol group. Clinical events (death, MI, or revascularization for worsening symptoms) occurred in 19% of patients assigned to conventional therapy compared with 7% in the lovastatin and colestipol group and 4% in patients assigned to receive niacin and colestipol. Stenosis severity was reduced by an average of 0.3% and 1.1% in the lovastatin plus colestipol group and niacin plus colestipol groups, respectively, whereas it increased by an average of 2.0% in the placebo group. For the two treatment groups combined, there was a 73% reduction in clinical events compared with placebo group.

The Regression Growth Evaluation Statin Study (REGRESS), a double-blind placebo-controlled multicenter study, assessed the effects of 2 years of treatment with pravastatin on progression and regression of coronary atherosclerosis in 885 male patients with serum cholesterol levels between 155 mg/dl and 310 mg/dl (51). At the end of the follow-up period there was less progression of atherosclerosis and fewer plaque rupture events in the treatment group [11% of the pravastatin treated patients and 19% of the placebo patients experienced new cardiovascular events].

The Multicenter Coronary Intervention Study (CIS) was a randomized, double-blind, placebo-controlled study of the effects of simvastatin on progression of CAD in 254 men with documented CAD and hypercholesterolemia (53). After a follow-up of 2.3 years, lesion progression occurred in 35% of subjects in the treatment arm compared with 56% in the placebo arm. Lesion regression was noted in 18% of subjects in the treatment arm compared with 13% of the placebo arm.

In the Lipoprotein and Coronary Atherosclerosis Study (LCAS), 429 men and women aged 35 to 75 years with CAD and mean LDL values of 115 mg/dl to 190 mg/dl were randomly assigned to fluvastatin or placebo and followed for 2.5 years (54). Lesions progressed in 29% of the treatment arm compared with 39% in the placebo arm. Lesions regressed in 15% of the treatment arm compared with 8% in the placebo arm. Beneficial but not statistically significant trends in clinical event rates were observed.

As summarized in Table 3, plaque progression is reduced ~50% with lipid lowering therapy as compared to placebo. Plaque regression is reported in about 7 to 15% of patients in the placebo arm and is roughly doubled to 15 to 30% in patients receiving lipid-lowering therapy. The average reduction in percent diameter stenosis achieved by active treatment was 1 to 2%. Surprisingly, these small improvements in angiographic stenosis are accompanied by a disproportionately large reduction in plaque rupture events. These observations implicate plaque stabilization rather than lesion regression as the likely mechanism responsible for the clinical benefit obtained from lipid-lowering therapy. In addition, the reduction in plaque rupture events occurs earlier than the time needed for plaque regression, suggesting plaque stabilization is a relatively rapidly occurring phenomenon.

VII. PLAQUE-STABILIZING MECHANISMS OF CHOLESTEROL REDUCTION

Although reduction in plaque rupture events has been observed with all effective forms of lipid-lowering therapy, beneficial effects on plaque stabilization independent of lipid lowering have been attributed to the statin drug class. However, if reduction in plaque rupture events is plotted against the cholesterol reduction achieved by statin therapy, the relationship is linear but not horizontal as would be expected if all benefit was due to nonlipid lowering mechanisms (Fig. 3).

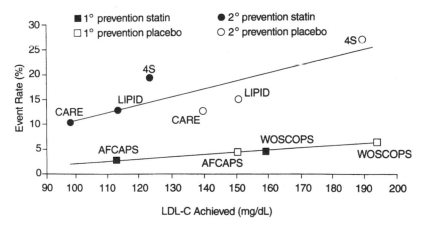

Figure 3 Relationship between low-density lipoprotein (LDL-C) levels and event rate in placebo-controlled secondary prevention trials. (Reprinted with permission from Am J Cardiol).

Table 4   Potential Mechanisms of Plaque Stabilization Achieved by Lipid Lowering

1. Depletion and physicochemical stability of lipid core
2. Increased fibrous cap stability
   a. Metalloproteinase inhibition
3. Anti-inflammatory effect
   a. Reduced endothelial-leukocyte interactions
   b. Reduced cytokine expression
   c. Reduced expression of major histocompatibility class II antigens by macrophages
4. Antithrombotic effect
   a. Improved platelet function
   b. Reduced tissue factor expression
   c. Decreased plasminogen activator inhibitor-1
5. Improvement of endothelial function

Thus, the predominant benefit of statin therapy seems to be mediated through the attainment of lower cholesterol levels. Nevertheless, in vitro and animal data suggest that there may also be synergistic beneficial effects of statins that are unrelated to lipid lowering. It must be emphasized that it is not proven that such effects are relevant in the intact human and that no conclusive data exist to suggest a cholesterol-independent effect of statins in humans. The potential plaque-stabilizing effects of cholesterol lowering are listed in Table 4 and discussed in the following.

VIII.   MODIFICATION OF PLAQUE STRUCTURE

As has been discussed in previous chapters, the vulnerable plaque tends to have a large lipid core covered by a thin fibrous cap. It is estimated that such plaques constitute about 15% of the total plaque burden (59). Because lesions, in general, do not regress significantly after lipid lowering, it is likely that lipid-lowering therapy structurally modifies this small but dangerous subgroup of lesions (59). By doing so, these lesions may be effectively stabilized, and the clinical event rate is accordingly decreased.

    Recent in-vitro and animal studies provide insight into the plaque-stabilizing changes achieved by lipid lowering. Specifically, cholesterol reduction has been associated with a diminution in extracellular lipid content and macrophage area. Macrophages that are resident in the atheroma synthesize and overexpress matrix metalloproteinase (MMP) enzymes, promoting destabilization and rupture of the atherosclerotic plaque by digesting the extracellular matrix and fibrous cap (60). Cholesterol reduction decreases expression of the collagenolytic enzyme

MMP-1 and reinforces the plaque's fibrous skeleton by preventing degradation of interstitial collagen (61, 62). These effects are manifested by an increase in the ratio of collagen area to macrophage area, which would tend to promote plaque stability.

IX. ANTITHROMBOTIC EFFECT

For plaque rupture to result in an acute ischemic event, thrombus must be able to form at the site of plaque rupture. Interventions that reduce the propensity for thrombus formation would be expected to ameliorate the clinical consequences of plaque rupture. Low-density lipoprotein augments platelet activation and increases platelet reactivity in patients with familial hypercholesterolemia, possibly by inhibition of the $Na+/H+$ antiport system (63). Thromboxane A_2 (TXA_2) biosynthesis is also increased in patients with hypercholesterolemia, leading to enhanced platelet thrombus formation in response to arterial injury. Cholesterol lowering causes significant reductions in TXA_2-mediated platelet aggregation in vivo, reduces serum fibrinogen and thrombin levels, decreases platelet aggregation and platelet-dependent thrombin generation, and reduces mural thrombus formation at both high and low shear rates (64–68). In patients with hypercholesterolemia, statins have been shown to increase the mean plasma concentration levels of tissue-type plasminogen activator while decreasing levels of plasminogen activator inhibitor-I and von Willebrand factor (69).

Tissue factor (TF) is a potent activator of the coagulation cascade, and TF antigen and activity are found in abundance in macrophages within human atherosclerotic plaques, as well as the lipid-rich plaque core (70,71). Statins inhibit TF expression in macrophages (72). Thus, cholesterol lowering has the potential to reduce acute coronary events despite plaque rupture by having a favorable impact on all phases of the coagulation process to limit thrombus formation and promote fibrinolysis (64).

X. ANTI-INFLAMMATORY EFFECT

An early step in atherogenesis involves monocyte adhesion to the endothelium followed by penetration into the subendothelial space. Ultimately, an inflammatory environment is established in which cytokines secreted by macrophages and T lymphocytes modify endothelial function, resulting in further recruitment of circulating monocytes that mature into resident macrophages with their matrix-degrading and prothrombotic phenotypes. The inflammatory nature of the atherosclerotic process is supported by the fact that high baseline C-reactive protein

(CRP) or elevated serum amyloid A (SAA) levels, both of which are markers of inflammation, are associated with an increased risk of coronary events.

In humans, statin treatment reduces CRP concentrations suggesting, but not proving, some direct anti-inflammatory effects of these drugs or of cholesterol reduction itself (73). In support of such a hypothesis, those patients with inflammation defined by elevated CRP or SAA levels receive more benefit from statins than those without inflammation (73, 74). Patients with severe coronary disease and the highest CRP levels receive the most benefit from statin therapy (75). In addition, the rate of plaque rupture events has been shown to be increased in patients with elevated baseline levels of CRP, and statin therapy may be effective in prevention of coronary events even among persons with relatively low lipid levels but with elevated levels of CRP (76).

Subjects with hypercholesterolemia have increased adhesiveness of their monocytes to endothelial cells in vitro, and this response is attenuated by cholesterol reduction. Specifically, in vitro and animal studies have shown that lipid lowering reduces monocyte CD11b expression and inhibits CD11b-dependent monocyte adhesion to endothelium and thereby lowers the number of plaque macrophages (62).

XI. ENDOTHELIAL DYSFUNCTION

The vasodilator function of vascular endothelium is impaired in hypercholesterolemia and atherosclerosis. Cholesterol lowering improves endothelium-dependent coronary artery vasomotion in response to intracoronary infusion of acetylcholine (77–79). Statins, by up-regulating endothelial nitric oxide synthase expression, augment nitric oxide–dependent vasodilator functions of the endothelium (80–82). That the benefits achieved by improving vasomotor function have some clinical significance is suggested by the fact that the improved coronary blood flow and vasodilatory response achieved by statin therapy reduces the number of ischemic episodes in patients with stable angina. In addition, single-photon emission computed tomography and positron emission tomography, after initiation of short-term statin therapy, have demonstrated improved myocardial perfusion in ischemic regions even before any anatomical regression of stenosis, suggesting that this improvement may be due to restoration of the nitric oxide–dependent vasodilatory functions of coronary endothelium (83, 84).

XII. SUMMARY

Elevations in cholesterol are strongly associated with the development of atherosclerotic plaque rupture events. Reduction of cholesterol reduces plaque rupture events without inducing significant regression of coronary arterial stenoses. The most likely mechanism by which lipid-lowering therapy reduces cardiovascular events is through prevention of progression and stabilization of the vulnerable atherosclerotic plaque. The mechanisms by which stabilization occurs are not completely understood but probably consist of a composite of the biochemical, mechanical, and biological sequelae of cholesterol reduction.

REFERENCES

1. Criqui MH, Golomb BA. Epidemiologic aspects of lipid abnormalities. Am J Med 1998; 105:48S–57S.
2. Lenzen G, Knauss K. Ueber Xanthoma multiplex planum, tuberosum, mollusciforms. Virchow's Arch Pathol Anat 1889; lxxvi:85.
3. Thannhauser SJ, Magendantz H. The different clinical groups of xanthomatous disease: a clinical physiological study of 22 cases. Ann Intern Med 1938; 11:1662–1746.
4. Muller C. Xanthomata, hypercholesterolemia, angina pectoris. Acta Med Scand 1938; suppl 89:75–84.
5. Kannel WB, Castelli WP, Gordon T, McNamara PM. Serum cholesterol, lipoproteins, and the risk of coronary heart disease. The Framingham study. Ann Intern Med 1971; 74:1–12.
6. Kannel WB, Castelli WP, Gordon T. Cholesterol in the prediction of atherosclerotic disease. New perspectives based on the Framingham study. Ann Intern Med 1979; 90:85–91.
7. Castelli WP. Cholesterol and lipids in the risk of coronary artery disease—The Framingham Heart Study. Can J Cardiol 1988; 4:5A–10A.
8. National Cholesterol Education Program. Second Report of the Expert Panel on Detection, Evaluation, and Treatment of High Blood Cholesterol in Adults (Adult Treatment Panel II). Circulation 1994; 89:1333–1445.
9. Natural history of myocardial infarction in the coronary drug project: long-term prognostic importance of serum lipid levels. Coronary Drug Project Research Group. Am J Cardiol 1978; 42:489–498.
10. Martin MJ, Hulley SB, Browner WS, Kuller LH, Wentworth D. Serum cholesterol, blood pressure, and mortality: implications from a cohort of 361,662 men. Lancet 1986; 2:933–936.
11. Wong ND, Wilson PW, Kannel WB. Serum cholesterol as a prognostic factor after myocardial infarction: the Framingham Study. Ann Intern Med 1991; 115:687–693.
12. Verschuren WM, Jacobs DR, Bloemberg BP, et al. Serum total cholesterol and long-term coronary heart disease mortality in different cultures. Twenty-five-year follow-up of the seven countries study. JAMA 1995; 274:131–136.
13. Isles CG, Hole DJ, Gillis CR, Hawthorne VM, Lever AF. Plasma cholesterol, coronary heart disease, and cancer in the Renfrew and Paisley survey. BMJ 1989; 298: 920–924.
14. Bengtsson C. Ischaemic heart disease in women. A study based on a randomized population sample of women and women with myocardial infarction in Goteborg, Sweden. Acta Medica Scandinavica 1973; 549:1–128.

15. Bush TL, Barrett-Connor E, Cowan LD, et al. Cardiovascular mortality and noncontraceptive use of estrogen in women: results from the Lipid Research Clinics Program Follow-up Study. Circulation 1987; 75:1102–1109.

16. Bush TL, Fried LP, Barrett-Connor E. Cholesterol, lipoproteins, and coronary heart disease in women. Clin Chem 1988; 34:B60–B70.

17. Aronow WS, Herzig AH, Etienne F, D'Alba P, Ronquillo J. 41-month follow-up of risk factors correlated with new coronary events in 708 elderly patients. J Am Ger Soc 1989; 37:501–506.

18. Barrett-Connor E. Hypercholesterolemia predicts early death from coronary heart disease in elderly men but not women. The Rancho Bernardo Study. Ann Epidemiol 1992; 2:77–83.

19. Benfante R, Reed D. Is elevated serum cholesterol level a risk factor for coronary heart disease in the elderly? JAMA 1990; 263:393–396.

20. Harris T, Cook EF, Kannel WB, Goldman L. Proportional hazards analysis of risk factors for coronary heart disease in individuals aged 65 or older. The Framingham Heart Study. J Am Ger Soc 1988; 36:1023–1028.

21. Klag MJ, Ford DE, Mead LA, et al. Serum cholesterol in young men and subsequent cardiovascular disease. NEJM 1993; 328:313–318.

22. Vaccaro O, Stamler J, Neaton JD. Sixteen-year coronary mortality in black and white men with diabetes screened for the Multiple Risk Factor Intervention Trial (MRFIT). Internat J Epidemiol 1998; 27:636–641.

23. Phillips AN, Shaper AG, Pocock SJ, Walker M, Macfarlane PW. The role of risk factors in heart attacks occurring in men with pre-existing ischaemic heart disease. BHJ 1988; 60:404–410.

24. A co-operative trial in the primary prevention of ischaemic heart disease using clofibrate. Report from the Committee of Principal Investigators. BHJ 1978; 40:1069–1118.

25. World Health Organization cooperative trial on primary prevention of ischaemic heart disease with clofibrate to lower serum cholesterol: final mortality follow-up. Report of the Committee of Principal Investigators. Lancet 1984; 2:600–604.

26. Steinberg D, Gotto AJ. Preventing coronary artery disease by lowering cholesterol levels: fifty years from bench to bedside. JAMA 1999; 282:2043–2050.

27. Hjermann I, Velve Byre K, Holme I, Leren P. Effect of diet and smoking intervention on the incidence of coronary heart disease. Report from the Oslo Study Group of a randomised trial in healthy men. Lancet 1981; 2:1303–1310.

28. The Lipid Research Clinics Coronary Primary Prevention Trial results. I. Reduction in incidence of coronary heart disease. JAMA 1984; 251:351–364.

29. LaRosa JC, Hunninghake D, Bush D, et al. The cholesterol facts. A summary of the evidence relating dietary fats, serum cholesterol, and coronary heart disease. A joint statement by the American Heart Association and the National Heart, Lung, and Blood Institute. The Task Force on Cholesterol Issues, American Heart Association. Circulation 1990; 81:1721–1733.

30. Anderson KM, Castelli WP, Levy D. Cholesterol and mortality. 30 years of follow-up from the Framingham study. JAMA 1987; 257:2176–2180.

31. Manninen V, Elo MO, Frick MH, et al. Lipid alterations and decline in the incidence of coronary heart disease in the Helsinki Heart Study. JAMA 1988; 260:641–651.

32. Shepherd J, Cobbe S, Ford I, et al. Prevention of coronary heart disease with pravastatin in men with hypercholesterolemia. West of Scotland Coronary Prevention Study Group. N Engl J Med 1995; 333:1301–1307.
33. Kumana C, Cheung B, Lauder I. Gauging the impact of statins using number needed to treat. JAMA 1999; 282:1899–1901.
34. Downs J, Clearfield M, Weis S, et al. Primary prevention of acute coronary events with lovastatin in men and women with average cholesterol levels: results of AFCAPS/TexCAPS. Air Force/Texas Coronary Atherosclerosis Prevention Study. JAMA 1998; 279:1615–1622.
35. Anonymous. Clofibrate and niacin in coronary heart disease. JAMA 1975; 231:360–381.
36. Canner PL, Halperin M. Implications of findings in the coronary drug project for secondary prevention trials in coronary heart disease. The coronary; drug project research group. Circulation 1981; 63:1342–1350.
37. Canner PL, Berge KG, Wenger NK, et al. Fifteen year mortality in Coronary Drug Project patients: long-term benefit with niacin. J Am Col Cardiol 1986; 8:1245–1255.
38. Carlson LA, Rosenhamer G. Reduction of mortality in the Stockholm Ischaemic Heart Disease Secondary Prevention Study by combined treatment with clofibrate and nicotinic acid. Acta Med Scand 1988; 223:405–418.
39. Buchwald H, Varco R, Matts J, et al. Effect of partial ileal bypass surgery on mortality and morbidity from coronary heart disease in patients with hypercholesterolemia. Report of the Program on the Surgical Control of the Hyperlipidemias (POSCH). N Engl J Med 1990; 323:946–955.
40. Randomised trial of cholesterol lowering in 4444 patients with coronary heart disease: the Scandinavian Simvastatin Survival Study (4S). Lancet 1994; 344:1383–1389.
41. Pedersen T, Olsson A, Faergeman O, et al. Lipoprotein changes and reduction in the incidence of major coronary heart disease events in the Scandinavian Simvastatin Survival Study (4S). Circulation 1998; 97:1453–1460.
42. Pedersen T, Wilhelmsen L, Faergeman O, et al. Follow-up study of patients randomized in the Scandinavian simvastatin survival study (4S) of cholesterol lowering. Am J Cardiol 2000; 86:257–262.
43. Sacks F, Pfeffer M, Moye L, et al. The effect of pravastatin on coronary events after myocardial infarction in patients with average cholesterol levels. Cholesterol and Recurrent Events Trial investigators. N Engl J Med 1996; 335:1001–1009.
44. Prevention of cardiovascular events and death with pravastatin in patients with coronary heart disease and a broad range of initial cholesterol levels. The Long-Term Intervention with Pravastatin in Ischaemic Disease (LIPID) Study Group. N Engl J Med 1998; 339:1349–1357.
45. Yusuf S, Wittes J, Friedman L. Overview of results of randomized clinical trials in heart disease. II. Unstable angina, heart failure, primary prevention with aspirin, and risk factor modification. JAMA 1988; 260:2259–2263.
46. Law M, Wald N, Thompson S. By how much and how quickly does reduction in serum cholesterol concentration lower risk of ischaemic heart disease? BMJ 1994; 308:367–372.

47. La Rosa J, He J, Vupputuri S. Effect of statins on risk of coronary disease: a meta-analysis of randomized controlled trials. JAMA 1999; 282:2340–2346.

48. Brensike J, Levy R, Kelsey S, et al. Effects of therapy with cholestyramine on progression of coronary arteriosclerosis: results of the NHLBI Type II Coronary Intervention Study. Circulation 1984; 69:313–324.

49. Watts G, Lewis B, Brunt J, et al. Effects on coronary artery disease of lipid-lowering diet, or diet plus cholestyramine, in the St Thomas' Atherosclerosis Regression Study (STARS). Lancet 1992; 339:563–569.

50. Brown G, Albers J, Fisher L, et al. Regression of coronary artery disease as a result of intensive lipid-lowering therapy in men with high levels of apolipoprotein B. N Engl J Med 1990; 323:1289–1298.

51. Jukema J, Bruschke A, van BA, et al. Effects of lipid lowering by pravastatin on progression and regression of coronary artery disease in symptomatic men with normal to moderately elevated serum cholesterol levels. The Regression Growth Evaluation Statin Study (REGRESS). Circulation 1995; 91:2528–2540.

52. Pitt B, Mancini G, Ellis S, Rosman H, Park J, McGovern M. Pravastatin limitation of atherosclerosis in the coronary arteries (PLAC I): reduction in atherosclerosis progression and clinical events. PLAC I investigation. J Am Col Cardiol 1995; 26: 1133–1139.

53. Bestehorn H, Rensing U, Roskamm H, et al. The effect of simvastatin on progression of coronary artery disease. The Multicenter Coronary Intervention Study (CIS). Eur Heart J 1997; 18:226–234.

54. Herd J, Ballantyne C, Farmer J, et al. Effects of fluvastatin on coronary atherosclerosis in patients with mild to moderate cholesterol elevations (Lipoprotein and Coronary Atherosclerosis Study [LCAS]). Am J Cardiol 1997; 80:278–286.

55. The effect of aggressive lowering of low-density lipoprotein cholesterol levels and low-dose anticoagulation on obstructive changes in saphenous-vein coronary-artery bypass grafts. The Post Coronary Artery Bypass Graft Trial Investigators. N Engl J Med 1997; 336:153–162.

56. Arntz H, Agrawal R, Wunderlich W, et al. Beneficial effects of pravastatin ($+/-$ colestyramine/niacin) initiated immediately after a coronary event (the randomized lipid-coronary artery disease). Am J Cardiol 2000; 86:1293–1298.

57. Effect of simvastatin on coronary atheroma: the Multicentre Anti-Atheroma Study (MAAS). Lancet 1994; 344:633–638.

58. Waters D, Higginson L, Gladstone P, et al. Effects of monotherapy with an HMG-CoA reductase inhibitor on the progression of coronary atherosclerosis as assessed by serial quantitative arteriography. The Canadian Coronary Atherosclerosis Intervention Trial. Circulation. 1994; 89:959–968.

59. Brown B, Zhao X, Sacco D, Albers J. Lipid lowering and plaque regression. New insights into prevention of plaque disruption and clinical events in coronary disease. Circulation 1993; 87:1781–1791.

60. Galis Z, Sukhova G, Lark M, Libby P. Increased expression of matrix metalloproteinases and matrix degrading activity in vulnerable regions of human atherosclerotic plaques. J Clin Invest 1994; 94:2493–2503.

61. Libby P, Aikawa M. New insights into plaque stabilization by lipid lowering. Drugs 1998; 56(suppl 1):9–13; discussion 33.

62. Weber C, Erl W, Weber K, Weber P. HMG-CoA reductase inhibitors decrease CD11b expression and CD11b-dependent adhesion of monocytes to endothelium and reduce increased adhesiveness of monocytes isolated from patients with hypercholesterolemia. J Am Col Cardiol 1997; 30:1212–1217.

63. Nofer J, Tepel M, Kehrel B, et al. Low-density lipoproteins inhibit the Na+/H+ antiport in human platelets. A novel mechanism enhancing platelet activity in hypercholesterolemia. Circulation 1997; 95:1370–1377.

64. Lacoste L, Lam J, Hung J, Letchacovski G, Solymoss C, Waters D. Hyperlipidemia and coronary disease. Correction of the increased thrombogenic potential with cholesterol reduction. Circulation 1995; 92:3172–3177.

65. Notarbartolo A, Davi G, Averna M, et al. Inhibition of thromboxane biosynthesis and platelet function by simvastatin in type IIa hypercholesterolemia. Arterioscler Thromb Vasc Biol 1995; 15:247–251.

66. Mayer J, Eller T, Brauer P, et al. Effects of long-term treatment with lovastatin on the clotting system and blood platelets. Ann Hematol 1992; 64:196–201.

67. Aoki I, Aoki N, Kawano K, et al. Platelet-dependent thrombin generation in patients with hyperlipidemia. J Am Col Cardiol 1997; 30:91–96.

68. Alfon J, Pueyo PC, Royo T, Badimon L. Effects of statins in thrombosis and aortic lesion development in a dyslipemic rabbit model. Thromb Haemost 1999; 81:822–827.

69. Wada H, Mori Y, Kaneko T, et al. Elevated plasma levels of vascular endothelial cell markers in patients with hypercholesterolemia. Am J Hematol 1993; 44:112–116.

70. Taubman M, Fallon J, Schecter A, et al. Tissue factor in the pathogenesis of atherosclerosis. Thromb Haemost 1997; 78:200–204.

71. Wilcox J, Smith K, Schwartz S, Gordon D. Localization of tissue factor in the normal vessel wall and in the atherosclerotic plaque. Proc Natl Acad Sci U S A 1989; 86: 2839–2843.

72. Colli S, Eligini S, Lalli M, Camera M, Paoletti R, Tremoli E. Vastatins inhibit tissue factor in cultured human macrophages. A novel mechanism of protection against atherothrombosis. Arterioscler Thromb Vasc Biol 1997; 17:265–272.

73. Ridker P, Rifai N, Pfeffer M, Sacks F, Braunwald E. Long-term effects of pravastatin on plasma concentration of C-reactive protein. The Cholesterol and Recurrent Events (CARE) Investigators. Circulation 1999; 100:230–235.

74. Ridker P, Rifai N, Pfeffer M, et al. Inflammation, pravastatin, and the risk of coronary events after myocardial infarction in patients with average cholesterol levels. Cholesterol and Recurrent Events (CARE) Investigators. Circulation 1998; 98:839–844.

75. Horne B, Muhlestein J, Carlquist J, et al. Statin therapy, lipid levels, C-reactive protein and the survival of patients with angiographically severe coronary artery disease. J Am Col Cardiol 2000; 36:1774–1780.

76. Ridker PM, Rifai N, Clearfield M, et al. Measurement of C-Reactive Protein for the Targeting of Statin Therapy in the Primary Prevention of Acute Coronary Events. N Engl J Med 2001; 344:1959–1965.

77. Anderson T, Meredith I, Yeung A, Frei B, Selwyn A, Ganz P. The effect of cholesterol-lowering and antioxidant therapy on endothelium-dependent coronary vasomotion. N Engl J Med 1995; 332:488–493.

78. Egashira K, Hirooka Y, Kai H, et al. Reduction in serum cholesterol with pravastatin improves endothelium-dependent coronary vasomotion in patients with hypercholesterolemia. Circulation 1994; 89:2519–2524.
79. Treasure C, Klein J, Weintraub W, et al. Beneficial effects of cholesterol-lowering therapy on the coronary endothelium in patients with coronary artery disease. N Engl J Med 1995; 332:481–487.
80. Laufs U, La FV, Plutzky J, Liao J. Upregulation of endothelial nitric oxide synthase by HMG CoA reductase inhibitors. Circulation 1998; 97:1129–1135.
81. Liao J, Shin W, Lee W, Clark S. Oxidized low-density lipoprotein decreases the expression of endothelial nitric oxide synthase. J Biol Chem 1995; 270:319–324.
82. O'Driscoll G, Green D, Taylor R. Simvastatin, an HMG-coenzyme A reductase inhibitor, improves endothelial function within 1 month. Circulation 1997; 95:1126–1131.
83. Eichstadt H, Eskotter H, Hoffman I, Amthauer H, Weidinger G. Improvement of myocardial perfusion by short-term fluvastatin therapy in coronary artery disease. Am J Cardiol 1995; 76:122A–125A.
84. Gould K, Martucci J, Goldberg D, et al. Short-term cholesterol lowering decreases size and severity of perfusion abnormalities by positron emission tomography after dipyridamole in patients with coronary artery disease. A potential noninvasive marker of healing coronary endothelium. Circulation 1994; 89:1530–1538.

20
Antibiotic Therapy to Stabilize Vulnerable Plaque

Enrique P. Gurfinkel
Favaloro Foundation, Buenos Aires, Argentina

Benjamin Scirica
Harvard Medical School, Boston, Massachusetts

At the turn of the century, infection was the leading cause of death in the world with pneumonia, tuberculosis, and diarrheal diseases being the most prevalent killers. Advances in sanitation and the introduction of antibiotics dramatically decreased the death toll of infection and heralded what was then considered the beginning of the end of the war against infectious diseases. As life expectancy lengthened, medical research turned away from infection and concentrated on the study of pathophysiology to battle the new scourges of the modern world— atherosclerosis and cancer. Research in the second half of this century led to the discoveries of hormonal, receptor, and most recently, genetic origins of disease. Just as we began to feel medicine was approaching the final frontier in the origin of disease, two of the most prevalent diseases, asthma and peptic ulcers, were unexpectedly discovered to have important infectious components. To further question our understanding of common diseases, a recent randomized trial of antibiotics in patients with coronary artery disease demonstrated a significant improvement in those treated with a macrolide antibiotic (1). Remarkably, atherosclerosis, the most deadly disease of the end of the twentieth century may indeed have an important infectious component that has been largely ignored for decades.

I. INTRODUCTION

Traditionally, several risk factors, such as hypercholesterolemia, arterial hypertension, diabetes mellitus, and tobacco abuse are associated with more advanced atherosclerotic disease. Close to 50% of patients who have an acute myocardial infarction, however, have no identifiable risk factor (2), and even patients sharing similar risk profiles experience varied disease courses. The known risk factors must not, then, entirely explain the pathogenesis of atherosclerosis. Recent research implicates inflammation as a critical component in the growth and development of atherosclerotic plaques. Inflammation is a final pathological pathway initiated by a myriad of stimulants with the trigger of the vascular inflammatory response largely remaining an enigma. Several possible causes, including elevated levels of homocysteine, autoimmune reactions, and infection are potentially linked to the initiation and eventual severity of atherosclerotic disease. In 1908, Sir William Osler suggested a link between infection and atherosclerosis (3). Except for several isolated reports, his theory was largely ignored for most of the century (4, 5). Research in atherosclerosis in the past half century has concentrated on modifying known risk factors such as hypercholesteremia and treating the sequelae of acute atherosclerotic events such as myocardial infarctions and strokes. Several intriguing associations, however, were noted in the epidemiology of coronary artery disease to suggest a potential infectious influence. For example, rates of myocardial infarction and cardiac death increase in the winter and after influenza epidemics (6, 7). Systemic bacterial infections have been associated with a 4% incidence of myocardial infarction and a 10% incidence of stroke (8). Patients with chronic dental disease were also noted to have higher rates of coronary artery disease (9). Increased use of antibiotics coincided with a decrease in cardiac deaths, and campaigns to end widespread use of broad-spectrum antibiotics for respiratory tract infections coincided with an increase in the number of patients with symptomatic coronary artery disease (10). Increased leukocyte counts also correlate with the severity of angiographically determined coronary artery disease (11). These observations suggested that infection might play a more important role in atherosclerosis beyond just increasing the metabolic stress on previously injured hearts.

II. CELLS AND INFECTION

Even after the Fabricants showed in 1978 (12), that germ-free chickens infected with a herpesvirus quickly had atherosclerotic lesions similar to human coronary artery disease develop, linking infection to atherosclerosis has proven difficult, largely because atherosclerosis and infectious diseases affect so many people. Small epidemiological studies with numerous confounding factors have offered conflicting results. Many of these microbes prove difficult to culture and lack adequate serological measurements. Despite these problems, now at the end of the twentieth century, there is a growing body of evidence to suggest that infection is an important component in the pathogenesis and development of atherosclerosis.

The primary cells involved in the development of atherosclerosis are the endothelial cells, vascular smooth muscle cells, monocytes, macrophages, lymphocytes, and platelets. The vascular endothelium is a monolayer of cells covering a basement membrane that completely lines the vasculature. Once considered a simple layer over the arterial basement membrane, it is now recognized as an integral element of vascular physiology. This monolayer of cells provides a selective barrier to circulating blood components and regulates permeability through receptors for a variety of compounds and cells. Endothelial cells prevent pathological thrombosis by inhibiting the coagulation cascade with membrane-bound heparin sulfate molecules and lysing fibrin-bound clots through the release of tissue plasminogen activator. Powerful vasoactive compounds like prostacyclin and nitric oxide diffuse out of endothelial cells to inhibit platelet aggregation and to stimulate vasodilation through smooth muscle cell relaxation. Endothelial cells transform the action of many vasoconstrictive elements, such as epinephrine and norepinephrine, into vasodilatory stimuli through nitric oxide production. Arteries lose a powerful vasodilatory stimulus without a healthy endothelial layer. Nitric oxide also inhibits macrophage adhesion and activation. The endothelium is also a rich source of growth factors such as platelet-derived growth factor (PDGF) (13).

The vasodilatory and antithrombotic properties of endothelial cells are constantly challenged by normal physiological events. Transient postprandial elevations in serum cholesterol and glucose, high blood pressure, and exposure to tobacco can all damage the endothelium. Alone, these have a minor effect, but over a lifetime of continual exposure, they can severely impair the normal function of the endothelium. Chronic, low-level injury begins the inflammatory process by attracting inflammatory cells and facilitating their passage through the endothelium into the vessel's intimal layer. More intense damage accelerates the inflammatory process. Many different forms of injury have been proposed. Because the first evidence of atherosclerosis is often at the bifurcation of artery branches, shear stress of blood flow is often implicated in endothelial damage. The traditional risk factors of hypertension, diabetes mellitus, cigarettes, and elevated cholesterol can all disturb cellular equilibrium and lead to endothelial injury. Elevated cholesterol, especially high levels of low-density lipoprotein (LDL), is closely linked with atherosclerosis. The endocytosis of LDL by specific endothelial receptors accounts for 75% of LDL clearance from serum. LDL, however, may undergo oxidation by endothelial cells, smooth muscle cells, and macrophages. Oxidated LDL (ox-LDL) plays an important role in atherosclerosis, in part because, in contrast to normal LDL receptors, the ox-LDL receptors are not down-regulated by high cholesterol concentrations. The exact mechanism of injury by LDL is not entirely clear but may result from an increase in the endothelial membrane concentration of cholesterol, which decreases membrane fluidity and makes endothelial cells more susceptible to shear stress. More work is needed to explain how homocysteine, apolipoproteins, and other newly discovered risk factors injure endothelium, but the work of Fabricant with germ-free chickens demonstrated the damage a viral infection can inflict on the vascular wall.

The damage to the endothelium is the basis of the most compelling theory on the pathogenesis of atherosclerosis, the "response-to-injury" hypothesis, first proposed by Ross and Glomset in 1976 (14). Modified several times, this theory builds on the initial ideas of Virchow and other early pathologists and incorporates more recent evidence of cell-cell interaction and inflammation. The hypothesis suggests that a first "injury" to the endothelium triggers a complex set of interactions between endothelial cells, smooth muscle cells, platelets, macrophages, and lymphocytes that eventually leads to the development and remodeling of atherosclerotic lesions in the vessel wall. The initial injury impairs the normal functions of the endothelial cells, leading to a condition known as "endothelial dysfunction" (14, 15).

Injury dramatically changes endothelial function. Damaged endothelial cells, for instance, produce less nitric oxide and prostacyclin, which facilitates vasoconstriction and platelet aggregation. Decreased nitric oxide and an increase in the production of superoxide anions activate transcription factors (e.g., NF-kB), promoting the expression of adhesion molecules such as vascular cell adhesion molecule-1 (VCAM-1) and intracelluar adhesion molecule-1 (ICAM-1) and the secretion of monocyte colony–stimulating factors, which together attract inflammatory cells (16).

Monocyte-derived macrophages are present in all atherosclerotic plaques, and their arrival heralds the beginning of the inflammatory process. After attaching to endothelial adhesion molecules, they migrate into the intima layer and scavenge free ox-LDL. Under certain circumstances, macrophages release inflammatory compounds such as interleukin-1, superoxide anions, and growth factors such as transforming growth factor-β (TGF-β) and PDGF. Macrophages turn into lipid-laden foam cells with increased ox-LDL ingestion and eventually undergo programmed cell death, spilling cholesterol and proteolytic enzymes. The release of extracellular matrix–degrading enzymes is important in plaque remodeling because they can weaken the plaque structure. There appears to be at least two morphologies of macrophages in plaques. One, the foam cell morphology, is dedicated to lipid scavenging, whereas another expresses the major histocompatibility complex molecule HLA-DR and costimulatory molecules necessary for a complete immune response (17). Perhaps the most interesting and least understood cell in atherosclerotic plaques is the T cell lymphocyte. Immunohistochemical analysis reveals both CD8+ and CD4+ lymphocytes present in all stages of plaque development, with CD4+ cells predominating in mature plaques and CD8+ cells in precursor lesions or in the periphery of mature plaques. CD4+ cells are usually found together with macrophages, and both express molecules (HLA-DR) suggesting a state of activation. Major histocompatibility molecules are a class of membrane-bound receptors that continually present peptides of different proteins to immune cells to protect against "foreign" pathogens. Class I molecules are present in all cells and present peptides largely from intracellular proteins to CD8+ T cells. Class II molecules are specific to antigen-presenting cells (e.g., macrophages) that interact with CD4+ T cells and present phagocytosed extracellular proteins. A greater percentage of T cells in atherosclerotic plaques are in a late stage of activation compared with peripheral T cells. In addition, a small population of atherosclerotic T cells expresses receptors for IL-2 and the proliferating-cell nuclear antigen, as well as costimulatory receptors necessary for complete activation, indicating they are responding to antigen stimulation (17). The nature of the stimulating antigen is still unclear, although there is evidence for both autoimmune and infectious origins.

III. SYMPTOMATIC ATHEROSCLEROSIS

Most atherosclerotic plaques are not clinically significant because even with years of gradual growth, they never critically occlude arterial blood flow. It was previously held that arterial-induced ischemia and distal necrosis were caused by lesions, that, through smooth muscle cell proliferation and increased lipid accumulation, eventually completely occluded the arterial lumen. The severity of disease was thought to be proportional to the degree of arterial stenoses. However, it has been questioned whether the degree of arterial stenoses is a valid prognostic indicator for acute ischemic events. For example, a completely occluded carotid artery does not correlate with the frequency or size of strokes. In the heart, coronary arteriography may reveal completely occluded arteries in asymptomatic patients and no lesions in patients with angina or myocardial infarction (20, 21).

This discrepancy between angiographic evidence of stenosis and a patient's clinical course led to a new theory that blamed acute ischemic events on the rupture of a subocclusive plaque resulting in an occlusive thrombus. The rapid thrombus formation accounts for the acute clinical presentation, often in previously asymptomatic patients who experience the most severe consequences of ischemia (22). Often the culprit atherosclerotic plaques appear to be "less severe" stenosises occupying 50 to 60% of the lumen and are not easily identified as vulnerable lesions by angiography (23). Plaques, however, do not need to rupture to trigger thrombosis. Severe endothelial damage may alone precipitate the release of prothrombotic factors (most importantly, tissue factor) that begin clot formation. Autopsy studies of patients with ischemic sudden death demonstrated that only 60% of arterial thrombosis had an underlying plaque rupture, whereas the remainder showed some type of erosion of the endothelial cells underlying the clot (23). In summary, angiographically determined "less severe" lesions that do not rupture are responsible for some of the most severe acute atherosclerotic events.

The most contemporary understanding of acute atherosclerotic events suggest that arterial thrombosis may develop as the result of several pathological processes of which plaque rupture is the most dramatic finale. Endothelial damage alone may stimulate a large release of tissue factor and other procoagulant compounds, which, if severe enough, can lead to cell death and the exposure of the thrombogenic subendothelium. The question again is what turns a stable atherosclerotic lesion into an unstable, "vulnerable" plaque, capable of triggering clot formation. The key appears to be in the composition of the plaque. Atherosclerosis, by its very name, implies a heterogeneous makeup of athero, or "gruel," referring to the soft lipid center, and sclerosis, describing the hard fibrous cap. The size of the lipid center and the thickness of the cap vary in different plaques. Plaques with large lipid centers and thin fibrous caps are considered more vulnerable than those with thick fibrous plaques and a small lipid center and are more likely to be the culprit lesion in arterial thrombosis. Plaques often rupture at the weak "shoulder" of the lesion, where the thin fibrous cap joins the intima (13, 24).

Inflammation again appears to be critical in changing a stable atherosclerotic lesion into a vulnerable plaque. Systemic markers of inflammation such as leukocyte count, interleukin-1 (25), C-reactive protein (26), and neopterin are elevated in patients with acute coronary ischemic events. Pathological studies reveal a greater number of macrophages and T-cell lymphocytes, increased lipid core, and fewer smooth muscle cells in thrombosed plaques compared with intact plaques (27, 28). More activated leukocytes are seen in cardiac sinus blood samples from patients with unstable angina compared with stable angina (29). Smooth muscle cells, previously thought to be the major pathological cell of atherosclerosis, may, in fact, provide plaque stability. Inflammatory and smooth muscle cells in these plaques express HLA-DR, indicating cell activation (30).

Plaques obtained from coronary catheter atherectomy procedures in patients with acute myocardial infarction or unstable angina demonstrate a higher percentage of macrophages compared with plaques in stable angina (31) with an even greater percentage of activated inflammatory cells in ruptured plaques (23). An elevated number of macrophages and activated immune cells are also seen at the site of superficial erosions, suggesting that just the inflammatory reaction may be sufficient to trigger thrombosis (30). The macrophage's ability to weaken plaques is likely due to the secretion of enzymes, specifically extracellular matrix–degrading metalloproteinases, which erode the fibrous cap (31). Not surprisingly, a large number of macrophages and a high concentration of these metalloproteinases (32) are found near the plaque's vulnerable shoulder. The other major

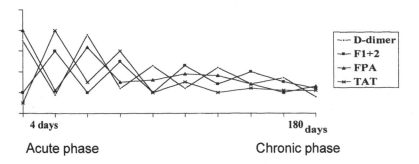

4 days   180 days

Acute phase   Chronic phase

Figure 1 Unstable angina. D-dimer, break-down degradation fibrin products; F1 + 2, fragment 1 + 2; FPA, fibrinopeptide A; TAT; thrombin antithrombin III complex.

component in weakening the plaque may be the T-cell lymphocytes that, through the release of cytokines such as interferon-γ, weaken the plaques by inhibiting smooth muscle cell proliferation and decreasing collagen and fibrin formation (33, 34).

The clinical presentation of an acute atherosclerotic event depends on the extent of thrombosis. A partial lumen obstruction or a total obstruction followed by clot lysis presents clinically as unstable angina or a transient ischemia attack. Complete obstruction with ischemia and cell death is the origin of myocardial infarctions, strokes, and sudden death. Acute ischemic syndromes, then, are a continuum of a single disease process—the thrombosis and lysis over an atherosclerotic plaque (Fig. 1).

Yet again, the most important question concerns the origin of the inflammatory reaction that converts stable atherosclerotic plaques into deadly "vulnerable" lesions. Active immunocompetent lymphocytes and macrophages suggest an immune response. Several potential antigens have been proposed, including ox-LDL and cellular heat shock proteins in autoimmune reactions, as well as various proteins from infectious agents. Antibodies to ox-LDL are elevated in patients with atherosclerotic disease, but their levels actually decrease during acute events (31). Antibody titers to heat shock proteins, molecules produced at times of stress to protect other cellular proteins, are also elevated in atherosclerosis, suggesting they may be antigens in a chronic inflammatory process. Anti-heat shock protein antibody titers, however, are not apparently related to disease severity (35, 36).

IV. INFECTION AND MECHANISM OF ATHEROGENESIS

The elevation of systemic inflammatory markers like leukocyte count, C-reactive protein, serum amyloid A, and cytokines in atherosclerosis suggests a possible immune or infectious inflammatory stimulant. Differentiating between either process is often difficult because of shared inflammatory patterns and the difficulty in identifying culprit antigens in arterial plaques.

Several mechanisms are postulated to explain how infection may contribute to both the chronic and acute phases of atherosclerosis. Both elevated leukocyte count and multiple sites of plaque formation suggest a systemic disease process. Infection may upset many normal physiological equilibria, which increases susceptibility to accelerated atherosclerosis even without direct endothelial damage by infectious pathogens. Infection alters metabolic pathways through increased glucose intolerance and changes in cholesterol metabolism. Macrophages activated by infection release interluekin-1, interleukin-6, interferon-γ, and tumor necrosis factor-α (TNF-α) (37). TNF, in particular, decreases lipoprotein lipase activity, thereby increasing triglyceride levels while decreasing levels of the cardioprotective high-density lipoprotein (HDL) and enhancing cholesterol uptake through up-regulated scavenger receptors (37, 38). Infection also creates a prothrombotic state through increased hepatic fibrinogen production and by circulating gram-negative bacterial lipopolysaccharide molecules that stimulate the release of both plasminogen activation inhibitor and the prothrombotic thromboxane A_2, which directly activates the clotting cascade (38).

Importantly, infectious agents have been identified within atherosclerotic plaques and can directly injure endothelial cells. In animal models, injected pathogens produce atherosclerotic lesions through direct endothelial damage. Viral infections of endothelial cells induce increased secretion of prothrombotic compounds such as tissue factor and thrombin and augmented ox-LDL uptake (39). Endotoxins and TNF-α severely impair endothelial nitric oxide and prostaglandin production in a condition called ''endothelial stunning,'' with a prolonged decrease in nitric oxide and prostaglandin synthesis. Infection may also stimulate an autoimmune reaction through molecular mimicry, which prolongs a chronic inflammatory process. Viral infections may contribute to atherogenesis in a novel manner by interacting with the p53 protein, which interferes with the normal cell cycle thereby disinhibiting cell proliferation (40). This is reminiscent of an older theory that suggested atherosclerotic cells were of monoclonal origin (41–43).

V.   POTENTIAL PATHOGENS

A.   Viruses

The first infectious agent directly associated with atherosclerosis was identified in 1978, when Fabricant inoculated germ-free chickens with an avian herpesvirus (Marek's disease herpesvirus) and fed half of the infected and control chickens a high-cholesterol diet (12). At autopsy, visible atherosclerotic lesions were found in the entire arterial wall in the infected chickens with the most severe lesions in chickens fed the cholesterol-rich diet. Microscopic examination again revealed many coronary atherosclerotic lesions in the infected chickens with more severe disease in those fed a high-cholesterol diet. The plaques were similar to human atherosclerosis lesions with a fibrous cap overlying an atheromatous core. Noninfected chickens had minimal lesions. Marek's disease herpsevirus–specific antigens were identified in lesions of several infected birds and in none of the virus-free birds. Fabricant and colleagues extended their findings (44, 45) to report that immunization of chickens with a turkey herpesvirus prevented the development of atherosclerosis. They also showed that cultured smooth muscle cells infected with the Mareck's disease and herpes simplex virus had increased cholesterol and cholesteryl ester accumulation (44, 46). Hajjar extended the observation of increased cholesterol ester accumulation in human smooth muscle cells infected by herpes simplex virus (47).

Although other viruses, namely coxsackie B, have been implicated in human atherosclerosis (48–50), the herpes viridae family, and specifically human cytomegalovirus are the most likely viral agents. Identifying specific viruses that increase the risk of atherosclerosis, however, has proven troublesome. Numerous studies examining different viruses offer conflicting results. These studies highlight several of the problems interpreting data concerning infection in atherosclerosis. There are few prospective trials, with most being case-control studies susceptible to bias by confounding factors. Also, because we all have atherosclerosis to some degree, "controls" may have significant atherosclerotic disease that is currently asymptomatic. The research in viral atherogenesis is complicated because much of it centers on heart transplant patients and postpercutaneous transluminal coronary angioplasty (PTCA) restenosis rather than on native artery atherosclerosis.

1. Cytomegalovirus

Cytomegalovirus, like other herpesviruses, is a common viral infection. In immunocompetent hosts, it remains in a latent phase and is largely asymptomatic. As many as 50% of people older than 35 and more than 70% of people older than 65 have antibodies to cytomegalovirus. In normal host cells, cytomegalovirus may undergo an "abortive" infection without viral replication. Reactivation, through immunosuppression for example, leads to renewed viral replication with severe systemic manifestations. In immunocompromised heart transplant patients, accelerated atherosclerosis is a well-recognized and important complication. Serological evidence of cytomegalovirus infection, associated with both high rates of rejection and accelerated heart transplant atherosclerosis, raises the possibility that cytomegalovirus may also be involved in native artery atherosclerosis (51, 52). Transplant atherosclerosis is not exactly similar to normal atherosclerosis, developing with more diffuse, concentric lesions and less plaque calcification than in native atherosclerotic plaques. Evidence of cytomegalovirus genomes within transplant atherosclerotic lesions has been contradictory (53, 54), but the florid nature of cytomegalovirus replication in the immunosuppressed heart may only offer a limited insight into native atherosclerosis, which lacks active viral replication.

a. Serological Evidence

Serological evidence of prior cytomegalovirus infection has generally shown a correlation with atherosclerosis, but the studies have been small and complicated by a high number of confounding factors (55, 56). Cytomegalovirus infection, however, has been more closely associated with carotid artery atherosclerosis (57, 58). Cytomegalovirus antigens and nucleic acid sequences are found in atherosclerotic plaques obtained from carotid endarterectomy specimens and may be more prevalent in thrombosed plaques (58). Patients with positive cytomegalovirus titers years later appear to have a higher risk of carotid arterial stenosis (57), although the high prevalence of cytomegalovirus infection and confounding risk factors makes a causal relationship difficult to prove. There is strong evidence to suggest that cytomegalovirus plays a role in postpercutaneous transluminal coronary angioplasty (PTCA) restenosis. A recent study demonstrated that patients seropositive for cytomegalovirus had a much higher rate of restenosis 6 months after angioplasty (43 vs. 8%, $p = 0.002$), with cytomegalovirus titers independently predictive of future restenosis (59). Restenosis correlated with high IgG levels and not IgM levels. There was no change in IgG levels between the initial angioplasty and follow-up angiography, suggesting a chronic cytomegalovirus infection rather than an acute infection after angioplasty.

b. Pathological Evidence

Cytomegalovirus is found in vessel walls throughout the arterial tree (60), although it is unclear whether the virus is more prevalent in atherosclerotic arteries than in normal appearing arteries. Disagreement may, in part, be due to different isolation methods. A meta-analysis of 16 pathological studies of native and transplant vessels revealed cytomegalovirus in only a slightly greater percentage of atherosclerotic arteries compared with nonatheromatous vessels (47 vs. 39%). When only using polymerase chain reaction (PCR) technique–based studies, the percentage of cytomegalovirus detected in atheromatous lesion was slightly greater at 57 vs. 36% in normal vessels (61). The more sensitive PCR technique identified cytomegalovirus more frequently in more developed atherosclerotic samples compared with less severe lesions (62). The failure to detect cytomegalovirus (63, 64) within lesions may be due to temporal sampling error, whereby a virus initiates cellular damage but does not persist as a latent infection. Evidence in chickens suggests that viral antigens may only be present in the early stages of lesions and in the periphery of old lesions (65).

c. Potential Mechanisms of Viral-Induced Atherosclerosis

Despite the often contradictory serological and pathological evidence, viruses offer several explanations for how infection may precipitate and accelerate atherosclerosis. Coxsackie virus, as well as the herpesviruses, upset normal cholesterol metabolism, decreasing cytoplasmic and lysosomal cholesterol ester hydrolytic activity, thereby facilitating cholesterol accumulation (44, 46, 47, 49). Increased smooth muscle cell uptake of ox-LDL appears to be mediated by a virus-induced up-regulation of ox-LDL scavenger molecules on smooth muscle cell surfaces (59). Herpesvirus and cytomegalovirus may also directly change the normally anticoagulant endothelium to a procoagulant surface through interfering with normal hemostasis (66). Infected endothelial cells increase thrombin expression (67) and decrease thrombomodulin expression (68). The secretion of von Willebrand factor (69) and a reduction in prostacyclin (67) production facilitates platelet adhesion. Most important to triggering coagulation may be the viral-induced secretion of the powerful coagulant, tissue factor (68). Herpes-infected endothelial cells also have impaired ability to bind to basement membrane components, which may contribute to endothelial erosion exposing underlying collagen and stimulating thrombosis (70). Smooth muscle cells infected by cytomegalovirus quickly activate the nuclear transcription factor NF-kB, increasing the expression of cytokines and inflammatory molecules and precipitating an inflammatory response.

d. Cytomegalovirus in Postangioplasty Restenosis

Epstein and Speir offer an interesting theory explaining the role of cytomegalovirus in coronary restenosis that may also be important in the development of systemic atherosclerosis (39, 40). Symptomatic restenosis is a common complication of coronary angioplasty, occurring in nearly 30% of patients not receiving stents. Restenosed lesions tend to have increased smooth muscle cell proliferation, causing a fibrotic occlusion of the arterial lumen. In immunocompetent hosts, latent cytomegalovirus rarely reactivates with active replication; however, it may undergo an "abortive infection," where only immediate early viral gene products are produced. Two immediate early gene products are IE72 and IE84. The IE72 protein stimulates smooth muscle cells' expression of scavenger ox-LDL receptors. Drawing from the monoclonal theory of atherogenesis, Epstein observed that smooth muscle cells in restenosis stained positively for the proto-oncogene p53, which is considered critical in controlling the cell cycles and inducing cell apoptosis. Although wild-type p53 has a very short half-life and cannot be identified by immunohistochemistry, mutated p53 is identifiable in properly stained cells. Nearly 40% of arterial restenosis samples stained positively for p53, suggesting impaired p53 activity with diminished inhibition of cell replication. Nearly 85% of the p53-positive samples contained cytomegalovirus DNA compared with only 27% of the p53-negative samples. They found that early gene product IE84, which was identified in the cytomegalovirus-infected smooth muscle cells, both binds and inactivates p53. Thus, an "abortive" infection with only limited viral activity can severely alter the host's cell cycle. Thus, restenosis may be an accelerated form of normal atherogenesis triggered by the intense damage of angioplasty, which activates latent cytomegalovirus. A non-uniform induction of "aborted" infection may explain the presence of cytomegalovirus throughout the arterial tree with only certain sites developing atherosclerosis.

B. Bacteria

1. *Helicobacter pylori*

The discovery that *H. pylori* was responsible for most peptic ulcer disease and chronic gastritis revolutionized the field of gastroenterology. *H. pylori*, a spiral-shaped, microaerophillic gram-negative bacillus can be identified in nearly 100% of duodenal ulcers, 60% of gastric ulcers, and 50% of nonulcer dyspepsia. Treatment with a combination of antibiotics and antacids often results in cure. It was perhaps logical to theorize that *H. pylori* might also be responsible for another major disease of the modern world—atherosclerosis. But investigating the link between *H. pylori* and atherosclerosis is difficult. *H. pylori* infections are acquired early in life with between 50 and 100% of the population demonstrating positive serological evidence for infection. Numerous confounding factors, often not considered, complicate study interpretations. At first glance, *H. pylori* infection appears independently associated with atherosclerosis, but more careful analysis often blurs any potential connections.

a. Serological Evidence

The studies that demonstrate an association between *H. pylori* and atherosclerosis tend to be case-control studies with a small number of patients (71–74). Several potential confounding factors, such as socioeconomic status, are closely linked with both *H. pylori* infection and atherosclerosis. Several small studies that controlled for cardiac risk factors showed an association between *H. pylori* and atherosclerosis (75), although one included only patients undergoing cardiac catheterization (76) and another was based on electrocardiographic evidence of coronary artery disease (77). The control patients could have had significant asymptomatic atherosclerosis. The association observed between positive serological findings for *H. pylori* and atherosclerosis is lost with larger studies that control for age, sex, cardiac risk factors, and socioeconomic status (78–80). Two

Table 1 *H. pylori*, CMV, Mycoplasma
Serology and Atherosclerosis

IgG	UA	CSA	PVD	HV
HP (%)	76	86	56	36
CMV (%)	92	91	94	50
MP (%)	49			39

UA, unstable angina; CSA, chronic stable angina; PVD, peripheral vascular disease; HV, healthy volunteers; HP, *Helicobacter pylori*; CMV, Cytomegalovirus; MP, *Mycoplasma pneumoniae*.

nested case-control studies do not demonstrate a relationship between *H. pylori* and atherosclerosis (81, 82). *H. pylori* infection is associated with social class, smoking, and other risk factors for atherosclerosis (Table 1) (81).

b. Pathological Evidence

Positive titers to *H. pylori* are associated with more severe angiographic coronary artery disease (76), but no bacteria have yet been identified in any atherosclerotic plaque (83), and it is uncertain whether *H. pylori* can survive in blood. Despite the lack of convincing epidemiological evidence for *H. pylori*, there are several potential indirect mechanisms that may contribute to atherogenesis. A few studies have suggested that fibrinogen levels (77, 84) are elevated in *H. pylori* infection, but this was not confirmed in a larger study (79). One theory (85) suggests a link between *H. pylori* and elevated levels of homocysteine. Chronic *H. pylori* infection of the stomach may lead to malabsorption syndromes and nutritional deficiencies, specifically folate and vitamins B_6 and B_{12}, which are essential cofactors for several of the enzymes needed to convert homocysteine to methionine. A *H. pylori*–induced vitamin B_{12} deficiency could lead to elevated homocysteine levels that significantly increase the risk of coronary artery disease. *H. pylori*, like *Chlamydia pneumoniae*, produces a heat shock protein (HSP) with close homology to human heat shock protein 60. High levels of antibodies to human HSP60 correlate with more severe and diffuse atherosclerotic disease, as well as with serological evidence of *H. pylori* infection (35).

2. *Mycoplasma pneumoniae*

Mycoplasma pneumoniae is a prevalent obligate intracellular pathogen that potentially could play a role in atherosclerosis. The only two studies to date testing a relationship between *Mycoplasma* antibody titers and coronary artery disease were negative (86, 87) (Table 1).

3. Chlamydia pneumoniae

C. pneumoniae was the last of the three known Chlamydia strains to be identified in 1986, when Grayston identified a new pathogen during an outbreak of respiratory tract infections (88). Originally called the TWAR strain after the initials of the first two isolates, TW-183 and AR-39, C. pneumoniae is now recognized as the second most prevalent bacterial cause after M. pneumoniae for atypical pneumonia, accounting for nearly 11% of cases (89). The first C. pneumoniae infection is usually acquired between 5 and 14 years of age (90) and reinfection is common. Up to 50% of the adult population have positive anti-C. pneumoniae antibody titers, which rise with age. Interestingly, more men than women have positive anti-C. pneumoniae titers (37).

The most fastidious of the Chlamydia species, C. pneumoniae has two developmental forms. The infectious extracellular elementary body attaches to cell membranes, perhaps by means of heparin sulfate molecules, and is incorporated through phagocytosis. C. pneumoniae mostly infects mucosal cells but, importantly, it is also found within monocytes. Once within the cytoplasm, C. pneumoniae transform into intracellular, uniquely "pear"-shaped, reticulate bodies that through binary fission fill a membrane-bound "inclusion body" with progeny. Within 24 hours, reticulate bodies condense and become elementary bodies that are released with cell rupture and infect adjacent cells. C. pneumoniae is responsible for acute pharyngitis, sinusitis, bronchitis, and pneumonia with a clinical presentation indistinguishable from many other "upper respiratory" pathogens.

Definitively diagnosing acute and chronic C. pneumoniae infections is troublesome because of a lack of reliable laboratory tests and its nonspecific clinical presentation. Because Chlamydia species share a similar lipopolysaccharide antigen, complement fixation techniques are nonspecific among Chlamydia species. The microimmunoflourescence technique to test for antibodies has been the most accepted method to show evidence of infection, but it is a difficult technique requiring skilled observers and is complicated by the tendency of positive titers to weaken years after an initial infection. Grayston has proposed serological guidelines for C. pneumoniae infection. An acute infection requires a fourfold increase in IgG titers, an IgM >1:16, or a single IgG titer >1:512. Patients with chronic or past infection should have titers of IgG >1:16 and IgM >1:512 for chronic infection (91). In new infections, the IgM elevation appears at 3 weeks, whereas IgG responds at 6 to 8 weeks. Reinfection may not have an increase in IgM titers with only an IgG response within 1 to 2 weeks of re-exposure (92). C. pneumoniae culture requires 3 to 7 days in specific mucosal cell lines with specific fluorescent-antibody staining for confirmation. C. pneumoniae can be cultured from nasopharyngeal swabs and bronchoalveolar lavage specimens, but the sensitivity of culture is much lower than for serological evidence of infection. PCR of specimens has not proven to be more sensitive than immunocytochemistry techniques, perhaps because handling techniques and specimen contamination with blood, mucus, or nucleases may inhibit DNA amplification (92).

a. Serological Evidence

Only 2 years after Grayston identified the TWAR strain, Saikku (93) noted that patients with acute myocardial infarction and angina pectoris had a significantly higher percentage of anti-*C. pneumoniae* IgG titers >1:128 compared with asymptomatic controls. There was no difference in the level of titers between patients with acute myocardial infarction compared with those with angina pectoris. Nearly 70% of the myocardial infarction patients, however, had positive titers to a different lipopolysaccharide antigen known to cross-react with all *Chlamydia* species, whereas none of the control or angina patients' serum reacted with this antigen. This suggests that acute myocardial infarction patients might have an active infection with circulating immune complexes, whereas the stable angina patients have a chronic infection with only elevated IgG titers. The antilipopolysaccharide titers in the myocardial infarction patients decreased after 3 months. This study linked *C. pneumoniae* to both chronic atherosclerosis and, potentially, acute ischemic events precipitated by an active infection.

Since Saikku's first report of an association between coronary heart disease and *C. pneumoniae*, numerous studies have also found serological links using *Chlamydia* genus–specific immune complexes suggesting active infection (94, 95), as well as *C. pneumoniae*–specific antigens as markers of infection (77, 87, 94–102). Most of these studies were either case control or retrospective analyses with potential confounding factors. The only prospective observational study, however, also found a correlation between *C. pneumoniae* antibody titers and coronary heart disease, although the association was attenuated when controlling for other risk factors (94). Concern that smoking was a confounder because of the higher prevalence of high anti-*C. pneumoniae* titers in smokers (103, 104) was not confirmed in another study that controlled for smoking as a risk factor (99). *C. pneumoniae* also appears to be linked with increased rates of cerebrovascular events (101, 105). Acute coronary and ischemic events such as acute myocardial infarction and stroke may be related to acute *C. pneumoniae* infection with serology patterns of higher IgG, IgM, and IgA titers (100, 101), although the failure to always identify IgM antibodies may suggest an acute reinfection as opposed to a newly acquired infection. One study that did not show a correlation between *C. pneumoniae* infection and acute myocardial infarctions had a very high prevalence of IgG seropositivity that might obscure any relationship (106). In addition to humoral-mediated immunity through antibodies, cell-mediated immunity is also up-regulated in *C. pneumoniae* infection. Lymphocytes from patients with coronary artery disease respond to *C. pneumoniae* antigen stimulation more intensely than lymphocytes from control patients (107).

Unfortunately, besides the difficulty of the microimmunofluorescence technique and the normal pattern of titer fluctuation, most studies have specified different antibody titers as positive or negative, making direct comparisons of studies difficult and questioning the clinical usefulness of this technique to identify patients at risk.

b. Pathological Evidence

There is convincing evidence linking *C. pneumoniae* directly to atherosclerotic lesions. Patients with positive IgG titers to *C. pneumoniae* have a greater likelihood of angiographically demonstrated coronary artery disease compared with patients without positive titers (108) and, independent of other risk factors, are more likely to have ultrasonographically detected carotid wall thickening, indicating atherosclerotic lesions (109). Autopsy studies of young adults who died of noncardiac causes found *C. pneumoniae* in atheromatous lesions in coronary arteries by immunocytochemistry and PCR but could not identify the bacteria in autopsy samples from normal-appearing arteries of patients with and without evidence of overt atherosclerosis (110). Other autopsy studies confirm a high prevalence of *C. pneumoniae* in atherosclerotic plaques with *C. pneumoniae* elementary bodies seen by electron microscopy in foam cells and in areas of tissue damage (111). Abdominal aorta samples also reveal *C. pneumoniae* by immunocytochemistry in cytoplasm of macrophages and smooth muscle cells (112). In addition to autopsy studies, advanced atherosclerotic lesions can be obtained from coronary atherectomy procedures and carotid endarterectomy operations. *C. pneumoniae* has consistently been identified by immunocytochemistry, PCR, and in one case (113) by culture in coronary arteries (113–115), in carotid arteries (58, 116, 117), in the abdominal aorta (83, 118) in peripheral arteries (118) and recently in a greater percentage of nonrheumatic stenosed aortic valves compared with normal age-matched valves (119). Both elementary and reticulate bodies were identified (114), suggesting active replication, with bacteria located within smooth muscle cells and macrophages (116). *C. pneumoniae* is rarely, if ever, detected in normal arterial samples. A combination of pathological study findings reveals that *C. pneumoniae* can be identified by at least one technique in 52% (257/495) of atheromatous lesions compared with only 5% (6/188) in control samples (61). One study that identified *C. pneumoniae* in only one atherectomy lesion did not use immunohistochemistry techniques and relied on the less-sensitive PCR, electron microscopy, and culture methods (120).

c. Potential Mechanisms of C. Pneumoniae-*Induced Atheosclerosis*

Even though serological and pathological evidence suggests an important role of *C. pneumoniae* in atherosclerosis, it does not prove a causal relationship. Laboratory studies have proposed several methods by which *C. pneumoniae* might promote atherosclerosis. In addition to macrophages, *C. pneumoniae* replicates in a variety of cells in vitro, including endothelial and smooth muscle cells (121).

C. pneumoniae lipopolysaccharide, although not as toxic as that of other gram-negative bacteria, is incorporated into the host cell wall and secreted into the bloodstream, where it can trigger the clotting cascade. In addition, circulating immune complexes and monocyte-released tissue factor also contribute to a pro-coagulant state. *C. pneumoniae* infection of macrophages stimulates release of interleukin-1, interleukin-6, TNF-α, and interferon-γ, which stimulate the inflammatory response and change lipid profiles (37).

d. Autoimmune Reaction

In ocular trachomas, *Chlamydia trachamotis* induces a chronic inflammatory response resulting in blindness from excessive fibrosis caused by macrophage and lymphocyte infiltration. A similar reaction might occur in chronic *C. pneumoniae* arterial infection, perhaps mediated through an autoimmune reaction involving heat shock proteins. Heat shock proteins are a family of about two dozen proteins, with a great homology among species, that are expressed in the cytoplasm and on cell walls in times of stress, such as infection and exposure to oxidants or high temperatures. Because they are not normally present, when expressed they may not be recognized as "self" by host immune cells and could initiate antibody production and an autoimmune reaction. A human 60 kDa heat shock protein (HSP60) has a close homology with a 65 kDa mycobacterial heat shock protein (HSP65). A common antibody against both human and mycobacterial heat shock proteins can damage and lyse macrophages, endothelial cells, and intimal cells through a humoral and cell-mediated immune reaction (122, 123). Elevated levels of the anti-HSP60/65 are associated with ultrasonographically determined carotid wall thickening (36). *C. pneumoniae* and *H. pylori* both express HSP60 (35). Simply exposing the eye to HSP60 in an animal previously infected with *C. trachamotis* will induce inflammation suggesting that HSP60 may be the sensitizing antigen in a delayed hypersensitivity reaction (124). Infertility rates are also elevated in patients with anti-HSP60 antibodies suggesting increased postinfection scarring (125, 126). Reaction to HSP60 may depend on HLA types making some people more susceptible to the autoimmune reaction. This susceptibility could explain why the patients that do not respond to current therapy for unstable angina have high anti-*Chlamydial* antibody titers (127).

e. Animal Models of C. pneumoniae-*Induced Atherogenesis*

A mouse model of *C. pneumoniae*-induced atherosclerosis was developed (128) by injecting *C. pneumonia* into infected Apo-E–deficient mice that spontaneously develop atherosclerosis and into another strain of mice that does not experience accelerated atherosclerosis. Persistent *C. pneumoniae* infection was found in the atheromatous lesions from the Apo E–deficient mice and a transient *C. pneumoniae* infection was found in the lesions of the other mouse strain. The most promising evidence, however, is derived from a recently described rabbit model of

C. pneumoniae–induced atherogenesis, (129). Pathogen-free rabbits were inoculated with purified *C. pneumoniae* by way of the nasopharynx and then compared with rabbits receiving placebo inoculations. Ten of the 11 infected rabbits demonstrated serological evidence of infection with the strongest reaction at 28 days. Several of the inoculated animals had evidence of atherosclerotic disease with "foamy" macrophages in one case and smooth muscle cell proliferation with periaortitis in another rabbit. Elementary bodies were seen in two aortas, and *C. pneumoniae* was cultured from one aortic arch. There was no evidence of *C. pneumoniae* infection or atherosclerosis in any of the control animals. This evidence contrasted with another rabbit model that did not reveal any arterial *C. pneumoniae* involvement (130).

A possible hypothesis linking *C. pneumoniae* to both the chronic and acute phase of atherosclerosis begins in the early teens with a *C. pneumoniae* respiratory tract infection. In this model, alveolar monocytes infected with *C. pneumoniae* pass into the bloodstream and attach to vascular endothelium at the site of transient endothelial dysfunction caused by injuries such as hypercholesterolemia or sheer stress. After migrating into the arterial intima, macrophages stimulated by *C. pneumoniae* prolong and amplify the inflammatory process. This chronic infection lasts for years, priming the cellular and humoral immune system and slowly contributing to smooth muscle cell proliferation and fibrosis. A reinfection by *C. pneumoniae* later in life stimulates the previously primed immune response, reactivating lymphocytes and macrophages within plaques, leading to an intense inflammatory response that changes plaque composition and creates a more vulnerable lesion. Plaque rupture or endothelial erosion in this newly vulnerable plaque causes thrombosis, that if severe enough, leads to an acute ischemic event.

VI. CLINICAL INTERVENTIONS

To date, three clinical trials, both in patients with coronary artery disease, have attempted to prove the value of antibiotic therapy in atherosclerotic disease. One study (131) screened 200 patients from South London recovering from an acute myocardial infarction for anti-*C. pneumoniae* antibodies. The 80 patients with titers $\geq 1:64$ were randomized to receive the macrolide antibiotic azithromycin 500 mg per day for 3 days, azithromycin 500 mg per day for 6 days, or placebo, with the primary end point being a reduction in anti-*C. pneumoniae* titers. After 6 months, anti-*C. pneumoniae* titers fell to $1:16$ or less in 43% of those patients receiving antibiotics compared with only 10% of the patients receiving placebo ($p = 0.02$). Analysis of secondary clinical end points revealed that patients with high anti-*C. pneumoniae* titers who did not receive antibiotics had an increased risk of adverse cardiac events compared with patients treated with antibiotics who had a similar outcome as patients with negative anti-*C. pneumoniae* antibodies (Fig. 2).

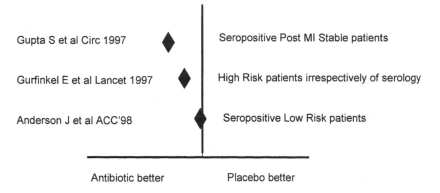

Figure 2 Interventional studies.

In the Randomised Trial of Roxithromycin in Non-Q-wave Coronary Syndromes: ROXIS Pilot Study (1), we designed the first clinical trial with a primary clinical end point to prove the benefit of antibiotics in coronary artery disease. More than 200 patients admitted with the diagnosis of unstable angina or non-Q-wave infarction were randomly assigned to receive either the macrolide roxithromycin (150 mg twice daily) or placebo for 30 days with primary end points of cardiac ishemic death, recurrent myocardial infarction, or severe recurrent angina. Patients were randomly assigned independently of basal anti-*Chlamydia* antibody titers, because there is no current evidence that IgG titers, as a marker of chronic infection, have any use in guiding treatment. It is, for instance, unknown whether a titer of 1:64 confers more or less risk than 1:32. Also, other ''*Chlamydia*-like'' proteins may activate the immune system and may also be sensitive to antibiotics, thereby falsely affecting antibody titers. These factors may make *Chlamydia* IgG titers less important in clinical decisions. Patients were enrolled in both private and public hospitals in different socioeconomic areas of Argentina to demonstrate the universal presence of this pathogen. Of the 202 patients initially enrolled, 196 completed 72 hours of treatment, with 129 finishing all 30 days of treatment. Patients who completed at least 72 hours of treatment with roxithromycin had a significantly lower rate of combined clinical end points (1 vs. 10%, adjusted $p = 0.032$) after 30 days of follow-up (Figs. 2, 3).

The ACADEMIC trial tested azithromycin in 300 patients with unstable angina. A very few numbers of events occurred during the study probably due to the low risk profile of this population. Results at 6 months fail to demonstrate a benefit of antibiotic treatment (Figs. 2, 3).

Azithromycin and roxithromycin were chosen because macrolides are active against *Chlamydia* and quickly reach a high intracellular concentration. Azithromycin achieves a cellular-to-extracellular concentration ratio of 300 after

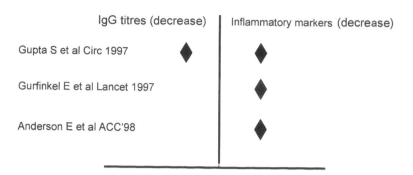

Figure 3   Interventional studies.

3 hours, whereas roxithromycin achieves a plateau slightly quicker, 30 to 60 minutes, but with a ratio of 100 (132). An important issue in both studies is the potential anti-inflammatory effect of macrolide antibiotics beyond their antimicrobial action. Azithromycin lowers the concentration of tissue factor (133). Long-term treatment of a chronic inflammatory respiratory disease with the macrolide erythromycin has improved patient outcome not through bactericidal activity but through a hypothesized inhibition of neutrophils and lymphocytes in bronchial tissue that reduced inflammation (134). Other antibiotics also have anti-inflammatory properties. Tetracycline drugs, for example, inhibit human collagenase activity (135), which could temper the degradation of the protective fibrous cap of atherosclerotic lesions mediated by active inflammation. Antibiotics may also act as free radical scavengers (136). These early results need confirmation by large-scale studies, not only to confirm the efficacy of antibiotic treatment but also to evaluate the use of serological evidence in identifying patients at higher risk and define the optimal treatment period. Two large-scale trials with greater power to detect a clinical difference between control are testing the efficacy of azithromycin therapy in patients with coronary artery disease.

VII.   CONCLUSIONS

Thus far, the most convincing evidence links both cytomegalovirus and *C. pneumoniae* to atherosclerosis. Extensive research into the relationship between viruses and atherosclerosis supports an epidemiological association. Cytomegalovirus may have a more important role in postangioplasty restenosis, although its role in natural atherosclerosis development cannot be discarded. There is sufficient epidemiological evidence with a growing body of pathophysiological research to implicate *C. pneumoniae* in both the prolonged gradual development of atherosclerosis and perhaps as a precipitant of acute atherothrombotic events.

The mainstay of treatment of acute events such as stroke, unstable angina, and acute myocardial injury centers on minimizing the damage of intra-arterial thrombosis formed after the onset of severe endothelial damage with urgent angioplasty, thrombolytics, antithrombotics, and antiplatelet therapy. Treatment is aimed at the consequences of the disease rather than at the causes. To date, the two most effective preventive treatments involve reducing plaque instability. Aspirin, in addition to an antiplatelet effect, may offer a weak anti-inflammatory component. Patients receiving aspirin therapy have lower C-reactive protein levels (139). The HMG CoA reductase inhibitor drugs also reduce the risk of a myocardial infection through theoretically reducing plaque lipid content and improving plaque stability.

Atherosclerosis and subsequent arterial thrombosis are likely the end result of various and diverse injuries to the arterial wall. All patients are not susceptible to the same injuries. Just as we do not treat all anemic patients with vitamin B_{12} injections, we may not need to treat all coronary patients with aggressive lipid-lowering agents (140). Treatment might become tailored to individual risk factors. Just as patients with hypercholesterolemia benefit from lipid-lowering drugs, patients with high serological titers to cytomegalovirus may benefit from postangioplasty antiviral treatment. Antibiotics may be appropriate for patients with evidence of acute or chronic *C. pneumoniae* infection. Considering the large burden that atherosclerotic disease inflicts on society, we should be open to new treatments to prevent the most severe consequences. The development of atherosclerosis remains largely an enigma, but infection may turn out to be a critical, but treatable, component.

REFERENCES

1. Gurfinkel E, Bozovich G, Daroca A, Beck E, Mautner B. Randomised trial of rox-ithromycin in non-Q-wave coronary syndromes: ROXIS Pilot Study. ROXIS Study Group. Lancet 1997; 350(9075):404–407.
2. Braunwald E. Shattuck Lecture—Cardiovascular medicine at the turn of the millennium: Triumphs, concerns, and opportunities. N Engl J Med 1997; 337(19):1360–1369.
3. Osler W. Diseases of the Arteries. In: Osler W, ed. Modern Medicine—Its Practice and Theory. Philadelphia: Lea & Febiger, 1908:429–447.
4. Ophuls W. Atherosclerosis and cardiovascular disease: their relation to infectious disease. JAMA 1921; 76(11):700–701.
5. Frothingham C. The relation between acute infectious diseases and arterial lesions. Arch Intern Med 1911:153–162.
6. Woodhouse PR, Khaw KT, Plummer M, Foley A, Meade TW. Seasonal variations

of plasma fibrinogen and factor VII activity in the elderly: winter infections and death from cardiovascular disease. Lancet 1994; 343(8895):435–439.

7. Tillet HE, Smith JWG, Gooch CD. Excess death attributable to influenza in England and Wales: Age at death and certified cause. Int J Epidem 1983; 12(3):344–352.

8. Valtonen V, Kuikka A, Syrjanen J. Thrombo-embolic complications in bacteraemic infections. Eur Heart J 1993; 14(Suppl K):20–23.

9. Mattila KJ, Nieminen MS, Valtonen VV, et al. Association between dental health and acute myocardial infarction. BMJ 1989; 298:779–782.

10. Anestad G, Scheel O, Hungnes O. Chronic infection and coronary artery disease. Lancet 1997; 350:1028.

11. Kostis JB, Turkevich D, Sharp J. Association between leukocyte count and the presence and extent of corornary atherosclerosis as determined by coronary arteriography. Am J Cardiol 1984; 53:997–999.

12. Fabricant CG, Fabricant J, Litrenta MM, Minick CR. Virus-induced atherosclerosis. J Exp Med 1978; 148(1):335–340.

13. Ross R. The pathogenesosis of atherosclerosis. In: Braunwald E, ed. The Heart—A Textbook of Cardiovascular Medicine. 5th ed. Philadelphia: W.B. Saunders Co., 1997:1105–1121.

14. Ross R, Glomset JA. The pathogenesis of atherosclerosis. N Engl J Med 1976; 295(7):369–377, 420–425.

15. Ross R. The pathogenesis of atherosclerosis: a perspective for the 1990s. Nature 1993; 363:801–806.

16. Cooke PJ. The role of endothelium in atherosclerosis. In: Schultheiss H, Schwimmbeck P, eds. The Role of Immune Mechanisms in Cardiovascular Disease. Berlin: Springer, 1997:194–204.

17. Gurfinkel E, Bozovich G. *Chlamydia pneumoniae*: Inflammation and the instability of the plaque. Atherosclerosis 1998; 140(Suppl 1):S31–S35.

18. Fuster V, Badimon L, Badimon JJ, Chesebro JH. The pathophysiology of coronary artery disease and the acute coronary syndromes. N Engl J Med 1992; 326:242–250, 310–318.

19. Mascri A. The variable chronic atherosclerosis background. Ischemic Heart Disease. New York: Churchill Livingstone, Inc., 1995:194–237.

20. Ambrose JA, Tannenbaum MA, Alexopoulos D, et al. Angiographic progression of coronary artery disease and the development of myocardial infection. J Am Coll Cardiol 1988; 12(1):56–62.

21. Hackett D, Davies G, Maseri A. Pre-existing coronary stenoses in patients with first myocardial infarction are not necessarily severe. Eur Heart J 1988; 9(12):1317–1323.

22. Davies MJ, Thomas A. Plaque fissuring—the cause of acute myocardial infarction, sudden ischemic death, and crescendo angina. Br Heart J 1985; 53:363–373.

23. Farb A, Burke AP, Tang AL, et al. Coronary plaque erosion without rupture into a lipid core. Circulation 1996; 93:1354–1363.

24. Libby P. Molecular basis of the acute coronary syndrome. Circulation 1995; 91(11):2844–2850.

25. Schwartz BS. Antigen-induced monocyte procoagulant activity. Requirement for

antigen presentation and histocompatibility leukocyte antigen-DR molecules. J Clin Invest 1985; 76(3):970–977.

26. Gurfinkel E, Scirica B, Bozovich G, Manos E, Mautner B. Neopterin levels and the aggressivenes of atherosclerosis. Am J Cardiol 1999; 83:515–518.

27. Lendon CL, Davies MJ, Born GV, Richardson PD. Atherosclerotic plaque caps are locally weakened when macrophages density is increased. Atherosclerosis 1991; 87(1):87–90.

28. Davies MJ, Richardson PD, Woolf N, Katz DR, Mann J. Risk of thrombosis in human atherosclerotic plaques: role of extracellular lipid, macrophage, and smooth muscle cell content. Br Heart J 1993; 69(5):377–381.

29. De Servi S, Mazzone A, Ricevuto G, et al. Clinical and angiographic correlates of leukocyte activation in unstable angina. J Am Coll Cardiol 1995; 26(5):1146–1150.

30. van der Wal AC, Becker AE, van der Loos CM, Das PK. Site of intimal rupture or erosion of thrombosed coronary atherosclerotic plaques is characterized by an inflammatory process irrespective of dominat plaque morphology. Circulation 1994; 89:36–44.

31. Moreno PR, Fallon JT. Inflammation in acute coronary syndromes. In: Schultheiss H, Schwimmbeck P, eds. The Role of Immune Mechanisms in Cardiovascular Disease. Berlin: Springer, 1997:213–229.

32. Galis ZS, Suhkova GK, Lark MW, Libby P. Increased expression of matrix mettalloproeinases and matrix degrading activity in vulnerable regions of human atherosclerotic plaques. J Clin Invest 1994; 94:2493–2503.

33. Warner SJC, Friedman GB, Libby P. Immune interferon inhibits proliferation and induces 2′-5′-oligoadenylate synthetase gene expression in human vascular smooth muscle cells. J Clin Invest 1989; 83:1174–1182.

34. Hansson GK, Jonasson L, Holm J, Clowes MM, Clowes AW. Gamma-interferon regulates vascular smooth muscle proliferation and Ia antigen expression in vivo and in vitro. Circ Res 1988; 63(4):712–719.

35. Birnie D, Holme E, McKay IC, Hood S, McColl KEL, Hillis WS. Correlation between antibodies to heat shock protein 65 and coronary atherosclerosis: possible role of *Helicobacter pylori* infection. Eur Heart J 1996; 18(suppl):231.

36. Xu Q, Willeit J, Marosi M, et al. Association of serum antibodies to heat-shock protein 65 with carotid atherosclerosis. Lancet 1993; 341:255–259.

37. Leinonen M. Pathogenetic mechanisms and epidemiology of *Chlamydia pneumoniae*. Eur Heart J 1993; 14(Suppl K):57–61.

38. Nieminen MS, Mattila K, Valtonen V. Infection and inflammation as risk factors for myocardial infarction. Eur Heart J 1993; 14(Suppl K):12–16.

39. Epstein SE, Speir E, Zhou YF, Guetta E, Leon M, Finkel T. The role of infection in restenosis and atherosclerosis: focus on cytomegalovirus. Lancet 1996; 348:s13–s16.

40. Speir E, Modali R, Huang ES, et al. Potential role of human cytomegalovirus and p53 interaction in coronary restenosis. Science 1994; 265(5170):391–394.

41. Benditt EP, Benditt JM. Evidence for a monoclonal origin of human atherosclerotic plaques. Proc Natl Acad Sci USA 1973; 70(8):1753–1756.

42. Benditt EP. Implication of the monoclonal character of human atherosclerotic plaques. Am J Pathol 1977; 86(3):693–702.

43. Benditt EP, Barrett T, McDougall JK. Viruses in the etiology of atherosclerosis. Proc Natl Acad Sci USA 1983; 80(20):6386–6389.
44. Fabricant CG, Hajjar DP, Minnick CR, Fabricant J. Herpesvirus infection enhances cholesterol and cholesteryl ester accumulation in cultured arterial smooth muscle cells. Am J Pathol 1981; 105:176–184.
45. Minick CR, Fabricant CG, Fabricant J, Litrenta MM. Atherosclerosis induced by infection with a herpesvirus. Am J Pathol 1979; 96:673–706.
46. Hajjar DP, Fabricant CG, Minick CR, Fabricant J. Virus-induced atherosclerosis. Herpesvirus infection alters aortic cholesterol metabolism and accumulation. Am J Pathol 1986; 122(1):62–70.
47. Hajjar DP, Pomerantz KB, Falcone DJ, Weksler BB, Grant AJ. Herpes simplex virus infection in human arterial cells. Implications in arteriosclerosis. J Clin Invest 1987; 80(5):1317–1321.
48. Griffiths PD, Hannington G, Booth JC. Coxsackie B virus infections and myocardial infarction. Results from a prospective, epidemiologically controlled study. Lancet 1980; 1(8183):1387–1389.
49. Ilback NG, Mohammed A, Fohlman J, Friman G. Cardiovascular lipid accumulation with Coxsackie B virus infection in mice. Am J Pathol 1990; 136(1):159–167.
50. Nicholls AC, Thomas M. Coxsackie virus infection in acute myocardial infarction. Lancet 1977; 1(8017):883–884.
51. McDonald K, Rector TS, Braulin EA, Kubo SH, Olivari MT. Association of coronary artery disease in cardiac transplant recipients with cytomegalovirus infection. Am J Cardiol 1990; 64(5):359–362.
52. Grattan MT, Moreno-Cabral CE, Starnes VA, Oyer PE, Stinson EB, Shumway NE. Cytomegalovirus infection is associated with cardiac allograft rejection and atherosclerosis. JAMA 1989; 261(24):3561–3566.
53. Wu T, Hruban RH, Ambinder RF, et al. Demostration of cytomegalovirus nucleic acids in the coronary arteries of transplanted hearts. Am J Pathol 1992; 140:739–747.
54. Gulizia JM, Kandolf R, Kendall TJ, et al. Infrequency of cytomegalovirus genome in coronary arteriopathy of human heart allografts. Am J Pathol 1995; 147(2):461–475.
55. Adam E, Melnick JL, Probtsfield JL, et al. High levels of cytomegalovirus antibody in patients requiring vascular surgery for atherosclerosis. Lancet 1987; 2(8554):291–293.
56. Cour MI, Lopez de Atalaya FJ, Palau L, Fernandez Contreras E, Perezagua C. Lack of serological association between herpesvirus and atherosclerosis. Lancet 1989; 1(8632):279.
57. Nieto FJ, Adam E, Sorlie P, et al. Cohort study of cytomegalovirus infection as a risk factor for carotid intimal-medial thickening, a measure of subclinical atherosclerosis. Circulation 1996;94(5):922–927.
58. Chiu B, Viira E, Tucker W, Fong IW. *Chlamydia pneumoniae*, cytomegalovirus, and herpes simplex virus in atherosclerosis of the carotid artery. Circulation 1997; 96(7):2144–2148.
59. Zhou YF, Leon MB, Maclawiw MA, et al. Association between prior cytomegalo-

virus infection and the risk of restenosis after coronary atherectomy. N Engl J Med 1996; 335:624–630.

60. Hendrix MG, Dormans PH, Kitslaar P, Bosman F, Bruggeman CA. The presence of cytomegalovirus nucleic acids in arterial walls of atherosclerotic and nonatherosclerotic patients. Am J Pathol 1989; 134(5):1151–1157.

61. Danesh J, Collins R, Peto R. Chronic infections and coronary heart disease: Is there a link? Lancet 1997; 350(9075):430–436.

62. Hendrix MG, Salimans MM, van Boven CP, Bruggeman CA. High prevalence of latently present cytomegalovirus in arterial walls of patients suffering from grade III atherosclerosis. Am J Pathol 1990; 136(1):23–28.

63. Pauletto P, Pisoni G, Boschetto R, Zoleo M, Pessina AC, Palu G. Human cytomegalovirus and restenosis of the internal carotid artery. Stroke 1996; 27:1669–1671.

64. Kol A, Sperti G, Shani J, et al. Cytomegalovirus replication is not a cause of instability in unstable angina. Circulation 1995; 91(7):1910–1913.

65. Petrie BL, Melnick JL, Adam E, Burek J, McCollum CH, DeBakey ME. Nucleic acid sequences of cytomegalovirus in cell cultured from human arterial tissue. J Infect Dis 1987; 155(1):158–159.

66. van Dam-Mieras MCE, Muller AD, van Hinsbergh VWM, Mullers WJHA, Bomans PHH, Bruggeman CA. The procoagulant response of cytomegalovirus infected endothelial cells. Thromb Haemost 1992; 68(3):364–370.

67. Visser MR, Tracy PB, Vercellotti GM, Goodman JL, White JG, Jacob HS. Enhanced thrombin generation and platelet binding on herpes simplex virus-infected endothelium. Proc Natl Acad Sci USA 1988; 85(21):8227–8230.

68. Key NS, Vercellotti GM, Winkelmann JC, et al. Infection of vascular endothelial cells with herpes simplex virus enhances tissue factor activity and reduces thrombomodulin expression. Proc Natl Acad Sci USA 1990; 87(18):7095–7099.

69. Etingin OR, Silverstein RL, Hajjar DP. von Willebrand factor mediates platelet adhesion to virally infected endothelial cells. Proc Natl Acad Sci USA 1993; 90:5153–5156.

70. Visser MR, Vercellotti GM, McCarthy JB, et al. Herpes simplex virus inhibits endothelial cell attachment and migration to extracellular matrix proteins. Am J Pathol 1989; 134(1):223–230.

71. Ponzetto A, La Rovere MT, Sanseverino P, Bazzoli F. Association of *Helicobacter pylori* infection with coronary heart disease. BMJ 1996; 312:251.

72. Martin-de-Argila C, Boixeda D, Canton R, Gisbert JP, Fuertes A. High seroprevalence of *Helicobacter pylori* infection in coronary heart disease. Lancet 1995; 346(8970):310.

73. Morgando A, Sanseverino P, Perotto C, Molino V, Gai V, Ponzetto A. *Helicobacter pylori* seropositivity in myocardial infarction. Lancet 1995; 345:1380.

74. Aceti A, Mazzacurati G, Amendolea M, et al. Relation of C reactive protein to cardiovascular risk factors. *H pylori* and *C pneumoniae* infections may account for most acute coronary syndromes. BMJ 1996; 313(7054):428–429.

75. Mendall MA, Goggin PM, Molineaux N, et al. Relation of *Helicobacter pylori* infection and coronary heart disease. Br Heart J 1994; 71(5):437–439.

76. Ossei-Gerning N, Moayyedi P, Smith S, et al. *Helicobacter pylori* infection is re-

lated to atheroma in patients undergoing coronary angiography. Cardiovasc Res 1997; 35(1):120–124.

77. Patel P, Mendall MA, Carrington D, et al. Association of *Helicobacter pylori* and *Chlamydia pneumoniae* infections with coronary heart disease and cardiovascular risk factors [published erratum appears in BMJ 1995 Oct 14;311(7011):985]. Br Med J (Clinical Research Ed.) 1995; 311(7007):711–714.

78. McDonagh TA, Woodward M, Morrsion CE, et al. *Helicobacter pylori* infection and coronary artery disease in the North Glasgow MONICA population. Eur Heart J 1997; 18:1257–1260.

79. Murray LM, Bamford KB, O'Reilly DPJ, McCrum EE, Evans AE. *Helicobacter pylori* infection: relation with cardiovascular risk factors, ischeamic heart disease, and social class. Br Heart J 1995; 74:497–501.

80. Niemela S, Karttunen T, Korhonen T, et al. Could *Helicobacter pylori* infection increase the risk of coronary heart disease by modifying serum lipid concentrations? Heart 1996; 75(6):573–575.

81. Whincup PH, Mendall MA, Perry IJ, Strachan DP, Walker M. Prospective relations between *Helicobacter pylori* infection, coronary heart disease, and stroke in middle aged men. Heart 1996; 75(6):568–572.

82. Wald NJ, Law MR, Morris JK, Bagnall AM. *Helicobacter pylori* infection and mortality from ischaemic heart disease: negative result from a large, prospective study. BMJ 1997; 315:1199–1201.

83. Blasi F, Denti F, Erba M, et al. Detection of *Chlamydia pneumoniae* but not *Helicobacter pylori* in atherosclerotic plaques of aortic aneurysms. J Clin Microb 1996; 34(11):2766–2769.

84. Mendall MA, Patel P, Ballam L, Strachan D, Northfield TC. C reactive protein and its relation to cardiovascular risk factors: a population based cross sectional study. BMJ (Clinical Research Ed.) 1996; 312(7038):1061–1065.

85. Sung JJ, Sanderson JE. Hyperhomocysteinaemia, *Helicobacter pylori*, and coronary heart disease. Heart 1996; 76(4):305–307.

86. Ponka A, Jalanko H, Ponka T, Stenvik M. Viral and mycoplasmal antibodies in patients with myocardial infarction. Ann Clin Res 1981; 13(6):429–432.

87. Gurfinkel EP, Rozlosnik J, Bozovich G, Duronto E, Dos Santos A, Mautner B. IgG antibodies to *Chlamydia* and *Mycoplasma* infection plus C reactive protein related to poor outcome in unstable angina. Arch Ins Cardiol Mex 1997; 67:462–468.

88. Grayston JT, Kuo C, Wang S, Altman J. A new *Chlamydia psittaci* strain, TWAR, isolated in acute respiratory tract infections. N Engl J Med 1986; 315(3):161–168.

89. Marrie TJ, Peeling RW, Fine MJ, Singer DE, Coley CM. Ambulatory patients with community acquired pneumonia: The frequency of atypical agents and clinical course. Am J Med 1996; 1010:508–515.

90. Aldous MB, Grayston JT, Wang A, Foy H. Seroepidemiology of *Chlamydia pneumoniae* TWAR in Seattle Families, 1966–79. J Infect Dis 1992; 166:646–649.

91. Grayston JT, Campbell LA, Kuo CC, et al. A new respiratory tract pathogen: *Chlamydia pneumoniae* strain TWAR. J Infect Dis 1990; 161(4):618–625.

92. Hammerschlag MR. Diagnostic methods of intracellular pathogens. Clin Microb Infect 1996; 1(suppl 1):s3–s8.

93. Saikku P, Leinonen M, Mattila K, et al. Serological evidence of an association of

a novel *Chlamydia*, TWAR, with chronic coronary heart disease and acute myocardial infarction. Lancet 1988; 2(8618):983–986.

94. Saikku P, Leinonen M, Tenkanen L, et al. Chronic *Chlamydia pneumoniae* infection as a risk factor for coronary heart disease in the Helsinki Heart Study. Ann Intern Med 1992; 116(4):273–278.

95. Linnamaki E, Leinomen M, Mattila K, M.S. N, Valtonen V, Saikku P. *Chlamydia pneumoniae*–specific circulating immune complexes in patients with coronary heart disease. Circulation 1993; 87:1130–1134.

96. Thomas GN, Scheel O, Koehler AP, Bassett DCJ, Cheng AFB. Respiratory Chlamydial infections in a Hong Kong teaching hospital and association with coronary heart disease. Scand J Infect Dis 1997; 104(suppl):30–33.

97. Thom DH, Grayston JT, Siscovick DS, Wang SP, Weiss NS, Daling JR. Association of prior infection with *Chlamydia pneumoniae* and angiographically demonstrated coronary artery disease. JAMA 1992; 268(1):68–72.

98. Miettinen H, Lehto S, Saikku P, et al. Association of *Chlamydia pneumoniae* and acute coronary heart disease events in non-insulin dependent diabetic and nondiabetic subjects in Finland. Eur Heart J 1996; 17(5):682–688.

99. Mendall MA, Carrington D, Strachan D, et al. *Chlamydia pneumoniae* Risk factors for seropositivity and association with coronary heart disease. J Infect 1995; 30: 121–128.

100. Blasi F, Cosentini R, Raccanelli R, et al. A possible association of *Chlamydia pneumoniae* infection and acute myocardial infarction in patients younger than 65 years of age. Chest 1997; 112(2):309–312.

101. Cook PJ, Honeybourne D, Lip GYH, Beevers DG, Wise R. *Chlamydia pneumoniae* and acute arterial thrombotic disease. Circulation 1995; 92(10):3148–3149.

102. Dahloff K, Maass M. *Chlamydia pneumoniae* pneumonia in hospitalized patients. Chest 1996; 110:351–356.

103. Hahn DL, Golubjatnikov R. Smoking is a potential confounder of the *Chlamydia pneumoniae*–coronary artery disease association. Arterioscler Thromb 1992; 12(8): 945–947.

104. Karvenon M, Tuomilehto J, Pitkaniemi J, Naukkarinen A, Saikku P. Importance of smoking for *Chlamydia pneumoniae* seropositivity. Int J Epidemiol 1994; 23(6): 1315–1321.

105. Wimmer ML, Sandmann-Strupp R, Saikku P, Haberl RL. Association of chlamydial infection with cerebrovascular disease. Stroke 1996; 27(12):2207–2210.

106. Kark JD, Leinonen M, Paltiel O, Saikku P. *Chlamydia pneumoniae* and acute myocardial infarction in Jerusalem. Int J Epidemiol 1997; 26(4):730–738.

107. Halme S, Syrjala H, Bloigu A, et al. Lymphocyte responses to *Chlamydia* antigens in patients with coronary heart disease. Eur Heart J 1997; 18(7):1095–1101.

108. Thom DH, Wang SP, Grayston JT, et al. *Chlamydia pneumoniae* strain TWAR antibody and angiographically demonstrated coronary artery disease. Arterioscler Thromb 1991; 11(3):547–551.

109. Melnick SL, Shahar E, Folsom AR, et al. Past infection by *Chlamydia pneumoniae* strain TWAR and asymptomatic carotid atherosclerosis. Atherosclerosis Risk in Communities (ARIC) Study Investigators. Am J Med 1993; 95(5):499–504.

110. Kuo CC, Grayston JT, Campbell LA, Goo YA, Wissler RW, Benditt EP. *Chlamydia*

pneumoniae (TWAR) in coronary arteries of young adults (15–34 years old). Proc Natl Acad Sci USA 1995; 92(15):6911–6914.

111. Kuo CC, Shor A, Campbell LA, Fukushi H, Patton DL, Grayston JT. Demonstration of Chlamydia pneumoniae in atherosclerotic lesions of coronary arteries. J Infect Dis 1993; 167(4):841–849.

112. Kuo CC, Gown AM, Benditt EP, Grayston JT. Detection of Chlamydia pneumoniae in aortic lesions of atherosclerosis by immunocytochemical stain. Arterioscler Thromb 1993; 13(10):1501–1504.

113. Ramirez JA. Isolation of *Chlamydia pneumoniae* from the coronary artery of a patient with coronary atherosclerosis. The *Chlamydia pneumoniae*/Atherosclerosis Study Group. Ann Intern Med 1996; 125(12):979–982.

114. Muhlenstein JB, Hammond EH, Carlquist JF, et al. Increased incidence of chlamydial species within the coronary arteries of patients with symptomatic atherosclerotic versus other forms of cardiovascular disease. J Am Coll Cardiol 1996; 37(7):1555–1561.

115. Jackson LA, Campbell LA, Kuo CC, Grayston JT. Detection of *Chlamydia pneumoniae* in atheroma specimens. J Infect Dis 1996; 174(4):893–896.

116. Grayston JT, Kuo CC, Coulson AS, et al. *Chlamydia pneumoniae* (TWAR) in atherosclerosis of the carotid artery. Circulation 1995; 92(12):3397–3400.

117. Jackson LA, Campbell LA, Kuo CC, Rodriguez DI, Lee A, Grayston JT. Isolation of *Chlamydia pneumoniae* from a carotid endarterectomy specimen. J Infect Dis 1997; 176(1):292–295.

118. Ong G, Thomas BJ, Mansfield AO, Davidson BR, Taylor-Robinson D. Detection and widespread distribution of *Chlamydia pneumoniae* in the vascular system and its possible implications. J Clin Pathol 1996; 49(2):102–106.

119. Juvonen J, Juvonen T, Laurila A, et al. Demonstration of *Chlamydia pneumoniae* in the walls of abdominal aortic aneurysms. J Vasc Surg 1997; 25(3):499–505.

120. Weiss SM, Roblin PM, Gaydos CA, et al. Failure to detect *Chlamydia pneumoniae* in coronary atheromas of patients undergoing atherectomy. J Infect Dis 1996; 173: 957–962.

121. Gaydos CA, Summersgill JT, Sahney NN, Ramirez JA, Quinn TC. Replication of *Chlamydia pneumoniae* in vitro in human macropages, endothelial cells, and aortic artery smooth muscle cells. Inf Immun 1996; 64(5):1614–1620.

122. Schett G, Xu Q, Amberger A, et al. Autoantibodies against heat shock protein 60 mediate endothelial cytotoxicity. J Clin Invest 1995; 96(6):2569–2577.

123. Metzler B, Schett G, Kleindienst R, et al. Epitope specificity of anti-heat shock protein 65/60 serum antibodies in atherosclerosis. Arterioscler Thromb Vasc Biol 1997; 17(3):536–541.

124. Morrison RP, Belland RJ, Lyng K, Caldwell HD. Chlamydial disease pathogenesis. The 57-kD chlamydial hypersensitivity antigen is a stress response protein. J Exp Med 1989; 170(4):1271–1283.

125. Arno JN, Yuan Y, Cleary RE, Morrison RP. Serologic responses of infertile women to the 60-kd chlamydial heat shock protein (hsp60). Fertil Steril 1995; 64(4):730–735.

126. Jones RB. *Chlamydia trachamotis*. In: Mandel GL, Bennet JE, Dolin R, eds. The

Principles and Practice of Infectious Diseases. New York: Churchill Livingstone, 1995:1679–1693.

127. Gurfinkel E, Duronto E, Cerda M, et al. Patients with unstable angina with C reactive protein and *Chlamydia pneumoniae* infection—Clinical outcome. Eur Heart J 1996; 17(suppl):S–578.

128. Moazed TC, Kuo C, Grayston JT, Campbell LA. Murine models of *Chlamydia pneumoniae* infection and atherosclerosis. J Infect Dis 1997; 175(4):883–890.

129. Fong IW, Chiu B, Viira E, Fong MW, Jang D, Mahony J. Rabbit model for *Chlamydia pneumoniae* infection. J Clin Microb 1997; 35(1):48–52.

130. Moazed TC, Kuo C, Patton DL, Grayston JT, Campbell LA. Experimental rabbit models of *Chlamydia pneumoniae* infection. Am J Pathol 1996; 148(2):667–676.

131. Gupta S, Leatham EW, Carrington D, Mendall MA, Kaski JC, Camm AJ. Elevated *Chlamydia pneumoniae* antibodies, cardiovascular events, and azithromycin in male survivors of myocardial infarction. Circulation 1997; 96(2):404–407.

132. Labro MT. Intracellular bioactivity of macrolides. Clin Microb Infect 1996; 1(suppl 1):s24–s30.

133. Gupta S, Leatham EW, Carrington D, et al. The effect of azithromycin in postmyocardial infarction (MI) patients with elevated *Chlamydia pneumoniae* antibody titres. J Am Coll Cardiol 1997; 29(suppl A):209A.

134. Kadota J. Non-antibiotic effect of antibiotics. Clin Microb Infect 1996; 1(suppl2):2s20–2s22.

135. Greenwald JA, Golub LM, Lavietes B, et al. Tetracyclines inhibit human synovial collagenase in vivo and in vitro. J Rheum 1987; 14(1):28–32.

136. Halliwell B. Chronic infection and coronary artery disease. Lancet 1997; 350:1030.

137. Libby P, Egan D, Skarlatos S. Roles of infectious agents in atherosclerosis and restenosis—An assessment of the evidence and need for future research. Circulation 1997; 96(11):4095–4103.

138. Marshall BJ. *Helicobacter pylori* in peptic ulcer: have Koch's postulates been fulfilled? Ann Med 1995; 27(5):565–568.

139. Ridker PM, Cushman M, Stampfer MJ, Tracy RP, Hennekens CH. Inflammation, aspirin, and the risk of cardiovascular disease in apparently healthy men. N Engl J Med 1997; 336(14):973–979.

140. Maseri A. Inflammation, atherosclerosis, and ischemic events: Exploring the hidden side of the moon. N Engl J Med 1997; 336(14):1014–1015.

21

Plaque Sealing
Mechanical Treatment to Stabilize Plaque

Willibald Maier
University Hospital Zurich, Zurich, Switzerland

Bernhard Meier
University Hospital, Bern, Switzerland

I. DEFINITION OF PLAQUE SEALING

Plaque sealing is defined as angioplasty of an angiographically nonsignificant coronary stenosis in a strategically important vessel without previous infarction (1). This is based on the following rationale: coronary angioplasty typically induces an extensive splitting of the atherosclerotic plaque. This splitting engenders proliferation of new tissue layers covering the former plaque area (i.e., plaque sealing). The smooth muscle–rich intima observed over the first few months after angioplasty transforms into a collagen-rich layer subsequently (2). Thus once the acute effect with its inherent risk of acute occlusion has passed, the subsequent risk of acute occlusion should be markedly reduced compared with that of an untreated plaque. The covering of the intimal wound by cell proliferation, caused by angioplasty, may well have the beneficial effect of plaque sealing, but it is also a major component of restenosis. Restenosis is a significant shortcoming of coronary angioplasty, but it can be dealt with effectively and is not irreversible. In contrast, acute occlusion caused by plaque rupture may cause irreversible myocardial damage or even death (3).

Several clarifications need to be made around this working hypothesis. The reasons for a patient to undergo coronary angiography, the assessment of stenosis severity versus the symptoms, the risk profile for coronary artery disease, and the anticipated clinical course of the disease require consideration. Plaque sealing serves to possibly prevent future rupture of a coronary plaque that has been identified by angiography. In a typical scenario, a patient is discovered to have a stenosis that is not flow-limiting—defined by morphological (angiography, intravascular ultrasonography) or physiological (coronary flow reserve, fractional flow reserve) assessment. Thus the patient does not have typical angina pectoris or objective signs of ischemia. If the patient has demonstrable angina pectoris (by stress test or scintigraphy), angioplasty of an angiographically borderline stenosis would represent standard therapeutic angioplasty and plaque sealing would be a welcome side product but not the primary intention. Small vessel disease with typically reduced coronary flow reserve also is another disease entity and will be addressed briefly for differentiation. The second crucial point for this concept is a pragmatic one: angiography has already been performed on the patient for whatever reason, there is vascular access, and a coronary catheter is in place. A lesion of <50% diameter stenosis by visual estimate or on-line quantitative coronary angiography has been identified in a proximal segment of the left anterior descending, left circumflex, or right coronary artery with a sufficiently large perfusion territory to cause a major myocardial infarction in case of plaque rupture and thrombotic occlusion. Given these circumstances, an immediate decision is warranted whether to proceed with a preventive angioplasty to transform this potentially vulnerable plaque mechanically into scar tissue by stimulating a healing response. Do we know anything about the potential of this specific plaque to undergo rupture? Do we know when it is likely to happen? Do we know about the natural course of nonsignificant plaques? Not really, because data are sparse (4). Positive data exist as to the presence of numerous angiographically inapparent plaques with growth toward the lamina elastica externa and enlargement of the vessel circumference (5) in apparently (luminographically) normal coronary arteries. Next, the potential risk of performing angioplasty in this lesion must be taken into account.

II. PLAQUE MORPHOLOGY: IMPACT FOR MECHANICAL STABILIZATION

Fig. 1 shows characteristics of the vulnerable and the stable plaque (6). Atherosclerotic plaques typically consist of a lipid-rich core in the central portion of the eccentrically thickened intima. The lipid core is bonded on its luminal side by a fibrous cap. The thickness of the fibrous cap is one of the determinants of the probability of the plaque to undergo rupture. Fig. 1 represents a non-pressure-fixed cross-section of a coronary artery with a thick fibrous cap in the upper right side and a thin fibrous cap in the lower left side (arrows). Clinical data suggest that stable plaques more often show luminal narrowing detectable by angiography than do vulnerable plaques (6). The central, lipid-rich core contains many lipid-laden macrophage foam cells derived from blood monocytes. In Fig. 1, the dark staining indicates CD 68–positive inflammatory macrophages, which extend close to the surface of the thin fibrous cap in the lower left margin. At the site of

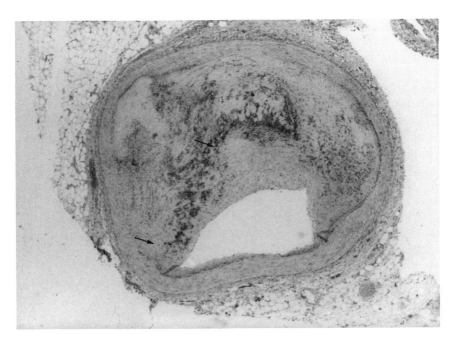

Figure 1 Characteristics of the vulnerable and the stable plaque. Non-pressure-fixed cross-section of a coronary artery with a thick fibrous cap in the upper right side and a thin fibrous cap in the lower left side (arrows). The dark staining indicates CD 68-positive inflammatory macrophages, which extend close to the surface of the thin fibrous cap in the lower left margin. (Courtesy of T. Schaffner, MD, Pathology, University Hospital, Bern.)

lesion disruption, smooth muscle cells are often activated, and the inflammatory reaction is pronounced. Disruption of fibrous caps occurs at points of ongoing inflammation, indicated by the presence of activated macrophages (7). Macrophages can degrade extracellular matrix by phagocytosis or by secreting proteolytic enzymes such as plasminogen activators and matrix metalloproteinases, all capable of weakening the fibrous cap (8). In this context, the concept of atherosclerosis as an inflammatory disease has emerged, and inflammatory processes have been shown to play a role even in very early stages of the disease characterized by endothelial dysfunction and mediated by leukocyte adhesion molecules (9). Several reports have shown an association between the incidence of atherosclerosis and the presence of infectious agents, among them *Chlamydia pneumoniae* (10). Interestingly, there are observations that chlamydial proteins can induce metalloproteinase production under experimental conditions and thus provide a link to plaque vulnerability (11). Several ongoing clinical studies address the role of infectious agents in acute ischemic syndromes and restenosis, which might elucidate the possible role of anti-inflammatory (antibiotic?) therapy in the context of pharmacological plaque passivation.

Only a minority of spontaneous plaque ruptures lead to total occlusion of the vessel and to infarction. Most heal and may contribute to a more severe stenosis by an overzealous coating with neointimal layers. In analogy to the mechanical plaque-sealing theory, it is unlikely that the very same site will fissure again in the future. Yet, these small fissures only lead to a very localized sealing of the plaque, and the remainder of the plaque may remain unsealed and therefore dangerous.

The mechanical approach by percutaneous transluminal coronary angioplasty (PTCA) intends to convert the thin fibrous cap of the lower left side into the thick fibrous septum of the upper right side in Fig. 1 by creating a stretch, tear, or even dissection of the vessel wall, thereby inducing wound-healing mechanisms.

III. FACTORS TRIGGERING PLAQUE RUPTURE

Considering mechanical aspects of plaque stabilization, possible factors triggering plaque rupture (8) and the respective therapeutic options will be taken into account. *Cap tension* is determined in part by the circumferential tension in the wall, which relates to blood pressure and luminal diameter according to Laplace's law. An additional important factor in this equation, however, is the tensile strength of the fibrous cap itself determined by its own consistency and that of the surrounding or underlying tissue (e.g., the atheromatous gruel of the lipid core). Although blood pressure easily can be treated medically, the lipid content of the plaque might be influenced by aggressive lipid-lowering. This is suggested by experimental studies (12,13) and the incidence of coronary events in large-scale statin (14,15) studies, although not yet ultimately proven by direct morphological evidence in humans. Mechanical plaque stabilization remains a treatment option to be considered on angiographic identification of a plaque in a strategically important location until final evidence of pharmacological passivation exists. *Heart contraction*, especially axial vessel bending and stretching might be another trigger mechanism with few possible inhibitors (beta-blockers?). *Vaso motion* and *vasospasm* are not within the scope of mechanical stabilization and might be influenced pharmacologically (nitrates and calcium antagonists). *Capillary bleeding* within the plaque has been suggested as a possible trigger for which no therapeutic option is evident except elimination of the plaque. *Wall shear stresses* are usually smaller than blood and pulse pressure, but exact calculation of regional wall stress within the human coronary arteries might represent a future option for determining *loci minoris resistentiae* within coronary segments containing extensive plaque.

IV. IDENTIFICATION OF THE VULNERABLE PLAQUE?

Identification of a coronary plaque prone to rupture would be the most desirable approach before intended mechanical stabilization. However, currently no method exists that reliably discriminates vulnerable and stable plaques. *Intravascular ultrasonogarphy* (IVUS) in the present two-dimensional mode detects coronary wall morphology (16,17) but has not been proven able to identify vulnerable plaques (18). In the future, complex approaches toward anatomically correct three-dimensional reconstruction of intravascular ultrasonography using image fusion of IVUS and angiography (19) might provide indirect indicators for plaques at risk by means of cap/plaque volume ratio and shear stress calculations. Current technology does not yet allow performance of these analyses routinely. Coronary angioscopy has been shown to provide some criteria for identification of unstable plaques (18,20–23), but the method has been abandoned because of unrealistic complexity for routine clinical purposes. Intracoronary temperature measurements, magnetic resonance imaging (MRI), or MR spectroscopy might offer theoretical potential for application in this respect, without any current clinical practicability, however. The development of a tool for intracoronary analysis of plaque vulnerability (detection of the inflammatory process?) would be most intriguing for the concept of mechanical plaque stabilization.

V. A MISSED CHANCE

Fig. 2 shows the coronary angiogram of a 54-year-old patient referred for primarily atypical angina. The stress tests (exercise electrocardiogram and thallium scintigraphy) were negative, but in the presence of risk factors cardiac catheterization was performed to exclude coronary artery disease. Angiography revealed a nonsignificant lesion of the proximal left anterior descending (LAD) artery. Left ventricular function was normal (Fig. 3). No current indication for an intervention was present. The patient was given aspirin and discharged. About 4 weeks later, the patient was seen in the emergency department with a large anterior myocardial infarction with severely compromised ventricular function (Fig. 4).

VI. CALCULATED PROBABILITIES OF MYOCARDIAL INFARCTION AND RESTENOSIS

The literature clearly indicates that about 80% or more of all infarctions result from acute thrombosis on a lesion, which by itself is not hemodynamically significant (4,24–26). This does not mean that a mild stenosis is more dangerous in terms of producing an acute infarction than a severe stenosis. It rather implies that there are commonly numerous mild stenoses to every single severe stenosis,

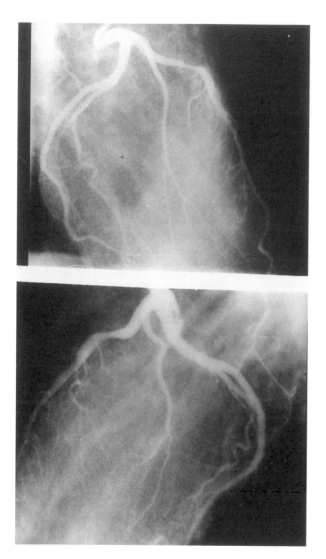

Figure 2 Biplane coronary angiogram of a 54-year-old patient referred for atypical angina. The stress tests (exercise ECG and thallium scintigraphy) were negative. Angiography reveals a nonsignificant lesion of the proximal LAD.

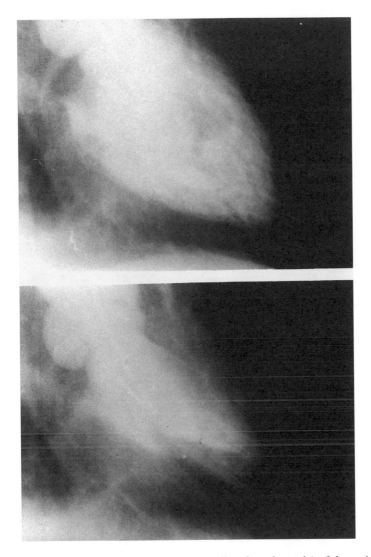

Figure 3 Left ventricular angiogram (diastole and systole) of the patient with the non-significant LAD stenosis shown in Fig. 2 at the time of first diagnostic catheterization. Normal left ventricular function without wall motion abnormalities.

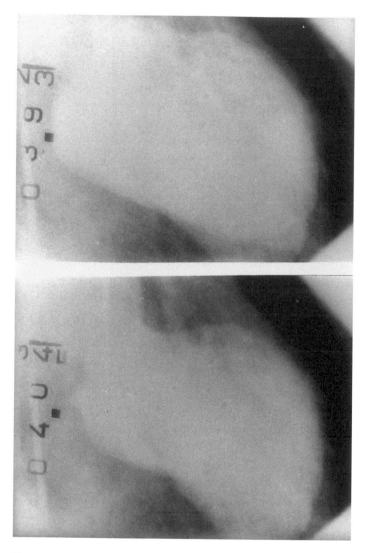

Figure 4   Left ventricular angiogram of the same patient 4 weeks later. Large anterior myocardial infarction with severely compromised ventricular function.

and it is the cumulative risk of all the nonsignificant stenoses that prevails (27). According to the Coronary Artery Surgery Study registry data, the risk of infarction over 3 years is 2% for a stenosis of less than 50%, 7% for a stenosis of 50 to 70%, 8% for a stenosis of 70 to 90%, 15% for a stenosis of 90 to 98%, and 7% for a functionally occlusive lesion (28). A number of other factors also influence the risk of subsequent occlusion and infarction, such as an irregular surface of the lesion or a lesion in a tortuous segment (28), a branching point stenosis (28,29), or a proximal location of the stenosis (25). The latter criterion may be misleading. The more proximal a lesion, the more likely it is that the resultant occlusion will become manifest to the clinician or the pathologist.

Let us direct our attention to the likely outcome of the mild or moderate lesion subjected to coronary angioplasty. Enough data have been accumulated to emphasize the fact that such lesions have a lower risk of acute occlusion and restenosis after angioplasty, which, nevertheless, must be taken into account. In the era of modern angioplasty equipment and techniques, particularly with the use of stents for suboptimal results and for impending or acute occlusions, infarctions should occur in less than 3% of procedures in the acute phase. To this we have to add roughly a 0.5% incidence of infarctions during the next year (including the risk carried by repeat angioplasty in about 20% of patients), if we count only the ones being unequivocally attributable to the dilated site (30). Beyond this period, spontaneous infarctions related to the dilated site are extremely rare. Even in case of restenosis, the highest incidence of related infarctions reported is 0.5% (31–34).

It has also been observed that the incidence of all late infarctions (related or unrelated to the dilated site) is independent of the occurrence of restenosis (35). This indicates that these infarctions are not related to the dilated site itself but predominantly to other diseased segments (unsealed plaques). Although occlusions at the dilated site do occur in a few percent of patients during long-term follow-up after angioplasty, these occlusions typically occur in previously occluded or collateralized vessels and rarely cause a clinical event (36). Although these data largely pertain to hemodynamically significant stenoses, the figures for nonsignificant stenoses are bound to be similar, if not lower. In fact, one study of 415 patients who underwent angioplasty for moderately severe stenoses reported only one case of myocardial infarction (37). Another small study addressing truly nonsignificant stenoses (<50% diameter stenosis assessed by quantitative coronary angiography), which had been dilated in the same session with a significant stenosis and had angiographic follow-up at 6 months, reported no major adverse cardiac events related to these stenoses during that period. However, no angiographic benefit was seen at 6 months, i.e., the same nonsignificant diameter stenosis was observed, albeit possibly with different plaque histology (38).

VII. CLINICAL EXAMPLES

On decision to perform angioplasty in a nonsignificant stenosis for preventive reasons, the method and the potential risk deserve consideration. Fig. 5 shows a plaque-sealing angioplasty of the mid LAD performed through the diagnostic 4F system with a Cordis Lightning 3.0-mm fixed wire balloon. This illustrates the underlying philosophy: keep the procedure as simple and as cost-effective as possible. In this example it is not even necessary to exchange the sheath, and the diagnostic 4F catheter can be easily advanced for a deep engagement to provide sufficient backup for balloon advancement, if necessary. Another important point is illustrated here as well: during balloon inflation, contrast was injected, which is trapped by the inflated balloon. There is no washout at 3 minutes of balloon inflation (Fig. 5), indicating no collateral perfusion at all for this nonsignificant

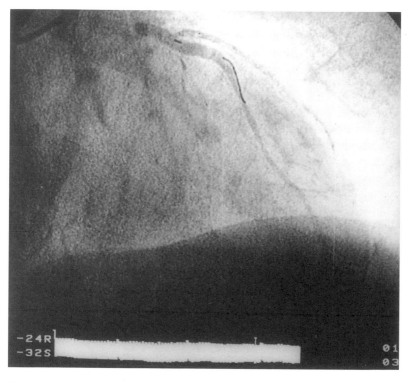

Figure 5   Plaque-sealing angioplasty of the mid LAD performed through the diagnostic 4F system with a Cordis Lightning 3.0-mm fixed wire balloon. During balloon inflation, contrast was injected, which is trapped by the inflated balloon. There is no washout at 3 minutes of balloon inflation indicating no collateral perfusion.

lesion. This is expected, but focuses attention on two aspects: first, if that plaque ruptured spontaneously, a large, possibly lethal myocardial infarction could ensue. Second, angioplasty is imposing a certain risk to the uncollateralized territory. However, mild lesions without calcification or complex anatomy rarely show serious dissections or acute closure. Stenting should be used only on a conditional basis to save cost and to avoid imposing the unsolved problem of a long in-stent restenosis on a physiologically noncritical lesion, which is dilated for preventive purposes.

VIII. PHYSIOLOGICAL ASSESSMENT AND SMALL VESSEL DISEASE

There is no rationale from flow dynamics or structure-function relationships to dilate nonsignificant stenoses, because lesions with diameter reduction of 45% or less have an almost normal coronary flow reserve (39). The concept of measuring coronary flow reserve or fractional flow reserve (40) only relates to functional lesion severity. The concept of plaque sealing is preventive and independent of functional relevance. Dilating nonsignificant stenoses with a reduced coronary flow reserve or fractional flow reserve means therapeutic angioplasty. Plaque

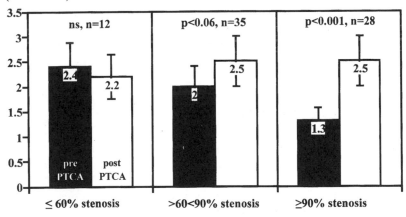

Figure 6 Coronary flow velocity reserve (CFVR) before and after PTCA from a series of routine coronary angioplasties. Coronary flow reserve is normal before PTCA in borderline lesions and unchanged after the procedure. Significant lesions show a reduced CFVR before intervention, which increases after PTCA.

sealing is still a by-product of the procedure, but it is not the principal reason for the procedure. This is illustrated in Fig. 6, which shows a series of patients from our institution in whom coronary flow reserve measurements have been performed during routine coronary angioplasty. Coronary flow reserve was normal before PTCA in borderline lesions and remained unchanged after angioplasty, whereas it was reduced in the significant lesions before intervention and increased thereafter.

Patients with small vessel disease or syndrome X represent a heterogenous population (41). Patients with microvascular dysfunction usually show an impaired coronary flow reserve (42). There might be symptom overlap between patients with classical syndrome X and patients with atypical angina and documentation of a coronary plaque. However, syndrome X resulting from pure microvascular dysfunction should show no distinct plaques. On the other hand, the presence of nonsignificant coronary artery disease in syndrome X can be dealt with using the plaque-sealing approach.

IX. THE ULTIMATE EQUATION

The ultimate equation balances the risk of a spontaneous infarction based on a moderate (hemodynamically nonsignificant) lesion of 7% over 3 years to a 3% infarction rate during coronary angioplasty to which 0.5% has to be added for the next 4 to 5 years in two thirds of patients without restenosis and 2.5% in the remaining third with restenosis (factoring in a 2% infarction risk during the repeat coronary angioplasty). This yields a pessimistically calculated overall infarction risk in the plaque-sealing angioplasty group of 5%, which represents a relative risk reduction of about 30% over 3 years and argues in favor of angioplasty for such lesions.

X. CLINICAL EXPERIENCE

We have followed 30 patients with plaque sealing for up to 66 months. Mean reference diameter assessed by quantitative coronary angiography was 3.0 ± 0.4 mm; the target vessels were predominantly LAD (65%) and right coronary arteries (22%). Before intervention, mean ejection fraction was $74 \pm 7\%$, and no wall motion abnormalities were documented. The lesions were dilated from $45 \pm 2\%$ to $15 \pm 2\%$ diameter stenosis. No cardiac death or myocardial infarction occurred. Seven follow-up angiograms were performed for recurrence of initial symptoms and resulted in one repeat angioplasty of the dilated plaque, and three dilatations of new lesions.

A randomized trial for plaque sealing should be performed with parallel aggressive chemical plaque passivation in both arms. The small absolute benefit to be expected from plaque sealing in the first 2 years would require an extremely large sample size to ultimately prove the hypothesis under these conditions. Smaller or shorter duration trials may show no difference or even a disadvantage of the interventional strategy (e.g., DEFER trial, N. Pijls, B. de Bruyne, W. Wijns, Aalst), but they are subject to both type I and type II errors.

XI. MECHANICAL AND CHEMICAL PLAQUE STABILIZATION AND CONCLUSIONS

The merits of lipid lowering in slowing the progression of coronary artery disease have already been established in studies of lifestyle changes and dietary modification in small, well-documented study groups (43). Convincing evidence has been provided by large-scale lipid-lowering studies that lipid lowering reduces the incidence of coronary events (44,45) and may induce plaque passivation (15,46). The effect may be more impressive with aggressive lipid lowering and lead to the conclusion that the need for coronary intervention might be postponed or even obviated pharmacologically according to data from the AVERT trial (47). However, there is no convincing proof that interventions for coronary artery disease are not just being deferred by a few years. Moreover, the reduction in events in the AVERT trial, which compares PTCA with conservative management under aggressive lipid lowering, is mainly due to reductions in minor events (e.g., repeat hospitalization) in the medically treated group and not to reduction in hard end points like death or myocardial infarction during the first 18 months of follow-up. It is no mystery that once an invasive strategy is engaged, it produces downstream medical attention and expenditure, in part because of the patient's enhanced awareness of the disease, because it could not be managed medically.

The need for plaque sealing is affected, but not eliminated, by aggressive lipid lowering. It simply provides a solid background. We do not call for screening everyone older than 50 with coronary angiography to detect functionally nonsignificant plaques and dilate them. But once a coronary angiogram has been performed for whatever reasons and there is documentation of a nonsignificant coronary stenosis in a strategically important location without previous infarction, it is justified to proceed to preventive angioplasty according to the plaque-sealing concept. In case of multiple borderline plaques, this concept is moot for obvious reasons. Diffuse nonsignificant coronary artery disease needs aggressive medical risk factor management. The plaque-sealing patient additionally deserves lipid-lowering agents to derive benefit from both the pharmacological and the mechanical approach. In conclusion, plaque sealing in a carefully selected group of patients is definitively an option to consider.

REFERENCES

1. Meier B, Ramamurthy S. Plaque sealing by coronary angioplasty. Cathet Cardiovasc Diagn 1995; 36:295–297.
2. Inoue K, Nakamura N, Kakio T, Suyama H, Tanaka S, Goto Y, Nakazawa Y, Yamamoto Y, Nagamatsu T. Serial changes of coronary arteries after percutaneous transluminal coronary angioplasty: histopathological and immunohistochemical study. J Cardiol 1994; 24:279–291.
3. Virmani R, Farb A, Burke AP. Coronary angioplasty from the perspective of atherosclerotic plaque: morphologic predictors of immediate success and restenosis. Am Heart J 1994; 127:163–179.
4. Little WC, Constantinescu M, Applegate RJ, Kutcher MA, Burrows MT, Kahl FR, Santamore WP. Can coronary angiography predict the site of a subsequent myocardial infarction in patients with mild-to-moderate coronary artery disease? Circulation 1988; 78:1157–1166.
5. Glagov S, Weisenberg E, Zarins CK, Stankunavicius R, Kolettis GJ. Compensatory enlargement of human atherosclerotic coronary arteries. N Engl J Med 1987; 316: 1371–1375.
6. Libby P. Molecular bases of the acute coronary syndromes. Circulation 1995; 91: 2844–2850.
7. Falk E, Shah PK, Fuster V. Coronary plaque disruption. Circulation 1995; 92:657–671.
8. Gronholdt ML, Dalager-Pedersen S, Falk E. Coronary atherosclerosis: determinants of plaque rupture. Eur Heart J 1998; 19 Suppl C:C24–29.
9. Ross R. Atherosclerosis—an inflammatory disease. N Engl J Med. 1999; 340:115–126.
10. Libby P, Egan D, Skarlatos S. Roles of infectious agents in atherosclerosis and restenosis: an assessment of the evidence and need for future research. Circulation 1997; 96:4095–4103.
11. Kol A, Sukhova GK, Lichtman AH, Libby P. Chlamydial heat shock protein 60 localizes in human atheroma and regulates macrophage tumor necrosis factor-alpha and matrix metalloproteinase expression. Circulation 1998; 98:300–307.
12. Williams JK, Sukhova GK, Herrington DM, Libby P. Pravastatin has cholesterol-lowering independent effects on the artery wall of atherosclerotic monkeys. J Am Coll Cardiol 1998; 31:684–691.
13. Libby P, Aikawa M. New insights into plaque stabilisation by lipid lowering. Drugs 1998; 56:9–13.
14. Kullo IJ, Edwards WD, Schwartz RS. Vulnerable plaque: pathobiology and clinical implications. Ann Intern Med 1998; 129:1050–1060.
15. Brown BG, Zhao XQ, Sacco DE, Albers JJ. Lipid lowering and plaque regression. New insights into prevention of plaque disruption and clinical events in coronary disease. Circulation 1993; 87:1781–1791.
16. Hodgson JM, Reddy KG, Suneja R, Nair RN, Lesnefsky EJ, Sheehan HM. Intracoronary ultrasound imaging: correlation of plaque morphology with angiography, clinical syndrome and procedural results in patients undergoing coronary angioplasty. J Am Coll Cardiol 1993; 21:35–44.

17. Ge J, Erbel R, Gerber T, Gorge G, Koch L, Haude M, Meyer J. Intravascular ultrasound imaging of angiographically normal coronary arteries: a prospective study in vivo. Br Heart J 1994; 71:572–578.

18. de Feyter PJ, Ozaki Y, Baptista J, Escaned J, Di Mario C, de Jaegere PP, Serruys PW, Roelandt JR. Ischemia-related lesion characteristics in patients with stable or unstable angina. A study with intracoronary angioscopy and ultrasound. Circulation 1995; 92:1408–1413.

19. Roelandt JR, di Mario C, Pandian NG, Wenguang L, Keane D, Slager CJ, de Feyter PJ, Serruys PW. Three-dimensional reconstruction of intracoronary ultrasound images. Rationale, approaches, problems, and directions. Circulation 1994; 90:1044–1055.

20. Bauters C, Lablanche JM, Renaud N, McFadden EP, Hamon M, Bertrand ME. Morphological changes after percutaneous transluminal coronary angioplasty of unstable plaques. Insights from serial angioscopic follow-up. Eur Heart J 1996; 17:1554–1559.

21. Lablanche JM, Van Belle E, McFadden E, Gautier L, de Groote P, Bauters C, Bertrand M. Coronary angioscopy. Arch Mal Coeur Vaiss 1997; 90(2):29–33.

22. Thieme T, Wernecke KD, Meyer R, Brandenstein E, Habedank D, Hinz A, Felix SB, Baumann G, Kleber FX. Angioscopic evaluation of atherosclerotic plaques: validation by histomorphologic analysis and association with stable and unstable coronary syndromes. J Am Coll Cardiol 1996; 28:1–6.

23. Kleber FX, Dopfmer S, Thieme T. Invasive strategies to discriminate stable and unstable coronary plaques. Eur Heart J 1998; 19(suppl C):C44–49.

24. Hackett D, Davies G, Maseri A. Pre-existing coronary stenoses in patients with first myocardial infarction are not necessarily severe. Eur Heart J 1988; 9:1317–1323.

25. Ambrose JA, Tannenbaum MA, Alexopoulos D, Hjemdahl-Monsen CE, Leavy J, Weiss M, Borrico S, Gorlin R, Fuster V. Angiographic progression of coronary artery disease and the development of myocardial infarction. J Am Coll Cardiol 1988; 12:56–62.

26. Brown BG, Gallery CA, Badger RS, Kennedy JW, Mathey D, Bolson EL, Dodge HT. Incomplete lysis of thrombus in the moderate underlying atherosclerotic lesion during intracoronary infusion of streptokinase for acute myocardial infarction: quantitative angiographic observations. Circulation 1986; 73:653–661.

27. Giroud D, Li JM, Urban P, Meier B, Rutishauser W. Relation of the site of acute myocardial infarction to the most severe coronary arterial stenosis at prior angiography. Am J Cardiol 1992; 69:729–732.

28. Ellis S, Alderman E, Cain K, Fisher L, Sanders W, Bourassa M. Prediction of risk of anterior myocardial infarction by lesion severity and measurement method of stenoses in the left anterior descending coronary distribution: a CASS Registry Study. J Am Coll Cardiol 1988; 11:908–916.

29. Taeymans Y, Theroux P, Lesperance J, Waters D. Quantitative angiographic morphology of the coronary artery lesions at risk of thrombotic occlusion. Circulation 1992; 85:78–85.

30. Ernst SM, van der Feltz TA, Bal ET, van Bogerijen L, van den Berg E, Ascoop CA, Plokker HW. Long-term angiographic follow up, cardiac events, and survival

in patients undergoing percutaneous transluminal coronary angioplasty. Br Heart J 1987; 57:220–225.

31. Guiteras P, Tomas L, Varas C, Auge JM, Masotti M, Crexells C, Oriol A. Five years of angiographic and clinical follow-up after successful percutaneous transluminal coronary angioplasty. Eur Heart J 1989; 10(suppl G):42–48.

32. Kober G, Vallbracht C, Kadel C, Kaltenbach M. Results of repeat angiography up to eight years following percutaneous transluminal angioplasty. Eur Heart J 1989; 10(suppl G):49–53.

33. Dimas AP, Grigera F, Arora RR, Simpfendorfer CC, Hollman JL, Frierson JH, Franco I, Whitlow PL. Repeat coronary angioplasty as treatment for restenosis. J Am Coll Cardiol 1992; 19:1310–1314.

34. Bottner RK, Green CE, Ewels CJ, Recientes E, Patrissi GA, Kent KM. Recurrent ischemia more than 1 year after successful percutaneous transluminal coronary angioplasty. An analysis of the extent and anatomic pattern of coronary disease. Circulation 1989; 80:1580–1584.

35. Vlietstra RE, Holmes DR, Jr., Rodeheffer RJ, Bailey KR. Consequences of restenosis after coronary angioplasty. Int J Cardiol 1991; 31:143–147.

36. Kitazume H, Kubo I, Iwama T, Ageishi Y. Long-term angiographic follow-up of lesions patent 6 months after percutaneous coronary angioplasty. Am Heart J 1995; 129:441–444.

37. Rozenman Y, Gilon D, Welber S, Sapoznikov D, Wexler D, Lotan C, Mosseri M, Weiss AT, Hasin Y, Gotsman MS. Total coronary artery occlusion late after successful coronary angioplasty of moderately severe lesions: incidence and clinical manifestations. Cardiology 1994; 85:222–228.

38. Hamon M, Bauters C, McFadden EP, Lablanche JM, Bertrand ME. Six-month quantitative angiographic follow-up of 50% diameter stenoses dilated during multilesion percutaneous transluminal coronary angioplasty. Am J Cardiol 1993; 71:1226–1229.

39. Gould KL. Coronary Artery Stenosis. New York: Amsterdam, London: Elsevier, 1991.

40. Pijls NH, De Bruyne B, Peels K, Van Der Voort PH, Bonnier HJ, Bartunek JKJJ, Koolen JJ. Measurement of fractional flow reserve to assess the functional severity of coronary-artery stenoses. N Engl J Med 1996; 334:1703–1708.

41. Wiedermann JG, Schwartz A, Apfelbaum M. Anatomic and physiologic heterogeneity in patients with syndrome X: an intravascular ultrasound study [see comments]. J Am Coll Cardiol 1995; 25:1310–1317.

42. Chauhan A, Mullins PA, Petch MC, Schofield PM. Is coronary flow reserve in response to papaverine really normal in syndrome X? Circulation 1994; 89:1998–2004.

43. Ornish D, Scherwitz LW, Billings JH, Gould KL, Merritt TA, Sparler S, Armstrong WT, Ports TA, Kirkeeide RL, Hogeboom C, Brand RJ. Intensive lifestyle changes for reversal of coronary heart disease. JAMA 1998; 280:2001–2007.

44. Randomised trial of cholesterol lowering in 4444 patients with coronary heart disease: the Scandinavian Simvastatin Survival Study (4S). Lancet 1994; 344:1383–1389.

45. Shepherd J, Cobbe SM, Ford I, Isles CG, Lorimer AR, MacFarlane PW, McKillop JH, Packard CJ. Prevention of coronary heart disease with pravastatin in men with

hypercholesterolemia. West of Scotland Coronary Prevention Study Group. N Engl J Med 1995; 333:1301–1307.

46. Effect of simvastatin on coronary atheroma: the Multicentre Anti-Atheroma Study (MAAS). Lancet 1994; 344:633–638.

47. Pitt B, Waters D, Brown WV, van Boven AJ, Schwartz L, Title LM, Eisenberg D, Shurzinske L, McCormick LS. Aggressive lipid-lowering therapy compared with angioplasty in stable coronary artery disease. Atorvastin versus Revascularization Treatment Investigators. N Engl J Med 1999; 341:70–76.

22

The Potential Role of Serine Proteinase Inhibitors for the Prevention of Plaque Rupture

Christian V. Zalai, Piers Nash, Erbin Dai, Li Ying Liu, and Alexandra Lucas
University of Western Ontario, London, Ontario, Canada

I. INTRODUCTION

The thrombotic cascade interacts with the thrombolytic cascade in a delicate physiological balance that is intended to control clot formation at sites of vascular injury (1–3). Both cascades consist of sequentially activated serine proteinase enzymes that form a catalytic chain. The balance between thrombosis, coagulation (Figs. 1, 2), and thrombolysis (Fig. 3) is thus dependent on the relative activation states of the serine proteinase enzymes in each cascade. The activation of the regulatory steps or enzymes in each cascade is controlled, at least in part, by serine proteinase inhibitors (serpins) that can alter the balance between coagulation and clot lysis (4–7). These interactions of enzyme and serpin in each system may act as the dominant players or simply as background, low-level activity, depending on the current activation states of each cascade, much as two soloists in a duet shift dominance with each other and the chorus throughout a musical composition.

The thrombotic cascade (Fig. 1) has long been known to accelerate clot formation at sites of plaque rupture, as well as activate platelets and inflammatory cell responses to injury (1, 5, 8). However, it is only very recent work that has implicated the counterbalancing thrombolytic cascade in inflammatory cell activation and plaque rupture (7–14). Plasminogen activators are found at the leading edge membrane of invading macrophages and can enhance cellular invasion

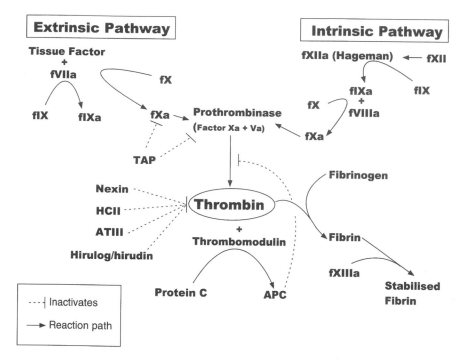

Figure 1 Schematic representation of the thrombotic cascade and the main regulatory serpins for coagulation. APC, activated protein c; f, factor; AT, antithrombic; HC, heparin cofactor; TAP, tick anticoagulant peptide.

through activation of matrix degrading enzymes that degrade and rupture the fibrous cap of vulnerable plaques (Fig. 4) (4, 7, 15). Once ruptured, the exposed collagen and lipid activate platelets and the extrinsic cascade, producing local thrombosis that, when excessive, will occlude the arterial lumen causing ischemic organ damage, myocardial infarction, cerebrovascular accident, or peripheral vascular occlusion (16–19). The thrombolytic cascade is concomitantly activated to control excess thrombus formation. Thus, both the thrombotic and thrombolytic systems play pivotal roles in the various stages of plaque rupture, thrombosis, and clot lysis; the thrombolytic cascade, initially, in plaque rupture, the thrombotic cascade next in clot formation and inflammatory responses, and finally the thrombolytic cascade to dissolve the clot. Manipulation of the activation levels of the thrombotic and the thrombolytic cascades through serine proteinase inhibitors may provide new approaches for controlling plaque rupture and associated thrombosis (4–11, 20).

    Both the coagulation and clot lysis systems are part of very ancient defense responses intended to prevent excess blood loss and subsequently excess clot

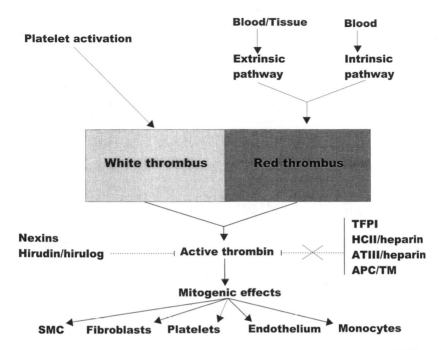

Figure 2 Diagram of the intrinsic and the extrinsic coagulation cascades. ATIII, antithrombin III; TFPI, tissue factor pathway inhibitor; APC, activated protein C; TM, thrombomodulin; SMC, smooth muscle cells.

formation in the event of injury to an artery wall (1–8). By logical extension, both systems would be expected to trigger wound healing responses with removal of residual clot, scar formation, and eventual regrowth of normal tissue. These systems are central mediators of such diverse processes as coagulation (1, 8), fibrinolysis (2–5, 8), complement activation (7, 21), ovulation (7, 22, 23), embryonic development (7, 8, 24, 25), neuromuscular remodeling (25), angiogenesis (7, 23), inflammation (7, 9–11, 21, 26), apoptosis (7, 21, 26, 27), neoplasia/malignancy (7, 23), and viral pathogenesis (23, 27). Beyond its role in regulating thrombotic responses, thrombin has been found to regulate inflammatory responses (4, 5, 8, 23), through triggering P selectin release in endothelial cells, stimulating monocyte activation, and accelerating cellular proliferation (DNA synthesis). Thrombin limits neurite extension in neuronal plasticity responses after injury or potentially during the acquisition of new skills (24). The serine proteinase thrombin inhibitor, protease nexin, has been reported to reverse neuronal extension in response to injury (24, 25). The thrombolytic cascade plasminogen activators are now known to be acute-phase reactants, activating growth factors (4, 27, 29, 30),

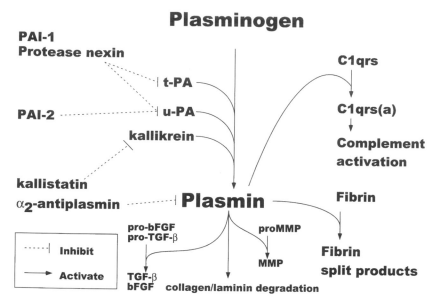

Figure 3 Schematic representation of the thrombolytic cascade. tPA, tissue-type plasminogen activator; uPA, urokinase-type plasminogen activator; PAI-1, plasminogen activator inhibitor-1; MMP, matrix metalloproteinase enzymes; C1q, complement component 1q; TGFβ, transforming growth factor β; bFGF, basic fibroblast growth factor.

accelerating inflammatory cellular responses in infections and in diseases such as rheumatoid arthritis (31) and inflammatory bowel disease, and again associated with neuronal responses to injury. The plasminogen activator inhibitors regulate acute inflammatory responses to injury, acute nervous system responses to injury and during development (25), as well as the metastasis of tumor cells (7, 8, 23, 26). These extended responses of the thrombotic and thrombolytic cascades are now believed to also play central roles in unstable plaque development and rupture.

The development of an unstable thrombotic plaque in the intimal layer of the arterial wall is a complex process. On the surface, the development of local thrombosis appears to be a simple process involving predominantly a thrombotic response to exposed lipid and connective tissue (32–34). As noted previously, recent data have, however, altered our perception of the thrombolytic cascade, which has, heretofore, been believed to play an entirely benign role in thrombotic vascular occlusion, preventing clot propagation, and opening occluded vessels. Elements of the thrombolytic system may in fact produce unstable or vulnerable plaque (4, 7–15, 35–37). Both the clot-forming and the clot-lysing pathways may initiate responses that lead to plaque rupture and acute vascular thrombosis. The

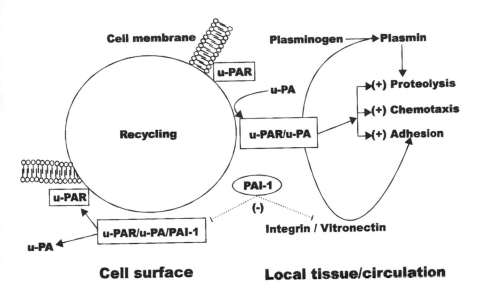

Figure 4 The uPA/uPAR complex cycle. Diagram outlining the effects of the uPA/uPAR complex on cellular adhesion, migration, and invasion at sites of inflammation as in the vascular wall after injury. tPA, tissue-type plasminogen activator; uPA, urokinase-type plasminogen activator; uPAR, urokinase-type plasminogen activator receptor; PAI-1, plasminogen activator inhibitor-1; MMP, matrix metalloproteinase enzymes.

plasminogen activators and plasmin itself activate inflammatory mononuclear cellular adhesion, migration, and invasion at sites of tissue damage (Fig. 4). Inhibition of the thrombolytic cascade therefore has the potential to prevent fibrous tissue degradation and inflammatory cell invasion, which are now believed to cause the initial breakdown and rupture of the fibrous cap in unstable plaque (15–18).

Serine proteinase enzymes in the thrombolytic cascade, tissue- (tPA) and urokinase- (uPA) type plasminogen activators, and plasmin activate matrix metalloproteinase (MMP) proenzymes that in turn degrade collagen and elastin, allowing inflammatory macrophages to invade the weakened fibrous shoulder of a lipid-filled plaque (7–9, 11–15, 35–37). Cellular invasion breaks down the fibrous cap leading to eventual plaque rupture, which exposes highly thrombotic substrates, lipid, and collagen. The thrombotic cascade is then triggered by activation of platelets and tissue factor complexed with factors VII and IX in the extrinsic cascade (1, 5, 17–19). Both the thombolytic and the thrombotic systems may thus play pivotal roles in acute thrombotic occlusion, the thrombolytic cascade in the early stages of plaque rupture (Fig. 4) and in later stages of clot dissolution

(Fig. 3) and the thrombotic cascade in subsequent arterial thrombosis and occlusion (Figs. 1, 2). These cascades are in turn regulated by specific inhibitors, the serine proteinase inhibitors (7, 23). The thrombotic and thrombolytic cascades also both interact to activate and, alternatively, to inhibit the clot lysis and formation pathways. It has now become increasingly evident that the serine proteinase systems and regulatory inhibitors actively control basic responses to arterial injury and are intimately involved in both the development of early atherosclerosis, plaque progression to an unstable state, and finally plaque rupture with acute vascular thrombosis.

In this chapter we will seek to review some of the mechanisms and key players in the thrombotic system and the currently accepted therapies for the prevention and treatment of unstable plaque. The biochemistry of known vascular serine proteinase inhibitors will be described first. Inhibitors of the thrombotic cascade and hence the prevention or reversal of arterial thrombotic occlusion will then be discussed. In addition, new avenues of intervention using serine protease inhibitors will also be explored in the hopes of gaining insight into possible future courses of antithrombotic strategies. Finally, a novel role for inhibitors of the thrombolytic cascade in the prevention of plaque progression to an unstable state or plaque rupture will be discussed. Overall, we wish to examine this hemostatic duet of vascular serine proteinase inhibitors, both as potential inhibitors of plaque rupture and acute vascular thrombosis.

II. THE BIOCHEMISTRY OF SERINE PROTEINASE INHIBITORS

A. Serpins

The serine proteinase inhibitors are classified according to the molecular mechanism of inhibition and are divided into groups as (1) serpins and (2) standard mechanism inhibitors. The serpins are a family of structurally related protein inhibitors of serine proteinases. The term "serpin" is itself an abbreviation of *ser*ine *p*roteinase *in*hibitor, although not all serpins have inhibitory activity (38). Serpins play a major regulatory role in a host of biological processes that involve proteinase activity, and serpin mutations have been associated with a host of human diseases relating to thrombosis, angioedema, hemorrhage, and emphysema (39). The mechanism by which serpins act to inhibit their specific target serine proteinase(s) is relatively well understood at both the molecular and biochemical level.

The conserved serpin structure takes the form of a compact globular protein composed of β-sheets connected by α-helices. A single exposed loop known as the reactive center loop (RCL) forms an arc above one pole of the protein (Fig. 5). The RCL is the business end of the serpin with which it interacts with the

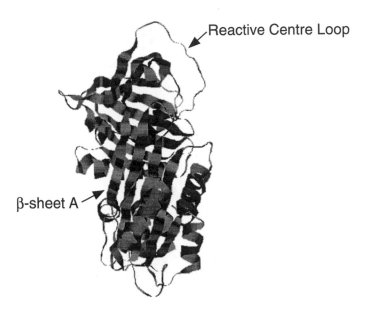

Figure 5 A ribbon diagram of α_1-antitrypsin showing the surface-exposed reactive center loop and the β-sheet A, which together form the serpin "mousetrap" mechanism for serine proteinase inhibition. Based on the structure by Elliott et al., 1998. (Refs. 40–45.)

target proteinase at a scissile P1–P1′ bond. Amino acids in the RCL are referred to according to their position relative to the P1–P1′ bond, with residues at the C-terminus assigned the designations of P1′–P2′–P3′ . . . etc., and N-terminal residues referred to as P1–P2–P3–P4 . . . etc., enumerated out from the active site (Fig. 6). In this form the serpin is in a strained or high-energy metastable conformation, very much like a set mousetrap (40). The current model for the mechanism of serpin inhibition of target proteinase(s) is relatively well defined. First, the serpin binds to its target proteinase to form a reversible complex analogous to a Michaelis complex between an enzyme and a substrate. Next, the proteinase cleaves the P1–P1′ reactive center peptide bond, resulting in the formation of a covalent acylenzyme intermediate (41, 42). The serpin therefore acts as a substrate, but a very poor substrate, for the target serine proteinase enzyme. The degree to which the serpin functions as an inhibitor or as a substrate for the target enzyme determines the ability of the serpin to act as an inhibitor. This cleavage releases the serpin from its strained state, releasing the "trap" and allowing a rapid folding or insertion of the reactive center loop into β-sheet A up to at least the P9 position. Thus, the entire serpin structure is important to the function of serine proteinase inhibition (43). The altered conformation of the serpin allows

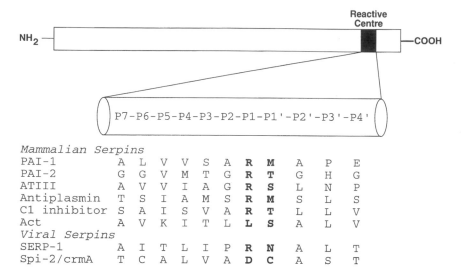

Figure 6 A schematic representation of a serpin. The reactive center loop (RCL) interacts with the active site of the proteinase and contains the critical P1-P1′ residues. The stable inhibited serpin-enzyme complex is believed to be an acyl-enzyme linked covalently at the P1 residue. The RCL sequence of a selection of mammalian and viral serpins are shown below. PAI-1, bovine plasminogen activator inhibitor-1; PAI-2, human plasminogen activator inhibitor-2; ATIII, human antithrombin III; Act, antichymotrypsin.

the peptide arm connected to the P1–P1′ active site to be folded into the β-sheet once cleaved. Because the enzyme and serpin are covalently bound, this results in a large-scale movement of the enzyme, which is effectively dragged across the face of the serpin (44, 45). The bound proteinase prevents full insertion of the RCL and the complex becomes locked. This resulting strain is transferred to the enzyme, distorting the active site and preventing deacylation of the acylenzyme intermediate, thus trapping the complex. This complex is extremely stable in solution with a half-life in the order of hours to days. Biologically this is ample time for the trapped enzyme to be degraded or removed from circulation.

Serpins comprise about 10% of all serum proteins (Table 1). See Fig. 6 for a comparison of the active site loop sequence of several widely studied serpins. Antithrombin III (ATIII), heparin cofactor II (HCII), and protein C inhibitor regulate thrombosis. Plasminogen activator inhibitor (PAI), α_2-antiplasmin, and potentially the protease nexins (PN) regulate thrombolysis. Outside of the coagulation and fibrinolytic systems are other regulators as with the C1q inhibitor, which is a serpin that blocks complement activation, and α_1-antitrypsin, α_1-antichymotrypsin, and aprotinin, which are serpins that regulate inflammatory responses.

Table 1 Serine Proteinase Inhibitors

Serine proteinase inhibitors	Target serine proteinase enzymes	Mechanism of action
Thrombotic cascade inhibitors		
TFPI 1 and 2	TF/VIIa complex, Xa	Standard
rTAP	Xa	Standard
rAST	Xa	Standard
ATIII	Thrombin, IXa, Xa, XIa, XIIa, plasmin	Serpin
HCII	Thrombin	Serpin
PN I and II	Thrombin, uPA, tPA, plasmin	Serpin
LICI	Thrombin, Xa, XIa, uPA, tPA, kallikrein plasmin, trypsin, chymotrypsin, elastase	Serpin
Hirudin, hirulog	Thrombin	Direct inhibitor
PPACK	Thrombin	Direct inhibitor
Thrombolytic cascade inhibitors		
Protein C inhibitor	Protein C	Serpin
PAI-1	uPA, tPA, thrombin	Serpin
PAI-2	uPA, plasmin	Serpin
α_2-antiplasmin	Plasmin	Serpin
SERP-1 (Spi-4)	uPA, tPA, plasmin	Serpin
PN I and II	Thrombin, uPA, tPA, plasmin	Serpin
LICI	Thrombin, Xa, XIa, uPA, tPA, kallikrein, plasmin, trypsin, chymotrypsin, elastase	Serpin
Complement		
C1 inhibitor	Complement	Serpin
Inflammation		
α_1-antitrypsin	Neutrophil elastase	Serpin
α_1-antichymotrypsin	Chymotrypsin	Serpin
Aprotinin	Kallikrein, trypsin, chymotrypsin XIIa, protein C	Serpin
Apoptosis		
Spi-1-3	II 1β-converting enzyme	Serpin
Noninhibitory		
Ovalbumin	NA	Serpin
Angiotensinogen	NA	Serpin
Thyroxin binding globulin	NA	Serpin
Cortisol binding globulin	NA	Serpin

TFPI, tissue factor pathway inhibitor; rTAP, recombinant tick anti-coagulant peptide; ATIII, antithrombin III; HCII, heparin cofactor II; PN, protease nexin; PPACK, D-phenylalanyl-L-prolyl-L-arginyl chloromethyl ketone; LICI, Limulus intracellular coagulation inhibitor; PAI, plasminogen activator inhibitor; uPA, urokinase type plasminogen activator; tPA, tissue type plasminogen activator; rAST, recombinant antistasin.

There are also proteins with classical serpin structures that do not function as inhibitors, such as ovalbumin, angiotensinogen, thyroxin-binding globulin, and cortisol-binding globulin.

The mechanism of inhibition of thrombin by ATIII, HCII, PN-1, and PN-2 occurs by means of a classical serpin-related mechanism. Substitution of residues in the P1 to P9 sites reduces inhibitory activity of antithrombin III (ATIII), a serpin that binds and inhibits thrombin (45). Similarly, deletion of helix A in the serpin reduces inhibitory function of heparin cofactor II, another thrombin-binding serpin (46). Inhibition of the thrombolytic serine proteinase enzymes, plasminogen activators, also occurs by means of a serpin, plasminogen activator inhibitor or PAI, related mechanism. PAI-1 is unique, however, in that this serpin, in addition to having "strained" and "relaxed" (sprung) states, can also exist in a latent form that can be converted back to the active or strained state (27).

B. Standard Mechanism Inhibitors

The standard mechanism inhibitors refer collectively to a number of families of small proteins, with the Kunitz and Kazal families being the best known (47). Like serpins, the standard mechanism inhibitors of serine proteinases use a surface loop or reactive site loop to bind to the active site of their target serine proteinase (48). The reactive site loop acts as a pseudosubstrate that docks into the active site. Structurally, the reactive site loop does not change on binding to the proteinase, and different members of this group exhibit the same structure despite sequence differences. This canonical structure is complementary to the active site of the enzyme. Unlike serpins, the entire inhibition mechanism is reversible (49).

Tissue factor pathway inhibitors, TFPI-1 and TFPI-2, are Kunitz-type inhibitors and have three protease-binding domains, the second of which binds near the active site of their respective serine proteases. Unlike for serpins, this reaction is 95% irreversible, with the remaining 5% proceeding in the opposite direction (45).

C. Viral Serpins

Given the critical role of proteinases in the regulation of biological responses to infections such as inflammation and apoptosis, it is not surprising that certain parasites have hijacked serpins to use for their own purposes. Both filarial parasites and large DNA viruses have been shown to produce serpins as part of their repertoire of defenses against the host immune response (50). The best-studied examples of viral serpins are in the poxvirus family. Members of this diverse and highly successful family of large double-stranded DNA viruses include variola virus, the causative agent of smallpox, and myxoma virus, an exceptionally efficient pathogen of rabbits (51). The poxviruses are complex viruses that encode virulence factors in the terminal inverted repeats of the viral genome. The poxvirus genomes encode seven serpins termed Spi 1 to Spi 7 and a newly recognized eighth serpin that has not yet been given a Spi notation (G. McFadden, University of Western Ontario, London, Ontario, Canada, personal communication). Among the serpins produced by poxviruses are SERP-1 (Spi 4) and crmA (27). These two serpins fulfill critical roles in viral strategies designed to evade or disable host responses to infection. The crmA protein, also known as Spi-2, is an intracellular poxviral (cowpox, rabbit pox, and orthopox) serpin capable of blocking the production of the proinflammatory cytokine, interleukin-1β, by inhibiting interleukin-1β–converting enzyme (ICE) (52). In addition, crmA is able to block apoptosis of infected cells in in vitro systems by inhibiting key caspases in the apoptotic signal cascade and by inhibiting the cytotoxic T-cell granule protein, granzyme B (53, 54). SERP-1 is one of many immunomodulatory proteins produced by myxomavirus (50, 55–57), but has the distinction of being the only secreted serpin produced by a virus. Other viral serpins discovered to date have been intracellular proteins. These include the orthopoxvirus serpins that prevent apoptosis (Spi 1 and 2) and cell-to-cell fusion (Spi 3), respectively (27). There are also two avipoxvirus serpins, Spi 5 and 6, and a suipox serpin, Spi 7 (27). Recent work from our laboratory has demonstrated a significant protective effect for this viral SERP-1 protein for angioplasty-induced atherosclerosis, allograft transplant vasculopathy, and arthritis in animal models (11, 31) (see Sec. IV).

III. THROMBOTIC CASCADE SERINE PROTEINASE INHIBITORS: ROLE IN PLAQUE RUPTURE AND THROMBOSIS

A. Overview of the Thrombotic Clotting Cascade

Plaque rupture, with associated thrombosis and arterial occlusion, often results in acute ischemic syndromes and is the leading cause of morbidity and mortality in North America, Europe, and Japan (58). Because treatment of thrombosis often proves difficult, the emphasis is shifting from treatment to prevention. Resistant thrombotic complications during thrombolytic therapy or mechanical intervention, such as balloon angioplasty, atherectomy, or endovascular stents, are potentially life threatening. In such a system, the role of serine proteinase inhibitors is underscored and plays a crucial role in maintaining the appropriate hemostatic balance.

In response to vascular damage, hemostasis is maintained by a complex series of interactions resulting in the formation of a clot and the initiation of tissue repair processes. Maintenance of vascular integrity by the coagulation cascade can be divided into separate stages. These stages, which include initiation of clot formation, propagation and amplification, termination, elimination, and vascular repair, are described in the following section. The key serine proteinase inhibitors known to play central roles in clot regulation in the vascular hemostatic response are antithrombin III (ATIII), heparin cofactor II (HCII), and tissue factor protein inhibitor (TFPI). There are other serine proteinase inhibitors (such as protease nexin, PN) whose role in the vascular system is still being studied. Several foreign or derived serine proteinase inhibitors, hirudin, hirulog, and aprotinin, have also been successfully used to reduce thrombosis. The stages of the thrombotic cascade, the regulatory serine protease inhibitors, and their function in vascular wound healing responses and potential therapeutic applications will be discussed in this section.

1. Initiation

On damage to the vascular endothelium, the normally anticoagulant surface becomes compromised, circulating blood cells are perturbed, and prothrombotic elements of the subendothelial space become exposed. Damage can occur by way of mechanical or inflammatory injury. Exposure of these prothrombotic spaces results in the accumulation of circulating blood cells, most notably platelets with concomitant expression of procoagulant receptors. The physiological balance shifts from an anticoagulant state to a procoagulant, activated state. It is on these surfaces that the components of the coagulation cascade are activated and initiate the formation of a clot (the first soloist in this hemostasis duet) (1, 59).

2. Propagation

Propagation can occur by two separate pathways that converge to form a common pathway resulting in thrombin (factor IIa) generation (Fig. 2). The intrinsic pathway is activated when factor XII contacts a negatively charged surface, in addition to prekallikrein and high-molecular weight kininogen (HMWK) (Fig. 1). This results in the activation of factor XI, followed by factor IX, which in turn activates the prothrombinase complex consisting of factor Xa and factor Va (1).

The extrinsic pathway is initiated when factor VIIa contacts tissue factor (TF), which is present on most extravascular cell surfaces (60). Increased exposure of TF during vascular damage results in contact with factor VIIa, present in low concentrations in the blood (61). The TF-factor VIIa–activated complex can then activate the prothrombinase complex. The common pathway then occurs, whereby the prothrombinase complex (consisting of factors Xa and Va) cleaves prothrombin (factor II) to release active thrombin. Active thrombin then catalyses the formation of fibrin from fibrinogen, resulting in the formation of a red clot (as opposed to a white clot, which is platelet-rich) (Fig. 2).

There is a positive feedback loop, whereby thrombin can accelerate the formation of the activated cofactors, factors Va and VIIIa, the zymogens, factors VIIa and XIa, and the fibrin-stabilizing enzyme, factor XIIIa. Propagation and amplification occur by both the extrinsic (TF-mediated) pathway, with its tissue- or cell surface–derived components, and the intrinsic (factor XII-mediated) pathway, with its plasma-derived components. The end result of propagation and amplification is the cessation of blood loss and the formation of a stable thrombus plug at the site of vascular injury.

3. Termination

Clot formation is restricted to the site of vascular injury to prevent uncontrolled, systemic clotting and subsequent cessation of blood flow. This is demonstrated in patients with clinical thrombotic disorders, who have deficiencies in anticoagulant pathway components. On activation of thrombin and clot formation, two constitutive inhibitory processes and a clotting-initiated anticoagulant system come into play (the second soloist in this hemostasis duet). Termination can occur by direct inhibition of thrombin itself or prevention of activation of prothrombin. The constitutive systems involve antithrombin III (ATIII), tissue-factor pathway inhibitor (TFPI), and heparin cofactor II (HCII). ATIII, TFPI, and HCII are all serine protease inhibitors present in blood plasma. Increasing amounts of thrombin on activation of the blood-clotting cascade also result, paradoxically, in increased anticoagulation by means of the protein C pathway. Thrombin can bind to thrombomodulin present on endothelial cell surfaces, which results in a change in affinity of thrombomodulin from fibrinogen to protein C. The thrombomodulin-thrombin complex cleaves protein C to form activated protein C (APC), which in turn inactivates the prothrombinase and the intrinsic "ten-ase" (consisting of factors IXa and VIIIa). This is accomplished by the cleavage and inactivation of the cofactors, factors Va and VIIIa by APC (62, 63). Factor XIIa (Hageman factor) also is known to up-regulate the thrombolytic cascade, in addition to activating the intrinsic cascade. Other anticoagulant systems have been discovered and these include TFPI-2, protease nexin-1 (PN-1), and PN-2. The physiological significance of these systems in plaque rupture and vascular thrombosis remains to be determined.

4. Elimination

Clot elimination is essential for tissue repair to occur and requires the activity of the fibrinolytic system (see Sec. IV, Fig. 3). The link between the thrombotic cascade and the fibrinolytic system occurs through protein C, which also inhibits plasminogen activator inhibitor-1 (PAI-1). Factors Va and Xa have been shown to enhance plasmin generation (64). Conversely, thrombin, which as described under the thombolytic cascade system, also up-regulates transcription of plasminogen activator inhibitor (PAI-1) and down-regulates tissue plasminogen activator (tPA) activity (4), would be expected to enhance further clot formation.

5. Repair

Thrombin, in addition to functioning as the key mediator in blood clotting, is also involved in tissue repair processes. It is a potent growth factor and chemokine, exerting activating effects on fibroblasts, smooth muscle cells, platelets, and macrophages (59, 65–68). Activation of these cell types results in secretion of growth factors, migration of cells into the wounded area, and clean-up of debris. The cells repopulate the damaged area and restore vascular integrity while recreating the endothelial surface required to maintain an antithrombotic tissue–blood interface.

In addition to its main function as a coagulant protein, thrombin has become the focus for recent research into its mitogenic properties. Thrombin has been shown to be a potent mitogen for vascular cells (67). The effects of thrombin on endothelial cells, monocytes, smooth muscle cells, fibroblasts, and platelets are slowly being characterized. Thrombin appears to induce secretion of growth factors from platelets, matrix proteins from fibroblasts, proliferation of smooth muscle cells and fibroblasts, migration of monocytes and smooth muscle cells, and differentiation of monocytes (68–71). Thus clot-bound thrombin may play a significant role in disease development because cells and repair mechanisms are activated in an aberrant manner.

B. Thrombotic Serine Proteinase Enzymes and Inhibitors as Plasma Markers of Unstable Plaque

The intima of atherosclerotic human aorta (postmortem) sections is rich in fibrinogen and derivatives as determined by immunohistochemical staining (72). Prior clinical studies have demonstrated a good correlation between increased blood levels of fibrinogen and later cardiovascular system–related deaths (73). In several studies, elevated fibrinogen levels have been found to be an independent risk factor for cerebrovascular accidents (strokes), myocardial infarctions (heart attacks), and reocclusion of an infarct-related artery, a predictive value comparable to other risk factors (73). There are essentially no studies that do not support fibrinogen as an independent risk factor. This is, however, an acute-phase reactant and is not used as a diagnostic tool, as of yet, for unstable angina. In patients with unstable coronary syndromes, factor XII and kallikrein-like activity are elevated early after onset of symptoms. Again fibrinogen and D dimer are increased as are factors VII and VIII, von Willebrand's factor (vWF), and platelet aggregation (74). Circulating thrombin/ATIII complexes are markers of coagulation activity and thrombotic potential in acute cardiac syndromes (33, 34, 75).

Whether these factors are true causal agents or simply secondary response markers, however, remains to be determined.

C. Serine Proteinase Inhibitors of the Thrombotic Cascade in the Prevention of Acute Thrombosis and Plaque Rupture

1. Antithrombin III

ATIII is the primary anticoagulant in the bloodstream, found at concentrations of about 2.4 µM, and is synthesized in the liver (1, 4, 5, 8, 9, 23). It is known to inhibit several of the serine proteinase clotting factors including thrombin, factors VIIa (when bound to TF), IXa, Xa, XIa, and XIIa, and kallikrein, as well as the central thrombolytic enzyme plasmin (Table 1, Figs. 1, 2) (76, 77). ATIII inhibits these factors by forming irreversible 1:1 complexes, which are eventually cleared by the liver. Its activity is enhanced 2000-fold in the presence of heparin and heparan-sulfate proteoglycans (HSPG) found on the surface of cells. Clinically administered heparin and cellular HSPG act as catalysts by facilitating the interaction between ATIII and thrombin, because both molecules have specific heparin-binding sites (78, 79). Heparin may thus be clinically useful in preventing plaque rupture by maintaining the anticoagulant balance in the bloodstream through its activity on ATIII. However, once rupture has occurred, heparin may not be useful, because heparin/ATIII complexes cannot penetrate blood clots and inactivate the thrombin found therein (80). Clot-bound thrombin acts as a nidus for further clot formation and other methods are called for to effect anticoagulation (81).

Inhibition of selected steps in the coagulation cascade has been associated with the inhibition of plaque growth after balloon-mediated arterial injury (82). In one study, the effects of inactivated factor VII (ifVII), recombinant tissue factor pathway inhibitor (rTFPI), recombinant tick anticoagulant protein (rTAP), or hirudin were assessed for their effects on neointimal hyperplasia in a cholesterol-fed rabbit model of air desiccation injury followed by angioplasty injury of the femoral artery (82) (see Table 2). Each of these proteins selectively inhibits steps in the extrinsic cascade; ifVII blocks factor VIIa/TF complex formation, rTFPI blocks factor VIIa/TF/Factor Xa complex formation, rTAP blocks factor Xa (even when part of the prothrombinase complex), and hirudin, as will be discussed in the following sections, is a specific thrombin inhibitor (Table 1). Intimal hyperplasia was significantly reduced by all four inhibitors with the greatest inhibition seen (as determined by contrast angiography and morphometric histological analysis of plaque area) with ifVII and rTFPI, which act at the earliest activation times in the extrinsic thrombotic cascade (Table 2). A second study confirmed these findings for rTAP and rAST (recombinant antistasin protein) in a similar rabbit arterial injury model (83). Although this model is not a model

Table 2 Animal Model Studies

Agent tested	Species	Number	Model	Outcome
Serine proteinase enzymes				
Tissue-type plasminogen activator[8,36]	tPA[−/−] mouse	32–56	Perivascular femoral artery injury	No effect
Tissue-type plasminogen activator[a]	Rat	12	Femoral balloon injury	Slight decrease
Urokinase type plasminogen activator[8,36]	uPA[−/−] mouse	32–56	Perivascular femoral artery injury	Reduced plaque
Elastase[128]	Quail	44	Cholesterol/corn oil diet	Reduced plaque
Protease (trypsin, bromelain, rutosid)[129]	Rat	16	Aortic allograft transplant	Reduced vasculopathy
Serine proteinase inhibitors				
Thrombotic cascade inhibitors				
iFVII[82]	Rabbit	16	Femoral desiccation/balloon injury	Reduced plaque
rTFPI[82]	Rabbit	17	Femoral desiccation/balloon injury	Reduced plaque
rTAP[82,83]	Rabbit	16	Femoral desiccation/balloon injury	Reduced plaque
rAST[82,83]	Rabbit	41	Carotid balloon injury	Reduced plaque
ATIII/heparin[86,87]	Rabbit, rat	54	Balloon injury	Reduced plaque
hirudin/hirulog[93–95]	Rabbit	36/27	Femoral desiccation/balloon injury	Reduced plaque
hirulog[96]	Pig	14	Carotid artery stent implant	No effect
Thrombolytic cascade inhibitors				
PAI-1[112]	Guinea pig/rat	20	Guinea pig/rat aortic xenograft	Reduced aneurysm rupture
PAI−[9]	PAI-1[−/−] mouse	32–56	Perivascular femoral artery injury	Increased plaque
SERP-1[11]	Rabbit	72	Aorta balloon injury	Reduced plaque
SERP-1[113]	Rat	98	Aortic allograft transplant	Reduced vasculopathy
SERP-1[a]	Rabbit	27	Aorta RVV/histamine, balloon injury	Reduced foam cells
SERP-1[a]	Swine	30	Iliofemoral arteries, balloon injury	Reduced plaque

uPA, urokinase type plasminogen activator; uPA[−/−], uPA knock out mouse; tPA, tissue type plasminogen activator; tPA[−/−], tPA knock out mouse; PAI-1, plasminogen activator inhibitor; PAI-1[−/−], PAI-1 knock out mouse; iFVII, inactivated factor VII; rTFPI, recombinant tissue factor pathway inhibitor; rTAP, recombinant tick anticoagulant peptide; ATIII, anti-thrombin III; rAST, recombinant antistasin; RVV, Russell viper venom.
[a] Unpublished observations.

for unstable plaque formation, this work does indicate a significant role for the thrombotic cascade in vascular responses to injury. This also suggests that selective serine protease inhibitors of elements of the thrombotic cascade may be developed as ancillary therapy for treatment of unstable plaque.

2. Heparin Derivatives and Hirudin

The pharmacological anticoagulant activity of heparin is derived from its ability to interact with specific inhibitors of members of the coagulation cascade and greatly increase the rate of inhibition of these serine proteases. Specifically, heparin interacts with ATIII (formerly known as heparin cofactor I), TFPI, and to some degree, HCII. Thus, rather than effecting direct anticoagulant activity, heparin and heparin derivatives indirectly activate specific protein inhibitors of the clotting cascade (84). The mechanism of activation usually involves formation of a ternary complex between heparin, protease inhibitor, and coagulant protease, with heparin acting as a catalyst to facilitate the reaction. In some instances, quaternary complexes are formed when coagulation cofactors are present. Heparin is clinically useful in preventing thrombosis in patients with unstable angina, but this beneficial effect is lost on cessation of heparin therapy (84). Heparin has also been shown to increase the activity of u-PA by about twofold, thus not only decreasing thrombosis, but even increasing thrombolysis (85). Heparin infusion in a rat model of arterial injury has been found to reduce intimal hyperplasia, but this finding is variable in animal models and has not been reproduced in clinical studies of restenosis (86, 87).

The use of heparin is not without risk, however; hemorrhage and heparin-induced thrombocytopenia (HIT), hypersensitivity reactions, elevated liver enzymes, and osteoporosis occur in a small percentage of patients (84). The severity of hemorrhage can range from minor bleeding to life-threatening hemorrhagic shock and appears to be dependent on the dose administered. In addition, heparin is not effective in blocking the activity of clot-bound thrombin, because of inability of ATIII/heparin complexes to penetrate the fibrin clot and displace fibrin-bound thrombin (80). Activated platelets, in addition to sequestering factor Xa and thus protecting it from inactivation, also secrete platelet factor 4, which inactivates heparin and increases coagulant potential (67). Alternative heparin derivatives were developed to address some of these problems.

Low-molecular-weight heparins (LMWH), which are approximately one third the molecular weight of unfractionated heparin, are increasingly being used in the treatment of unstable angina and other cardiovascular complications. The increased efficiency of LMWH stems from the fact that only 20 to 30% of "standard" heparin is biologically active, whereas nearly 100% of LMWH is biologically available (84). The anticoagulant activity of LMWH is less than that of heparin because it interacts with ATIII in a 1:2 to 1:4 ratio (heparin interacts in a 1:1 ratio), however, it binds with higher affinity to ATIII and may be associated with a reduced risk of hemorrhage. Thus, neutralization of factor Xa (but not thrombin) by ATIII proceeds more efficiently than with heparin; however, an increased dose is required (88). LMWH is clinically effective but, in addition to interaction with ATIII, the release of sequestered pools of TFPI may be a significant contributor to the anticoagulant effects of LMWH (84). The primary use of LMWH is in the prophylaxis of deep vein thrombosis. However, it is also indicated for the initial treatment of thromboembolism and unstable angina (84, 88, 89).

Native hirudin is a mixture of closely related polypeptides secreted by the medicinal leech, *Hirudo medicinalis*. All of the hirudin polypeptides inhibit thrombin. In fact, hirudin is the most potent known inhibitor of thrombin with Ki values below the picomolar range. Hirudin is a direct thrombin inhibitor, unlike heparin, with a C-terminal domain that binds the fibrinogen-binding site of thrombin and an N-terminal domain that blocks the active site. Hirulog-1 was designed as an analog of hirudin, a 20 amino acid peptide that binds to the anion-binding site of thrombin and effectively blocks the active site for substrate activation. Hirulog-1 reduces the time for clot lysis when administered together with tPA and reduces the risk of ischemic events in patients with unstable angina (90–92).

As noted in the preceding section, several investigators have demonstrated that both hirudin and hirulog reduce plaque growth after arterial injury in rabbit models (Table 2) (93–95). Work with the hirudin analog, hirulog-1, has also demonstrated a reduction in plaque growth in a rat model of balloon injury–induced intimal hyperplasia. However, a swine stent implant model demonstrated no reduction in intimal hyperplasia with hirudin treatment (96). Thus the data in animal models do not consistently demonstrate effective reduction of plaque growth with thrombin inhibitor treatment in animal models of restenosis. This suggests that there are other factors involved in the initial events that lead to atherosclerotic plaque growth after vascular injury.

3. Heparin Cofactor II

HCII is a member of the serpin family of serine proteinase inhibitors, shows 25% homology to ATIII (Table 1, Fig. 7), and is present in the plasma at a concentration of 1.2 µM (76). Like ATIII, it is involved in effecting anticoagulation. Unlike ATIII, however, HCII interacts primarily with dermatan sulfate proteoglycans (DSPG), in addition to heparin and HSPG. Its specificity is restricted to the coagulant properties of thrombin only, with which it forms a 1:1 stoichiometric complex (97). The mitogenic properties of thrombin remain unaffected. Because DSPG are found primarily in the extracellular matrix, thrombin inhibition by HCII is thought to occur primarily on fibroblasts and smooth muscle cells (98). Hypothetically, HCII/dermatan sulfate (DS) may play a role in limiting further

THROMBOSIS	THROMBOLYSIS	CYTOKINES	GROWTH FACTORS	OTHER
Fibrinogen	t-PA / u-PA	bFGF	IL-1	LDL / VLDL
Protein C	Plasminogen	PDGF	IL-4	Lp(a)
Thrombin	PAI-1	EGF	TNF-α	Bradykinin
	Plasmin	TGFβ	IFN-γ	Angiotensin / RAA
	α2-antiplasmin			

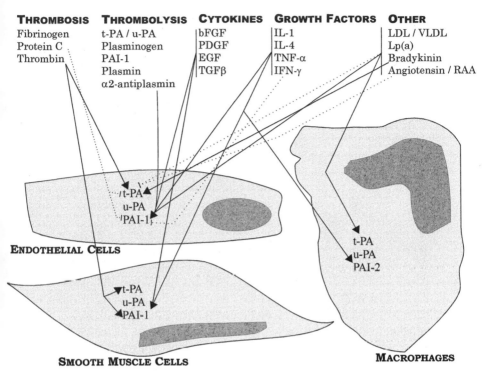

ENDOTHELIAL CELLS

t-PA
u-PA
PAI-1

t-PA
u-PA
PAI-1

t-PA
u-PA
PAI-2

SMOOTH MUSCLE CELLS

MACROPHAGES

Figure 7 Plasminogen activator and inhibitor regulation in endothelial cells, smooth muscle cells, and macrophage cells in the vessel wall. tPA, tissue-type plasminogen activator; uPA, urokinase-type plasminogen activator; PAI-1, plasminogen activator inhibitor-1; MMP, matrix metalloproteinse enzymes; TGFβ, transforming growth factor β; bFGF, basic fibroblast growth factor; EGF, epidermal growth factor; PDGF, platelet-derived growth factor; IL-1, interleukin-1; IL-4, interleukin-4; TNFα, tumor necrosis factor-α; IFNγ, interferon γ; RAA, renin angiotensin aldosterone system.

thrombus formation once plaque rupture has occurred and a thrombus has formed, because it is more efficient at inactivating the coagulant properties of clot-bound thrombin than ATIII/heparan sulfate (99).

The physiological significance of HCII/DS and HCII/DSPG anticoagulation is still unclear. Decreased levels of HCII do not appear to be a strong risk factor for thrombotic events, yet there have been some reports of increased venous thrombosis in individuals with low HCII levels (100,101). However, when HCII and/or DS levels are increased, such as in ATIII deficiency or pregnancy, HCII may be essential for maintenance of the appropriate hemostatic balance and adequate thrombin inhibition (76). There are, to date, no animal studies assessing the effect of HCII in models of vascular injury and atherosclerotic plaque development.

4. Tissue Factor Pathway Inhibitor (TFPI)

TFPI is a member of the Kunitz family of serine protease inhibitors (102). Normally, the largest pool of TFPI is bound to the endothelial cell surface, in association with glycosaminoglycans, whereas most of what remains is found in the plasma in association with lipoproteins. Increased levels of TFPI have been found in the aorta of cholesterol-fed rabbits and atherosclerotic human carotid arteries at sites colocalized with invading macrophages (103). It is an extrinsic pathway inhibitor, because it simultaneously binds to and inactivates factors VIIa/TF and Xa (104). Unlike ATIII and HCII, which inhibit activated thrombin in a reaction catalyzed by heparin, HSPG, or DS/DSPG (for HCII), TFPI blocks the activation of the prothombinase complex, thus preventing the formation of activated thrombin. Heparin injections have been shown to release TFPI from the endothelial pool (85, 102). TFPI may thus prove clinically useful in the prevention of unstable plaque rupture; however, it has no effect on clot-bound, active thrombin.

Even though TFPI used alone may not be the ideal clinical therapy for stabilization of unstable plaque, recombinant TFPI (rTFPI) has successfully been used in rabbit models of sepsis and various vascular diseases, including disseminated intravascular coagulation (DIC) (1, 76, 82). After successful thrombolytic therapy, exposure of TF in the lipid- and collagen-rich subendothelium of atherosclerotic plaque can lead to reocclusion of the artery. rTFPI in this case may be useful in preventing reocclusion and has been evaluated in a preliminary study using a canine model of femoral artery thrombosis (104, 105) and in a rabbit model of balloon injury–induced atheroma development (82) (Table 2).

5. Protease Nexin 1 (PN1)

A link between the thrombotic and thrombolytic cascades is formed by the activity of protease nexin 1 (PN1). PN1 is a serpin sharing approximately 30% sequence homology with ATIII and containing a high-affinity heparin-binding site (Table 1, Fig. 6) (106). PN1 is an effective inhibitor of thrombin, in addition to inhibiting the thrombolytic enzymes, uPA and tPA (107). Human plasma contains very low quantities of this protein (about 1 ng/ml), thus PN1 may not be a physiologically important anticoagulant in the blood (76, 107).

In the extravascular matrix, PN1 may play a significant role in limiting thrombosis and protecting the extravascular matrix from degradation by uPA and tPA. It is postulated that PN1 binds to collagen type IV, thus altering the enzyme's binding ability to uPA and tPA, but not thrombin (107). It is synthesized, however, by a wide range of cell types, including fibroblasts, skeletal and smooth muscle cells, neuronal and glial cells, and platelets (76). Clearance of PN1/thrombin complexes is thought to occur on the surface of endothelial cells and fibroblasts, mediated by the tight association of PN1 with the surface-bound glycosaminoglycans, heparan-sulfate, and chondroitin-sulfate. Thus, rather than having blood-based anticoagulant properties, PN1 is thought to promote cell- or extracellular matrix–based coagulation inhibition by attenuating the adverse effects of thrombin outside the vasculature. Whether this extends to the mitogenic properties of thrombin remains to be explained. No studies have examined the use of PN1 or PN2 as treatment for restenosis or unstable plaque formation.

6. Activated Protein C

Another important anticoagulant mechanism restricted to the surface of endothelial cells is the one mediated by protein C. Once thrombin is activated, mechanisms exist to keep its activity confined to the site of arterial injury. Present on the surface of endothelial cells is thrombomodulin (TM), an acidic proteoglycan, which acts as a high-affinity receptor for thrombin. Thrombin bound to TM undergoes a conformational change and loses its procoagulant properties as its specificity changes from fibrinogen to protein C. Protein C then becomes activated by thrombin to activated protein C (APC), which is a potent anticoagulant serine protease. Endothelial cell surface–bound APC (in association with a cofactor protein, protein S) cleaves the coagulant cofactors, factor Va and factor VIIIa, thus preventing the activation of the prothrombinase complex (76). Furthermore, APC destroys PAI-1, thus producing a net fibrinolytic effect at the endothelial cell surface (107). Deficiencies in APC and/or protein S have been associated with clinical thrombotic syndromes (108).

IV. THROMBOLYTIC SERPINS: ROLE IN PLAQUE RUPTURE AND CLOT LYSIS

A. Overview of the Thrombolytic Cascade

On the basis of the recent discoveries surrounding plasminogen activator activity in inflammatory responses, theoretical considerations would predict a protective role for thrombolytic serpins in unstable plaque rupture (2–4, 7–9). The matrix metalloproteinase (MMP) enzymes that degrade connective tissue, releasing smooth muscle cells bound in matrix or providing paths for invading circulating monocytes, are activated by the thrombolytic enzymes, tPA, uPA and plasmin (Figs. 3, 4) (10, 12–15, 35–37). Further, uPA binds to uPAR (the uPA receptor) that is found at the leading edge of invading macrophages associated with the degradation of the fibrous cap overlying an unstable plaque. Degradation of the fibrous tissue leads to rupture of the cap and exposure of the underlying lipid core and connective tissue (Fig. 4). The uPA/uPAR complex is believed to be instrumental in directing cellular adhesion through vitronectin interactions, cellular migration through chemotactic activity, and cellular invasion through activation of matrix metalloproteinase enzymes (MMP) proenzymes (Figs. 3, 4) (15, 35). The uPA/uPAR complex is involved in local tissue responses to injury, inflammatory responses, and infection. Inhibition by plasminogen activator inhibitors-1 or -2 (PAI-1 or PAI-2) the two most active vascular thrombolytic serpins, can be either through direct binding to circulating tPA and uPA (109) or through binding of PAI-1 to the uPA/uPAR complex (1, 4, 7). The uPA/uPAR complex is subsequently internalized and degraded. PAI-1 is believed to play a dominant role in the regulation of the thrombolytic cascade in the vascular system. Inhibition of the thrombolytic system would therefore be predicted to interfere with cellular adhesion and migration in the process of fibrous cap rupture, and PAI-1 would provide a protective role, preventing the fibrous cap rupture that initiates the chain of events leading to vascular thrombosis and total arterial occlusion.

Consistent with a role for the thrombolytic cascade in mononuclear cell invasion at sites of vessel damage are the results reported recently by Carmeliet's group demonstrating that plasminogen-deficient and, uPA-, but not tPA-, deficient knock out mice have reduced plaque growth after arterial injury (8, 36, 110, 111). This suggests a proactive role for the uPA/uPAR system in accelerating scar tissue formation and plaque growth after vascular trauma. Elegant studies by Carmeliet et al. have also demonstrated that PAI-1 does, indeed, have a central protective role in vascular wound healing. Knock out (KO) mice that lack PAI-1 have accelerated intimal hyperplasia in response to injury, whereas uPA KO mice have reduced plaque formation after vascular injury (9, 35–37). The PAI-1 protection or inhibition of intimal hyperplasia was restored in the PAI-1$^{-/-}$ (knock out) mice by the infusion of adenovirus that secretes PAI-1 in excess (9). Clowes et al. have demonstrated a protective role for aneurysm formation with the seeding of cells that overexpress tissue inhibitor of matrix metalloproteinase (TIMP) and PAI-1 in Guinea pig to rat aortic xenograft models (Table 2) (112). In our own work we have demonstrated a marked reduction in plaque growth and inflammatory cell invasion in rabbit (11) and rat models of angioplasty-mediated balloon injury and in a rat aortic allograft transplant model following serine protease inhibition (113).

Two central questions remain: First, does the thrombolytic cascade have greater impact through prevention and removal of clot (e.g., dissolution of thrombus and reduction of plaque bulk which will reduce arterial occlusion and end-organ ischemia), or through activation of matrix degrading enzymes and increased inflammatory cellular invasion at sites of unstable plaque? Second, is the role of the thrombolytic inhibitor, PAI-1, of greater importance in enhancing further clot formation by inhibiting plasminogen activation and clot lysis or as an antagonist that reduces inflammatory cellular invasion at sites of unstable plaque? It is also possible that plasmin and the plasminogen-activating enzymes have a greater detrimental role in areas of unstable plaque initiating macrophage invasion and plaque rupture, whereas the thrombolytic cascade may subsequently have a greater protective role at sites where the plaque has already ruptured and a thrombus is forming and threatening to cause arterial occlusion. In the following sections, the thrombolytic cascade and thrombolytic serine proteinase inhibitors, their role in plaque rupture and fibrinolysis, and potential therapeutic insights or applications will be reviewed.

B. Thrombotic Serine Proteinase Enzymes and Inhibitors as Plasma Markers of Unstable Plaque

Differentiation of stable and unstable angina by current parameters relies heavily on nonspecific criteria such as a history of crescendo angina and coronary angiography or possible intravascular ultrasonography (IVUS) or angioscopic detection of thrombosis. Clinical history can be notoriously inexact. Similarly, angiography and IVUS are both invasive and not particularly sensitive for the detection of ulcerated, lipid-filled, ruptured, or thrombotic plaque (114, 115). A simple blood test for a serum component would allow rapid triage of patients needing urgent catheterization and intervention, and might allow unnecessary tests to be avoided.

Elevated serum tPA and PAI-1 levels have been correlated with vessel restenosis after percutaneous transluminal coronary angioplasty (116, 117) or with the development of transplant vasculopathy after heart transplant (118). More specifically, assessment of coagulation, fibrinolytic, and kallikrein-kinin systems has detected altered circulating levels of these factors in patients with unstable coronary syndromes (33). Increased thrombin/ATIII complexes ($p <$ 0.05), increased D dimer ($p =$ NS), increased tPA ($p <$ 0.01), and increased PAI-1 ($p =$ NS) were detected in one study of unstable patients. There was also elevated kallikrein-like activity and kininogen ($p <$ 0.01) (33). In other studies tPA levels have been depressed or normal (119), but in general PAI-1 levels have been increased in studies of patients with unstable angina (33, 116).

Many investigators have interpreted the elevated PAI-1 levels to be symptomatic of a prothrombotic state that will be conducive to further thrombosis. The precise role of PAI-1 elevation has, however, not been determined. Whether the plasminogen activator inhibitory activity acts as a protective mechanism enhancing vascular healing and reducing inflammatory responses as discussed in the following sections or more simply as a procoagulant causing increased thrombosis and vascular occlusion remains to be determined.

C. Serine Proteinase Inhibitors of the Thrombolytic Cascade

1. The Thrombolytic Cascade

With formation of clot on the luminal surface of a ruptured plaque, there is activation of platelets and formation of fibrin networks as described in the preceding section (Sec. III). To balance the formation of thrombus and prevent excessive clot formation, these activated enzymes, in turn, activate the thrombolytic system (1, 2). Plasminogen is activated to the lytic form, plasmin, that proteolytically cleaves fibrin, thus dissolving fibrin-based clots and activating several other proteins such as the proforms of the matrix metalloproteinases (MMP) (Fig. 3) (7, 35, 111). Plasminogen is synthesized in the liver and then released to circulate in the bloodstream and other body fluids (4, 8).

Plasmin is regulated by the tissue- and urokinase-type plasminogen activators (tPA and uPA). Both endothelial cells and smooth muscle cells in the vascular walls secrete tPA and uPA, and their specific serpin inhibitor plasminogen activator inhibitor (PAI). uPA is also synthesized by macrophages, fibroblasts, ductal epithelial cells, granulosa and thecal cells, and several tumor cell lines in addition to vascular endothelial and smooth muscle cells (4). tPA is a 70-kDa protein transcribed from chromosome 8, whereas uPA is a 53-kDa protein transcribed from chromosome 10 (4). Each plasminogen activator contains a kringle structure, a growth factor–like domain, and a protease domain. Thrombin and fibrin activate uPA and tPA that convert plasminogen into the active thrombolytic enzyme plasmin.

The urokinase-type plasminogen activator receptor, uPAR, is now known to play a leading role in cellular invasion during inflammatory responses as noted in the preceding introductory section. Increased uPAR is found in areas of atherosclerotic plaque growth as are increased amounts of uPA and tPA (7, 8, 35, 109, 111, 120). Epidermal growth factor (EGF), basic fibroblast growth factor (bFGF), transforming growth factor-β (TGFβ), and platelet-derived growth factor increase transcription of uPA mRNA (Fig. 7). The cytokine interferon-γ (IFNγ) and angiotensin have, to the contrary, been found to decrease uPA mRNA transcription (Fig. 7) (121, 122).

2. Thrombolytic Serpins

The plasminogen activator inhibitors are serine proteinase inhibitors binding the target plasminogen activators 1 : 1 and acting as very poor substrates for the plasminogen activators, which allows the PAI molecule to effectively block the serine proteinase active site. There are four known naturally occurring mammalian inhibitors of tPA and uPA called PAI-1, PAI-2, protease nexin, and PAI-3 in order of the reaction rate constants (123). There are, in addition, eight known viral serine proteinase inhibitors, Spi 1–8. PAI-1 is a 52-kDa glycosylated protein that effectively inhibits both tPA and uPA to equivalent extents with a rate constant of 10^7L/mol.s. PAI-1 also reacts with protein-C, but PAI-1 is inactivated by this interaction. PAI-1 is mainly secreted by endothelial cells and platelets but is also produced by vascular smooth muscle cells, fibroblasts, and several tumor cell lines. PAI-2 exists in two forms, a 46.6-kDa nonglycosylated protein and a 60-kDa glycosylated protein that primarily inhibit two chain uPA. PAI-2 reacts weakly with plasmin and does not react at all with single-chain uPA, tPA, or kallikrein. PAI-2 is secreted by monocytes, polymorphonuclear leukocytes, and trophoblastic epithelial (placental) cells. Both PAI-1 and PAI-2 have arginine in their P1–P1' active sites. PAI-3 inhibits tPA and uPA poorly but also inhibits protein-C. PAI-1 and PAI-2 have only 25% sequence homology, whereas PAI-1 and 2 have 33 to 38% homology with other serpins. These two proteins, with similar inhibitory ranges in the thrombolytic cascade, may have evolved separately to perform similar basic functions (123). Protease nexin is a 47-kDa glycoprotein with a broad spectrum of action. Besides uPA (Ki = 10^5 L/mol.s) and two-chain tPA (Ki = 3 × 10^4 L/mol.s), nexin rapidly inhibits thrombin in the presence of heparin (Ki = 10^8 L/mol.s), trypsin (Ki = 4 × 10^6 L/mol.s), plasmin (Ki = 10^5 L/mol.s), and factor Xa (Ki = 7 × 10^3 L/mol.s). Protease nexin is known to inhibit thrombin as described in the preceding sections but also inhibits uPA. PAI-3 is a 51-kDa protein that reacts with two-chain uPA and thrombin (Ki = 10^4 − 10^5 L/mol.s) and more slowly with tPA (Ki = 10^3 L/mol.s). PAI-1 is the dominant vascular antithrombolytic agent. All these naturally occurring inhibitors function as classical serpins, binding and inhibiting the respective substrates in 1:1 complexes, functioning as poor substrates that bind the serine proteinase active site, and inhibiting enzyme activity. There is, in addition, a circulating plasmin inhibitor α_2-antiplasmin, which is the most active serum inhibitor of plasmin. There have not been any studies examining the role of this serpin in atheroma formation or in unstable plaque.

a. PAI-1

PAI-1 is a fascinating protein that has apparently evolved from a role as a regulator of the thrombolytic cascade in basic response reactions to injury to play a pivotal role in controlling other basic response reactions as an acute-phase reactant. In the central nervous system PAI-1 is up-regulated after injury or seizure activity (124). In the vascular system PAI-1 has been found to be up-regulated in patients with unstable atherosclerosis and has been put forward as a serum marker for unstable plaque (116, 117, 132) as noted in Sec. IV.B. Increased PAI-1 is also found in areas of developing atherosclerotic plaque.

PAI-1 is regulated by multiple factors in the vessel wall, many of which are directly related to vessel injury or substances that can damage the endothelial surface or activate inflammatory responses (Fig. 7). Thrombin the central regulatory protein in the thrombotic cascade up-regulates PAI-1 transcription in vascular endothelial cells and smooth muscle cells (125). Thrombin is also believed to form a complex with PAI-1, inactivating PAI-1 and cleaving PAI-1 in the extracellular matrix, which increases the release of PAI-1 from the matrix (126). Oxidized Lp(a) and LDL both also up-regulate PAI-1 (127). Several cytokines, specifically interleukin-1β and tumor necrosis factor-α (TNFα) also up-regulate PAI-1 transcription (124). Basic fibroblast growth factor (bFGF), transforming growth factor beta (TGFβ), and epidermal growth factor (EGF) upregulate PAI-1 (123). Conversely PAI-1 activates the proforms of the TGFβ and bFGF growth factors to their active forms. PAI-1 activity is also regulated by glucocorticoids and endotoxin (4, 7).

b. Viral Serpins

Eight viral serine proteinase inhibitors are currently known. The discovery of the poxviral serpins is relatively new, first reported in the 1980s (27). SERP-1 is one of many immunomodulatory proteins produced by myxomavirus (50, 53, 55) but has the distinction of being the only virus-encoded secreted serpin. SERP-1 serves to dampen the in vivo inflammatory response to viral infection (11, 53, 56, 113). Biochemically, SERP-1 has been shown to inhibit enzymes of the plasminogen cascade such as tissue-type plasminogen activator (t-PA), urokinase (u-PA), and plasmin (55–57). It is not clear yet whether these are in fact the biological targets or whether SERP-1 is targeting other, yet unidentified, proteinases.

D. Serine Proteinase Inhibitors of the Thrombolytic Cascade in the Prevention of Plaque Growth and Rupture

1. PAI-1—A Native Vascular Serpin

Aortic xenografts used in a model of aneurysm development (guinea pig to rat aortic transplant) have been seeded with endothelial cells that overproduce PAI-1. In this rat model, PAI-1 markedly inhibited aneurysm formation (112). Because many of the mechanisms related to aneurysm formation with connective tissue remodeling and inflammatory response may mimic events leading to unstable plaque formation, this work may indicate that PAI-1 or a similar serpin may eventually be developed as a stabilizing agent for the prevention of plaque rupture.

2. SERP-1—A Viral Anti-inflammatory Serpin

We have tested SERP-1 protein, isolated and purified from vaccinia virus vectors or CHO cells (11, 55, 57) in both rabbit (11) and rat (113) models of balloon angioplasty–induced atherosclerosis and in a rat aortic allograft model of transplant vasculopathy (113). In both atherosclerosis models we have detected marked reductions in plaque growth at 28 days follow-up after treatment with SERP-1 infusions given immediately after surgery. We have also tested SERP-1 infusions in a cholesterol-fed Yucatan microswine model of repeat (triple) balloon angioplasty injury model in iliofemoral arterial branches. SERP-1 reduced plaque size as determined by morphometric analysis (unpublished data). Figure 8 shows histological cross sections taken from the iliac arteries after three balloon

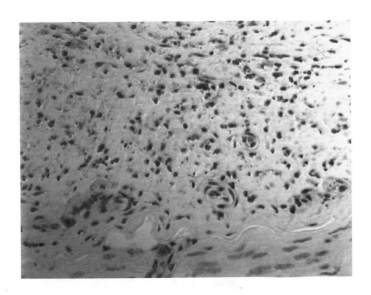

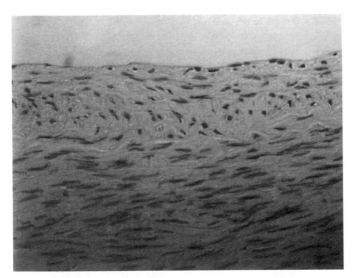

Figure 8   Iliac arteries from Yucatan microswine after three angioplasty balloon injuries. A marked reduction in intimal plaque growth is detected after treatment with the viral serpin, SERP-1, in the lower panel when compared to the saline treated control (top panel) at 28 days follow-up.

injuries and infusions, after the third injury, of either control saline (Fig. 8, top panel) or SERP-1 (Fig. 8, bottom panel) by means of a Wolinsky perforated balloon (11). As can be seen in this figure, there is a reduction in plaque size and invading hemosiderin-laden macrophages after SERP-1 treatment and the third arterial balloon injury.

SERP-1 is similar to PAI-1 in that this viral serine proteinase inhibitor binds to and inhibits tPA and uPA. SERP-1, however, also binds to plasmin, thrombin, and C1q; however, only plasmin is inhibited. SERP-1 serves as a good substrate for thrombin, and SERP-1 binds C1q very weakly and hence is not an inhibitor of either enzyme (53, 55–57).

In each of the animal models tested, associated with this reduction in plaque size produced by this viral serpin is a significant reduction in early macrophage invasion at 24 hours after balloon injury (11) and at 12 to 48 hours after aortic transplant (113). This suggests that SERP-1 may be inhibiting cellular invasion through regulation of uPA-mediated cellular adhesion, migration, and invasion. This inhibition of the plasminogen activator pathway may be either direct through binding of circulating tPA and uPA or through binding to the uPA/uPAR complex. SERP-1 may also act through regulation of mRNA transcription of the thrombolytic cascade activators or the native vascular serpins (113). We have detected, in preliminary work, a reduction in early tPA mRNA and an increase in early PAI-1 and uPAR mRNA levels in the rat aorta after balloon injury and SERP-1 treatment (113). This alteration in mRNA levels is mimicked when HUVEC (human umbillical vein endothelial cells) cells are incubated with SERP-1, but not with smooth muscle cells. These studies point to a potential gold mine of therapeutic agents that we have yet to harness from viruses.

V. CONCLUSIONS

We have reviewed the current known roles of vascular serpins in unstable atherosclerotic plaque development and rupture. The serpins that direct the activation of the thrombolytic and the thrombotic cascade play central roles in plaque rupture. These serpin-based inhibitory regulators may have variable effects, depending on the developmental stage of the plaque. The thrombolytic cascade may potentially have greater impact on lipid-filled, vulnerable plaque through acceleration of macrophage invasion, whereas the thrombotic cascade may play a central role once rupture has occurred with thrombosis formation. Thus, serine proteinase inhibitors may be capable of altering the course of events that lead to plaque rupture and acute vascular occlusion. The efficacy of these serine proteinase inhibitors may, however, depend on the state of the vulnerable plaque at the time of intervention, much as the roles of the soloists in a duet change throughout a concert (to complete our analogy). The serine proteinase inhibitors are a rich source of potentially therapeutic agents for both thrombotic and inflammatory disorders that have been in many cases minimally investigated or virtually untouched. The investigation of these proteins may well provide new and highly effective treatments for prevention and containment of labile plaque in unstable cardiovascular syndromes.

REFERENCES

1. Jenny NS, Mann KG. Coagulation cascade: an overview. In: Loscalzo J, Shafer AI, eds. Thrombosis and Hemorrhage. Baltimore: Williams & Wilkins, 1998: 3–24.
2. Vassalli JD, Sappino AP, Belin D. The plasminogen activator/plasmin system. J Clin Invest 1991; 88:1067–1072.
3. Farrehi PM, Ozaki K, Carmeliet P, Fay WP. Regulation of arterial thrombolysis by plasminogen activator inhibitor-1 in mice. Circulation 1998; 97:1002–1008.
4. Shen GX. Vascular cell-derived fibrinolytic regulators and atherothrombotic vascular disorders [review]. Int J Mol Med 1998; 1:399–408.
5. Royston D. Serine protease inhibition prevents both cellular and humoral responses to cardiopulmonary bypass. J Cardiovasc Pharm 1996; 27(suppl 1):S42–S49.
6. Potempa J, Korzus E, Travis J. The serpin superfamily of proteinase inhibitors: structure, function, and regulation: Review. J Biol Chem 1994; 269:15957–15960.
7. Stefansson S, Haudenschild CC, Lawrence DA. Beyond fibrinolysis: The role of plasminogen activator inhibitor-1 and vitronectin in vascular wound healing. Trends Cardiovasc Med 1998; 8:175–180.
8. Carmeliet P, Collen D. Genetic analysis of the plasminogen and coagulation system in mice. Haemostasis 1996; 26(suppl 4):132–153.
9. Carmeliet P, Moons L, Lijnen R, Janssens S, Lupu F, Collen D, Gerard RD. Inhibitory role of plasminogen activator inhibitor-1 in arterial wound healing and neointima formation. A gene targetting and gene transfer study in mice. Circulation 1997; 96:3180–3191.
10. Hasenstab D, Forough R, Clowes AW. Plasminogen activator inhibitor type-1 and tissue inhibitor of metalloproteinases-2 increase after arterial injury in rats. Circ Res 1997; 80:490–496.
11. Lucas A, Liu L, Macen JL, Nash PD, Dai E, Stewart M, Yan W, Graham K, Etches W, Boshkov L, Nation PN, Humen D, Hobman M, McFadden G. A virus-encoded serine proteinase inhibitor, SERP-1, inhibits atherosclerotic plaque development following balloon angioplasty. Circulation 1996; 94:2890–2900.
12. Lupu F, Heim DA, Bachmann F, Hurni M, Kakkar VV, Kruithof EKO. Plasminogen activator expression in human atherosclerotic lesions. Arterioscler Thromb Vasc Biol 1995; 15:1444–1455.
13. Raghunath PN, Tomaszewski JE, Brady ST, Caron RJ, Okada SS, Barnathan ES. Plasminogen activator system in human coronary arteriosclerosis. Arterioscler Thromb Vasc Biol 1995; 15:1432–1443.
14. Romer J, Bugge TH, Pyke C, Lund LR, Flick MJ, Degen JL, Dano K. Plasminogen and wound healing. Nature Med 1996;2:725.
15. Nikkari ST, Welgus HG, O'Brien KD, Alpers CE, Ferguson M, Clowes AW, Hat-

sukami T. Interstitial collagenase (MMP-1) expression in human carotid atherosclerosis. Circulation 1995; 92:1393–1398.

16. Fuster V. Human lesion studies. Ann NY Acad Sci 1997; 811:207–224.

17. Lassila R. Inflammation in atheroma: implications for plaque rupture and platelet collagen interaction. Eur Heart J 1993; 14(suppl K):K94–K97.

18. Gronholdt MLM, Dalager-Pedersen S, Falk E. Coronary plaque rupture: determinants of plaque rupture. Eur Heart J 1998; 19(suppl C):C24–C29.

19. Lewis JC, Bennett-Cain AL, DeMArs CS, Doellgast GJ, Grant KW, Jones NL, Gupta M. Procoagulant activity after exposure of monocyte-derived macrophages to minimally oxidized low density lipoprotein: co-localization of tissue factor antigen and nascent fibrin fibers at the cell surface. Am J Pathol 1995; 147:1029–1040.

20. Turpie AG, Weitz JI, Hirsh J. Advances in antithrombotic therapy: novel agents. Thromb Haemost 1995; 74:565–571.

21. Carreer FMJ. The C1 inhibitor deficiency: A review. Eur J Clin Chem Clin Biochem 1992; 30:793–807.

22. Bugge TH, Suh TT, Flick MJ, Daugherty CC, Romer J, Solberg H, Ellis V, Dano K, Degen JL. The receptor for urokinase-type plasminogen activator is not essential for mouse development or fertility. J Biol Chem 1995; 270:16886–16894.

23. Chai KX, Che LM, Chao J, Chao L. Kallistatin: A novel human serine proteinase inhibitor. J Biol Chem 1993; 268:24498–24505.

24. Turgeon VL, Houenou LJ. The role of thrombin-like (serine) proteases in the development, plasticity and pathology of the nervous system. Brain Res Rev 1997; 25:85–95.

25. Masos T, Miskin R. mRNAs encoding urokinase-type plasminogen activator and plasminogen activator inhibitor-1 are elevated in the mouse brain following kainate-mediated excitation. Mol Brain Res 1997; 47:157–169.

26. Rubin H. Serine protease inhibitors (SERPINS): where mechanism meets medicine. Natur Med 1996; 2:632–633.

27. Turner PC, Musy PY, Moyer RW. Poxvirus Serpins. In: McFadden, G. ed. Viroceptors, Virokines and Related Immune Modulators Encoded by DNA Viruses. Austin, TX: R. G. Landes Co., 1995:67–88.

28. Komiyama T, Ray CA, Pickup DJ, Howard AD, Thornberry NA, Peterson EP, Salvesen G. Inhibition of interleukin-1 beta converting enzyme by the cowpox virus serpin CrmA—An example of cross-class inhibition. J Biol Chem 1994; 269:19331–19337.

29. Herbert JM, Lamarche I, Carmeliet P. Urokinase and tissue-type plasminogen activator are required for the mitogenic and chemotactic effects of bovine fibroblast growth factor and platelet-derived growth factor-BB for vascular smooth muscle cells. J Biol Chem 1997; 272:23585–23591.

30. Riccio A, Pedone PV, Lund LR, Olesen T, Olsen HS, Andreasen PA. Transforming growth factor β1-responsive element: Closely associated binding sites for USF and CCAAT-binding transcription factor-nuclear factor I in the type 1 plasminogen activator inhibitor gene. Mol Cell Biol 1992; 12:1846–1855.

31. Maksymowych WP, Nation N, Nash PD, Macen J, Lucas A, McFadden G, Russell AS. Amelioration of antigen-induced arthritis in rabbits treated with a secreted viral serine proteinase inhibitor. J Rheumatol 1996; 23:878–882.

32. Depre C, Wijns W, Robert AM, Renkin JP, Havaux X. Pathology of unstable plaque: Correlation with the clinical severity of acute coronary syndromes. J Am Coll Cardiol 1997; 30:694–702.

33. Hoffmeister HM, Jur M, Wendel HP, Heller W, Seipel L. Alterations of coagulation and fibrinolytic and kallikrein-kinin systems in patients with unstable angina pectoris. Circulation 1995; 91:2520–2527.

34. Gurfinkel E, Bozovich G, Cerda M, Mejail I, Oxilia A, Mautner B. Time significance of acute thrombotic reactant markers in patients with and without silent myocardial ischemia and overt unstable angina pectoris. Am J Cardiol 1995; 76:121–124.

35. Lijnen HR, VanHoef B, Lupu F, Moons L, Carmeliet P, Collen D. Function of the plasminogen/plasmin and matrix metalloproteinase systems after vascular injury in mice with targeted inactivation of fibrinolytic system genes. Arterioscler Thromb Vasc Biol 1998; 18:1035–1045.

36. Carmeliet P, Moons L, Dewerchin M, Mackman N, Luther T, Breier G, Ploplis V, Muller M, Nagy A, Plow E, Gerard R, Edgington T, Risau W, Collen D. Insights in vessel development and vascular disorders using targeted inactivation and transfer of vascular endothelial growth factor, the tissue factor receptor, and the plasminogen system. Ann N Y Acad Sci 1997; 811:191–206.

37. Loskutoff DJ. PAI-1 inhibits neointimal formation after arterial injury in mice: A new target for controlling restenosis. Circulation 1997; 96:2772–2774.

38. Potempa J, Korzus E, Travis J. The serpin superfamily of proteinase inhibitors: structure, function, and regulation: Review. J Biol Chem 1994; 269:15957–15960.

39. Stein PE and Carrell RW. What do dysfunctional serpins tell us about molecular mobility and disease? Review. Nature Structural Biol 1995; 2:96–113.

40. Whisstock J, Skinner R, Lesk AM. An atlas of serpin conformations. Trends Biochem Sci 1998; 23:63–67.

41. Lawrence DA, Olson ST, Palaniappan S, Ginsburg D. Serpin reactive center loop mobility is required for inhibitor function but not for enzyme recognition. J Biol Chem 1994; 269:27657–27662.

42. Wilczynska M, Fa M, Ohlsson PI, Ny T. The inhibition mechanism of serpins. J Biol Chem 1995; 270:29652–29655.

43. Cunningham MA, Blajchman MA, Sheffield WP. Impact of mutations at the P4 and P5 positions on the reaction of antithrombin with thrombin and elastin. Thromb Res 1997; 88:171–181.

44. Stratikos E, Gettins PG. Major proteinase movement upon stable serpin-proteinase complex formation. Proc Natl Acad Sci USA 1997; 94:453–458.

45. Wilczynska M, Fa M, Karolin J, Ohlsson PI, Johansson L, Ny T. Structural insights into serpin-protease complexes reveal the inhibitory mechanism of serpins. Nature Structural Biol 1997; 4:354–356.

46. Sheffield WP, Blajchman MA. Deletion mutagenesis of heparin cofactor II: defining the minimum size of a thrombin inhibiting serpin. FEBS Lett 1995; 365:189–192.

47. Laskowski M, Kato I. Protein inhibitors of proteinases. Annu Rev Biochem 1980; 49:593–626.

48. Stone SR, Whisstock JC, Bottomley SP, Hopkins PC. SERPINS: a mechanistic class of their own. Adv Exp Med Biol 1997; 425:5–15.

49. Bode W, Huber R. Natural protein proteinase inhibitors and their interaction with proteinases. Eur J Biochem 1992; 204:433–451.

50. Nash P, Lucas A, McFadden G. SERP-1, a poxvirus-encoded serpin, is expressed as a secreted glycoprotein that inhibits the inflammatory response to myxoma virus infection. In: Church FC, Cunningham DD, Ginsburg D, Hoffman M, Stone SR, Tollefse DM, eds. Chemistry and Biology of Serpins. New York: Oxford University Press, 1997:195–205.

51. Moss B. Poxviridae and their replication. In: Fields BN, Knipe DM, eds. Virology. New York: Raven Press, Ltd., 1990:2079–2111.

52. Komiyama T, Ray CA, Pickup DJ, Howard AD, Thornberry NA, Peterson EP, Salvesen G. Inhibition of interleukin-1 beta converting enzyme by the cowpox virus serpin CrmA—An example of cross-class inhibition. J Biol Chem 1994; 269: 19331–19337.

53. Macen JL, Garner RS, Musy PY, Brooks MA, Turner PC, Moyer RW, McFadden G, Bleackley RC. Differential inhibition of the Fas- and granule-mediated cytolysis pathways by the orthopoxvirus cytokine response modifier A/SPI-2 and SPI-1 protein. Proc Natl Acad Sci USA 1996; 93:9108–9113.

54. Quan LT, Caputo A, Bleackley RC, Pickup DJ, Salvesen GS. Granzyme B is inhibited by the cowpox virus serpin cytokine response modifier A. J Biol Chem. 1995; 270:10377–10379.

55. Nash P, Barrett J, Cao J, Hota-Mitchell S, Lalani A, Everett H, Xu X, Robichaud J, Hnatiuk S, Ainslie C, Seet B, McFadden G. Immunomodulation by viruses: the myxoma virus story. Immunol Rev 1999; 168:103–120.

56. Macen JL, Upton C, Nation N, McFadden G. SERP1, a serine proteinase inhibitor encoded by myxoma virus, is a secreted glycoprotein that interferes with inflammation. Virology 1993; 195:348–363.

57. Nash P, Whitty A, Handwerker J, Macen J, McFadden G. Inhibitory specificity of the anti-inflammatory myxoma virus serpin, Serp-1. J Biol Chem 1998; 273:20982–20991.

58. Fuster V, Badimon L, Badimon JJ, Chesebro JH. The pathogenesis of coronary artery disease and the acute coronary syndromes. N Engl J Med 1992; 326:310–318.

59. Libby P, Schwartz D, Brogi E, Tanaka H, Clinton SK. A cascade model for restenosis: A special case of atherosclerosis progression. Circulation 1992; 86(suppl III): III-47–III-52.

60. Drake TA, Morrissey JH, Edgington TS. Selective cellular expression of tissue factor in human tissues. Implications for disorders of hemostasis and thrombosis. Am J Pathol 1989; 134:1087–1097.

61. Morrissey JH, Macik BG, Neuenschwander PF, Comp PC. Quantitation of activated Factor VII levels in blood plasma using a tissue factor mutant selectively deficient in promoting factor VII activation. Blood 1993; 81:734–744.

62. Eaton D, Rodriguez H, Vehar GA. Proteolytic processing of human factor VIII. Correlation of specific cleavages by thrombin, factor Xa and activated protein C

with activation and inactivation of Factor VIII coagulant activity. Biochem 1986; 25:505–512.

63. Esmon CT, Esmon NL, Le Bonniec BF, Johnson AE. Protein C activation. Methods Enzymol 1993; 222:359–385.

64. Pryzdial EL, Bajzar L, Nesheim ME. Prothrombinase components can accelerate tissue plasminogen activator-catalyzed plasminogen activation. J Biol Chem 1995; 270:17871–17877.

65. Kable EP, Monteith GR, Roufogalis BD. The effect of thrombin and serine proteases on intracellular Ca2+ in rat aortic smooth muscle cells. Cell Signal 1995; 7: 123–129.

66. Cirino G, Cicala C, Bucci MR, Sorrentino L, Maraganore JM, Stone SR. J Exp Med 1996; 183:821–827.

67. Badimon L, Meyer BJ, Badimon LL. Thrombin in arterial thrombosis. Haemostasis 1994; 24:69–80.

68. Varela O, Martinez-Gonzalez J, Badimon L. The response of smooth muscle cells to "alpha"-thrombin depends on its arterial origin: comparison among different species. Eur J Clin Invest 1998; 28:313–323.

69. Bar-Shavit R, Benezra M, Sabbah V, Bode W, Vlodavsky I. Thrombin as a multifunctional protein: induction of cell adhesion and proliferation. Am J Respir Cell Mol Biol 1992; 6:123–130.

70. Kanthou C, Benzakour O. Cellular effects of thrombin and their signalling pathways. Cell Pharmacol 1995; 2:293–302.

71. Pearson JD. Endothelial cell function and thrombosis. Baill Clin Haematol. 1994; 7:441–452.

72. Valenzuela R, Shainoff JR, DiBello PM, Urbanic DA, Anderson JM, Matsueda GR, Kudryk BJ. Immunoelectrophoretic and immunohistochemical characterizations of fibrinogen derivatives in atherosclerotic aortic intimas and vascular prosthesis pseudointimas. Am J Pathol 1992; 141:861–880.

73. Ernst E. Fibrinogen as a cardiovascular risk factor—interrelationship with infections and inflammation. Eur Heart J 1993; 14(suppl K):K82–K87.

74. Koenig W. Haemostatic risk factors for cardiovascular diseases. Eur Heart J 1998; 19(suppl C):C39–C43.

75. Fareed J, Hoppensteadt DA, Leya F, Iqbal O, Wolf H, Bick R. Useful laboratory tests for studying thrombogenesis in acute cardiac syndromes. Clin Chem 1998; 44:1845–1853.

76. Bombeli T, Mueller M, Haeberli A. Anticoagulant properties of the vascular endothelium. Thromb Haemost 1997; 77:403–423.

77. Rao LVM, Rapaport SI, Hoang AD. Binding of factor VIIa to tissue factor permits rapid antithrombin III/heparin inhibition of factor VIIa. Blood 1993; 81:2600–2607.

78. Cannon CP. Thrombin inhibitors in acute myocardial infarction. Card Clin 1995; 13:421–433.

79. Hirsh J. Heparin. N Engl J Med 1991; 324:1565–1574.

80. Weitz JI, Hudoba M, Massel DR, Maraganore J, Hirsh J. Clot-bound thrombin is protected from inhibition by heparin-antithrombin III but is susceptible to inactivation by antithrombin III-independent inhibitors. J Clin Invest 1990; 86:385–391.

81. Badimon L, Lassila R, Badimon JJ, Vallabhajosula S, Chesebro JH, Fuster V. Residual thrombus is more thrombogenic than severely damaged vessel wall. Circulation 1988; 78:II-119.

82. Jang Y, Guzman A, Lincoff M, Gottsauner-Wolf M, Forudi F, Hart CE, Courtman DW, Ezban M, Ellis SG, Topol EJ. Influence of blockade at specific levels of the coagulation cascade on restenosis in a rabbit atherosclerotic femoral artery injury model. Circulation 1995; 92:3041–3050.

83. Ragosta M, Gimple LW, Gertz SD, Dunwiddie CT, Vlasuk GP, Haber HL, Powers ER, Roberts WC, Sarembock IJ. Specific factor Xa inhibition reduces restenosis after balloon angioplasty of atherosclerotic femoral arteries in rabbits. Circulation 1994; 89:1262–1271.

84. Jeske W, Messmore, HL Jr., Fareed J. Pharmacology of heparin and oral anticoagulants. In: Loscalzo J, Shafer AI, eds. Thrombosis and Hemorrhage. Baltimore: Williams & Wilkins, 1998:3–24.

85. Dosne AM, Bendetowicz AV, Kher A, Samama M. Marked potentiation of the plasminogenolytic activity of pro-urokinase by unfractionated heparin and a low molecular-weight heparin. Thromb Res 1988; 51:627–630.

86. Timms ID, Tomaszewski JE, Shlansky-Goldberg RD. Effect of nonanticoagulant heparin (Astenose) on restenosis after balloon angioplasty in the atherosclerotic rabbit. J Vasc Intervent Radiol 1995; 6:365–378.

87. Edelman ER, Adams DH, Karnovsky MJ. Effect of controlled adventitial heparin delivery on smooth muscle cell proliferation following endothelial injury. Proc Natl Acad Sci 1990; 87:3773–3777.

88. Messmore HL, Wehrmacher WH. Therapeutic use of low molecular weight heparins. Sem Thromb Hemost 1993; 19(suppl 1):97–100.

89. Anonymous. Low molecular weight heparin is an effective and safe treatment for deep vein thrombosis and pulmonary embolism (Abst). The Columbus Investigators. Blood 1996; 88(suppl 1):626a.

90. Ren S, Fenton JW, Maraganore JM, Angel A, Shen GX. Inhibition by hirulog-1 of generation of plasminogen activator inhibitor-1 from vascular smooth-muscle cells induced by thrombin. J Card Pharmacol 1997; 29:337–342.

91. Sharma GV, Coccio E, Lapsley D, Adelman B, Vita JA, Loscalzo J, Sharma S. Usefulness and tolerability of hirulog, a direct thrombin-inhibitor, in unstable angina pectoris. Am J Cardiol 1993; 72:1357–1360.

92. Antman EM. Hirudin in acute myocardial infarction. Thrombolysis and Thrombin Inhibition in Myocardial Infarction (TIMI) 9B trial. Circulation 1996; 94:911–921.

93. Barry WL, Wiegman PJ, Gimple LW, Gertz SD, Powers ER, Owens GK, Sarcmbock IJ. A new single-injury model of balloon angioplasty in cholesterol-fed rabbits: beneficial effect of hirudin and comparison with double-injury model. Lab Invest 1997; 77:109–116.

94. Sarembock IJ, Gertz SD, Thome LM, McCoy KW, Ragosta M, Powers ER, Maraganore JM, Gimple LW. Effectiveness of hirulog in reducing restenosis after balloon angioplasty of atherosclerotic femoral arteries in rabbits. J Vasc Res 1996; 33:308–314.

95. Ragosta M, Barry WL, Gimple LW, Gertz SD, McCoy KW, Stouffer GA, McNa-

mara CA, Powers ER, Owens GK, Sarembock IJ. Effect of thrombin inhibition with desulfatohirudin on early kinetics of cellular proliferation after balloon angioplasty in atherosclerotic rabbits. Circulation 1996; 93:1194–1200.

96. Muller DW, Gordon D, Topol EJ, Levy RJ, Golomb G. Sustained-release local hirulog therapy decreases early thrombosis but not neointimal thickening after arterial stenting. Am Heart J 1996; 131:211–218.

97. Struss DJ, Storck RE, Zimmermann P. The inhibition of thrombin and chymotrypsin by heparin cofactor II. Thromb Res 1992; 68:45–56.

98. McGuire EA, Tollefsen DM. Activation of heparin cofactor II by fibroblasts and vascular smooth muscle cells. J Biol Chem 1987; 262:169–175.

99. Bendayan P, Boccalon H, Dupouy D, Boneu B. Dermatan sulfate is a more potent inhibitor of clot-bound thrombin than unfractionated and low molecular weight heparins. Thromb Haemost 1994; 71:576–582.

100. Tran TH, Marbet GA, Duckert F. Association of hereditary heparin co-factor II deficiency with thrombosis. Lancet 1985; 2:413–414.

101. Sie P, Dupouy D, Pichon J, Boneu B. Constitutional heparin co-factor II deficiency associated with recurrent thrombosis. Lancet 1985; 2:414–416.

102. Sandset PM. Tissue factor pathway inhibitor (TFPI)—an update. Haemostasis 1996; 26:154–165.

103. Drew AF, Davenport P, Apostolopoulos J, Tipping PG. Tissue factor pathway inhibitor expression in atherosclerosis. Lab Invest 1997; 77:291–298.

104. Haskel EJ, Torr SR, Day KC, Palmier MO, Wun T-C, Sobel BE, Abendschein DR. Prevention of arterial reocclusion after thrombolysis with recombinant lipoprotein-associated coagulation inhibitor. Circulation 1991; 84(suppl II):II–32.

105. Harker LA. New antithrombotic strategies for resistant thrombotic processes. J Clin Pharm 1994; 34:3–16.

106. Baker JB, Low DA, Simmer RL. Protease nexin: a cellular component that links thrombin and plasminogen activator and mediates their binding to cells. Cell 1980; 21:37–45.

107. Preissner KT. Anticoagulant properties of the endothelial cell membrane components. Haemostasis 1988; 18:271–306.

108. Bauer KA. Inherited and hypercoagulable states. In: Loscalzo J, Shafer AI, eds. Thrombosis and Hemorrhage. Baltimore: Williams & Wilkins, 1998:863–900.

109. Bugge TH, Flick MJ, Danton MJ, Daugherty CC, Romer J, Dano K, Carmeliet P, Collen D, Degen JL. Urokinase-type plasminogen activator is effective in fibrin clearance in the absence of its receptor or tissue-type plasminogen activator. Proc Natl Acad Sci USA 1996; 93:5899–5904.

110. Carmeliet P, Moons L, Ploplis V, Plow E, Collen D. Impaired arterial neointima formation in mice with disruption of the plasminogen gene. J Clin Invest 1997; 99:200–208.

111. Carmeliet P, Collen D. Molecular analysis of blood vessel formation and disease. Am J Physiol 1997; 273:H2091–2104.

112. Allaire E, Hasenstab D, Kenagy RD, Starcher B, Clowes MM, Clowes AW. Prevention of aneurysm development and rupture by local overexpression of plasminogen activator inhibitor-1. Circulation 1998; 98:249–255.

113. Lucas A, Dai E, Liu LY, Guan HY, Nash P, McFadden G, Miller L. Transplant

vasculopathy: viral anti-inflammatory serpin regulation of atherogenesis. J Heart Lung Transplant. (In press).

114. Flotte TJ. Pathology correlations with optical biopsy techniques. Ann N Y Acad Sci 1998; 838:143–149.

115. Nissen SE, DeFranco AC, Tuzco EM, Moliterno DJ. Coronary intravascular ultrasound: diagnostic and interventional applications. Coron Art Dis 1995; 6:355–367.

116. Weiczorek I, Ludlam CA, Fox KAA. Tissue-type plasminogen activator and plasminogen activator inhibitor activities as predictors of adverse events in unstable angina. Am J Cardiol 1994; 74:424–429.

117. Woodhouse PR, Meade TW, Khaw KT. Plasminogen activator inhibitor-1, the acute phase response and vitamin C. Atherosclerosis 1997; 133:71–76.

118. Garvin MR, Walley VM, Labinaz M, Mizgala HF, Pels K, O'Brien ER. Arterial expression of the plasminogen activator system early after cardiac transplantation. Card Res 1997; 35:241–249.

119. Zalewski A, Shi Y, Nardone D, Bravette B, Weinstock P, Fischman D, Wilson P, Goldberg S, Levin DC, Bjornsson TD. Evidence for reduced fibrinolytic activity in unstable angina at rest: Clinical, biocehmical, and angiographic correlates. Circulation 1991; 83:1685–1691.

120. Dewerchin M, Nuffelen AV, Wallays G, Bouch A, Moons L, Carmeliet P. Generation and characterization of urokinase-deficient mice. J Clin Invest 1996; 97:870–878.

121. Vaughan DE. The renin-angiotensin system and fibrinolysis. Am J Cardiol 1997; 79:12–16.

122. Andreasen PA, Georg B, Lund LR, Riccio A, Stacey SN. Plasminogen activator inhibitors: hormonally regulated serpins. Mol Cell Endocrin 1990; 68:1–19.

123. Kruithof EKO. Plasminogen activator inhibitors—A review. Enzyme 1988; 40:113–121.

124. Faber-Elman A, Miskin R, Schwartz M. Components of the plasminogen activator system in astrocytes are modulated by tumor necrosis factor-a and interleukin 1 b through similar signal transduction pathways. J Neurochem 1995; 65:1524–1535.

125. Ren S, Cockell KA, Fenton JW, Angel A, Shen GX. G proteins and phopholipase C mcdiate thrombin-induced generation of plasminogen activator inhibitor-1 from vascular smooth muscle cells. J Vasc Res 1997; 34:82–89.

126. Shen GX, Ren S, Fenton JW. Transcellular signaling and pharmacological modulation of thrombin-induced production of plasminogen activator inhibitor-1 in vascular smooth muscle cells. Semin Thromb Haemast 1998; 24:151–156.

127. Ren S, Man RYK, Angel A, Shen GX. Oxidative modification enhances lipoprotein(a)-induced overexpression of plasminogen activator inhibitor-1 in cultured vas cular endothelial cells. Atherosclerosis 1997; 128:1–10.

128. Toda T, Hokama S, Nagamine M, Takei H. Promotive effect of elastase on regression of aortic atherosclerosis in cholesterol-fed quails. Exp Pathol 1989; 36:201–209.

129. Gaciong Z, Paczek L, Bojakowski K, Socha K, Wisniewski M, Heidland A. Beneficial effect of proteases on allograft arteriosclerosis in a rat aortic allograft model. Nephrol Dial Transplant 1996; 11:987–989.

23
Gene Therapy to Stabilize Atherosclerotic Plaque

Carl M. Fier and Jonathan D. Marmur
Mount Sinai School of Medicine, New York, New York

Major advances in the fields of recombinant DNA technology, cell biology, and percutaneous angioplasty have established the scientific and technical basis for the transfer of genetic information to the vessel wall (1). Although gene therapy was initially proposed as a means to treat inherited disorders, whereby transfer of a normal copy of a single defective gene would prevent the development of disease, most of ongoing and planned human gene therapy trials have been developed to treat acquired diseases. The concept of gene therapy at present encompasses the transfer of genetic information using genetically modified cells, chromosomes, portions of genes, or nucleic acids in a variety of forms (e.g., viral vectors, DNA oligonucleotides, RNA ribozymes) for therapeutic intent (2). Thus, in its broadest sense, gene therapy may be defined as the genetic-based treatment of inherited and acquired diseases.

Despite the high prevalence of cardiovascular disease, disorders of the vascular system have been represented to date in a relatively small proportion of the approved human gene therapy protocols (3). In light of recent advances in the understanding of the molecular biology of the cardiovascular system, especially at the level of the vessel wall, however, the time may now be appropriate for the introduction of gene therapy to the management of a broad array of vasculopathies. However, several problems related to the delivery, integration, and regulation of the therapeutic gene constitute an obstacle to the broader application of the concepts of gene therapy. Further advances in the application of gene therapy to human vascular disease will depend on advances in the methods of gene delivery to the targeted cell, the achievement of stable gene expression at a defined level within the target cell, and the design of vectors that are not deleterious to the patient or to the public health.

Certain features of the vessel wall favor and others impede the development of effective strategies to deliver exogenous genetic material. Favorable characteristics include the accessibility of a large portion of the vascular tree to catheter-based delivery devices, the relative simplicity of the vessel wall architecture and paucity of cell types, and the availability of a plethora of both simple and sophisticated technologies (e.g., quantitative angiography, intravascular ultrasonography, and angioscopy) to assess the effects of an intervention. Unfavorable characteristics include the slow replication rate of endothelial and vascular smooth muscle cells, possibly rendering the vessel wall impenetrable to vectors such as retroviruses that require cell division for successful gene transduction, and the presence of acellular, fibrous, and dense extracellular matrix in segments obstructed by atherosclerotic plaque that may be an important target for gene therapy.

In an initial attempt to overcome the obstacles to gene delivery inherent to the arterial wall, studies used a cell-mediated approach in which cultured vascular cells were transduced ex vivo and then introduced to the vessel wall by means of a double balloon catheter (1). As reviewed by Nabel et al. (4), an advantage of cell-mediated gene transfer is that the effects of gene transfer in a particular cell type can be evaluated (e.g., endothelial vs. smooth muscle cell). Disadvantages include the requirement for syngeneic cell lines and the transfection of cells in culture that necessitates a time delay between cell harvest and implantation. Despite these technical difficulties, ex vivo gene transfer has been demonstrated in several animal models, including seeding of genetically modified endothelial or vascular smooth muscle cells on canine prosthetic grafts (5) and denuded porcine (6) and rat arteries (7), as well as seeding of stents with sheep endothelial cells (8) and seeding of autologous transduced endothelial cells onto rat skeletal muscle capillaries (9).

In contrast to the ex vivo approach, the direct introduction of genetic material into the vessel wall represents a conceptually attractive alternative to the instillation of genetically altered cells and has been demonstrated in a number of animal models using a variety of gene transfer vectors. Direct delivery requires both a delivery system and a gene transfer vector. Sophisticated technologies to deliver genetic vectors in vivo, including autoperfusion multichamber catheters (10) and micromechanical devices incorporated into intravascular stents (11), have been developed and are undergoing refinement to ensure safe, site-specific delivery of transfer vectors.

Gene transfer vectors play a critical role in the successful implementation of gene therapy. Studies demonstrate that the degree of gene transfer (transfection efficiency) and the stability of gene expression over time are influenced in large part by the nature of the gene transfer vector. Thus, much of the work in the field of gene therapy has focused on the development of these gene transfer vectors. The transfer of genes into the vascular cells of adult animals has been achieved using a variety of vectors including viral vectors (retrovirus, adenovirus, adeno-associated virus) and nonviral vectors (cationic liposomes, receptor-mediated molecular conjugates, and "naked" DNA gel delivery systems) (12).

I. VIRAL VECTORS

Recombinant viral vectors exploit the mechanisms that viruses have evolved to achieve efficient gene transfer. The common strategy for the design of these vectors involves the replacement of elements of the parent viral genome that are essential for replication with heterologous DNA sequences such that the recombinant virion is capable of effective transfer of the insert gene but incapable of replication. This is the so-called replication-deficient virus. By use of this basic paradigm, a variety of DNA and RNA viruses have been used in gene therapy applications.

II. RETROVIRUS

Retroviral vectors were the first viral vectors to be used for in vivo arterial gene transfer studies (1). A mature retrovirus is made up of an inner core enclosed in a phospholipid envelope. The envelope is a phospholipid bilayer derived from the plasma membrane of the virus-producing cell and is covered with glycoproteins that appear as surface projections on electron microscopy. The retroviral core consists of an icosahedral protein shell, the capsid, which contains two copies of the positive sense viral mRNA genome including 5' cap and 3' poly (A) structures (13). Also contained within the capsid are the virally encoded protease, reverse transcriptase, and integrase enzymes.

On addition of the retroviral particles to a culture of cells, the viral particle binds to the cell, the retroviral vector enters the cell, and the vector sequence is subsequently integrated into the host cell genome. Because the retroviral vector is lacking several genes needed for replication, this transfer procedure is termed "transduction" to distinguish it from "infection," which is reserved for replication-competent viruses (14). After integration of the retroviral vector, its internal sequences are expressed, resulting in the expression of a novel RNA molecule and protein in the transduced cell. Integration into the target cell genome confers the potential for stable long-term gene expression but is associated with the risk of insertional mutagenesis (15).

The advantages of retroviral vectors include the ability to infect a wide range of cell types in vitro, the integration of genetic material transported by the vector into the target cell genome, the lack of toxicity of these viruses in transduced cells, and the lack of vector spread or production of viral proteins after transduction. These properties have been exploited successfully in a number of human gene therapy protocols involving ex vivo modification of target cells followed by reimplantation of the genetically modified cells (16).

Despite these advantages, a number of features may limit the usefulness of retroviral vectors with regard to the vasculature. A characteristic feature of retroviruses is that replication of target cells is necessary for proviral integration (17). This presents a major limitation for direct arterial retroviral gene transfer because vascular cells have a low proliferation rate in vivo (18). Moreover, murine retroviral vectors are rapidly inactivated by human complement (19) and therefore may be unsuitable for direct gene delivery to human tissues in vivo. Finally, standard retroviruses are produced in relatively low titer because replication-deficient viruses are collected as supernatants from the producer cell line and cannot be concentrated. This has important implications for in vivo gene delivery, where efficient gene transfer requires a high multiplicity of infection. Strategies to overcome these limitations include the use of producer cell lines as delivery vehicles and attempts to alter the lability and tropism of the vector through genetic engineering of the glycoproteins on the lipid envelope of the retroviral particle (20).

III. ADENOVIRUS

Early studies using retroviral vectors and liposomes for arterial gene transfer reported low efficiencies, generally <1% of vascular cells in vivo (21–24). Adenoviral vectors transfer genes efficiently in a broad spectrum of eukaryotic cells, and therefore more current studies have concentrated on the use of the adenovirus as a vector for gene transfer to the vessel wall (25–27). Wild-type adenoviruses target primarily the epithelial cell and produce clinical illnesses that are usually mild and rarely life-threatening. The basic structure of the adenovirus is a nonenveloped icosahedral (20 facets and 12 vertices) protein capsid enclosing an inner DNA-protein core.

The adenoviral vector system possesses a number of favorable characteristics. Unlike retroviruses, adenoviruses infect both replicating and nonreplicating cells, including terminally differentiated cells. In addition, adenoviral vectors are not inactivated by human complement and are stable in vivo, permitting direct gene delivery in a variety of contexts (28), including the arterial wall (27). After entry into the target cell nucleus, adenoviral DNA sequences remain in an extrachromosomal form and rarely integrate into the host cell chromosome, thereby diminishing the likelihood of insertional mutagenesis and dysregulation of cellular genes. Arteries infected with adenoviral vectors achieve higher levels of reporter gene expression with transduction efficiencies 10- to 100-fold greater than those reported for retroviral and liposome vectors (12, 25, 29, 30).

Despite these advantages, there are limitations to currently available adenoviral vectors. In several models, adenoviral-mediated gene expression is transient, and an inflammatory reaction is detectable in target tissues (31, 32). These problems also apply to the vascular system; in most studies arterial reporter gene expression is diminished or undetectable by 28 days (12, 25, 33). The lack of persistent gene expression may be due to the development of an immune response to adenoviral proteins and/or acute adenovirus-associated tissue toxicity, as demonstrated by medial smooth muscle cell loss and neutrophilic infiltrates (34).

Adenovirus-based strategies to achieve arterial gene transfer may also be limited by the apparent impermeability of the endothelial layer to this vector, thereby necessitating mechanical disruption of the intima before gene transfer that is targeting medial smooth muscle (20). The presence of significant plaque accumulation has also presented a concern. Finally, each of the approximately 20 serotypes of human adenovirus may generate neutralizing antibody, potentially limiting the possibility of repeated administration of a particular vector.

Counter to these arguments is the recent work of Luo et al. who showed one model of effective adenoviral gene transfer unaffected by immunologic priming, supporting the possibility of repeat transfection to achieve therapeutic intent (35). With regard to plaque burden and the need for endothelial disruption, Rehter et al. explained some of the critical issues (36). This group found that successful transfection was possible in endothelial, adventitial, and intimal smooth muscle cells in a variety of human vessels, including internal mammary, native coronary, and saphenous vein in tissue culture. Furthermore, atherosclerotic plaques were transfected with a similar efficiency. Interestingly, areas with plaque rupture and thrombus showed a predilection toward effective gene expression, identifying them as particularly good targets for directed gene therapy. Treatment of the vessels with collagenase and elastase improved gene transfection, indicating that surrounding extracellular matrix does indeed play an important role in the successful deployment of gene therapies.

IV. ADENO-ASSOCIATED VIRUS

Another viral vector that has been used in human gene therapy trials is the adeno-associated virus (AAV). AAV is a single-stranded DNA virus and a member of the parvovirus family (37). Unlike the adenovirus, it is not associated with known pathological conditions in humans or animals, despite high levels of silent infection in vivo. Adeno-associated viruses are described as replication-defective, because either adenovirus or herpesvirus (defined in this setting as helper virus) is needed to provide adjunctive helper function to establish viral replication and complete an AAV life-cycle (38). The defective nature of AAV may be a useful feature for gene therapy, where replication and spread of the virus vector is not desirable. The defective nature of AAV does not represent an impediment to the gene-transferring capacities of recombinant adeno-associated virions; it has been demonstrated both wild-type and recombinant AAV integrate into the host genome efficiently and establish a latent infection in the absence of the helper virus (39). Transduction of a variety of primary human cells has been reported, including hepatocytes (40), bronchial epithelial cells (41), and peripheral blood mononuclear cells (42). The wild-type virus efficiently integrates into the host genome and usually does so preferentially in a small region of chromosome 19 (43–45). Such site-specific integration could diminish the likelihood of insertional mutagenesis, a major concern of gene therapy when using viruses that integrate indiscriminately into the genome.

When targeting the media of elastic arteries, the small size of AAV (18–26 nm) relative to adenovirus (65–80 nm) (37) may represent an advantage. Penetration of particles from the lumen into the media of these arteries varies as a function of particle size (46). Theoretically, the small size of AAV may allow it to penetrate the subendothelium and reach the media without the need for mechanical disruption of the intima before infection.

V. NONVIRAL VECTORS

Although viruses constitute highly efficient gene transfer vehicles, the risks, costs, and limitations associated with recombinant viral vectors have led investigators to develop a variety of synthetic chemical nonviral vector systems. To mediate gene transfer effectively, these systems must overcome the same cellular barriers encountered by viruses: transport across the cell membrane, transfer from cytoplasm to nucleus, and persistence within the host cell nucleus (47). Recombinant viral vectors take advantage of the mechanisms that viruses have evolved to facilitate each of these steps. Because synthetic vectors require analogous mechanisms to achieve gene transfer, the development of nonviral vectors initially focused on methods to achieve effective eukaryotic membrane transition (47). These methods have involved encapsulation of DNA into lipid membrane vesicles (liposomes) that fuse with the target cell membrane or precipitation of DNA into particles that are taken up by endocytosis.

Liposomes are artificial lipid bilayers that deliver nucleic acid to cells through fusion with cell membranes or through receptor-mediated endocytosis (48). The lipid bilayer may have a neutral or positively charged (cationic) surface. Cationic liposomes condense spontaneously with negatively charged DNA to form liposome-polynucleotide complexes. After entering the cell, these complexes are partially degraded in lysosomes, and the portion of plasmid DNA released in the cytoplasm translocates to the nucleus by means of unknown mechanisms, where it remains in an extrachromosomal location (49). Advantages of liposomes include the ease of preparation, the lack of viral sequences that may pose a safety hazard, and the absence of any DNA/RNA size constraint in vector construction. Disadvantages include low efficiency of gene transduction and the transience of gene expression. These limitations may be minimized by chemical modification of the liposome; for example, complexing the heat-inactivated hemagglutinating virus of Japan with cationic liposomes improves transfection efficiency of the vessel wall in vivo (50). The proliferative state of the cell population targeted by cationic liposomes also appears to effect in vivo arterial transfection efficiency. Balloon dilatation of rabbit iliac artery before gene transfer increases liposome-mediated gene delivery, presumably because of the resultant intimal smooth muscle cell proliferation (51).

VI. ANTISENSE OLIGONUCLEOTIDES

In most human gene therapy trials, the objective is to generate high levels of a particular protein to produce a desired therapeutic effect. An alternate gene therapy approach is to block the production or function of a protein that plays a critical role in disease pathogenesis. To block or ''knock out'' the synthesis of a protein, investigators have used antisense oligonucleotides, short pieces of RNA or DNA that are complementary to specific sequences of a target gene (52).

Antisense therapeutics exploit the specificity of nucleic acid base pairing and take advantage of the natural tendency of DNA and RNA to bind complementary strands in solution. By constructing an oligonucleotide with a sequence that is complementary to the target gene, antisense technology may be used to inhibit gene expression at several potential sites along the information flow from DNA to protein: (a) at the level of transcription, by triple helix formation with uncoiled DNA or by hybridization to nascent RNA; (b) at the level of RNA splicing through hybridization at intron-exon junctions; and (c) at the level of translation, through the inhibition of the binding of initiation factors, inhibition of the assembly of ribosomal subunits at the start codon, or inhibition of ribosome sliding along the coding sequences of the mRNA. Research pertinent to the stabilization of plaque done by Pickering showed that chimeric antisense oligonucleotides to human proliferating cell nuclear antigen can significantly inhibit the protein content in vascular smooth muscle cells, thereby inhibiting their proliferation and potentially mediating their deleterious effects on plaque destabilization (53).

VII. RIBOZYMES

Despite their conceptual elegance, antisense oligonucleotides may have limited efficacy (54). Inhibition of vascular gene expression by these molecules may be constrained by a number of variables including the stability of the oligonucleotide in vivo, the ability of the oligonucleotide to enter and be retained by the target cell, and the ability of the oligonucleotide to interact in a nonsequence-specific manner with other molecules, such as charged glycosaminoglycans present in the connective tissue of the vessel wall. An alternative to the use of antisense oligonucleotides, strategies have been developed on the basis of the use of ribozymes, which are short catalytic RNAs possessing specific endoribonuclease activity (55–56).

Ribozymes exist in several forms and are classified on the basis of their primary and secondary structures. The best characterized type of ribozyme is the hammerhead, found in vivo in certain plant viruses (57). Their discovery, in the early 1980s, answered previously perplexing questions related to the processing of mRNA and indicated that there was a time when biological reactions were catalyzed in the absence of protein based enzymes (58). In nature, these enzymes cleave intramolecularly (i.e., in cis) and cut 3′ to the sequence GUC. However, with the appropriate manipulations, they can be made to cut intermolecularly (i.e., in trans) at virtually any cleavage site (59).

Hammerhead ribozymes contain two separable functions: a catalytic core region containing several conserved bases, which cleaves the target RNA, and flanking regions, which, by nucleic acid complementarity, direct the ribozyme core to a specific target site. By attaching the core to sequences complementary to those flanking the target site GUC, ribozymes can be designed to specifically cleave almost any target RNA molecule (60). The conformational geometry of the hammerhead, which had previously been problematic in terms of describing its in vivo function was recently explained by the identification of an intermediate crystalline form (61). A major advantage of ribozymes is that a single ribozyme is able to cleave a large number of mRNA molecules (i.e., ribozymes are catalytic, making them attractive tools by which to bring about molecular changes). It has been estimated that some ribozymes cleave an RNA molecule every 2 minutes (61).

VIII. STABILIZATION OF ATHEROSCLEROTIC PLAQUE

Several studies with ribozymes with direct relevance to vascular biology and plaque stability have been reported. Smooth muscle cell proliferation has been inhibited by ribozymes that cleave c-myb mRNA. Jarvis et al. synthesized three ribozymes that were delivered to rat aortic smooth muscle cells (62). All three inhibited serum-stimulated cell proliferation and demonstrated excellent target specificity. In addition, ribozymes inhibit porcine and human smooth muscle cell proliferation effectively. In a related study, Frimerman et al. were able to show that a chimeric DNA-RNA hammerhead ribozyme to proliferating cell nuclear antigen inhibited porcine vascular smooth muscle cell growth (63). Smooth muscle cell proliferation is involved in neointimal growth and the expression of matrix metalloproteinases, which decrease plaque fibrous cap stability. The inhibition of smooth muscle cell proliferation is therefore one potentially effective target in the improvement of plaque stability.

In another interesting use of this technology, ribozymes were constructed to selectively inhibit apolipoprotein Lp(a), a mediator of atherogenesis (64). Concerns with the use of this technology existed, however, because of the approximate 80% homology with plasminogen and the potential for increasing the risk of thrombosis. In a study by Morishita et al. (64), cotransfection of cells with an apo(a)-producing gene and the inhibiting ribozyme led to a marked decrease in apo(a) mRNA and Lp(a). Importantly, there was no decrease in the production of plasminogen, revealing excellent target specificity, even in the presence of high gene homology. Thus, the use of ribozyme technology may provide an effective and safe strategy in the protection against plaque instability.

As alluded to earlier, gene therapy in its earliest phases was envisioned as a tool to correct disorders caused by single gene defects in an attempt to correct the physiological consequences of the lacking gene product. This attractive strategy would thus correct a problem at its most basic level and render the individual cured. This theoretical construct has gained new impetus with regard to disorders of the vascular system with the increasing fund of genetic knowledge and the recognition of the ubiquitous nature of disorders caused by errors in gene expression. Since the discovery of the high prevalence of the polymorphism-driven procoagulant disorder characterized by resistance of activated factor V to protein-C, estimated to be the most common inborn explanation for hypercoaguability, major research has been undertaken to define the genetic basis for similar disorders.

Several polymorphisms with significance to vascular biology and plaque development and stability have recently been explored. The acknowledgment of these genetic coding variations and their consequences make them attractive targets for patient-specific genetic therapy to correct the resultant effects. The near future may be defined by the routine screening for known polymorphisms associated with atherosclerosis and plaque instability with the goal of rectifying the aberrant gene product expression. One model for this was a retrospective subgroup analysis within a large population-based cohort that identified subjects with a history of myocardial infarction (MI) and matched them with controls (65).

Subjects were screened for an insertion/deletion polymorphism in intron h in the t-PA gene. In this study, homozygosity for the insertion allele was independently associated with the risk of nonfatal MI.

Recently two other polymorphisms with relevance to plaque stability and subsequent thrombus formation have been reported. The first, described by Moshfegh et al., concerns two silent, linked polymorphisms in the glycoprotein Ia/IIa receptor. This platelet receptor is critical in the linking of collagen and platelets, and this polymorphism was linked to receptor density and function. In a case-controlled review of subjects with MI, the prevalence of the homozygous genotype was 2.9 times higher in subjects with MI. The odds ratio of the association of homozygosity and MI was 3.3. The homozygous genotype was found to be an independent risk factor for MI after logistic regression adjusting for other major risk factors (66).

Finally, Zhang and colleagues (67) identified a matrix metalloproteinase, gellatinase B, whose activity was found to vary according to a genetic variation involving the promoter region. In this elegant study, a naturally occurring genetic variation was identified, caused by a single allele transition. This allelic transition led to higher promoter activity. No significant difference was found in the frequency of this allele in an age-matched sample of men with and without MI. However, on review of available angiographical data, of those with one or two copies of the allele transition, 26% had triple vessel coronary artery disease as compared with only 15% without the transition, thereby implicating this functional variation for more advanced atherosclerotic disease.

The stabilization of plaque through the use of gene therapy conceivably targets three critical periods in the prevention of an acute coronary syndrome. The strategies are tailored either to a systemic effect or to local tissue expression. The first target involves the modification of systemic characteristics that influence the development and progression of plaque, mainly the genetic modification of the lipid profile. The second target seeks to impede the degradation of existing plaque to allow for the intrinsic stabilizing properties associated with plaque maturation, in effect allowing the body to regain a homeostatic condition. Much of this strategy focuses on the interaction between the macrophage, the atheromatous plaque, and the vessel wall. A third target involves the local expression of factors that decrease the thrombogenicity of plaques undergoing early rupture to promote lamination of ruptured plaque rather than allowing the propagation of the thrombotic cascade with ensuing vessel occlusion. Any or all of these strategies could be used in an individual patient, depending on the plaque volume and other parameters of plaque stability.

A critical issue on which much of the therapeutic strategy hinges is the ability to effectively identify the target lesion. Inherent to the understanding of the problem is that it is plaque existing largely within the vessel intima and thus inapparent to standard imaging modalities, especially angiography, that are perhaps most prone to rupture. Although various modalities are being investigated, including dynamic computed tomographic scanning with quantification of calcium, magnetic resonance imaging with enhancement techniques, and more experimental ones such as the identification of thermal heterogeneity between stable and unstable plaque (68), the identification of rupture-prone plaques remains a challenge.

IX. LIPIDS AS A TARGET

Dyslipidemia is well recognized as a risk factor for atherosclerotic disease. Elevated levels of low-density lipoprotein and depressed levels of high-density lipoproteins contribute to the dynamic accumulation of lipid content in atheromatous core. There is abundant evidence to suggest that the normalization of lipid parameters can decrease both the morbidity and mortality associated with their presence when abnormal. This is true in patients before and after a primary vascular event.

The ability to genetically alter the lipid profile in a dyslipidemic individual holds promise for a potential solution to the disorder, rather than its palliation through drug therapy. Feldman and Isner have reviewed the history of LDL and HDL targeted gene therapy, with the first trials being performed on individuals with familial hypercholesterolemia (69). The use of ex vivo and in vivo techniques has been shown to be effective in the transfection of cells and the production of gene products that have a favorable impact on the cholesterol profile. This systemically modifiable property remains a central target in the prevention and passivation of atheromatous plaque.

X. MATRIX METALLOPROTEINASES AS A TARGET

Recently, a great deal of interest has been focused on the production of matrix metalloproteinases (MMP) by macrophages that accumulate in atherosclerotic plaque. The MMP are a group of enzymes that appear to play a role in the degrading of plaque collagen, thereby providing other inflammatory cells access into the inner layers and lipid core of the atheromatous plaque. In addition, it is postulated that these MMP-producing macrophages may contribute to the degradation and eventual weakening of the protective fibrotic cap overlying the highly thrombogenic core, leading finally to rupture of the vulnerable plaque. These macrophages appear to align themselves at points of maximal stress in atheromatous plaque, especially at the shoulder region, the luminal interface between healthy intima and plaque.

Shah et al. investigated the relationship between macrophage MMP and atheromatous fibrous caps in vitro (70). In this study, fibrous caps were isolated from human aortic and carotid plaques and allowed to incubate with monocyte-derived macrophages. Levels of MMP-1 and MMP-2 were ascertained by immunocytochemistry in cell culture and an assessment of MMP activity in the culture supernatant. This model established a relationship between MMP expression and function with respect to the ability to induce collagen degradation in the human atherosclerotic fibrous cap. Similar relationships linking the up-regulation of MMP with surgical preparative injury of saphenous veins has been noted by Kranzhofer and George (71, 72), helping to clarify the mechanism of basement membrane degradation that allows the influx of smooth muscle cells and intimal hyperplasia in patients undergoing coronary artery bypass grafting.

Tissue inhibitors of metalloproteinases (TIMPs) are a family of closely related secreted proteins that antagonize the effects of the MMP (73). Normally, a homeostasis exists that allows for the effective remodeling of collagen networks. Plaque vulnerability, however, implies a disequilibrium between these opposing forces, allowing the degradation of collagen at the fibrous cap to overshadow fibrotic strengthening at the plaque surface. Fabunmi et al. was able to suggest that the TIMPs (specifically 1, 2, and 3) were involved in plaque stabilization and that macrophages were able to express TIMP-3 (74). This group showed that smooth muscle cells associated with atheroma constituitively expressed TIMP 1,2, and 3 proteins and that the presence of these inhibitors (TIMPs 1 and 3) were augmented by other local factors including platelet-derived growth factor and transforming growth factor-β. They suggested that the presence of the TIMPs counteracts MMP activity in vivo. Thus, a strategy for reducing the vulnerability of a given plaque could be to suppress the expression of MMP (for example, by using ribozymes designed against MMP mRNAs), or conversely to bring about gene-mediated overexpression of the TIMPs. These strategies have been studied extensively in a related arena.

The collagen-degrading mechanisms of the MMPs are implicated in the pathogenicity of not only plaque destabilization but also with neointimal formation after balloon injury of aortic tissue and vascular invasion of metastatic tumors. The common pathway involves the degradation of collagen as the underlying source of pathogenicity. Much of the knowledge gained in the understanding of these mechanisms comes from experimentation aimed at the inhibition of neointimal proliferation after balloon angioplasty. The common end point, however, the inhibition of collagen degradation by the overexpression of TIMPs or the suppression of MMPs, delivers the requisite effect.

Baker et al. were able to induce high levels of expression of TIMPs 1 and 2 (as well as MMP-9) through the use of a replication-deficient adenovirus, driven by the cytomegalovirus major immediate early promoter (75). Protein production was identified by immunofluorescence, and secretion of the gene product by gelatin zymography. This model defined an efficient gene transfer system for high-level expression of potentially therapeutic products.

Because of a similar strategy, George et al. were able to decrease neointimal proliferation through the expression of TIMP-1 in a human saphenous vein model (76). An adenoviral vector was used to tranfect the saphenous vein tissue in culture, which significantly increased levels of TIMP-1 expression. Specific MMP inhibition was also shown using in situ zymography. Similar results were shown in another study by the same group expressing in this instance TIMP-2 (77). Cheng and colleagues were able to overexpress TIMP-2 both in vitro and in an in vivo model involving rat carotid artery injured with balloon withdrawal (78). By delivery of the adenoviral vector directly to the vessel at the time of balloon injury, neointimal proliferation was significantly inhibited 8 days. Whether the goal remains neointimal retardation or the stabilization of the fibrotic plaque cap, these studies demonstrate the potential for gene therapeutics to alter macrophage-mediated events in the vessel wall.

Recently, several studies have suggested a mechanism for the previously observed reduction in plaque instability through modification of the lipid profile. The link between cholesterol and the matrix metalloproteinases has been suggested to explain the alteration of atherogenic risk with lipid reduction. Aikawa et al. (79) and Libby et al. (80) were able to show that lipid lowering by diet significantly correlated with reduction in macrophage number, MMP level, and proteolytic activity in the lesions of rabbit aorta. Xu and colleagues established the inverse relationship, showing that macrophages in tissue culture that were exposed to oxidized LDL exhibited increased MMP-9 mRNA expression, protein synthesis, and gelatinolytic activity (81). In addition, oxidized LDL decreased TIMP-1 expression. HDL abrogated the oxidized LDL up-regulation of MMP-9. Thus, a putative mechanism for the role of dyslipidemia in plaque destabilization has been established.

XI. THROMBOSIS AS A TARGET

Plaque rupture involves the exposure of a highly thrombogenic core material to flowing blood, which leads to local thrombus formation and impairment of distal blood flow. Therapies aimed at reducing the thrombogenic response on core exposure may limit the extent of thrombus propagation and allow the intrinsic thrombolytic system to prevent myocardial damage. The demonstration that site-specific gene transfer to the vascular endothelium is feasible has stimulated the development of genetic strategies to prevent thrombosis that may complicate spontaneous or iatrogenic atherosclerotic plaque disruption. Gene therapy is particularly attractive in this setting in that local, tissue-specific expression of fibrinolytic agents may prevent the morbidity and mortality associated with systemic delivery of these agents, such as intracranial hemorrhage. Strategies relying on gene therapeutics to limit thrombus formation have focused on the prostacyclin synthetic pathway, nitric oxide synthase, plasminogen activators, and hirudin (82).

Tissue-type plasminogen activator (t-PA) is a naturally occurring protease that remains in dynamic equilibrium with the mediators of thrombus formation. The engineered overexpression of t-PA by endothelial cells within and surrounding areas of plaque may limit thrombosis after plaque rupture. Several models now exist in which both retrovirus- and adenovirus-mediated transfer of t-PA has been successful in producing high levels of local expression of t-PA with subsequent thromboresistance.

Dunn et al. were able to transduce sheep endothelial cells with a retroviral vector ex vivo, which coded for human t-PA (83). Dichek et al. (84) transduced cultured baboon endothelial cells with a retroviral vector carrying the human cDNA for tissue plasminogen activator (t-PA). These cells were seeded onto collagen-coated vascular grafts that were interposed in exteriorized arteriovenous femoral shunts. By measuring ^{111}In-platelet deposition and [128]I-fibrin accumulation, a focal antithrombotic effect, presumably caused by local enhancement of thrombolysis, was demonstrated in vivo.

By use of an adenoviral vector, various groups have been able to achieve high levels of t-PA expression. Carmeliet et al. were able to show that in plasminogen activator inhibitor 1–overexpressing mice, as well as t-PA–deficient mice, the intravenous administration of adenovirus vectors could cause liver gene transfer with subsequent t-PA synthesis and secretion into plasma (85). Various parameters measuring the effectiveness of this strategy, including clot lysis, were assessed revealing an approximately 1000-fold increase above normal levels. In addition, in this model, t-PA expression was seen in as little as 4 hours after transfection. Waugh and coworkers were also able to induce t-PA expression using an adenovirus delivered to rabbit femoral artery (86). Without perturbing systemic coagulation parameters, this construct was able to effectively prevent arterial thrombosis in a stasis/injury model.

In an intriguing model developed by Riesbeck et al., immortalized porcine endothelial cells and pituitary secretory cells were transfected with transgenes expressing hirudin fusion proteins (87). The endothelial cells were able to prolong the clotting times associated with this procoagulant phenotype in human plasma. Most interestingly, the pituitary secretory cells accumulated the fusion protein into granules that remained intracellular until activation by a stimulatory signal that caused the hirudin to be relocated to the outer membrane of the cells. This ability to selectively express a desired antithrombotic product adds another dimension to the use of gene-tailored therapy to the field of thromboresistance in atherosclerotic plaque rupture.

In a related study, the antagonism of tissue factor was shown to bring about decreased plaque thrombogenicity. Tissue factor, an abundant component in the lipid core of atherosclerotic plaque (88), has been postulated to be a major mediator of plaque thrombogenicity on exposure of the core material to flowing blood (89). Tissue factor (TF) may be synthesized by almost all cells present in an atherosclerotic plaque, including macrophages (90). Badimon et al. were able to show that the use of a recombinant tissue factor inhibitor was associated with decreased plaque thrombogenicity (89). Drew et al. showed that in areas of high TF expression, tissue factor pathway inhibitor was also elevated and colocalized with macrophages (90). High levels of TFPI protein and mRNA were also found in fatty streak lesions of 18 of 19 rabbits fed with high-cholesterol diets. The ability to successfully transfect either endothelial or smooth muscle cells in a target region of unstable plaque with tissue factor inhibitor could provide a potent strategy to diminish thrombus accumulation after plaque disruption.

XII. SUMMARY

Gene therapy is a rapidly advancing field that, hinging on the progress made in the fields of molecular and cellular biology, has made the transfer of genetic material to the vessel wall possible using a variety of vectors and delivery strategies. These techniques provide the means with which to either produce proteins not normally present or to deter the production of proteins that are normally synthesized by the cellular elements of the vasculature to stabilize plaque. Targeting three stages in the evolution of the fatty streak to atheromatous plaque and eventual nidus for thrombosis, gene therapy may become broadly applied to the cardiovascular system.

Several challenges remain before gene therapy can be more commonly used in the treatment of cardiovascular disorders. Improved, noninvasive, in vivo delivery to intimal tissue, more predictable gene transfection and more durable protein expression, and the development of an inducible system all represent challenges to the use of this technology in clinical practice. Further, the assurance that this therapeutic strategy supersedes the efficacy of current practice, yet is without increased risk to the patient remains crucial. Once these goals are met, however, a new paradigm for disease modification targeting the most elemental level of the disease process may be realized.

REFERENCES

1. Nabel EG, Plautz G, Boyce FM, Stanley JC, Nabel GJ. Recombinant gene expression in vivo within endothelial cells of the arterial wall. Science 1989; 244:1342–1344.
2. Curiel DT, Pilewski JM, Albelda SM. Gene therapy approaches for inherited and acquired lung diseases. Am J Respir Cell Mol Biol 1996; 14:1–18.
3. Sobel RE. Scanlon KJ: Clinical Protocols. Cancer Gene Ther 1995; 2:137–145.

4. Nabel EG, Pompili VJ, Plautz GE, Nabel GJ. Gene transfer and vascular disease. Cardiovasc Res 1994; 28:445–455.
5. Wilson JM, Birinyi LK, Salomon RN, Libby P, Callow AD, Mulligan RC. Implantation of vascular grafts lined with genetically modified endothelial cells. Science 1989; 244:1344–1346.
6. Plautz G, Nabel EG, Nabel GJ. Introduction of vascular smooth muscle cells expressing recombinant genes in vivo. Circulation 1991; 83:578–583.
7. Lynch CM, Clowes MM, Osborne WR, Clowes AW, Miller AD. Long-term expression of human adenosine deaminase in vascular smooth muscle cells of rats: a model for gene therapy. Proc Natl Acad Sci USA 1992; 89:1138–1142.
8. Dichek DA, Naville RF, Zwiebel JA, Freeman SM, Leon MB, Anderson WF. Seeding of intravascular stents with genetically engineered endothelial cells. Circulation 1989; 80:1347–1353.
9. Messina LM, Podrazik RM, Whitehill TA, Ekhterae D, Brothers TE, Wilson JM, Burkel WE, Stanley JC. Adhesion and incorporation of lacZ-transduced endothelial cells into the intact capillary wall in the rat. Proc Natl Acad Sci USA 1992; 89: 12018–12022.
10. Tahlil O, Brami M, Feldman LJ, Branellec D, Steg PG. The Dispatch catheter as a delivery tool for arterial gene transfer. Cardiovasc Res 1997; 33(1):181–187.
11. Reed ML, Wu C, Kneller J, Watkins S, Vorp DA, Nadeem A, Weiss LE, Rebello K, Mescher M, Smith AJ, Rosenblum W, Fedman MD. Micromechanical devices for intravascular drug delivery. J Pharm Sci 1998; 87(11):1387–1394.
12. Nabel EG. Gene therapy for cardiovascular disease. Circulation 1995; 91:541–548.
13. Vile RG, Russell SJ. Retroviruses as vectors. Br Med Bull 1995; 51:12–30.
14. Morgan RA, Anderson WF. Human gene therapy. Annu Rev Biochem 1993; 62: 191–217.
15. Cone RD, Mulligan RC. High-efficiency gene transfer into mammalian cells: Generation of helper-free recombinant retrovirus with broad mammalian host range. Proc Natl Acad Sci USA 1984; 81:6349–6353.
16. Grossman M, Raper SE, Kozarsky K, Stein EA, Engelhardt JF, Muller D, Lupien PJ, Wilson JM. Successful ex vivo gene therapy directed to liver in a patient with familial hypercholesterolacmia. Nat Genet 1994; 6:335–341.
17. Miller DG, Adam MA, Miller AD. Gene transfer by retrovirus vectors occurs only in cells that are actively replicating at the time of infection. Mol Cell Biol 1990; 10:4239–4242.
18. Clowes AW, Reidy MA, Clowes MM. Kinetics of cellular proliferation after arterial injury. I. Smooth muscle growth in the absence of endothelium. Lab Invest 1983; 49:327–333.
19. Welsh RM, Cooper NR, Jensen FC, Oldstone MBA. Human serum lyses RNA tumour viruses. Nature 1975; 257:612–614.
20. Miller N, Vile R. Targeted vectors for gene therapy. FASEB J 1995; 9:190–199.
21. Nabel EG, Plautz G, Nabel G. Site-specific gene expression in vivo by direct gene transfer into the vessel wall. Science 1990; 249:1285–1288.
22. Lim CS, Chapman GD, Gammon RS, Muhlestein JB, Bauman RP, Stack RS, Swain JI. Direct in vivo gene transfer into the coronary and peripheral vasculatures of the intact dog. Circulation 1991; 83:2007–2011.

23. Leclerc G, Gal D, Takeshita S, Nikol S, Weir L, Isner JM. Percutaneous arterial gene transfer in a rabbit model. J Clin Invest 1992; 90:936–944.

24. Flugelman MY, Jaklitsch MT, Newman KD, Casscells W, Bratthauer GL, Dichek DA. Low level in vivo gene transfer into the arterial wall through a perforated balloon catheter. Circulation 1992; 85:1110–1117.

25. Lee SW, Trapnell BC, Rade JJ, Virmani R, Dichek DA. In vivo adenoviral vector-mediated gene transfer into balloon-injured rat carotid arteries. Circ Res 1993; 73: 797–807.

26. Ohno T, Gordon D, San H, Pompili VJ, Imperiale MJ, Nabel GJ, Nabel EG. Gene therapy for vascular smooth muscle cell proliferation after arterial injury. Science 1994; 265:781–784.

27. Willard JE, Landau C, Glamann B, Burns D, Jessen ME, Pirwitz MJ, Gerard RD, Meidell RS. Genetic modification of the vessel wall. Comparison of surgical and catheter-based techniques for delivery of adenovirus. Circulation 1994; 89:2190–2197.

28. Nevins JR. Mechanism of activation of early viral transcription by the adenovirus E1A gene product. Cell 1981; 26:213–220.

29. Lemarchand P, Jones M, Yamada I, Crystal RG. In vivo gene transfer and expression in normal uninjured blood vessels using replication-deficient recombinant adenovirus vectors. Circ Res 1993; 72:1132–1138.

30. Guzman RJ, Lemarchand P, Crystal RG, Epstein SE, Finkel T. Efficient and selective adenovirus-mediated gene transfer into vascular neointima. Circulation 1993; 88: 2838–2848.

31. Simon RH, Engelhardt JF, Yang Y, Zepeda M, Weber-Pendleton S, Grossman M, Wilson JM. Adenovirus-mediated transfer of the CFTR gene to lung of non-human primates: toxicity study. Hum Gene Ther 1993; 4:771–780.

32. Gerard RD, Herz J. Adenovirus-mediated low density lipoprotein receptor gene transfer accelerates cholesterol clearance in normal mice. Proc Natl Acad Sci USA 1993; 90:2812–2816.

33. Barr E, Carroll J, Kalynych AM, Tripathy SK, Kozarsky K, Wilson JM, Leiden JM. Efficient catheter-mediated gene transfer into the heart using replication-defective adenovirus. Gene Ther 1994; 1:51–58.

34. Schulick AH, Newman KD, Virmani R, Dichek DA. In vivo gene transfer into injured carotid arteries. Optimization and evaluation of acute toxicity. Circulation 1995; 91:2407–2414.

35. Luo Z, Sata S, Nguyen T, Kaplan JM, Akita GY, Walsh K. Adenovirus-mediated delivery of Fas ligand inhibits intimal hyperplasia after balloon injury in immunologically primed animals. Circulation 1999; 14:1776–1779.

36. Rekhter MD, Simari RD, Work CW, Nabel GJ, Gordon D. Gene transfer into normal and atherosclerotic human blood vessels. Circ Res 1998; 82(12):1243–1252.

37. Berns KI. Parvovirus replication. Microbiol Rev 1990; 54:316–329.

38. Berns KI, Bohenzky RA. Adeno-associated viruses: an update. Adv Viral Res 1994; 32:243–306.

39. Samulski RJ, Chang LS, Shenk T. Helper-free stocks of recombinant adeno-associated viruses: normal integration does not require viral gene expression. J Virol 1989; 63:3822–3828.

40. Muzyczka N. Use of adeno-associated virus as a general transduction vector for mammalian cells. Curr Topic Microbiol Immunol 1992; 158:97–129.

41. Flotte TR, Solow R, Owens RA. Gene expression from adeno-associated virus vectors in airway epithelial cells. Am J Respir Cell Mol Biol 1992; 7:349–356.

42. Philip R, Brunette E, Kilinski L, Murugesh D, McNally MA, Ucar K, Rosenblatt J, Okarma TB, Lebkowski JS. Efficient and sustained gene expression in primary T lymphocytes and primary and cultured tumor cells mediated by adeno-associated virus plasmid DNA complexed to cationic liposomes. Mol Cell Biol 1994; 14:2411–2418.

43. Kotin RM, Siniscalco M, Samulski RJ, Zhu XD, Hunter L, Laughlin CA, McLaughlin S, Muzyczka N, Rocchi M, K. I. Berns KI. Site-specific integration by adeno-associated virus. Proc Natl Acad Sci USA 1990; 87:2211–2215.

44. Kotin RM, Menninger JC, Ward DC, Berns KI. Mapping and direct visualization of a region-specific viral DNA integration site on chromosome 19q13-qter. Genomics 1991; 10:831–834.

45. Samulski RJ, Zhu X, Xiao X, Brook JD, Housman DE, Epstein N, Hunter LA. Targeted integration of adeno-associated virus (AAV) into human chromosome 19. EMBO J 1991; 10:3941–3950.

46. Rome JJ, Shayani V, Flugelman MY, Newman KD, Farb A, Virmani R, Dichek D. Anatomic barriers influence the distribution of in vivo gene transfer into the arterial wall. Modeling with microscopic tracer particles and verification with a recombinant adenoviral vector. Arterioscler Thromb 1995; 14:148–161.

47. Curiel DT. Gene transfer mediated by adenovirus-polylysine-DNA complexes. In: Vos J-MH, ed. Viruses in Human Gene Therapy. Durham, NC: Carolina Academic Press, 1995:179–212.

48. Felgner PL, Gadek TR, Holm M, Roman R, Chan HW, Wenz M, Northrop JP, Ringold GM, Danielsen M. Lipofection: a highly efficient, lipid-mediated DNA-transfection procedure. Proc Natl Acad Sci USA 1987; 84:7413–7417.

49. Malone RW, Felgner PL, Verma IM. Lipofectin mediated RNA transfection. Proc Natl Acad Sci USA 1989; 86:6077–6081.

50. Morishita R, Gibbons GH, Kaneda Y, Ogihara T, Dzau VJ. Novel and effective gene transfer technique for study of vascular renin angiotensin system. J Clin Invest 1993; 91:2580–2585.

51. Takeshita S, Gal D, Leclerc J, Pickering JG, Riessen R, Weir L, Isner JM. Increased gene expression after liposome-mediated arterial gene transfer associated with intimal smooth muscle cell proliferation. J Clin Invest 1994; 93:652–661.

52. Milligan JF, Jones RJ, Froehler BC, Matteucci MD. Development of antisense therapeutics. Implications for cancer gene therapy. Ann N Y Acad Sci 1994; 716:228–241.

53. Pickering JG, Isner JM, Ford CM, Weir L, Lazerovits A, Rocnik EF, Chow LH. Processing of chimeric antisense oligonucleotides by human vascular smooth muscle cells and human atherosclerotic plaque. Implications for antisense therapy of restenosis after angioplasty. Circulation 1996; 92(4):772–780.

54. Stein CA, Cheung Y-C. Antisense oligonucleotides as therapeutic agents-is the bullet really magic? Science 1993; 261:1004–1012.

55. Cech TR. The chemistry of self-splicing RNA and RNA enzymes. Science 1987; 236:1532–1539.
56. Pyle AM. Ribozymes: a distinct class of metalloenzymes. Science 1993; 261:709–714.
57. Buzayan JM, Gerlach WL, Bruening G. Satellite tobacco ringspot virus RNA: a subset of the RNA sequence is sufficient for autolytic processing. Proc Natl Acad Sci USA 1986; 83:8859–8862.
58. Phylactou LA, Kilpatrick MW, Wood MJ. Ribozymes as therapeutic tools for genetic disease. Hum Mol Genet 1998; 7(10):1649–1653.
59. Ruffner DE, Stormo GD, Uhlenbeck OC. Sequence requirements of the hammerhead RNA self-cleavage reaction. Biochemistry 1990; 29:10695–10702.
60. Uhlenbeck OC. A small catalytic oligoribonucleotide. Nature 1987; 328:596–600.
61. Doudna J. Ribozymes: The hammerhead swings into action. Curr Biol 1998; 8: R495–R497.
62. Jarvis TC, Alby LJ, Beudry AA, Wincott FE, Beigelman L, McSwiggen JA, Usman N, Stinchcomb DT. Inhibition of vascular smooth muscle cell proliferation by ribozymes that cleave c-myc mRNA. RNA 1996; 2(5):419–428.
63. Frimerman A, Welch PJ, Jin X, Eigler N, Tei S, Forrester J, Honda H, Makkar R, Barber J, Litvack F. Chimeric DNA-RNA hammerhead ribozyme to proliferating cell nuclear antigen reduces stent-induced stenosis in a porcine coronary model. Circulation 1999; 99(5):697–703.
64. Morishita R, Yamada S, Yamamoto K, Tomita N, Kida I, Sakurabayashi I, Kikuchi A, Kaneda Y, Lawn R, Higaki J, Ogihara T. Novel therapeutic strategy for atherosclerosis: ribozyme oligonucleotides against apolipoprotein(a) selectively inhibit apolipoprotein(a) but not plasminogen gene expression. Circulation 1998; 98(18): 1898–1904.
65. van der Bom JG, de Knijff P, Haverkate F, Bots ML, Meijer P, de Jong PT, Hofman A, Kluft C, Grobbee DE. Tissue plasminogen activator and risk of myocardial infarction. The Rotterdam Study. Circulation 1997; 95(12):2623–2627.
66. Moshfegh K, Wuillemin WA, Redondo M, Lammie B, Beer JH, Licchti-Gallati S, Meyer BJ. Association of two silent polymorphisms of platelet glycoprotein Ia/II a receptor with risk of myocardial infarction: a case-control study. Lancet 1999; 353(9150):351–354.
67. Zhang B, Ye S, Herrmann S, Eriksson P, De Maat M, Evans A, Arveiler D, Luc G, Cambien F, Hamsten A, Watkins H, Henney A. Functional polymorphism in the regulatory region of gelatinase b gene in relation to severity of coronary atherosclerosis. Circulation 1999; 99:1788–1804.
68. Stefanadis C, Diamantopoulos L, Vlachopoulos C, Tsiamis E, Dernellis J, Toutouzas K, Stefanadi E, Toutouzas P. Thermal heterogeneity within human atherosclerotic coronary arteries detected in vivo. A new method of detection by application of a special thermography catheter. Circulation 1999; 99: 1965–1971.
69. Feldman LJ, Isner JM. Gene therapy for the vulnerable plaque. J Ann Coll Cardial 1995; 26(3):826–835.
70. Shah PK, Falk E, Badimon JJ, Fernandez-Ortiz A, Mailhac A, Villareal-Levy G, Fallon JT, Regnstrom J, Fuster V. Human monocyte-derived macrophages induce collagen breakdown in fibrous caps of atherosclerotic plaques. Potential role of ma-

trix-degrading metalloproteinases and implication for plaque rupture. Circulation 2995; 92(6):1565–1569.

71. Kranzhofer A, Baker AH, George SJ, Newby AC. Expression of tissue inhibitor of metalloproteinase-1, -2, and -3 during neointima formation in organ cultures of human saphenous vein. Arterioscler Thromb Vasc Biol 1999; 19(2):255–265.

72. George SJ, Zaitsman AB, Newby AC. Surgical preparative injury and neointima formation increase MMP-9 expression and MMP-2 activation in human saphenous vein. Cardiovasc Res 1997; 33(2):447–459.

73. Baker AH, Zaitsman AB, George SJ, Newby AC. Divergent effects of tissue inhibitor of metalloproteinase -1,-2, or -3 overexpression on rat vascular smooth muscle cell invasion, proliferation, and in vitro TIMP-3 promotes apoptosis. J Clin Invest 1998; 10(6):1478–1487.

74. Fabunmi RP, Sukhova GK, Suglyama S, Libby P. Expression of tissue inhibitor of metalloproteinase-3 in human atheroma and regulation in lesion-associated cells: a potential protective mechanism in plaque stability. Circ Res 1998; 83(3):270–278.

75. Baker AH, Wilkinson GW, Hembry RM, Murphy G, Newby AC. Development of recombinant adenoviruses that drive high level expression of the human metalloproteinase-9 and tissue inhibitor of metalloproteinase-1 and -2 genes: characterization of their infection into rabbit smooth muscle cells and human MCF-7 adenocarcinoma. Matrix Biol 1996; 15(6):383–395.

76. George SJ, Johnson JL, Angelini GD, Newby AC, Baker AH. Adenovirus-mediated gene transfer of the human TIMP-! gene inhibits smooth muscle cell migration and neointimal formation in human saphenous vein. Hum Gen Ther 1998; 9(6):867–877.

77. George SJ, Baker AH, Angelini GD, Newby AC. Gene transfer of tissue inhibitor of metalloproteinase-2 inhibits metalloproteinase activity and neointima formation in human saphenous veins. Gene Ther 1998; 5(11):1552–1560.

78. Cheng L, Mantile G, Pauly R, Nater C, Felici A, Monticone R, Bilato C, Gluzband YA, Crow MT, Stetier-Stevenson W, Capogrossi MC. Adenovirus-mediated gene transfer of human tissue inhibitor of metalloproteinase-2 blocks vascular smooth muscle cell invasiveness in vitro and modulates neointimal development in vivo. Circulation 1998; 98(20):2195–2201.

79. Aikawa M, Rabkin E, Okada Y, Voglie SJ, Clinton SK, Brinckerhoff CE, Sukhova GK, Libby P. Lipid lowering by diet reduces matrix metalloproteinase activity and increases collagen content of rabbit atheroma: a potential mechanism of lesion stabilization. Circulation 1998; 97(24):2433–2444.

80. Libby P, Aikawa M. New insights into plaque stabilization by lipid lowering. Drugs 1998; 56(suppl 1):9–13; discussion 33.

81. Xu XP, Meisel SR, Ong JM, Kaul S, Cercek B, Rajavashisth TB, Sharifi B, Shah PK. Oxidized low-density lipoprotein regulates matrix metalloproteinase-9 and its tissue inhibitor in human monocyte-derived macrophages. Circulation 1999; 99(8): 993–998.

82. Vassalli G, Dichek DA. Gene therapy for arterial thrombosis. Cardiovasc Res 1997; 35(3):459–469.

83. Dunn PF, Newman KD, Jones M, Yamada I, Shayani V, Virmani R, Dichek DA. Seeding of grafts with genetically modified endothelial cells. Secretion of recombi-

nant TPA results in decreased seeded cell retention in vitro and in vivo. Circulation 1996; 93(7):1439–1446.

84. Dichek DA, Anderson J, Kelly AB, Hanson SR, Harker LA. Enhanced in vivo antithrombotic effects of endothelial cells expressing recombinant plasminogen activators transduced with retroviral vectors. Circulation 1996; 93:301–309.

85. Carmeliet P, Stassen JM, Vas Vlaenderen I, Meidell RS, Collen D, Gerard RD. Adenovirus mediated transfer of tissue-type plasminogen activator augments thrombolysis in tissue-type activator deficient and plasminogen activator inhibitor-1 -overexpressing mice. Blood 1997; 90(4):1527–1534.

86. Waugh JM, Kattash M, Li J, Yuskel E, Kuo MD, Lussier M, Weinfeld AB, Saxena R, Rabinovsky ED, Thung S, Woo SL, Shenaq SM. Gene therapy to promote thromboresistance: local overexpression of tissue plasminogen activator to prevent arterial thrombosis in an in vivo rabbit model. Proc Natl Acad Sci USA 1999; 96(3): 1065–1070.

87. Riesbeck K, Chen D, Kemball-Cook G, McVey JH, George AJ, Tuddenham EG, Durling A, Lechler RI. Expression of hirudin fusion proteins in mammalian cells: a strategy for prevention of intravascular thrombosis. Circulation 1998; 98(24):2744–2752.

88. Marmur JD, Thiruvikraman SV, Fyfe BS, Guha A, Sharma SK, Ambrose JA, Fallon JT, Nemerson Y, Taubman MB. The identification of active tissue factor in human coronary atheroma. Circulation 1996; 94:1226–1238.

89. Badimon JJ, Lettino M, Toschi V, Fuster V, Berrozpe M, Chesebro J, Badimon L. Local inhibition of tissue factor reduces the thrombogenicity of disrupted human atherosclerotic plaques. Effects of tissue factor pathway inhibitor on plaque thrombogenicity under flow conditions. Circulation 1999; 99:1780–1787.

90. Drew AF, Davenport P, Apostolopoulos J, Tipping PG. Tissue factor pathway inhibitor expression in atherosclerosis. Lab Invest 1997; 77(4):291–298.

Index

About the Editor

DAVID L. BROWN is an Associate Professor of Medicine (Cardiology, Epidemiology, and Social Medicine), the Associate Director of the Division of Cardiology, the Chief of Clinical Cardiology, and the Director of the Cardiovascular Translational Research Unit at the Albert Einstein College of Medicine and Montefiore Medical Center, Bronx, New York. The author of numerous publications, he is a Fellow of the American College of Cardiology; the American Heart Association Council on Arteriosclerosis, Thrombosis, and Vascular Biology; and the Society of Coronary Angiography and Interventions. A member of the American Medical Association, the American Association for the Advancement of Science, the American Federation of Clinical Research, and the American Heart Association Clinical Cardiology Council, among others, Dr. Brown received the B.A. degree (1977) from the University of Texas, Austin, and the M.D. degree (1982) from the Baylor College of Medicine, Houston, Texas.